Principles
of
Clinical
Cardiology
An Analytical Approach

ARTHUR SELZER, M.D.

Chief of Cardiology and Director of Cardiac Laboratories,
Presbyterian Hospital of Pacific Medical Center, San Francisco;
Clinical Professor of Medicine, University of California
(San Francisco), and Stanford University Schools of Medicine

W. B. SAUNDERS COMPANY
Philadelphia • London • Toronto

W. B. Saunders Company: West Washington Square
Philadelphia, Pa.   19105

1 St. Anne's Road
Eastbourne, East Sussex BN21 3UN, England

833 Oxford Street
Toronto, M8Z 5T9, Canada

Library of Congress Cataloging in Publication Data

Selzer, Arthur.

Principles of clinical cardiology.

Includes index.

1. Cardiology.   I. Title. [DNLM: 1. Heart diseases—
   Diagnosis.   2. Heart diseases—Therapy. WG200 S472p]

RC667.S44   616.1'2   74–17762

ISBN 0–7216–8060–7

Principles of Clinical Cardiology   ISBN 0-7216-8060-7

Last digit is the print number: 9   8   7   6   5   4   3   2

Preface

L.B., a 39-year-old executive, considered himself in excellent health. He was active in many sports, including golf, tennis, and mountain climbing, and performed above average in all. He underwent a routine annual checkup required by his company and, among the many tests, an electrocardiographic treadmill stress test. A computer printout reported the results of the test as follows: "Electrocardiographic response to exercise suggests ischemia; coronary arteriography should be considered." He was immediately sent to a radiologist, who performed coronary arteriography and interpreted the findings as showing a 50 per cent narrowing of the proximal portion of the right coronary artery. He was then sent to a cardiovascular surgeon who advised a prophylactic aortico-coronary bypass operation. Thus our young man, who had never had an ache or pain, sailed through the "assembly line" untouched by a clinician's hand until he found himself recovering from the operation, nursing a painful median sternotomy scar. He returned to work after 2½ months, but it took him another 3 months before he could resume fully his recreational activities. The following year he underwent another routine checkup. An electrocardiographic stress test was performed and the computer printout read: "Electrocardiographic response to exercise suggests ischemia; coronary arteriography should be considered. . . ."

This is a fictional case summary, but it could have been a real one; in some institutions, the overall philosophy exemplified here is being followed. It is presented here as an example of cardiology at its very worst: automation, gadgetry, assembly-line medicine, and over-reliance on laboratory findings may become substitutes for clinical judgment, particularly if the key figure is bypassed—the cardiologist-clinician.

In looking at cardiology from the perspective of nearly four decades the changes that have taken place have been, indeed, dramatic. Cardiac diagnosis and cardiac therapy exploded with a broad range of new methods: cardiac surgery and physiological and angiocardiographic methods of study were initiated and blossomed out into fully developed specialties and subspecialties. A gamut of powerful new cardiac drugs was developed. An obvious question to be asked is: How much better care do cardiac patients receive now, in the light of all these new developments?

Admittedly, the view of the cardiac consultant may be biased, for the cases he sees are weighted toward unusual and difficult problems. Nevertheless, it is my considered judgment that the care of cardiac patients today is suboptimal. It is so in part because the recent advances in the field of cardiology aren't well enough known, but even more so because they are too well known. More patients appear to be over-diagnosed and overtreated than underdiagnosed and undertreated.

Thus we see a significant fraction of patients with cardiac disease admitted to acute care hospitals suffering from drug intoxication. Cardiac catheterization laboratories, angiocardiographic units, and open-heart surgical teams have become "status symbols"; the trend to develop them in too many hospitals invites overutilization and inferior performance. Coronary care units are organized even in the smallest hospitals under the mistaken notion that buying the hardware ensures good patient care.

These are the considerations that have stimulated me to undertake the task of writing a book on cardiology. I have often been referred to as a conservative cardiologist and have received invitations for participation in various debates, always representing the negative aspects of a given problem. I would prefer to describe myself as taking a middle-of-the-road approach, which can be defined as early acceptance of promising new methods of diagnosis or treatment but cautious and critical application of them. It is my firm belief that good medicine cannot be practiced unless critically examined clinical judgment is applied to each individual patient. The logical choice of a person who can apply critical clinical judgment to a cardiac problem is the clinician, not the physiologist, the radiologist, or the cardiovascular surgeon.

The objectives of this book, which represent my personal "overview" of cardiology, are presented in the Introduction (Chapter 1). It is fully realized that some of the statements contained in this book will be objected to by some and may be the subject of controversy. Furthermore, the world of cardiology is changing so rapidly that by the time the book appears in print some statements may have become obsolete, and some views may have changed. However, if the analytical approach to problem solving, expounded in the book, is valid, details are of secondary importance: every reader can substitute his own listings for those submitted in this book. It is the validity of this concept upon which the book will stand or fall.

In closing, I wish to acknowledge the assistance of the many friends in medicine who patiently answered my persistent questioning, reviewed portions of the manuscript, and helped in many other ways. There are too many of them to be listed here. Thanks are due also to Mr. James Brodale for the excellent drawings and diagrams and to Mr. George Vilk, Associate Medical Editor of the W. B. Saunders Company, for his personal interest and editorial assistance.

ARTHUR SELZER

Contents

vii

Section II: Therapy

*Section III: Disturbances of Cardiac Performance
and Rhythm*

*PART TWO — DISEASES OF THE HEART AND
CIRCULATION*

Section IV: Acute Diseases of the Heart

Section V: Diseases Primarily Increasing Cardiac Workload

1

Introduction

A textbook dealing with a medical subject traditionally involves an orderly presentation of the factual material. The many excellent textbooks of cardiology presently available differ from each other in their approaches: some take an encyclopedic standpoint of presenting all reasonable viewpoints and supplying exhaustive bibliographic support; others concentrate on the presentation of the most widely accepted views; still others submit personal viewpoints of the author. Books vary in the clarity of their presentation, in the completeness of their coverage, and in their emphasis. The present trend of using almost exclusively multi-authored books often leads to some unevenness from chapter to chapter. The clinician learns to consult some books in order to find small details or facts about rare syndromes, others to obtain better comprehension of the underlying basic process, still others to find practical hints. However, missing from most textbooks, or chapters, is some help in the individual problem-solving process that confronts the physician when facing a patient. The complexity of present-day medicine in general, and cardiology in particular, can easily lead to clinical chaos, unless orderly thinking is insisted upon. A major step in this direction is the recent introduction and popularity of the Problem-Oriented-Record system of chart-keeping in which clinicians are encouraged to identify each critical clinical point and carry it through independently of other issues.

This book was written in the hope of aiding the clinician in his process of thinking, when confronted with a diagnostic or therapeutic problem in a patient with cardiac disease.

THE APPROACH

The ability to formulate well a clinical problem and to proceed in an orderly manner to its solution comes into the purview of *clinical judgment.* Clinical judgment is difficult to define and to measure. The subject of an interesting and thoughtful book by Feinstein, clinical judgment is a composite of many features and attributes of a clinician: the knowledge of facts is only one of them. Recently, an attempt to present clinical judgment in a quantitative form by means of a mathematical formula was suggested by Schwartz *et al.* and applied to the subject of renal failure (Gorry *et al.*). At the present time, insufficient data are as yet available to apply this interesting approach widely. In cardiology, only limited and circumscribed problems might be suitable to this type of analysis. The broad field of cardiology has to be approached more from the qualitative and semi-quantitative standpoint. Looking at clinical judgment in more general terms, the author believes that its most important ingredients are the following:

1. A critical appraisal of the "facts";

2. The definition of goals for each diagnostic or therapeutic decision;

3. The setting of priorities in regard to each decision.

The importance of a critical approach to diagnosis and treatment should be self-evident. The clinician is under constant pressure from enthusiasts within and without the medical profession to adopt new methods of diagnosis and treatment. Conversely, he may be unduly influenced by his conservative colleagues against trying any new methods. Only a critical and impartial—if possible—judgment will permit the separation of real advances from minor modifications of diagnosis or therapy and from prematurely touted techniques that later turn out to be dangerous or worthless. The history of cardiac transplantation illustrates well premature enthusiasm generated by a not sufficiently critical approach to a new method. To be sure, critical evaluation of the various methods of diagnosis or treatment is still at an early stage: a good deal of medical judgment still has to be based on the art of medicine rather than on scientifically demonstrated facts. Lacking quantification, controlled studies, and statistically validated approaches, we have to use educated guesses in our everyday clinical decisions. However, in doing so, let us at least base these guesses upon reasonably established probabilities rather than solely on someone's biases and dictums.

In defining goals and objectives for each diagnostic or therapeutic step to be undertaken, one can avoid the commonest error perpetrated in today's medical practice: making clinical decisions based on reflexes, or on the association of certain conditions with certain actions. As a result, superfluous tests are being performed, patients subjected to unnecessary risks or to unneeded restrictions, worthless drugs are administered, operations performed without appropriately thought out indications. For example, in some clinicians' minds, anterior chest pain is automatically associated with coronary arteriography, pleural type of chest pain or hemoptysis with anticoagulant therapy, mitral stenosis with open-heart surgery. The quality of medical care would greatly improve and its cost be reduced if a clinician asked himself the question: "What is the purpose of this action?" before undertaking each clinical step.

Next in the analytical approach to problem solving is the recognition of the fact that each decision-making step has to be weighed in terms of its importance and its priority in achieving the overall objective. In diagnosis, certain findings are more essential and more informative than others; results obtained from some tests may make others super-fluous—thus the order of their performance may be of crucial importance. In the cases of contradictory results, priorities have to be established: which findings need to be accepted and which should be rejected. In therapy, the setting of priorities combined with acceptance of realistic goals may help us to make the necessary treatment tolerable to the patient and acceptable by him. Ample examples are available of the treatment being worse than the disease.

Thus the design of this book places form before factual information. The analytical approach is based on the three principles discussed above. It was felt that the presentation of the factual material in great detail might detract from the problem-solving approach and therefore be undesirable. One may therefore consider the presentations of many subjects as a broad overview of cardiology rather than a detailed text-book of it. More emphasis is placed upon the commonest and the most important points in each subject than on the completeness and compre-hensiveness of the presentation.

ORGANIZATION OF THE BOOK

Textbooks of cardiology often suffer from either repetition or omission as a result of the fact that many manifestations of disease (e.g., cardiac failure or arrhythmias) are common to most conditions. Without claiming a satisfactory solution to this problem, but in an ef-fort to minimize it, this book was divided into two separate parts: *General Cardiology*—dealing with subjects overlapping all diseases—and *Diseases of the Heart and Circulation*—presenting systematically the various entities included in cardiology. While some repetition is inevita-ble, care has been exercised to minimize it as much as possible.

Certain assumptions had to be made. It was assumed that the reader possesses some familiarity with the basic aspects of cardiology: circulatory physiology, basic electrocardiography, cardiac roentgenol-ogy, hemodynamics. References are supplied for those wishing to con-sult other more detailed texts and reviews in these areas. This book is not intended to replace such texts but instead to offer useful practical clinical information to a wide audience already familiar with fundamentals, from the medical student to the fully trained cardiologist. Its slant is largely clinical, but in the broadest sense of the term, i.e., including the most sophisticated methods for diagnosis and therapy. Basic subjects are discussed only as a means of defining and clarifying the author's position, or when necessary to provide background information, particularly in areas that are thought to be widely misunderstood.

Bibliography fulfills two roles: first, it serves to provide references in support of certain statements that may appear not to be in the mainstream of cardiological thinking. Second, it lists general review articles and books for the reader who wishes to get more factual information than that provided in the book or who needs more basic introduction to some of the chapters. Since this is a somewhat subjective and personal account of cardiology, the number of references from our own department needs no apology.

The organization of Part II of the book differs from the traditional presentation of cardiac diseases. The conventional presentation by a sequential discussion of *Etiology, Pathology, Pathophysiology, Diagnosis, Course, Prognosis,* and *Treatment* is often modified. The pivotal point of the discussion is the natural history of the disease. When warranted, stages of a disease are discussed as separate syndromes. In the diagnostic part of the discussion, emphasis is placed upon the reliability of various methods. Modes and sequences of evaluation are presented. In the therapeutic part, goals and objectives of therapy are defined.

The number of illustrations is rather small. The decision not to include reproductions of electrocardiograms, roentgenograms, pressure curves, and other material from the various disease entities is in line with the overall objectives of the book, which is, of course, not designed as an atlas of cardiology. Rather, diagrammatic drawings are included that may help the reader review at a glance the basic pathophysiologic principles of many disease processes and that illustrate certain points in the discussion.

NOMENCLATURE AND TERMINOLOGY

Physicians are individualists and find it difficult to agree upon medical terms. Many diseases go under more than one name, sometimes with divisions along geographical lines. For example, "idiopathic hypertrophic subaortic stenosis" on this side of the Atlantic becomes "obstructive cardiomyopathy" on the other side of it. Starling's law of the heart becomes in some quarters Frank-Starling's law. Graves' disease in the English-speaking countries becomes Basedow's disease in the German-speaking countries and Flaiani's disease in Italy. Eponyms are especially ephemeral. It seems that the most durable ones are those with unusual names, e.g., Eisenmenger or Lutembacher.

The selection of the names of diseases, syndromes, and other terms used in the book has been made by using those with the broadest recognition. Some difficulties are inevitable. It has long been apparent that the commonest form of heart disease has a most "unstable" name: there is little uniformity in the designation of the clinical consequences of occlusive disease of the coronary arteries. The official term forced upon the cardiologist, but never really accepted — arteriosclerotic heart disease — is both illogical and obsolete, but still widely used. "Coronary heart disease" is awkward; "coronary artery disease" does not adequately describe the clinical situations. The term "ischemic heart disease" has some justifiable objections and is avoided by some; nevertheless, it comes closest to describing the clinical syndromes included in the overall concept of occlusive diseases of the coronary arterial system. It has, furthermore, the official sanction of the World Health Organization. Thus, the term "ischemic heart disease" has been selected for use in this book.

Names of chapters have been selected by their widest application to all conditions included in the discussion. Thus, the term "inflow obstruction" or "outflow obstruction" is used in preference to "stenosis" of the various orifices.

Many factors influenced the decision to use certain terms in preference to others. In general, the use of eponyms has been avoided unless their acceptance is universal and uniform (e.g., Wolff-Parkinson-White syndrome). Certain terms (e.g., in connection with mitral regurgitation) used in earlier writings have been retained. An effort has been made to define terms that may not be well known or self-explanatory.

Bibliography

Feinstein AR: CLINICAL JUDGMENT. The Williams and Wilkins Co., Baltimore, 1967.

Gorry GA, Kassirer JP, Essig A, Schwartz WB: Decision analysis as the basis for computer-aided management of acute renal failure. Amer. J. Med. 55:473, 1973.

Schwartz WB, Gorry GA, Kassirer JP, Essig A: Decision analysis and clinical judgment. Amer. J. Med. 55:459, 1973.

Part one

General Cardiology

2

Approach to Diagnosis

Two or three decades ago diagnostic evaluation of a patient with cardiac disease consisted of four principal components:

- History,

- Physical examination,

- Radiographic examination,

- Electrocardiographic examination.

Supplemented by a few simple laboratory tests, these four components constituted a "routine" upon which the cardiac diagnosis was based. Today, the clinician has at his disposal a large number of diagnostic techniques, some of which require special facilities and skills and entail some risk to the patient. The diagnostic process has thus become one consisting of several decision-making steps: when, where, by whom, and how far to go. The complexity of the diagnostic process should be viewed from the proper perspective. In order to permit the full grasp of this process, its various components have to be discussed in some detail.

THE TARGET

The patient represents the target of the diagnostic process. The range of patients in need of cardiac diagnostic evaluation is wide: from neonates to very old persons, from asymptomatic patients to extremely ill ones, from those with simple problems in whom the diagnosis can be made at a glance to complex diagnostic challenges.

The initiation of the diagnostic evaluation is usually prompted by one of three situations:

- Discovery of cardiac disease or awakening of suspicion that heart disease may be present,
- Decision to evaluate details of a known cardiac disease, usually elective, often resulting from new symptoms or signs,
- Evaluation of progress of a chronic cardiac disease (often seriatim).

Today, in an era of many mass surveys of the population, of periodic health examinations, of routine pre-employment examinations, suspicious findings suggesting the possibility of cardiac disease are often uncovered in seemingly healthy, asymptomatic individuals. Such case-finding is most often based upon the detection of one of the following:

- Abnormal physical findings, such as murmurs or arrhythmias,
- Abnormal findings on radiographic examination,
- Abnormal electrocardiographic tracings,
- Abnormal elevation of blood pressure.

Symptomatic patients consult physicians, sometimes concerned about their hearts, sometimes suspecting other diseases, sometimes merely reporting their symptoms. Symptoms may or may not be related to the heart; a certain number of cardiac problems are discovered as accidental findings in patients undergoing diagnostic evaluation for diseases of other organs or systems.

The evaluation of a known case of cardiac disease most often involves a chronic lesion present since childhood, e.g., congenital or rheumatic heart disease. A "definitive" diagnosis may await the optimal age in children, the development of certain new findings, appearance of symptoms, or may even be prompted by the patient coming under the care of another physician.

Longitudinal studies are frequently performed in patients with stable or slowly progressive chronic cardiac disease. Simpler diagnostic evaluation often involves periodic series of non-invasive tests to assess the progress of the disease. Complete evaluation may be advisable in patients who are either candidates for surgical treatment or subjects of postsurgical follow-up.

The various modes of initiation of the diagnostic process emphasize the wide variety of circumstances under which patients come to the attention of the clinician. Each patient requires an individual approach, weighing the various steps, one at a time, and establishing goals for each step.

THE FACILITIES

The facilities include the diagnostic teams, the physical setup and the equipment used for the performance of the various procedures. The diagnostic teams constitute the most critical factor in determining excellence. The number of individuals participating in the diagnostic process varies; potentially a large number may be needed. The principal team components include the following:

- The primary physician,
- The clinical consultant,
- Laboratory technicians and their supervisory experts (clinical pathologist, bacteriologist),
- Radiographic technicians and the radiologist-consultant,
- Electrocardiographic technician and the electrocardiographic reader,
- Technicians and physician-interpreters of the various other graphic tests used in cardiac diagnosis,
- The cardiac catheterization technical team and the clinical cardiac physiologist,
- The angiocardiographic technical team and the angiocardiographer.

It should be noted that each component part of the overall team consists of the technical part and the physician who interprets the findings. Only very few tests stand on their own merits, contingent solely upon correct technical execution. Here results are numerical (e.g., serum enzyme determination). In most others, the element of human judgment comes into the interpretation. It is, therefore, evident that in a complex diagnostic problem that requires a number of tests, the final opinion is, in reality, a conglomerate of opinions of many consultants. With apologies for the use of a worn-out cliché, the diagnostic chain is only as good as its weakest link. The difficulties in the interpretation of some apparently simple findings of the various diagnostic tests will be elaborated upon in the following chapters.

The quality control of diagnostic evaluation is thus contingent upon two approaches:

1. Either the clinician has enough expertise to evaluate and, if necessary, to reinterpret the findings of the various diagnostic procedures, or

2. He must be confident that every consultant partaking in the diagnostic process has the necessary training and experience to render a reliable report.

The first approach is obviously the preferable one; but practical necessity calls for the frequent application of the second approach.

The sequence of the diagnostic evaluation often involves three levels of medical care. The patient's primary physician—a family practitioner or an internist—is most often the first contact. If the situation warrants it, the patient may then be seen by a consultant—a local cardiologist or internist who may take the problem a step farther and may reach a solution. In some cases, the need may arise to refer the patient to a Cardiac Center where all the diagnostic facilities are available. There are, of course, variations of this sequence: the primary physician may elect to channel the patient to the Center directly. Some patients present themselves to a Center cardiologist on their own.

The primary physician, with the help of the electrocardiographic and radiological consultants, may solve the problem. It should be emphasized, however, that the seriousness of the patient's cardiac condition is not necessarily the criterion for its complexity. For example, the evaluation of cardiac murmurs in asymptomatic individuals ranks high among difficult problems and may require the "ultimate" in evaluation in terms of consultative facilities.

Among the critical issues in the diagnostic sequence, the reliability of the Cardiac Center ranks high. In spite of the fact that the Intersociety Commission for Heart Disease Resources has spelled out optimal criteria for the various facilities in cardiology with emphasis upon experience and adequate case load, there are many cardiac laboratories in which neither the personnel nor the caseload assures reliable and critically reviewed diagnostic tests. Diagnostic facilities of this type could lead astray the diagnostic chain of events, as a result of which either an incorrect diagnosis may be reached or the necessity may arise for having a major invasive diagnostic test repeated elsewhere.

RELIABILITY

Earlier in this discussion, the importance of the interpretation of the findings in diagnostic tests was stressed. It is now necessary to define the quality of the best tests. Assuming perfection in technique and the best expertise in interpretation, are results of various tests 100 per cent reliable? The obvious answer to this question is that all tests have some limitations. Awareness of these limitations is essential in the overall evaluation of each patient.

Results of a given test may be quantitative (e.g., P-R interval in the electrocardiogram, cardiac output, left atrial pressure), semiquantitative (size of a cardiac chamber radiographically evaluated, valvular regurgitation estimated angiocardiographically), or qualitative (presence or absence of a murmur, presence or absence of a small intracardiac shunt).

The differentiation between a normal and abnormal finding is easy if the abnormality is far from the norm; the closer the findings are to the normal range, the more difficult the interpretation becomes. Every biological phenomenon — including each measurement and finding used in cardiac diagnosis — has a distribution that can be fitted into a frequency curve — the Gaussian curve (Fig. 2–1). Normality, by generally accepted criteria, is defined as all the values within two standard deviations from the mean, the latter being the "ideal" value. Thus in the normal population only 96 per cent of each measurement lies within the accepted normal zone: 2 per cent reaches into the abnormal zone on each end of the curve. Such abnormal findings in normal individuals constitute the unusual "normal variants." Conversely, definite abnormalities far out in the abnormal zone of findings also fit in an appropriate frequency curve which will overlap with the normal curve. Thus there are for each measurement a normal zone, an abnormal zone, and a borderline zone, in which the two overlap. Occasionally, a normal offshoot can be found deep in the abnormal zone. Distribution curves of various measurements used in diagnostic procedures can be drawn for all quantitative results, provided normality and abnormality can be defined by an independent method (see below). If an alternate

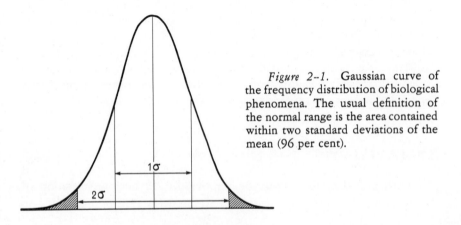

Figure 2–1. Gaussian curve of the frequency distribution of biological phenomena. The usual definition of the normal range is the area contained within two standard deviations of the mean (96 per cent).

method is not available, a normal distribution curve for a given measurement is assumed to contain the normal range within the area of two standard deviations of the mean. In actuality, only a few measurements in cardiology have such curves available, namely those in which large normal populations have been measured (e.g., some electrocardiographic criteria).

What represents the yardstick against which correctness of a clinical diagnosis is measured? Traditionally, the pathologist is the final arbiter, the judge of a clinical-pathological conference. More recently, the cardiovascular surgeon has assumed this role in inspecting the heart *in vivo*. Yet, the morphological yardstick has important limitations:

- Certain morphological abnormalities are difficult to detect, occasionally requiring special techniques as well as expertise;

- Obstruction to flow in the form of valvular stenosis, occlusive coronary artery disease, etc. can only be estimated in very rough terms;

- Abnormal flows through incompetent valves or abnormal communications are even more difficult to assess and their margin of error is great;

- Cardiac function and performance cannot be judged at all;

- Many physiological concepts—increased pressure, disturbances of rhythm—have no morphological substrate whatsoever.

Thus it is clear that other methods than morphological inspection are necessary to serve as "check" upon the diagnostic accuracy of the various techniques. Among these are the following:

- Physiological studies performed during cardiac catheterization,

- Angiographic studies,

- Electrocardiography as a means of analyzing arrhythmias,

- Echocardiography, in selected areas (e.g., valve motion).

In the following chapters, values and limitations of the various techniques will be presented. It will become apparent that in some areas an independent method of "checking" the diagnosis cannot be obtained at all; in many areas it has to be accepted with some reservations. The "black and white" answer of the traditional clinical-pathological conference now applies only to selected areas of cardiology.

It is obvious that if cardiovascular diagnosis is to attain any scientific basis, each method, even each clinical sign or criterion, has to be defined in terms of its reliability. This has been defined mathematically by assessing the frequency with which a given test (or sign) introduces an error, either by being absent in a condition for which it is supposed to be characteristic ("false negative") or by being present without the underlying condition ("false positive"). *Sensitivity* of a test is an index of false-negative results; *specificity,* of false-positive results. In order to define these two terms, it is necessary to study two groups of cases:

1. Patients who are known to have the findings which the diagnostic test is aimed at, e.g., pathologically determined presence of left ventricular hypertrophy in 100 cases whose electrocardiograms are being examined for criteria of left ventricular hypertrophy;

2. Patients who are known *not* to have left ventricular hypertrophy by pathological examination (using the same example).

Sensitivity then represents the number of patients in group 1 in whom the electrocardiogram shows the presence of left ventricular hypertrophy. A 90 per cent sensitivity, therefore, means that in 10 per cent the electrocardiogram missed the diagnosis.

Specificity represents the number of patients in group 2 in whom the electrocardiogram *did not* show left ventricular hypertrophy. Thus, a 95 per cent specificity indicates that there was a 5 per cent false-positive incidence of left ventricular hypertrophy.

Expediency and practical consideration have led to an alternative approach for the determination of the number of false-positive diagnoses: rather than examining a group of patients known not to have the feature to be tested, the number of false-positive findings is sought by determining independently how many patients in a series show a given criterion (e.g., electrocardiographic pattern of left ventricular hypertrophy), in whom the diagnosis was not confirmed (by pathological examination).

It should be obvious that specificity and sensitivity for a given test are inversely related to each other. If one were to set lenient criteria for a diagnostic test (e.g., increased QRS voltage for left ventricular hypertrophy), the sensitivity would be increased at the expense of specificity (few patients with left ventricular hypertrophy would be missed, but many false-positives would be pulled in). Conversely, if one requires for the diagnosis of left ventricular hypertrophy high voltage, prolonged QRS duration, and T-wave abnormalities, there might be no false-positives, but many cases of left ventricular hypertrophy would be missed. This reciprocal relationship between sensitivity and specificity of a test makes it futile to look for the perfect criterion. Each test can be expressed in terms of a diagnostic score. Holt suggested that a "performance score" be calculated as follows:

$$\frac{\%\ \text{sensitivity} + \%\ \text{specificity}}{2}$$

Calculation of a performance score of some diagnostic tests would show that some tests are of much higher diagnostic value than others. While perfect tests with a 100 per cent sensitivity and 100 per cent specificity do not exist, there are some that approach it, e.g., the hydrogen inhalation test for the detection of left-to-right intracardiac shunts.

The diagnostic capabilities of a given test can be utilized to advantage, if the overall objectives for its use are defined. Thus, criteria emphasizing high sensitivity may be used, in spite of the inherent low specificity, in case-finding surveys, where later the false-positives can be weeded out. Conversely, in the diagnostic process of the individual patient, higher specificity needs to be emphasized. The aim of the diagnostic process is to rely upon tests with reasonable specificity. A combination of several tests with moderate specificity may increase the diagnostic accuracy so as to make the diagnosis virtually certain. For example, the combination of clinical, electrocardiographic, and radiologic findings in a patient with atrial septal defect often establishes a definitive clinical diagnosis. However, inasmuch as each component criterion loses some cases by its moderately low sensitivity, the overall sensitivity of the combination of findings will be only fair (i.e., many less typical atrial septal defects will be missed).

As already stated, actual figures of sensitivity and specificity of

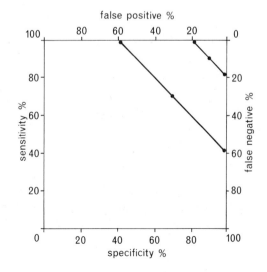

Figure 2-2. Relationship between specificity and sensitivity of a hypothetical test showing two examples of "isoperformance lines." The lower line indicates that the test ranges from a sensitivity of 60 per cent with a specificity of 100 per cent to a sensitivity of 100 per cent with a specificity of 60 per cent. The upper isoperformance line demonstrates a more reliable diagnostic test: at a sensitivity of 100 per cent the specificity is 80 per cent and vice versa. (Modified from Holt et al., Circulation, 40:697, 1969; by permission. American Heart Association, Inc.)

diagnostic tests are available only for relatively few procedures. In most, only approximate estimates are provided. Such estimates can be attempted even in semiquantitative tests (such as ones reported in terms of normal; slightly, moderately, or grossly abnormal; or O, +, ++, +++, ++++), as has been done in many of the diagnostic procedures reported in later chapters.

THE OBJECTIVES

At each level of the diagnostic process, the physician should have clearly defined goals and objectives of his efforts. It has already been mentioned that each diagnostic step should be defined in terms of its specific goal. The same attitude is often necessary in the overall assessment of a diagnostic problem. This can best be illustrated by citing some examples of disease entities in which different diagnostic approaches should be taken depending upon the circumstances:

1.   Diagnostic evaluation of a 40-year-old man who is found to have diastolic hypertension may be different from that in a 65-year-old patient with elevated systolic pressure.

2.   An asymptomatic patient with signs of aortic stenosis requires an approach different from that toward one with this disease who suffers from syncopal attacks and cardiac failure.

Given a clinical diagnosis or a series of findings suggestive of a certain cardiac disease, the evaluation may have as its objective a "final" diagnosis based upon reasonable probabilities derived by simple, noninvasive means in one case, but in another it may be necessary to clarify the minutest details of the patient's structural abnormalities and physiological derangements. This difference in approach will be discussed in more detail in Chapter 9.

Two further examples, both representing authentic cases, illustrate diagnostic abuses brought on by bad clinical judgment:

1.   A 14-year-old boy in apparent good health complained of sharp pain in the side of the chest, described as a "stitch," occurring occasionally while running fast; the pain was related to deep respiration. The anxious parents consulted a physician who detected a soft systolic ejection murmur in the pulmonary area and referred the boy to a cardiac center. The cardiologist found a normal roentgenogram and electrocardiogram, but nevertheless proceeded with catheterization of the right and left sides of the heart and performed selective coronary arteriography, *then* reassuring the parents about absence of cardiac disease.

2. A 50-year-old woman was treated for five years for "arterio-

sclerotic heart disease" with atrial fibrillation. When the patient no longer responded to cardiac therapy and persisted in intractable cardiac failure, she was referred to a cardiac center, but died before any studies could be performed. Necropsy showed severe mitral stenosis.

The first example shows how a patient can be subjected to an unnecessary risk and expense, when the diagnosis should have been made on the basis of adequate clinical history, physical examination, and a few simple laboratory tests. It represents the abuse of invasive diagnostic tests *ad absurdum*. The second illustrates the unawareness of a physician of atypical aspects of some surgically correctable lesions and his failure to ask for consultative help until the terminal stages of the disease.

Bibliography

Bennet G: Scientific Medicine? Lancet 2:453, 1974.

Holt JH Jr, Barnard ACL, Lynn MS: a study of the human heart as a multiple dipole electrical source: II. Diagnosis and quantification of left ventricular hypertrophy. Circulation 40:697, 1969.

Tumulty PA: The Effective Clinician. WB Saunders Co., Philadelphia, 1973.

3
History

GENERAL APPROACH

In cardiology, the contribution of the clinical history to the final diagnosis in a given patient varies widely: in a few cases the information gained is negligible, in some the entire diagnosis may be based on the history alone. It constitutes the initial part of the diagnostic evaluation and is always of paramount importance. History taking requires skill and judgment as well as experience. These attributes are so often missing from the "routine" history recorded by a house officer in the average teaching hospital, in which length may serve as a substitute for relevance. The recent introduction of the "problem oriented record" is a major step in the right direction.

Recently some tendency developed to experiment with the delegation of history taking to questionnaires to be answered by the patient, or to physician assistants. In the field of cardiology this appears ill-advised: the experienced physician-interviewer subjects the patient to a cross-examination comparable to that of a trial attorney; the latter would certainly never consider delegating this function to anyone else.

History taking involves two simultaneous functions:

1. The gathering of facts,

2. The assessment of the patient's credibility.

While the patient's symptoms are being discussed, the interviewer has to probe for answers to the following questions:

1. Is the patient observant and intelligent enough to give an accurate account of his symptoms?

2. Is his self-assessment objective or is he likely either to exaggerate or to minimize his symptoms?

3. Is there a possibility of the patient's benefiting either from withholding facts or from reporting fictitious symptoms?

The technique of history taking varies a great deal and is highly individual. In trying to provide guidelines, one can suggest that it is better to ask the patient a few directed questions rather than "let him loose" to relate his medical history entirely in his own words and according to his own sequential preference. The critical issues related to each symptom should not be asked directly in the form of leading questions, but the patient should be guided to volunteer them.

The history of a symptomatic patient with cardiac disease should include three areas:

1. An account of all symptoms ("problems"),

2. An assessment of the patient's disability,

3. A review of background facts.

In traditional terms, the first two points are included in the conventional "history of present illness"; the third one incorporates the past history, family history, social history, and systemic review.

The assessment of disability is probably the most difficult part of the history, the one most often varying from interviewer to interviewer. It need not be, if a few simple guidelines are followed and if one keeps in mind the natural history of most cardiac diseases. The guiding principles of disability assessment should take into consideration the following points:

1. In most cases of chronic cardiac disease, symptoms are likely to develop during stress and exercise; consequently they affect the effort tolerance.

2. In order to assess the patient's effort tolerance, a detailed knowledge of the patient's mode of living is needed.

3. History is the principal, often the only, means of assessing whether disability is stable or progressive. Specific questions to this effect are necessary to elicit this information.

PRINCIPAL CARDIAC SYMPTOMS

Dyspnea. Shortness of breath is the commonest symptom of cardiac disease, the one most often producing disability. Its two principal forms are:

- Dyspnea on effort,

- Dyspnea at rest (paroxysmal dyspnea, orthopnea).

When directing an inquiry into shortness of breath as the principal complaint of a patient, it is necessary to take into account the fact that effort dyspnea is a physiological phenomenon. Dyspnea is *subjective*, i.e., it represents the patient's consciousness of increased respiratory effort. Such consciousness in health occurs when a subject nears the limit of his physical endurance; in disease it is merely brought on at a lower level of exercise. The decline of effort tolerance — as indicated by dyspnea's occurring with lesser effort — can be abrupt or gradual. Sudden onset of symptoms often involves an obvious precipitating factor, e.g., a change from sinus rhythm to atrial fibrillation. The recognition of a major and sudden change in effort tolerance usually can be achieved without difficulty. On the other hand, the gradual onset of dyspnea requires detailed questioning in order to avoid pitfalls. In general the following points require probing:

1.   What is the patient's physical conditioning? An inventory of his daily activities is helpful and should involve not only work habits but recreational activities as well.

2. Is the alleged reduction of effort tolerance reproducible and consistently present?

3.   Is there a possible noncardiac factor, such as a respiratory infection, in the background?

4.   Is the phenomenon the patient calls "shortness of breath" really effort dyspnea? Patients often confuse dyspnea with anterior chest pain (tightness across the chest may give the patient the feeling that he is unable to take a deep breath); sometimes dyspnea is preceded by anginal pain.

Dyspnea at rest requires a detailed questioning in order not to confuse it with hyperventilation. Paroxysmal nocturnal dyspnea usually presents itself in a characteristic form — namely, the patient awakens with a feeling of suffocation; it may be associated with cough and orthopnea; at times it merges with acute pulmonary edema. Wheezing during nocturnal attacks of dyspnea may also occur, accounting for the term (now less often used than in the past) of "cardiac asthma." Wheezing produced by bronchospasm secondary to acute left ventricular failure may present diagnostic difficulties, inasmuch as it may be confused with true bronchial asthma developing in a patient with cardiac disease. Paroxysmal nocturnal dyspnea most often occurs unprovoked and unassociated with an obvious cause; at times, however, a precipitating factor may be identified and could be perceived by the patient. A common precipitating cause is nocturnal paroxysmal tachyarrhythmia; thus, directive questioning about sensations accompanying or preceding shortness of breath may yield important diagnostic information (history of chest pain, of palpitations). It should be noted that paroxysmal nocturnal dyspnea produced by an attack of tachyarrhythmia is as a rule less ominous than a spontaneously occurring left ventricular failure.

A special form of nocturnal dyspnea is that produced by Cheyne-Stokes respiration. Nocturnal periodic breathing often causes the patient to doze off during the apneic stage and to wake up with respiratory distress during hyperpnea. The patient is unlikely to note such a relationship, but a member of the family witnessing it may give the appropriate description of this phenomenon.

Hyperventilation and "sighing" respiration of the patient with anxiety neurosis may often be recognized by the patient's description of it. It is usually characterized by compulsion to take a deep breath "as if there were not enough air." The patient should be encouraged to demonstrate the type of respiratory distress he is referring to: he may be able to show "panting" as opposed to "sighing."

Orthopnea, by definition, is a breathing discomfort experienced by the patient lying down, which is relieved by his sitting up or lying propped on several pillows. This type of dyspnea is often misunderstood in the process of history taking and may be misrepresented:

- Patients often sleep propped up not because of experiencing discomfort when lying down, but following physician's recommendation — a fact easy to miss unless specifically inquired about;

- All too frequently a patient sleeping on two pillows is considered to be suffering from orthopnea, but this is a normal sleeping habit of many healthy subjects which does not necessarily constitute elevation of the thorax.

Thus, when inquiring about nocturnal respiratory discomfort, it is more important to note *changes* in the sleeping habits than the habits themselves. The type of position-related discomfort, the possible reasons for it and its response to therapy should all be considered before accepting this symptom as an important sign of left ventricular failure.

Chest Pain.   Anterior thoracic pain — along with dyspnea — represents a cardinal symptom of cardiac disease. Chest pain is obviously abnormal at all times and the problem of distinguishing a physiological from a pathological symptom does not come into consideration. The assessment of chest pain revolves around three questions:

1.   Is chest pain likely to be of cardiac origin?

2.   If it is cardiac, is it ischemic in nature?

3.   If it is ischemic, does it represent an anginal attack, myocardial infarction, or one of the intermediate forms between these two?

The differentiation of ischemic pain from noncardiac pain may be very easy, if either of the two appears in its most typical form. Ischemic pain is usually located in the substernal region, or across the upper anterior thorax, and is most frequently described as constricting or burning. It is radiated to the neck, shoulders and arms; sometimes to the sides of the face, the forearms down to the fingers and to the back of the thorax. "Typical" noncardiac pain occurs most often in the left side of the thorax, underneath the left breast, and is sharp or sticking in character, though it may also radiate to the left arm. Noncardiac pain often consists of a sharper component of short duration followed by a persistent dull ache located in the left submammary area.

Atypical forms of cardiac and noncardiac pain cause a considerable overlap between the ischemic and the innocent varieties of chest pain. A careful history taking often permits a reasonable differentiation. Yet, present-day coronary arteriography has demonstrated that occasionally false-positive as well as false-negative diagnoses of ischemic pain will be made even after the most careful assessment of symptoms. Each feature of the pain should be weighed in terms of the probability of its representing ischemic pain, especially when differentiation between it and the innocent chest-wall pain is being undertaken (Table 3–1).

It is important to be aware of the variations and peculiarities of ischemic cardiac pain. The painful sensation may be of such low inten-

TABLE 3–1. SOME FEATURES DIFFERENTIATING CARDIAC FROM NONCARDIAC CHEST PAIN

Favoring ischemic origin	Against ischemic origin
1. Character of pain	
constricting	dull ache
squeezing	"knife-like," sharp, stabbing
burning	"jabs" aggravated by respiration
"heaviness," "heavy feeling"	
2. Location of pain	
substernal	in the left submammary area
across mid-thorax, anteriorly	in the left hemithorax
in both arms, shoulders	
in the neck, cheeks, teeth	
in the forearms, fingers	
in the interscapular region	
3. Factors provoking pain	
exercise	pain *after* completion of exercise
excitement	provoked by a specific body motion
other forms of stress	
cold weather	
after meals	

sity that some patients refuse to call it pain and deny the presence of chest pain when asked, but insist on referring to the symptom they experience during exercise or otherwise as "unusual sensation," "pressure in the chest," or "burning in the chest." The possible confusion in the mind of the patient between pain and shortness of breath has already been mentioned. One should also be aware that not too infrequently patients may experience attacks of ischemic pain (or abovementioned pain-equivalent) located not in the thorax but in the areas of secondary radiation, i.e., the arms, the forearms, the neck, the shoulders, the teeth, and the interscapular region. Pain in one or more of these secondary areas may be associated with a delayed, often minor pain in the anterior thorax; occasionally no thoracic pain occurs at all.

In considering the probability of ischemic origin of chest pain one should include in the questioning a specific inquiry into certain factors capable of reducing the pain threshold and acting as precipitators of anginal attacks. Among these are:

- Walking after meals,

- Performance of any form of exercise in cold weather,

- Performance of the first exercise in the morning.

The last of these three factors is rather frequently seen in stable angina: Patients get an anginal attack when walking to work, but get no pain later while performing activities much more strenuous than the morning walk. Wenckebach referred to this phenomenon as acquiring the "second wind" after performance of the initial exercise.

There are many pitfalls in the differential diagnosis of chest pain. Whereas exercise is probably the most consistent and important provoking factor of ischemic chest pain, musculoskeletal pain, particularly originating in the costochondral and sternoclavicular junctions, also induces pain during exercise related to the motion of the arm concomitant with walking. Conversely, pain provoked by a specific body motion (moving the arms, bending down) may occasionally be ischemic in origin, although with such characteristics of the pain the questioner might be tempted to dismiss the pain as noncardiac.

The relief of pain by nitroglycerin is occasionally used as a therapeutic test aimed as identifying chest pain as ischemic in origin if relieved by the administration of this drug. This diagnostic approach may be useful but requires important qualifications:

1. Nitroglycerin, when properly taken (sublingually), should relieve the pain within $1/2$ to 3 minutes.

2. If the patient experiences side effect (headaches, throbbing), the relief of pain should roughly coincide with the timing of the side effect.

3. Failure of nitroglycerin to relieve the pain is a weak point against ischemic origin of the pain.

Even in observing these precautions, nitroglycerin as a therapeutic test may lead to false-positive and false-negative diagnoses.

The nonischemic varieties of anterior thoracic pain which should be differentiated from anginal pain include the following:

1. Left submammary pain of the neurotic and anxious individual,

2. Pain originating in the gastrointestinal tract (hiatus hernia, esophagitis, peptic ulcer, gallbladder disease, etc.),

3. Pleural pain, pain of pulmonary infarct and of pulmonary embolism,

4. Pain of aortic dissection,

5. Pain of pericarditis,

6. Pain of pneumothorax, mediastinal emphysema.

Ischemic pain appears in various forms: as effort angina, as angina at rest, as myocardial infarction with transitional forms in between. Except for the relationship to exercise or other exciting factors and for the difference in the duration, the features of the ischemic pain described above apply to all forms. The severity of pain may be higher in myocardial infarction than in pain associated with reversible myocardial ischemia, but not necessarily so. As a rule, the character of the pain tends to be repetitive: patients who suffer anginal attacks and then develop myocardial infarction often recognize the pain in the latter as resembling previous attacks, though it may be more intense and show wider radiation. A second myocardial infarction most frequently is associated with pain retaining the same characteristics as the first one. This constancy may be of considerable help in trying to reconstruct the natural history of ischemic disease in a given patient. Nevertheless the specificity of this feature is only fair: enough patients report differences in the type of pain between various ischemic episodes to advocate some caution in the interpretation of this relationship.

Nonischemic pain of cardiac origin involves two varieties: that originating in the pericardium and that associated with pulmonary hypertension. Pericardial pain overlaps partially with ischemic pain in regard to the location upon the thoracic wall. It does, however, often present sharp, stabbing components and is frequently influenced by changes in body position and by respiration (e.g., pain may be relieved by sitting up and leaning forward and may recur on resumption of recumbency).

Pain associated with pulmonary hypertension also has many similarities to ischemic pain. It is rare and its mechanism is not entirely clear. It is more often found in connection with acute pulmonary hypertension (i.e., massive pulmonary embolism) than in its chronic forms.

Differentiation of ischemic pain in particular or cardiac pain in general from other types of pain can be made with a reasonable probability on the basis of a carefully taken history. Pain of dissecting aneurysm will be discussed in Chapter 43. Pleural type pain (including that of pulmonary infarction) seldom presents diagnostic difficulties. Mediastinal emphysema may produce pain similar to that of myocardial infarction; it is, however, a very rare condition: its presence should be recognized by characteristic physical findings (e.g., subcutaneous emphysema) and by radiographic examination of the thorax. The similarity between the pain originating in the gastrointestinal tract (including hiatus hernia) and that produced by gallbladder disease and ischemic cardiac pain is overemphasized; an appropriate questioning should permit easy differentiation in most cases.

Thus the commonest and most important problem in the diagnosis of ischemic cardiac pain is its differentiation from thoracic wall pain of undetermined (and varied) origin. Details of the differentiation have been discussed in detail. Inasmuch as a definitive differentiation is not always possible, the classification of chest pain suggested by Hancock provides a useful way of presenting the *probability* of the nature of pain:

1. Typical ischemic chest pain

2. Atypical chest pain, probably ischemic in origin

3. Atypical chest pain, probably noncardiac

4. Noncardiac pain.

Palpitations.   The third common cardiac symptom is represented by palpitations, defined as the patient's consciousness of a forceful or unusual action of the heart. It should be emphasized that there is a wide individual variation regarding the awareness of one's cardiac action. Some patients are aware each time a premature contraction occurs; other cannot recognize the most chaotic cardiac action. Like dyspnea but unlike chest pain, palpitations represent a symptom that may be physiologically present in the normal population: excitement, fear, exercise make most normal subjects perceive some unusual cardiac action, often described as "pounding." Many also experience throbbing in the chest or the neck, when lying in bed.

Palpitations are perceived by patients with cardiac disease under a variety of circumstances and fall generally into two categories:

1. Perception of change in cardiac rate or rhythm,

2. Perception of a forceful cardiac action.

Palpitations as a symptom associated with arrhythmia often provide an important clue in the patient's history. Observant patients can describe the development of ectopic beats occurring singly or in series (e.g., bigeminy), can account for tachyarrhythmias or bradyarrhythmias, and can distinguish paroxysms of tachycardia or flutter (characterized by regular cardiac action) from atrial fibrillation (irregular cardiac action). A history of palpitations becomes of particular importance if arrhythmias occur in brief paroxysms that are often otherwise unwitnessed. It is necessary to question the patient regarding unusual heart action by asking for a description of the action and the mode of onset and termination (abrupt vs. gradual). It is often helpful to explain to the patient the significance of the various arrhythmias, thereby encouraging his more accurate observations. Patients who can reliably recount changes in their cardiac action often provide important diagnostic points regarding other aspects of the history (e.g., paroxysms of arrhythmia as a basis for ischemic pain at rest, syncope, dyspnea — otherwise unexplained).

The perception of the force of cardiac action may be present in overanxious normal subjects as well as in those with cardiac neurosis. ("Palpitations" are among the commonest symptoms in neurotic patients.) Some hypercirculatory states, such as hypertension, hyperthyroidism, and fever, may offer a background for "palpitations"; more important, however, are conditions in which cardiac overactivity is pathological, such as in states with volume overloading of the heart. The entity most consistently associated with subjective feeling of forceful cardiac action is aortic regurgitation, in which some patients find a constant throbbing barely tolerable.

An intermediate position between the two types of palpitations mentioned above is the consciousness of excessive cardiac action during exercise. Here the following conditions overlap and should be differentiated:

- Physiological tachycardia of a poorly conditioned individual during exercise;

- The same mechanism brought on prematurely by a cardiac malfunction, with the patient's attention drawn more easily to "pounding" than to dyspnea as the limiting factor during exercise;

- Excessive tachycardia developing in response to exercise (often minor) in patients with poorly controlled atrial fibrillation.

Fatigability. Tiredness is a detail in the clinical history to which very low specificity is attached. Yet, it often represents an important manifestation of impaired cardiac function. It is generally assumed that "fatigue" is more often due to causes other than cardiac disease and this is probably correct. However, the following qualifications should be taken into account:

1. Patients with poor powers of observation tend to lump all factors interfering with their locomotion as "fatigue." This can include dyspnea, chest pain, intermittent claudication and other symptoms. Detailed questioning usually permits some differentiation and identification of the components of "fatigue."

2. Fatigability is a specific cardiac symptom in patients whose circulatory malfunction involves primarily low cardiac output with an inadequate response to exercise, unaccompanied by excessively high filling pressures. It is most consistently observed in patients with cardiac failure who have involvement of the tricuspid valve (stenosis or regurgitation) in whom dyspnea is frequently minimized.

Dizziness.   As a clinical sign dizziness more often suggests abnormalities of the cerebral circulation or of the inner ear than cardiac disease. However, as a manifestation of cardiac disease it has the following implications:

1. As a symptom-equivalent of certain disturbances of cardiac rhythm: extremes of cardiac rate, i.e., bradyarrhythmia or very rapid tachyarrhythmias.

2. As a precursor of cardiac syncope, e.g., in ischemic heart disease, in quinidine toxicity, in aortic stenosis, or in heart block.

Some differential points can often be gathered from appropriate questioning: Dizziness associated with sudden change of posture is less significant in terms of a cardiac mechanism than that occurring during activity. Patients may also occasionally be aware of associated palpitations preceding or occurring simultaneously with an attack of dizziness.

Loss of Consciousness.   Syncope, like dizziness, may be associated with a variety of mechanisms, many of which are noncardiac. A careful questioning of the patient and—if available—of an eyewitness to the attack of "fainting" may provide diagnostic information. Such questioning may help in differentiating three conditions:

1. Simple faint (vasovagal attack or the like)

2. Cardiac syncope

3. Syncope due to a central nervous system mechanism.

The following points should be considered in questioning the patient:

• Suddenness of onset—the patient with true cardiac syncope

often falls to the ground without warning, possibly receiving injuries from the fall.

- In cardiac syncope loss of consciousness is the rule; upon termination of the attack consciousness is regained promptly.

- Observations may confirm the presence of an abnormal cardiac action (palpitations prior to the attack, slow or absent pulse during an attack).

These points, if present, throw the weight of evidence toward a cardiac mechanism of the syncopal attack. Vasovagal faint, also often associated with a bradycardia, tends to occur more gradually than cardiac syncope: the patient seldom falls to the ground fast enough to sustain injury; faint rarely leads to loss of consciousness, but rather to obtundation of senses. Neurological syncope may be followed by a prolonged semiconscious state and residual motor abnormalities. Nevertheless, the various forms of loss of consciousness have some similarities, and their causes may not always be readily determined; only tentative conclusions may be obtained from the history.

Fluid Retention. Fluid retention, one of the cardinal sequels to cardiac failure, produces a set of signs and symptoms that require consideration when a patient's history is being taken. Among clinical manifestations of fluid retention are the following:

- anasarca, most frequently manifested as dependent edema,

- pleural effusion and its consequences,

- various forms of dyspnea, as discussed above,

- epigastric "fullness," abdominal pain, ascites.

Cardiac edema is characteristically symmetrical. In questioning the patient it is necessary to probe into his concept of the meaning of the term "swelling." Observations of patients in this respect are often faulty, exaggerated, and have to be accepted with caution. Details, such as inability to put on a shoe or development of swelling in the evening and disappearance in the morning, add weight to the history of "swelling."

Many patients are aware of the importance of monitoring their body weight even before being instructed by the physician to do so. Variation in body weight represents an important historical point confirming the presence of fluid retention. In general, the following details should be elicited from the inquiry:

- relation of the variation of body weight to the administration of diuretics, if such drugs are used,

- variation of the body weight in relation to dietary salt intake, particularly sudden weight gain after a salty meal,

- relationship between body weight and cardiac symptoms such as dyspnea and abdominal fullness, particularly their disappearance after a diuresis.

Hemoptysis. Patients expectorating blood require detailed questioning regarding the following critical points:

- Does hemoptysis start with an attack of cough or develop late during a coughing spell?

- Is there pain associated with it?

- Does expectoration consist of pure blood, of blood-tinged sputum, or of foamy pink fluid?

- Is hemoptysis a single episode or is it repetitive?

- Is there a precipitating factor in evidence?

This analysis of factors associated with hemoptysis based on directed questioning of the patient may help identify the underlying cause, which varies greatly: it may be caused by pulmonary venous hemorrhage in mitral stenosis, by pulmonary hypertension, by pulmonary infarction, by acute pulmonary edema, as well as by hemorrhage from noncardiac causes, such as lung tumor, tuberculosis, pneumonia, bronchitis, or simply a rupture of a small vessel in the pharynx.

Embolic Phenomena. Systemic or pulmonary emboli play an important role in the course of various forms of cardiac disease. Specific questions should be directed toward events that could be interpreted as thromboembolism. This is of particular importance if the disease is known to be associated with a tendency to thrombus formation, e.g., mitral stenosis, infective endocarditis, acute myocardial infarction. A history of strokes, weakness of extremities, disturbances of speech, and lapses of memory represent items consistent with cerebral embolism, particularly in the association with conditions listed above. Other historical points include unexplained sudden pain in an extremity, abdominal colic, attacks of painful hematuria, all in the appropriate setting. Pulmonary emboli and infarcts may be suspected from a history of hemoptysis, attacks of "pneumonia," and attacks of chest pain of pleural type.

Other Clinical Symptoms. *Cyanosis* may be perceived by patients or their families. It is, however, a notoriously unreliable sign: history of cyanosis should be taken with caution and skepticism.

Abdominal pain, particularly that located in the right upper quadrant, may be related to hepatomegaly. This type of pain is often provoked by exercise; in older writings "intermittent swelling of the liver capsule" was occasionally mentioned as a symptom of cardiac failure. Today the widespread use of powerful diuretics makes this symptom less commonly encountered.

Upper respiratory infections occur in many forms of cardiac disease with higher frequency than in the general population. This is particularly true for patients with mitral valve disease and for children with large left-to-right intracardiac shunts.

Weight loss may occur in patients with chronic congestive cardiac failure. Some patients accumulate fluid inconspicuously, replacing body weight with fluid. When cardiac failure is diagnosed and diuretics administered patients can lose 10 kg. even though their original body weight remained the same while they accumulated the fluid. Extreme weight loss (cardiac cachexia) is rare; it occurs occasionally in patients with longstanding poorly controlled cardiac failure.

BACKGROUND HISTORY

The background history often provides important, even essential points permitting a more adequate interpretation of the patient's condition. It is most rewarding to focus the questioning upon areas likely to yield useful information in the light of clues obtained from the "history of the present condition." A lengthy, detailed inventory of *all* aspects of the patient's social, personal, and family history not only may be a waste of time but may detract from the pertinent questioning in the target area. In general, the goals of the background history include the following:

1. To provide information regarding the etiology of heart disease (e.g., rheumatic fever, lues).

2. To elicit the presence of risk factors (e.g., in ischemic heart disease)

3. To discover certain familial disease patterns.

4. To date the onset of cardiac disease (acute rheumatic fever, infective endocarditis), or determine the length it is known to have been present (history of cardiac murmur in childhood).

5. To probe for the possibility of erroneous past diagnoses with relationship to the heart, which in retrospect may be reinterpreted (e.g., attacks of "pneumonia" representing congestive cardiac failure, myocardial infarction mistaken for gastrointestinal upset).

The importance of the various bits of information obtained from the patient's past history varies considerably. For example, history of acute rheumatic fever in childhood is considered an important point in patients with valvular heart disease. Yet, the potential value of such a history is weakened by two aspects:

1. Somewhere between 25 and 50 per cent of patients with pathologically proven rheumatic heart disease give no history of rheumatic

fever. Various rheumatic fever "equivalents" are often inquired about: growing pains, frequent sore throats, nosebleeds, prolonged febrile illnesses in childhood. Yet the specificity of such details in the past history is so low as to make them practically valueless.

2. In the great majority of patients with a well-documented history of acute rheumatic fever no permanent valve damage results from it.

Thus, in an adult patient with a history of rheumatic fever a cardiac murmur, when present, is assumed to represent rheumatic heart disease; yet in some patients the murmur represents congenital heart disease; coincidental rheumatic fever in them may have left no sequels.

A history of a "heart murmur" in childhood may be of some assistance in suggesting congenital heart disease or rheumatic heart disease in an adult patient with cardiac disease. Yet it should always be remembered that this probability is weakened by the fact that a high proportion of normal children and adolescents have innocent systolic ejection murmur, the significance of which is often exaggerated.

In general, a past history of cardiac disease or of cardiac signs and symptoms should be regarded with caution, unless documented evidence is available. In addition to the rheumatic and congenital lesions discussed above, this applies to histories of "heart attacks," "endocarditis," "high blood pressure," and other illnesses.

The value of the *family history* is also variable, although in some conditions it may be of great assistance, even of critical importance. For example, in a young patient with ischemic heart disease a history of several cardiac deaths in the family at a young age may acquire ominous significance. Similarly, a history of severe hypertension in the family of a young hypertensive patient is of importance. In congenital heart disease the inquiry into the family history may provide aid in the differentiation between malformations caused by chromosomal abnormalities and genetic factors and those produced by "accidents" — noxious and teratogenic exposures — of the mother during early pregnancy.

There are some conditions in which a family history is of such importance that detailed inquiry regarding even distant relatives is in order. Among these are: hypertrophic subaortic stenosis, the syndrome of prolapsing mitral cusp, supravalvular aortic stenosis, and Marfan's syndrome. These clinical entities occur in both familial and sporadic forms, the latter being as a rule more benign than the former.

A SUMMARY OF GUIDELINES IN HISTORY TAKING

The guiding principle of the foregoing discussion is that a reliable and accurate history (perhaps better defined as the most accurate and reliable history a given individual is capable of providing under appropriately directed questioning) can be obtained, if specific objectives for each group of questions can be defined. One can best organize the process of history taking by starting the interview with some scouting around the patient's principal complaints until a list of possible diagnoses can be established. Then one can approach the patient with specifically directed questions in depth and detail. It is important not to neglect a supplementary history after the physical examination brings out new facts (e.g., if chest pain suggested ischemic heart disease and the questioning concentrated upon this diagnosis, but the physical examination revealed the presence of aortic stenosis, new questions specifically related to aortic stenosis should be asked after the examination).

Whenever the patient's activities are limited by symptoms, an attempt should be made to place the patient into a functional class. It is also of great importance to evaluate stability vs. progression of symptoms as well as the rapidity of progression.

The use of a problem-oriented system of record keeping renders itself well to history taking in a cardiac patient. Each symptom of note can be considered a "problem" that is pursued separately and analyzed independently from the others. By using this system one would be less likely to find a hospital chart with a 5-page history reporting every detail of the patient's life, listing every minor operation, but dismissing his principal problem with one sentence: "This patient suffers from shortness of breath (S.O.B.) of three months' duration."

Thinking in terms of the various problems, priorities might be set by asking the question, "Which part of the history is likely to contribute most to the diagnosis?" When the primary areas are identified, then the lower priority items can be handled more briefly, or even delegated to an assistant, or reviewed with the aid of a questionnaire. After all, it is hardly necessary to spend a great deal of time on a detailed family history and social history of a 75-year-old patient who suffers from angina of effort.

Bibliography

Hancock EW: Personal communication.

Rapaport E: Dyspnea; pathophysiology and differential diagnosis. Prog. Cardiovasc. Dis. *13*:532, 1971.

Wood P: The chief symptoms of heart disease. *In* DISEASES OF THE HEART AND CIRCULATION, 3rd Edition. Eyre and Spottiswoode, London, 1968, pp. 1–24.

Wright KE Jr, McIntosh HD: Syncope—A review of pathophysiological mechanisms. Prog. Cardiovasc. Dis. *13*:580, 1971.

4

Physical Examination

After completion of the clinical history, physical examination represents the next step in the orderly process of the diagnostic evaluation. Information gathered from the history usually permits one to focus upon the critical points of the examination.

The facilities and circumstances under which the examination is performed may have an important bearing upon the soundness of the conclusions that are to be reached: quiet surroundings insure better opportunity for accurate auscultation of the heart; proper setting and temperature may help the patient to attain better relaxation—a point that may significantly affect many findings (e.g., level of arterial pressure).

Physical examination of a patient with suspected or actual cardiac disease focuses upon three areas:

1. General status of the heart and circulation;

2. The presence or absence of signs indicative of cardiac failure ("congestion");

3. Overall observations pertaining to the etiology of cardiac disease, background features, and the presence of accompanying abnormalities of other organ-systems.

The traditional approach to the cardiac examination, one advocating inspection, percussion, palpation, and auscultation, performed sequentially, is now obsolete, for the following reasons:

First, percussion, as applied to the heart, has such a low reproducibility and variability from individual to individual that the time has come to retire its use.

Second, heart sounds and murmurs—the key to cardiac examination—need to be examined by both auscultation and palpation. These two approaches should obviously be performed together and not separately.

Third, all pulsatile phenomena require examination by palpation and inspection (occasionally auscultation as well). These, too, should be combined into one procedure.

In the following discussion the major emphasis will be placed upon the heart sounds, cardiac murmurs, and the various pulsatile phenomena. These components of the physical examination represent the principal sources of diagnostic information. Brief comments will be made regarding some of the remaining signs, many of which will be discussed in appropriate chapters.

The plan for an orderly performance of the physical examination of a patient with cardiac disease is highly individual. The following schema might be suggested:

1. General appearance: This part of the examination is largely performed by inspection, supplemented by palpation (e.g., temperature of the extremities). The following details should be considered:

   - color of skin and mucous membranes (cyanosis, pallor, icterus)

   - vasomotor status of the skin and extremities

   - body build, with special attention to hereditary syndromes

   - associated congenital malformation (cleft palate, etc.)

   - skeletal system (spinal and thoracic deformities)

   - extremities (joints, shape of fingers, clubbing)

2. Signs of congestion:

   - pulmonary rales

   - signs of pleural effusion

   - hepatomegaly

   - ascites

   - edema

3. Examination of the cardiovascular system:

   - arterial pulse

   - venous pulse

   - cardiac impulses and precordial motion

- cardiac sounds and murmurs
- funduscopic examination

HEART SOUNDS AND MURMURS

The principal tool for the examination of cardiac sounds and murmurs is the stethoscope. It is essential that two types of endpieces be available and used, namely the bell and the membrane. The former transmits better and amplifies low frequency vibrations, the latter higher frequencies. The areas of auscultation are well defined and include the apical and periapical area, the entire left sternal border, and the upper right sternal border. It is advisable to "inch" one's way from one area to another in order to explore the entire precordium. When murmurs are found, the secondary areas of the radiation should be determined over a wider area, including areas above and below both clavicles, the xiphoid area, the axilla, and the back of the thorax. Unusual radiation of a murmur may occur: murmurs should be traced and followed whenever they may be audible. In patients with poorly audible sounds and murmurs one can often hear the cardiac auscultatory phenomena better in the epigastrium or in the supraclavicular fossa, particularly if their poor audibility is caused by hyperinflation of the lungs.

Auscultation should be performed in the three standard body positions:

1.   With the patient recumbent,

2.   With the patient sitting, either straight or leaning forward,

3.   With the patient turned 45 to 60° into the left position, recumbent.

The First Sound

The first heart sound is a low frequency vibration heard in the apical region, but normally audible in all auscultatory areas. Though its origin is still subject to some controversy, it appears reasonable to accept the thesis that the principal components of this sound are generated by the tensing and closure of the atrioventricular valve apparatus, predominantly contributed by the mitral valve.

The normal splitting of the first sound — its separation into tricuspid and mitral components — is not nearly as regularly heard as that of the second sound. It is often uncertain whether a double first sound represents its normal splitting or merely its mitral component and an ejection sound.

Abnormalities of the first sound consist primarily of a change in its intensity. Occasionally the first sound is broad and reverberating, in which case it can easily be mistaken for a presystolic murmur. *Diminished* intensity of the first sound (also its "muffling") is traditionally linked with myocardial disease and cardiac failure. While this relationship undoubtedly exists, in practical terms the low intensity of the first sound is more often caused by poor transmission of the sound due to hyperinflation of the lungs, which provide an insulating cushion between the heart and chest wall. Consequently, low intensity of the first sound is a sign of very low specificity. Unless change in intensity can be observed in a day-to-day examination, this sign is unreliable.

Increased intensity of the first sound is, on the other hand, a sign of considerable importance. It is likely to occur when an altered atrioventricular pressure gradient is present in the left side of the heart (in mitral stenosis) or when atrial systole is delayed (short P-R interval). Other conditions that increase the intensity of the first sound (usually of the second sound as well) are various hypercirculatory states (tachycardia of fever, hyperthyroid state, anemia, and others).

The presence of an accentuated first sound is often the first finding drawing the attention of the examiner to the possibility of cardiac disease and encouraging him to search for other telltale findings that may be less apparent (e.g., diastolic murmur of mitral stenosis) and might be missed on a perfunctory clinical examination. Occasionally, none of the conditions mentioned are found, in which case one has to assume that the accentuated first sound represents an unusual variant of the norm.

The Second Sound

This sound consists of two sharp, high-frequency vibrations which are generated by the tightening and closure of the two semilunar valves. The first component normally represents aortic valve closure; the second one, pulmonic closure. The distance between the two components varies in relation to phases of respiration. During inspiration caval inflow of blood into the right side of the heart increases in response to the negative pressure inside the thorax: as a consequence of an increase in stroke volume, right ventricular systole lasts longer. At the same time there is a slight but definite inspiratory shortening of left ventricular systole. The reverse occurs during expiration. Thus, the variability of the splitting is related primarily to the pulmonary components moving away from the aortic component during inspiration. The inspiratory split is 0.03 to 0.05 sec, the expiratory 0.01 to 0.03. In most normal individuals the expiratory split is not perceived, hence the impression that a single sound is heard in expiration. How often normal inspiratory splitting is heard in healthy individuals depends largely upon the physician's auscultatory habits and training. The average examiner should be able to hear inspiratory splitting in the great majority of children and adolescents, with the frequency of perception of the split decreasing with age to about 40 per cent of healthy individuals over 50. Normally, the aortic component has an intensity two to three times that of the pulmonary component.

Abnormalities of the second sound rank high in importance in the diagnosis of cardiac disease. They include the following (Fig. 4–1):

1. *Reversed splitting* (paradoxical respiratory variation) occurs when a delay in left-sided ejection is present and/or left-sided systole is prolonged. As a consequence of this, the stable component — aortic valve closure — falls later than pulmonic valve closure and the normal respiratory shift of the pulmonic component brings the two close in inspiration, and farther away in expiration. The common conditions producing left-sided delay in valve closure are as follows:

- aortic stenosis

- left bundle-branch block

- left-to-right shunt bypassing the right ventricle (aorto-pulmonary communications)

- impairment of left ventricular function

There are adequate theoretical reasons for the presence of re-

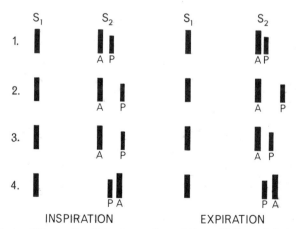

Figure 4–1. Diagrammatic presentation of the splitting of the second heart sound under normal and abnormal conditions: *1*, normal splitting; *2*, wide, fixed splitting; *3*, wide splitting with a normal respiratory variation; *4*, reversed splitting with a paradoxical respiratory variation.

versed splitting in the various conditions listed above. In reality, however, only a fraction of patients with these conditions show easily audible paradoxical respiratory variation. In aortic stenosis aortic valve closure may be poorly audible, or the pulmonary component may be overridden by the ejection murmur. Consequently reversed splitting is most commonly heard in young patients with aortic stenosis, or in the presence of pulmonary hypertension, when the pulmonic component is accentuated. In left bundle-branch block electromechanical dissociation may occur, i.e., delayed activation of the left ventricular musculature does *not* produce a mechanical delay in left ventricular contraction; hence reversed splitting is not always present. Thus, reversed splitting is a clinical sign of good specificity (within the context of the conditions producing it) but of low sensitivity.

2. *Widened interval* between the two components develops largely when right-sided ejection is prolonged or delayed. An additional factor may be increased capacitance of the pulmonary vascular tree (Shaver). Here the following are included:

- right bundle-branch block

- pulmonary stenosis

- left-to-right shunts at the intracardiac level (atrial and ventricular septal defect)

Right bundle-branch block—like its left-sided counterpart—does not always prolong the mechanical systole, hence wide splitting may be absent. In pulmonary stenosis widened splitting occurs regularly; one can even relate the severity of stenosis to the distance between the two components of the second sound. The pulmonary component of the second sound is of still lower intensity than normal and occasionally may be inaudible to auscultation, and demonstrated only by phonocardiography. When pulmonary stenosis is associated with considerable reduction of pulmonary flow (e.g., in tetralogy of Fallot) the late component of the second sound may disappear altogether, becoming unrecordable as well.

3. *Fixed splitting* implies the normal relationship of the two components but the absence of respiratory variation (actually some respiratory variation is present but cannot be perceived clinically). This occurs in atrial septal defect, in which the principal contribution of right ventricular stroke volume arrives from the left atrium rather than from outside the thorax, hence the influence of the variation in intrathoracic pressure is minimized. The two components are then more widely separated than usual. The intensity of the pulmonary component may be increased to match that of the aortic component.

4. *Increased intensity* of either component of the second sound occurs commonly when pressure or flow is increased in the respective circuits. Accentuation of the earlier component may occur in systemic hypertension, the second sound often acquiring a tambour-like quality. The pulmonary component, when accentuated, may become of equal intensity to the aortic. This occurs in pulmonary hypertension or with increase in pulmonary stroke volume.

5. *Disappearance of the second sound* may occur when aortic valve closure becomes inaudible and the pulmonary component is poorly transmitted. This occurs frequently in calcific aortic stenosis.

6. *Absence of the pulmonary component* alone produces a single second sound. Inasmuch as both components are heard consistently only in children and young adults, the finding of a single second sound is of importance in this age group only. This occurs when the pulmonary valve is absent (truncus arteriosus), when it is hypoplastic (tetralogy of Fallot and a variety of complex congenital defects), or in malposition of the pulmonic valve (in the various forms of transposition of the great arteries).

The diagnostic evaluation of the second sound requires careful auscultatory examination. Splitting is normally heard best at the left sternal border in the third and fourth intercostal spaces. Auscultation should be performed in recumbency and in the sitting position during quiet breathing and with breath-holding in inspiration and in expiration. The various abnormalities of the second sound listed above are of good specificity, therefore of diagnostic importance. The most common source of error is confusion between a fixed, widely split second sound of atrial septal defect and the opening snap of mitral stenosis. The similar frequency range of these two auscultatory findings may make the differentiation difficult, especially since their location upon the chest wall also overlaps to a considerable degree.

There are rare occasions when wide splitting of the second sound or other abnormalities of the relationship between its two components occur without any other detectable pathologic condition. This situation presumably represents an unusual normal variant.

The Third Sound

This sound occurs in early diastole toward the end of the rapid filling phase. Its origin is also the subject of some controversy. A widely held view is that the third sound is related to the re-tensing of the mitral valve apparatus (or tricuspid apparatus) occurring at the end of atrioventricular filling. The third sound is physiologically present in health and may become audible on the left side of the circulation as a low-frequency sound, resembling the first sound, located at the apical region. Its low intensity makes it easily audible only in children and thin-chested young adults. In the general population only an *accentuated* third sound is easily heard: it is termed an S3 gallop sound, or ventricular gallop sound (the older term "protodiastolic gallop sound" is rarely used now).

An S3 gallop sound develops when the flow through the mitral valve is increased or when an abnormal diastolic pressure relationship accelerates the atrioventricular filling. This includes:

- Mitral regurgitation

- Left-to-right shunts involving the left ventricle (ventricular septal defect and patent ductus arteriosus)

- Left ventricular failure

A special variety of an early diastolic sound similar in timing and acoustical quality to the S3 gallop sound, but different in mechanism, is the *pericardial sound,* which is thought to be generated by deceleration of the blood filling a ventricle when, in the presence of pericardial constriction, it suddenly reaches the limit of ventricular capacity. This sound is of value in confirming a clinical suspicion of pericardial constriction.

When abnormal pressure or flow relationship develops within the right ventricle, an S3 gallop sound originating in the right side of the heart may develop: this sound is usually heard along the left sternal border.

The diagnostic value of the S3 gallop sound is high in patients in the middle and older age groups. Even though it is occasionally possible to detect an S3 gallop sound in patients in these age ranges without evidence of underlying cardiac disease, the specificity of this sign, primarily as evidence of left ventricular failure, is still good and its sensitivity fair.

The Fourth Sound

The fourth heart sound occurs in the presystolic phase of diastole. Its origin, too, is not entirely clear: a valvular mechanism (re-tensing of the atrioventricular valve apparatus) is accepted by many. It occurs immediately after the atrial contraction and is contingent upon its presence; it disappears in atrial fibrillation and becomes misplaced in conditions in which the atrium contracts out of phase with ventricular contraction—remaining in constant relationship to the P wave of the electrocardiogram and the *a* wave of the venous pulse. It can be faintly heard in normal subjects over the entire age range but is particularly common in the older age group. As in the case of the third sound, the fourth sound acquires some diagnostic significance when accentuation of it takes place (S4 gallop sound, atrial gallop sound). Abnormally prominent S4 is related to lowered compliance of the left or right ventricle, respectively, i.e., when higher filling pressure is needed to "kick off" ventricular contraction and ejection. As a consequence, the S4 gallop sound occurs usually in association with an exaggerated *a* wave in the respective atrial pressure curves and with corresponding elevations of end-diastolic pressures. These phenomena can be recorded in the apexcardiogram and may be palpable; in fact an S4 gallop may occasionally be easier to perceive by palpation than by auscultation.

The diagnostic value of the S4 gallop sound is reduced by the fact that it is found in normal subjects as well as in patients with cardiac disease. Yet it is a very useful diagnostic sign when the S4 gallop is characterized by unusual loudness and supported by an abnormal apexcardiogram, or if it appears intermittently (e.g., during attacks of chest pain suspected of being ischemic in nature).

The S4 gallop sound thus may be an auscultatory equivalent of large *a* waves; its presence and prominence is expected in conditions characterized by the following:

- Pulmonary stenosis and pulmonary hypertension on the right side of the circulation,

- Left ventricular hypertrophy (particularly with outflow obstruction), acute forms of mitral regurgitation, ischemic heart disease — on the left side.

In patients with mitral or tricuspid stenosis, *a* waves are often prominent but an S4 gallop sound does *not* occur because of the slow rate of presystolic filling.

There are situations in which both S3 and S4 sounds become audible. When all four sounds are distinctly audible, the term "quadruple rhythm" has occasionally been used. More often, the two diastolic sounds merge into one, forming a "summation gallop" sound. This occurs either with excessive heart rates (usually above 120 beats per minute), or in cases with an abnormally long P-R interval, when the fourth sound moves away from the first sound.

The Mitral Opening Snap

Under normal conditions the mitral valve opens without producing an audible noise. The opening snap of the mitral valve is caused by the "doming" of the two mitral leaflets fused together by disease. It occurs at the moment the fused leaflets reach the maximum excursion permitted by their fusion as they attempt to open and move toward the ventricle. Thus, the requirement for the presence of a mitral opening snap is:

1. Sufficient fusion of the two leaflets to prevent complete opening,

2. Reasonable mobility of the mitral leaflets.

The opening snap disappears when heavy calcifications restrict the motion of this valve. The sound generated by this doming is one of high frequency, sharp; it is similar to the semilunar valve closure sounds. The opening snap occurs early during the diastolic phase of the cycle; its distance from the aortic component of the second sound is related to the height of left atrial pressure: the higher the pressure in the left atrium during early diastole, the closer is the opening snap to the second sound (Fig. 4–2). The opening snap of the mitral valve is best heard medially to the apical region and along the left sternal border. Loud opening snaps may be heard over the entire precordium. Inasmuch as the mitral opening snap usually initiates the rumbling diastolic murmur of mitral stenosis and is often merged with the murmur, its presence has to be established by careful auscultation in areas where the mitral diastolic murmur is no longer present but the snap may be audible.

The opening snap of the mitral valve, if correctly identified, is a highly specific diagnostic sign; it has good sensitivity in patients with mitral stenosis, in whom fluoroscopic examination does not show the presence of mitral valve calcifications. The mitral opening snap often is the more obvious clinical sign of mitral stenosis that may first draw attention to the presence of this valvular lesion.

The Systolic Ejection Sound

An early systolic sound occurring shortly after the first heart sound is present in a variety of conditions and is often of considerable diagnostic importance. It may be generated by one of two unrelated mechanisms:

1. It may represent an opening snap of a stenotic semilunar valve.

2. It may be related to the dilatation of either the aorta or the pulmonary artery above the semilunar valves. The production of this second variety of the ejection sound is not adequately explained.

An opening snap of a stenotic aortic valve is analogous to the mitral opening snap. It, too, requires valve mobility and fusion; it disap-

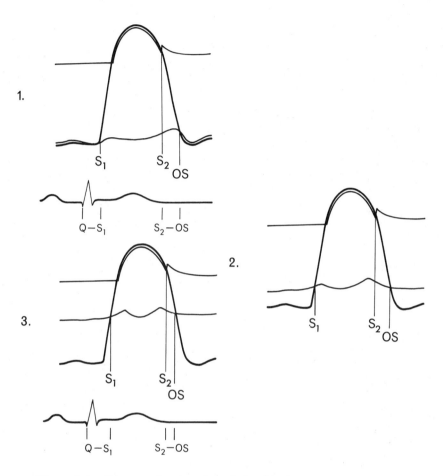

Figure 4-2. Diagram showing the relationship between the location of the mitral opening snap and the height of the left atrial pressure, as well as the delay of the first sound produced by elevation of left atrial pressure: *1*, normal, potential location of the opening snap (not heard in healthy subjects); *2*, mild delay of the first sound (in relation to the Q wave of the electrocardiogram) and the appearance of the mitral opening snap slightly closer to aortic valve closure in the presence of mild elevation of left atrial pressure; *3*, considerable delay of the first sound and still earlier appearance of the opening snap in the presence of high left atrial pressure. (See also Chapter 32.)

pears if the valve becomes heavily calcified and stiff. It occurs 0.04 to 0.08 sec after the first heart sound; it has a sharp, high-frequency quality and is usually heard along the left sternal border. The opening snap of the pulmonary valve occurs in valvular pulmonary stenosis and is in all respects similar to that originating at the aortic valve.

The diagnostic value of the ejection sound lies in the fact that it is generated by valve leaflets, hence proves the valvular origin of outflow obstruction. In aortic stenosis (before valve calcifications set in) the systolic ejection sound differentiates valvular from subvalvular and supravalvular varieties of stenosis. In pulmonary stenosis it separates valvular from infundibular stenosis. In this context it represents a good diagnostic sign in terms of sensitivity and specificity.

The ejection sound produced by dilatation of the great arteries is found in pulmonary hypertension, in large left-to-right shunts (particularly in atrial septal defect), in systemic hypertension, and in aortic aneurysm or other diseases of the aortic root. Its diagnostic contribution is only fair, especially since normal children and adolescents occasionally have systolic ejection sounds (presumably as normal variants).

The Midsystolic Click

This sound, also called non-ejection systolic sound or click, has been in the past associated with extracardiac events, particularly as a residual from pericarditis. In recent years this sound has been identified as originating in the mitral valve and generated by a midsystolic and late systolic prolapse of a valve cusp that is enlarged and associated with stretched chordae tendineae. This mechanism also produces the late systolic murmur. Midsystolic clicks associated with late systolic murmurs can be assumed as originating in the prolapsing mitral valve. Those present alone may be of either extracardiac or valvular origin (extracardiac sounds include not only those produced by pericarditis but also some associated with mediastinal shifts, e.g., in pneumothorax). Occasionally, two or more clicks may be heard in midsystole. The significance of these findings will be discussed in connection with mitral regurgitation.

Prosthetic Valve Sounds

Many patients today have prosthetic valves that generate sounds unlike those occurring naturally. The most widely used artificial valve is a ball valve or its modification. It generates a loud clicking sound of high frequency that is louder than physiological or pathological sounds. The prosthetic valve sounds correspond to the opening and closing of the prosthesis, which come close to, but are not identical in timing with, the opening and closure of the valve they replaced. The mitral valve prosthesis produces its closing sound at the time usually occupied by the first sound. The opening of the mitral prosthesis corresponds in timing to the opening snap of the mitral valve. Along with the semi-lunar valve closure, the mitral valve prosthesis produces a loud triple sound for each cardiac cycle. The aortic valve prosthesis opens, generating a click timed at a point corresponding to an ejection sound; its closure replaces the second sound (drowning out the pulmonary component). With the valve opening sound often drowning out the first sound, the aortic valve prosthesis produces a *double sound* with each cardiac cycle. A homograft valve placed in the aortic position produces soft sounds analogous to those of the normal aortic valve. A homograft or heterograft valve placed in the mitral position and artificial valves built of fascia lata generate sounds ranging from soft and near-normal to loud clicks similar to those produced by ball valves.

Auscultation of the artificial valve sounds may provide important clues regarding its malfunction. A decrease in the intensity of one or both sounds or a malposition within the cardiac cycle (delayed opening or closure) should be considered with suspicion as a possible sign of ball valve variance or of thrombus formation.

CARDIAC MURMURS

Murmurs originating within the heart and great vessels are customarily classified as systolic, diastolic, and continuous.

Murmurs in general are generated by vibrations of the valve and adjacent structures produced by periodic fluctuations of blood flow when passing obstacles (Bruns). They become audible if the flow is of high velocity and the obstacle (stenosis) of significant severity. Murmurs show wide variation in sound frequencies, covering most of the audible range. Some murmurs have symmetrical (harmonic) qualities, producing sounds of musical pitch; the majority show a mixture of frequencies audible as nonmusical noises. Murmurs showing predominance of low frequencies, when of appreciable intensity, produce vibration of the chest wall that can be palpated as *thrills*.

Systolic Murmurs

Murmurs occurring during systole are customarily divided into two principal varieties (Leatham) (Fig. 4–3):

- Ejection systolic murmurs, produced by abnormalities of blood flow passing through existing cardiac orifices in normal directions;

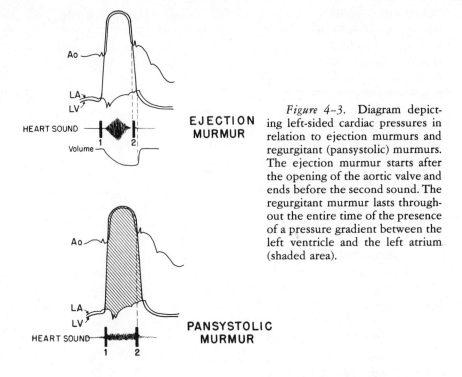

Figure 4-3. Diagram depicting left-sided cardiac pressures in relation to ejection murmurs and regurgitant (pansystolic) murmurs. The ejection murmur starts after the opening of the aortic valve and ends before the second sound. The regurgitant murmur lasts throughout the entire time of the presence of a pressure gradient between the left ventricle and the left atrium (shaded area).

- Regurgitant systolic murmurs (holosystolic, pansystolic), caused by flow of blood through abnormal channels or in abnormal directions.

Ejection systolic murmurs are generated when the flow of blood ejected into a great vessel is altered by one or more of the following:

- orifice stenosis

- increased stroke volume

- increased flow velocity

- decrease in blood viscosity

- a combination of these factors

Ejection murmurs start after the first sound, separated by an interval composed of the isovolumetric contraction period plus the earliest portion of the ejection period when not enough velocity of flow develops to produce the critical vibration. The murmur terminates before the second sound, at a point when the flow velocity drops below the level of audible vibrations. The murmur, furthermore, builds up higher intensity with the increase of flow velocity during the first half of systole, then drops off in intensity with the fall in velocity, hence its characteristic diamond shape (crescendo-decrescendo character). The ejection murmur is best heard at the upper part of the projection of the heart upon the thorax (the "base"). It may be conducted above the clavicles, to the back of the thorax, toward the apical area. Loud ejection murmurs, such as those in aortic stenosis, may be conducted far away from the precordium.

It is clear from the foregoing discussion that the ejection murmur occurs both with and without organic cardiac disease. Among causes of ejection type systolic murmurs are the following conditions:

- Left ventricular outflow obstruction (aortic stenosis, subvalvular aortic stenosis, supravalvular aortic stenosis, hypertrophic subaortic stenosis)

- Right ventricular outflow obstruction (valvular pulmonary stenosis, infundibular right ventricular stenosis, supravalvular pulmonary artery stenosis)

- Physiological hypercirculatory state of children and adolescents (increased stroke volume and flow velocity)

- Pathological hypercirculatory states ("high output states," e.g., hyperthyroidism)

- Regional increase in blood flow — pulmonary ejection murmur in atrial septal defect

- A combination of increased flow and reduced blood viscosity — severe anemia

The wide range of causes of systolic ejection murmurs requires a careful differentiation between clinically important and unimportant murmurs. Certain guidelines are helpful in the differential diagnosis, although consideration of other clinical findings as well as the murmurs is usually required. The following observations are helpful in the initial approach to the interpretation of the significance of an ejection murmur:

- The intensity of the ejection murmur is often helpful in the diagnosis: low intensity murmurs (grades I and II on the scale of I to VI) are seldom organic in nature. Conversely, loud murmurs (grades V and VI) are almost always due to organic outflow stenosis (but do not necessarily signify severe obstruction).

- The duration of the murmur is also of some significance: short midsystolic murmurs are likely to be innocent; long murmurs (starting close to the first sound and terminating just before the second sound) are usually due to organic disease.

- Given a murmur of organic outflow obstruction, late peaking of the "diamond-shaped" murmur signifies a higher degree of stenosis than in early-peaking murmurs of similar intensity.

- Being dependent upon the volume of flow, ejection murmurs vary with changes in cardiac output. They become louder with exercise (regardless of cause); their reproducibility from day to day is often variable, especially in the case of nonorganic murmurs. A murmur well heard during an outpatient examination may become faint or absent when the patient is re-examined under basal conditions (e.g., early morning examination in the hospital).

The *innocent cardiac murmur* ("functional" murmur) often presents a diagnostic challenge. Innocent murmurs fall into the category of ejection murmurs (with the sole exception of the venous hum) and, as noted in the discussion above, overlap widely with organic cardiac murmurs. At the extremes of the spectrum of loudness of murmurs a reasonable separation of innocent from organic murmurs can be made; in the center of the spectrum the two overlap. Among innocent murmurs there are some with special features:

- A low-frequency musical murmur, occasionally referred to as a "groaning murmur," "twanging string murmur," or "Still's murmur," located at the left sternal border, is frequently heard in older children and adolescents. It is occasionally quite loud (grade III or IV).

- Vascular bruit—a short, often loud midsystolic ejection murmur is usually heard loudest above the right clavicle, but may be audible far enough below the clavicles to overlap with a murmur of mild aortic stenosis; this murmur is thought to originate at the aorto-innominate junction.

These two murmurs, as well as noncharacteristic ejection murmurs heard at both sides of the sternum in the second, third and fourth intercostal spaces, overlap with those caused by cardiac disease. The following conditions need to be differentiated from innocent systolic ejection murmurs:

- mild aortic stenosis

- mild pulmonary stenosis

- atrial septal defect

- hypertrophic subaortic stenosis

The first two entities produce murmurs that are actually indistinguishable from innocent murmurs except by invasive diagnostic studies, inasmuch as in mild valvular diseases no effect upon other physical findings, upon the radiographic findings, and upon the electrocardiogram is detectable. In the latter two conditions, associated findings often, though not always, permit clinical differentiation.

When confronted with an ejection murmur loud enough to suggest a high probability of organic origin, the differentiation between pulmonary and aortic stenosis can usually be made on the basis of the location of the loudest point of the murmur. Occasionally murmurs are head in atypical locations, and this presents diagnostic difficulty. In such cases the associated clinical findings permit differentiation:

- characteristics of the second sound

- chamber enlargement, if any, as demonstrated in the radiograph

- electrocardiographic findings of hypertrophy of either ventricle.

There are cases in which differentiation between ejection murmurs and regurgitant murmurs presents diagnostic difficulty. The following situations exemplify possible points of confusion:

- Mitral regurgitation due to isolated rupture of chordae tendineae to the posterior mitral cusp often produces a diamond-shaped holosystolic murmur best heard at the base of the heart; it may be conducted above the clavicles, thus masquerading as aortic stenosis.

- Murmur of supracristal ventricular septal defect is also well heard at the base of the heart and may show diamond configuration.

- Murmur of calcific aortic stenosis may be best heard at the apical region; with both sounds often faint or inaudible, the guidelines for separation of the ejection from the regurgitant type of murmur are obliterated.

- In aortic stenosis the murmur may be widely conducted and acquire different acoustic qualities in its transmission to the apical area, thus making it difficult to decide whether one hears a single murmur or whether mitral regurgitation is present in addition.

Regurgitant systolic murmurs, produced by flow of blood through abnormal channels or in abnormal directions, are, as a rule, related to organic cardiac disease. They do not necessarily, however, carry serious connotations; some, in fact, may have a prognosis as favorable as an innocent murmur. The principal regurgitant murmurs are the following:

- regurgitation through an incompetent mitral valve

- regurgitation through an incompetent tricuspid valve

- flow through a ventricular septal defect

- flow through other abnormal communication occurring only in systole (e.g., left-ventricular–right-atrial communication, some aortocardiac fistulae)

Regurgitant murmurs start simultaneously with the closure of the atrioventricular valves and extend beyond the second sound up to the opening of the atrioventricular valve on the respective side. In practice, however, audible vibrations appear to terminate *with* the second sound. Murmurs of this variety as a rule show even intensity (with exceptions noted previously). Their location on the chest wall shows wider variation than that of ejection murmurs. As a rule they are heard best at the lower part of the cardiac projection upon the thorax.

While, as stated, regurgitant murmurs and holosystolic (pansystolic) murmurs are used interchangeably as synonyms, not all regurgitant murmurs are heard throughout systole: either the early systolic or the late systolic part of the murmur may be absent. They are never, however, midsystolic, a feature characteristic for ejection murmurs. Nonholosystolic regurgitant murmurs are produced by one of two mechanisms:

- The velocity of regurgitant flow may drop below the critical point of production of vibrations during a part of systole.

- The valve may be incompetent (or a septal defect open) only during a portion of the systole.

Thus, early systolic murmurs or late systolic murmurs have been observed in patients with mitral regurgitation as well as with ventricular septal defect. Some regurgitant murmurs present unusual acoustical features:

- high-frequency musical murmurs (whistling, "seagull" murmurs)

- low-frequency musical murmurs (honks, whoops)

Murmurs with these characteristics may be holosystolic or late systolic; some show an extraordinary variability in intensity from minute to minute and may change in character and loudness in relation to the patient's position.

The three principal regurgitant murmurs—those of mitral

regurgitation, tricuspid regurgitation, and ventricular septal defect — may present difficulties of differential diagnosis. In brief, the following distinguishing features are considered characteristic for these murmurs:

- Mitral regurgitant murmurs are apical with preponderant radiation to the axilla and the left infrascapular region.
- Tricuspid regurgitant murmurs are best heard in the xiphoid area and become louder during inspiration.
- Murmurs of ventricular septal defect are best heard at the lower left sternal border and are often fairly localized.

Murmurs of mitral regurgitation, as described above, account for the majority of patients with chronic (usually rheumatic) mitral valve disease. Some special forms of mitral regurgitation are characterized by murmurs different from the "classical" variety:

- Murmurs associated with partial prolapse of the posterior cusp, imitating aortic stenosis (see above);
- Murmurs associated with partial prolapse of the anterior leaflet, often conducted to the back of the thorax and the spine, and occasionally audible at the top of the head;
- Murmurs associated with "billowing" of the mitral valve — late systolic murmur, often initiated by a midsystolic click;
- Mitral "honks" and "whoops," mentioned above, also caused by billowing mitral leaflet; they may be late systolic or holosystolic.

Diastolic Murmurs

As in the case of systolic murmurs, diastolic cardiac murmurs may be produced either by altered flow conditions through normal orifices or by flow through abnormal channels (usually incompetent semilunar valves). By analogy, these two varieties deserve the terms "stenotic" and "regurgitant" murmurs; yet their acoustical qualities are not sufficiently characteristic to label them as such.

The principal diastolic murmurs are the following:

- murmur of organic mitral stenosis,
- murmur of "functional" mitral stenosis associated with increased velocity or volume of flow through the mitral orifice,

- murmur of organic tricuspid stenosis,

- murmur of "functional" tricuspid stenosis,

- murmur of aortic regurgitation,

- murmur of primary pulmonary regurgitation,

- murmur of secondary pulmonary regurgitation.

Murmurs of *mitral stenosis* are usually initiated by a mitral opening snap, if one is present; in any event, they are separated from the second sound by at least 0.06 sec. The mitral murmur is localized to the apical area, occasionally heard only in the left lateral position; it is a low-frequency vibration producing a "rumbling" quality. In patients with a normal rhythm the murmurs decrease slightly toward middiastole, then become accentuated with a crescendo terminating in the accentuated first sound of the next cardiac cycle. In the presence of atrial fibrillation the presystolic phase of the murmur is usually absent. The traditional view holds the presence of atrial systole to be a prerequisite of the presystolic part of the murmur, but recently mechanisms other than atrial systole have been implicated in the causation of the presystolic murmur.

The classical murmur of mitral stenosis occurs in organic mitral stenosis. Other low-frequency apical diastolic murmurs obviously originating in the mitral valve are found in conditions of altered flow through that valve:

- severe mitral regurgitation (without concomitant stenosis)

- patent ductus arteriosus

- ventricular septal defect

In these three conditions a large volume of blood passes through the mitral orifice, making the normal mitral valve "relatively stenotic" for the given flow. In addition, increased flow velocity without increase in the volume of flow may produce mitral diastolic rumbling murmurs. This occurs occasionally in left ventricular failure as a result of abnormal pressure relationships. These functional murmurs do not extend into presystole.

A specific mechanism of production of a nonorganic mitral diastolic murmur operates in patients with significant aortic regurgitation. Here the regurgitant jet of blood from the aorta and the atrial blood inflowing through the mitral orifice, both directed toward the apex of the left ventricle, produce vibration of the anterior leaflet of the mitral valve caught between the two streams. (Fluttering of that cusp can be shown in the echocardiogram.) This murmur—the Austin Flint murmur—may be indistinguishable from the murmur of organic mitral stenosis, as it often extends into the presystolic phase of diastole.

Functional mitral diastolic murmurs, with the exception of the Austin Flint murmur, are shorter than the organic murmurs (even in atrial fibrillation) and often are initiated by an S3 gallop sound.

The murmur of organic mitral stenosis, with the qualifications noted above, constitutes one of the most specific signs in cardiac diagnosis; its sensitivity is good too, especially if a most thorough physical examination is performed in a patient suspected of having rheumatic heart disease. (For further details see Chapter 32.)

The murmur of *tricuspid stenosis* differs from that of mitral stenosis in its auscultatory characteristics as well as in its location upon the chest wall. The murmur is basically of somewhat higher frequency than the mitral "rumble." Its relationship to respiration, already mentioned, is pathognomonic for it — as it is for right-sided hemodynamic events in general. The murmur is usually heard best at the lower end of the sternum. It should be noted that, whereas in mitral stenosis the diastolic murmur has a good sensitivity, the murmur of tricuspid stenosis has a low sensitivity, often being completely absent in organic tricuspid stenosis.

In atrial septal defect a tricuspid flow murmur is often present, representing a functional diastolic murmur originating at the tricuspid valve. This murmur is located to the left of the sternum (usually 4th to 6th costal cartilages), may have still higher frequency, and sometimes may acquire a "scratching" quality. It, too, varies with respiration, becoming louder in inspiration.

In *aortic regurgitation* the diastolic murmur begins with the closure of the aortic valve and extends into the diastole to a variable degree, never encroaching upon atrial systole, though. Characteristically, the murmur is of very high frequency, often of whispering quality, resembling breath sounds. Occasionally it acquires a twanging musical tinge. Its location upon the chest wall is at the lower part of the left sternal border and it is usually better conducted to the apical region than to the "aortic" area proper. Aortic diastolic murmur that shows maximum loudness at the right upper sternal border ("aortic area") should be suspected of being caused by unusual forms of aortic regurgitation.

Murmurs of aortic regurgitation have good specificity except in differentiation from secondary pulmonary regurgitation; sensitivity of such murmurs is very good (with careful auscultation).

Mitral and aortic diastolic murmurs often occur in the same patient, the bivalvular lesion being a common sequel to rheumatic fever. Inasmuch as the locations of the two murmurs upon the chest wall overlap, the differentiation may present some difficulties. In differentiation of the two murmurs — or in reaching the decision that both coexist — the most discriminating features in the differential diagnosis are, in the order of importance:

- the timing of onset of each murmur (aortic: early diastolic; mitral: delayed diastolic)

- the pitch of the murmur (aortic: high frequency; mitral: low frequency)

- distribution and radiation on the chest wall (aortic: left sternal border; mitral: apical conducted to axilla or localized)

Pulmonary regurgitation, as stated, occurs in a primary and in a secondary form, each producing a different sounding murmur:

1. Organic pulmonary regurgitation—found as an isolated congenital lesion or one produced by surgical manipulation upon the pulmonary valve—is characterized by a murmur slightly delayed, i.e., starting a brief interval after pulmonary valve closure and showing medium sound frequencies. This murmur may also present a diamond-shaped crescendo-decrescendo quality.

2. Secondary pulmonary regurgitation, occurring more frequently than the primary form, is produced when the pulmonary valve is exposed to unaccustomed high pressure in diastole, i.e., in severe pulmonary hypertension (from any cause). The murmur produced by this mechanism is acoustically indistinguishable from that of aortic regurgitation, though it may be located higher at the left sternal edge, at the level of the second or third costal cartilage. These murmurs obviously overlap in location with those of aortic regurgitation; the differentiation often depends upon demonstration of significant pulmonary hypertension, the *sine qua non* of the secondary pulmonary diastolic murmur. In mitral stenosis associated with high pulmonary vascular resistance this murmur is known by the eponym "Graham Steell murmur."

Continuous Murmurs

Intracardiac murmurs as a rule are limited to a single phase of the cardiac cycle (regurgitant systolic murmurs override the second sound, but appear, in auscultation, to be limited to systole). Murmurs widely overriding change of phase in the cardiac cycle originate—in part at least—outside the heart, usually in the arterial system. *Continuous murmurs* are murmurs that last throughout the entire cycle without interruption, showing some variation in pitch and intensity. *Venous hum* also presents a continuous noise; it can be distinguished from the continuous murmur by a more even intensity and somewhat higher pitch.

Loud continuous murmurs are truly continuous and are usually described as "machinery murmurs" because of their quality. They are as a rule accentuated in late systole, have their highest intensity at the time of semilunar valve closure, and then run decrescendo toward the first sound. Softer continuous murmurs show a similar configuration when recorded; however, part of the murmur falls below the threshold of audibility. Consequently, the murmurs are heard during most of systole, reach crescendo toward the second sound, and fade out in mid-diastole. Continuous murmurs are of high and medium frequencies. Their location upon the chest wall varies, depending upon their origin. Continuous murmurs are produced by one of two mechanisms:

1. The escape of blood from the high-pressure arterial system into a low-pressure system (a pressure gradient between the two systems has to be present both in systole and in diastole). The following entities fall in this category:

- patent ductus arteriosus
- aortic-pulmonary window
- aortic-right heart fistula (e.g., ruptured aneurysm of the sinus of Valsalva)
- arteriovenous fistula in the systemic circulation
- coronary artery — pulmonary artery fistula.
- coronary artery — right ventricular or coronary sinus fistula

2. Flow of blood through a stenotic segment within the arterial system with an adequate volume of flow to produce pressure gradient in diastole and in systole. Examples:

- coarctation of the aorta
- branch stenosis of the pulmonary artery (in the presence of pulmonary hypertension)
- various forms of collateral supply vessels from the systemic arterial circulation to the pulmonary circulation in complex forms of congenital heart disease

Continuous murmurs sufficiently loud to be audible throughout the cycle can be recognized relatively easily. Yet, some diagnostic difficulties may arise in separating them from certain combinations of systolic and diastolic murmurs of similar frequency and related areas of audibility. Among these are:

- ventricular septal defect with aortic regurgitation
- mitral regurgitation and aortic regurgitation

Other diagnostic difficulties may be posed by the following:

- venous hum, especially when conducted to and well audible in the subclavicular areas

- softer "continuous" murmurs that are audible mostly through systole which can be confused with systolic ejection murmurs

Other Precordial "Noises"

In addition to sounds and murmurs, the following acoustical phenomena heard in the precordial region and synchronous with cardiac action should be noted:

1. *Pericardial friction rub.* This noise is present in various stages of acute pericarditis, or, occasionally, in conditions in which the pericardium is involved in a pathological process (e.g., tumor invasion). In its typical form pericardial rub is characterized by its different acoustical features, described as "leathery, squeaky" noise, and by the fact that it occurs in more than one phase within each cycle — usually two in systole and one in diastole. Atypical friction rubs may acquire features that more closely resemble those of murmurs. In general the relationship of the rub to the heart sound is less constant than that of intracardiac murmurs.

2. *Extracardiac "murmurs."* Various noises may originate in the structures adjacent to the heart and become synchronous with cardiac motion. Among those in which a point of origin is tentatively established are the following:

- sterno-xiphoid crunch

- cardiorespiratory murmurs

- noise associated with mediastinal emphysema

3. *Tumor "plop"* is heard occasionally if the intracardiac tumor is pedunculated (usually atrial myxoma) whereby wide motion of the tumor is possible. This appears usually as an early diastolic sound somewhat resembling the S3 gallop sound but with a less constant relationship to the second sound.

AUSCULTATORY RECAPITULATION

Auscultation is often the key to the physical examination of patients with cardiac disease (Fig. 4–4). It is a difficult part of the examination, requiring experience and training. However, the information

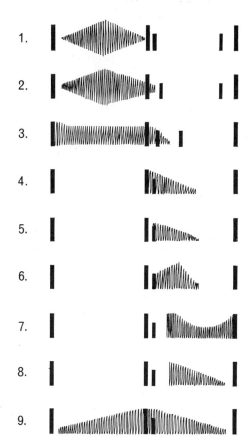

Figure 4-4. Diagrammatic presentation of some cardiac murmurs and their timing and "shape": *1,* ejection murmur originating in the left ventricle (aortic stenosis); *2,* ejection murmur originating in the right ventricle (pulmonary stenosis); *3,* regurgitant murmur originating in the left ventricle (mitral regurgitation or ventricular septal defect); *4,* early diastolic murmur of aortic regurgitation; *5,* early diastolic murmur of secondary pulmonary regurgitation; *6,* early diastolic murmur of primary pulmonary regurgitation; *7,* "rumbling" diastolic murmur of mitral stenosis in the presence of sinus rhythm; *8,* rumbling diastolic murmur of mitral stenosis in the presence of atrial fibrillation; *9,* continuous murmur (patent ductus arteriosus and the like).

gained from it often has the highest specificity of any part of the physical examination. Adequate cardiac auscultation requires the examiner to analyze each finding critically and to assure himself of its full diagnostic impact. Clinical judgment should dictate reasonableness of time investment: it is obviously unnecessary to perform as detailed an examination in a healthy subject undergoing routine check-up as in a patient with cardiac symptoms or with prior suspicion of cardiac disease. Yet, potentially serious cardiac lesions may be overlooked in seemingly healthy individuals subjected to brief perfunctory physical examinations. The analytic approach to auscultatory examination can be exemplified by the following points:

1. The examination should be approached in the light of the information gained from the history and should focus upon the most critical points likely to yield diagnostic leads. If the history is entirely negative, special attention should be directed toward subtle findings suggesting potential abnormalities.

2. Distinction should be made between findings that are definitely abnormal (diastolic murmurs, regurgitant systolic murmurs) and those with only quantitative margins separating the normal from the abnormal (abnormalities of heart sounds, ejection type systolic murmurs).

3. Given a finding with a good specificity, one should concentrate on concurrent diagnostic findings and on signs capable of amplifying the diagnostic information (e.g., finding a murmur of mitral stenosis establishes the diagnosis; additional presence of a mitral opening snap signifies that good mobility of the mitral valve exists).

4. Standard examination should be implemented by special maneuvers designed to amplify subtle abnormalities; furthermore, one should be aware of the various conditions that may modify auscultatory findings. This can often provide significant help in diagnosis. The following are especially worth noting:

- Carotid sinus stimulation may slow excessively rapid heart rates and permit a more reliable appraisal of auscultatory findings.

- Cardiac murmurs and abnormal sounds originating on the left side of the heart can often be differentiated from those on the right side of the heart by the fact that the latter become louder with inspiration, the former do not.

- The presence of an arrhythmia may greatly assist in the differentiation between ejection and regurgitant systolic murmurs; the former vary in loudness with the cycle length, becoming louder after longer pauses. Regurgitant murmurs show little variation associated with unequal cycle length.

- Exercise increases cardiac output and velocity of blood flow; its alteration of auscultatory findings may be important in bringing out previously inaudible murmurs (e.g., mitral stenosis). Furthermore, it augments ejection murmurs more than regurgitant murmurs.

- The Valsalva maneuver may help in the differentiation of some murmurs, particularly that of hypertrophic subaortic stenosis which becomes louder during the straining period.

- Drugs may alter murmurs in a predictable direction and help in their differentiation. The most widely used drug for this purpose is amyl nitrate, which reduces both the preload and the afterload of ventricular contraction: ejection murmurs may decrease in intensity, while regurgitant murmurs remain unchanged.

- Some auscultatory findings appear intermittently, yet their temporary presence may be of diagnostic importance. One can include in this category gallop sounds and murmurs appearing during attacks of ischemic chest pain; the murmur of mitral stenosis is heard only immediately after exercise.

- Day-to-day variability for some auscultatory findings has to be taken into consideration. The dependence of the intensity of systolic ejection murmurs upon time and place of the examination has already been mentioned. Murmurs of aortic regurgitation may be heard on some occasions but not on others. This points to the low specificity of the "changing murmurs" that are alleged to be characteristic for infective endocarditis and acute rheumatic fever.

CARDIOVASCULAR MOTION

The second part of the physical examination of the cardiovascular system is the examination of the various manifestations of motion: precordial motion, the arterial pulse and the venous pulse.

Precordial Impulses

The normal *apical impulse* is located in the fifth intercostal space in the midclavicular line, with the patient recumbent. It is palpable in about 40 per cent of normal individuals lying flat on the back; in another 30 to 40 per cent it becomes palpable when they are turned in the left lateral position. In the latter position the location of the impulse is shifted to the left. The impulse, when visible, is perceived as a short outward thrust; upon palpation it is felt as a light tap occurring during the early part of systole, characterized by a short duration and very little force. The location of the apical impulse represents the most important bedside approach to the recognition of cardiac enlargement. Abnormalities of precordial motion include the following:

1. Left ventricular hypertrophy (concentric type) is evidenced by a localized yet forceful and sustained apical impulse. The force with which the palpating finger is displaced and the duration of the displacement, together, correlate reasonably well with the degree of left ventricular hypertrophy, particularly when produced by pressure overload. The classification of the apical impulse regarding the degree of left ventricular hypertrophy as + to ++++ is reasonable.

2. Left ventricular hypertrophy associated with volume overload also produces a sustained and forceful apical impulse. It differs from

the first variety by a more diffuse pulsation involving often the entire left precordium. Both in severe aortic regurgitation and in mitral regurgitation of an appreciable degree, the entire precordium may be involved in what appears to be a rocking motion synchronous with the heart beat.

3. Right ventricular hypertrophy presents itself as a pulsation along the left sternal border ("left parasternal lift"). Such pulsation may be faintly palpable in children and young adults with thin chest walls who have no heart disease, but in average adults it is absent. The parasternal lift represents a forceful and sustained outward thrust of this region that is most frequently found in right ventricular hypertrophy produced by systolic overload (pulmonary hypertension, pulmonary stenosis); a broad motion of a wider parasternal area and adjacent parts of the thorax occurs in right ventricular hypertrophy resulting from diastolic overload (atrial septal defect: its effect upon the precordium was termed by Wood "tumultuous precordial pulsation"). In this condition the force and duration of the pulsation may not be increased unless pulmonary hypertension is present as well.

4. Abnormal chest wall pulsations occur frequently in patients with ischemic heart disease. These involve:

- The abnormal motion of ventricular dyskinesia and aneurysm,

- A temporary abnormal motion during anginal attacks.

In both of these, the direction of the motion, its force and duration overlap with that produced by ventricular hypertrophy, particularly left. The differentiation may be aided by the following:

- Involvement of areas other than the apical and parasternal region,

- Perception of a double pulsation—that of the normal or hypertrophied heart, separated from pulsations of the ischemic area.

Information gained from cardiac pulsation is usually considered important, especially when differentiating normal findings from those produced by heart disease. Differential points in the diagnosis, such as described above, have a fair specificity but only when the various abnormal pulsations are in their typical forms. There are, however, a few pitfalls that are worthy of mentioning in the interpretation of pulsatory precordial motion:

- In mitral regurgitation the entire heart may be propelled forward against the sternum, producing a false parasternal lift, which is, however, of shorter duration than one produced by right ventricular hypertrophy.

- In extreme degrees of right ventricular hypertrophy, such as is present in some congenital cardiac lesions, the right ventricle may form the cardiac apex. The exaggerated apical impulse then represents evidence for *right* rather than left ventricular hypertrophy.

In addition to the overall abnormalities of precordial motion, inspection and palpation of the thorax often permits the recognition of some of the lesser abnormalities of cardiac motion—e.g., S3 gallop sound—that have their counterpart in the form of abnormal precordial pulsations; a bifid apical impulse may be seen and felt in cases of hypertrophic subaortic stenosis.

The Arterial Pulse

Examination of the arterial pulse involves the inspection and palpation of the quality of the pulse, the rate and rhythm, the determination of the blood pressure in the arterial system, and a search for possible differences in amplitude and timing between various regions of the body.

The normal pulse consists of a rapid upstroke and a somewhat gentler downstroke interrupted by the dicrotic notch. It is equally well palpable over all exposed arteries; all beats under normal conditions have the same amplitude and are spaced equidistantly. Blood pressure measured by the indirect-cuff method is usually recorded in an arm; it should also be checked in the other arm and in one leg. The use of a correct-sized blood pressure cuff is a prerequisite for a reliable reading of pressure in the leg. In a normal, relaxed individual a casual reading of the blood pressure should not exceed 150/85, although the normal range can vary considerably between the sexes and among different age groups.

Abnormalities of the arterial pulse include the following (Fig. 4–5):

1. *Bounding pulse;* this involves a quick-rising arterial pulse, often but not always associated with widened pulse pressure. It is not necessarily indicative of heart disease. It is often associated with hypercirculatory states, and occasionally may be a normal variant. Among cardiac diseases moderate aortic regurgitation (or other conditions listed under 2, following) and mitral regurgitation may produce such pulses.

2. *Collapsing (water-hammer) pulse:* This is a characteristic pulse occurring in conditions with a run-off from the arterial system: aortic

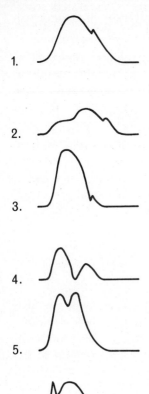

Figure 4–5. Diagrammatic presentation of arterial pulses: *1*, normal pulse; *2*, small pulse (pulsus parvus) with an anacrotic notch; *3*, collapsing pulse of aortic regurgitation; *4*, dicrotic pulse; *5*, bisferiens pulse of combined aortic stenosis and regurgitation; *6*, bisferiens pulse of hypertrophic subaortic stenosis.

regurgitation, patent ductus arteriosus, arteriovenous fistula, and other similar conditions. The size of the run-off has to be appreciable to alter the pulse contour.

3. *Small pulse (pulse parvus)* denotes low amplitude of the pulse wave and is frequently associated with a slow-rising upstroke. Low amplitude alone is found in conditions associated with abnormally low cardiac output, in vasconstricted states, and in shock. A small pulse with slow-rising upstroke is characteristic for aortic stenosis.

4. *Bifid pulse* occurs in three varieties:

    a. *Dicrotic pulse* shows the second "hump" separated from the first by the normal dicrotic notch (of exaggerated depth). It may be found in some hypercirculatory states with low peripheral resistance (e.g., fever).

    b. *Pulsus bisferiens* occurs in hypertrophic aortic stenosis with an initial thin spike ("percussion wave"), separated from the main systolic wave by a shallow notch; in another form it occurs in combined aortic stenosis and regurgitation as a rapidly rising tall pulse wave with two equal peaks separated by a deep notch with a rapid descent that often does not show a dicrotic notch.

   c. *Anacrotic pulse* represents an exaggeration of the normal small hump on the upstroke. It often occurs in aortic stenosis and is also characterized by a slow upstroke (see above).

   5. *Pulsus alternans* occurs in conditions associated with serious myocardial damage. While the pulse waves remain equidistant, alternate beats vary in their amplitude. Pulsus alternans is often exaggerated by the patient's standing up motionless; occasionally the weaker pulse beat may then become impalpable, producing a pulse rate that is half the cardiac rate. In addition, premature contractions may exaggerate or elicit pulsus alternans for a few cycles following them.

   6. *Pulsus paradoxus* occurs primarily in cardiac tamponade. Occasionally, mild pulsus paradoxus may be present in chronic constrictive pericarditis as well. It consists of the reduction in pulse amplitude during inspiration (which is merely an exaggeration of the normal respiratory effect upon the arterial pulse). The specificity of pulsus paradoxus is low, except in cases where it is particularly striking; it may also occur in congestive heart failure without pericardial involvement.

Examination of the arterial pulse should be performed by palpatory examination of the carotid, brachial, radial, and femoral pulses. The carotid pulse most closely resembles the central aortic pulse; the femoral pulse exhibits most of the distortion produced by secondary standing waves and reflected waves; the femoral pulse exaggerates and makes easier to recognize such abnormalities as the collapsing pulses. The detection of pulsus alternans and pulsus paradoxus can be facilitated by means of blood pressure measurement with auscultation of the artery during deflation of the cuff to about 20 mm. Hg below the systolic level.

Included in the examination of the arterial pulse is a comparison of the amplitude of pulses in the various regions in order to detect reduced or absent pulse. Conditions such as coarctation of the aorta, dissecting aneurysm, aortic arch syndrome, and occlusive disease of the lower aorta are all characterized by stenosis of large arteries whereby the arterial pulse is dampened and/or delayed in a region. Unimportant variants due to hypoplasia of some arteries need to be differentiated from significant signs of disease. Slight differences between pulses can be verified by differential blood pressure determination.

The Venous Pulse

Examination of the jugular venous pulse is one of the more critical parts of the physical examination in patients with cardiac disease, especially when the question of cardiac failure is being considered. The venous pulse provides means of direct assessment of right ventricular competence by estimation of its filling pressure—the left-sided equivalent of which is not available, short of invasive techniques.

The goals of the examination of the venous pulse are:

- to assess the height of venous pressure,

- to detect qualitative alteration of venous pulse waves.

Longstanding tradition encourages the estimation of the venous pressure by noting the angle at which the patient is reclining when the external jugular veins become "distended." This method is fraught with potential errors, inasmuch as factors other than elevated right atrial pressure may cause neck vein distention, e.g., hyperinflation of the thorax due to lung disease, compression of the veins by the clavicles or by muscles, and so on. In general it is safest to ignore the distention of the external jugular veins unless a definite venous pulse is seen involving either the entire venous column or its top. The reliability of visual estimation of venous pressure is greatly enhanced if major attention is paid to the pulsation of the *internal* (deep) jugular vein system, which is located underneath the sternocleidomastoid muscle.

The pulsation of an internal jugular vein produces motion of the central and posterior portion of that muscle (the arterial pulse moves the anterior part of the sternocleidomastoid).

The normal jugular venous pulse is seen in recumbency; when the patient is elevated above 30° the pulse disappears. Borderline elevation of central venous pressure can be diagnosed when a visible pulse is observed with the patient inclined at 45 to 60°. A clearly visible venous pulse present in a patient sitting up indicates abnormally high venous pressure. The venous pressure can be estimated by measuring the distance between the level of the right atrium (in the sitting position, 5 cm. below the sternal angle) and the highest point of the pulsating venous column.

Venous pressure rises slightly in normals in response to pressure upon the upper abdomen (Wood). This response is exaggerated in right ventricular failure and its recognition is considered helpful before the venous pressure rises permanently. As such, the diagnostic value of this "hepatojugular reflux" has been overestimated, since its specificity is low; therefore the differential value in discriminating between normals and patients with right ventricular failure is limited.

In the presence of considerable elevation of venous pressure the jugular venous pulse may be not only visible but also palpable; difficulty may arise as to whether pulsation in the neck represents arterial or venous pulsation. The following points are helpful in the differentiation:

- The arterial pulse is located more anteriorly, the venous pulse more posteriorly (see above).

- The upstroke of the arterial pulse represents the rapid—therefore the most prominent—motion visible; in the venous pulse the inward motion (*x* or *y* descent) is the more abrupt and more striking part of the pulse wave.

- The venous pulse can be eliminated by pressure upon the soft structures above the sternoclavicular junction; the arterial cannot.

The normal venous pulse consists of two positive waves—the *a* wave and the *v* wave—and of two negative parts—the *x* descent and the *y* descent. A notch in the *x* descent can frequently be noted, representing the *c* wave.

The *a* wave is presystolic and is related to atrial contraction. In the presence of arrhythmias in which atrial contraction is absent or is out of phase, corresponding changes in the *a* wave are noted: it is absent in atrial fibrillation or in atrial standstill; in various forms of atrioventricular block the *a* wave is found immediately following each atrial contraction. Separation of *a* waves from the *v* waves (and arterial pulse waves) constitutes the basis for the bedside diagnosis of conduction disturbances.

Abnormally tall *a* waves ("giant *a* waves") represent an important clinical sign which is found in the following conditions:

1. Increase of inflow resistance to the right ventricle (tricuspid stenosis or atresia, Ebstein's anomaly).

2. Increased outflow resistance from the right ventricle (pulmonary hypertension, pulmonary stenosis, and various related congenital cardiac syndromes).

3. Atrial contractions occurring out of phase, namely at the time when the tricuspid valve is closed (atrioventricular junctional rhythm, certain beats in atrioventricular dissociation). These waves are often referred to as "cannon waves"; they may be audible when auscultating over the neck.

Giant *a* waves in categories *1* and *2* are associated with abnormally tall P waves in the electrocardiogram.

Prominent *v* waves occur in right ventricular failure, particularly when it is accompanied by tricuspid valve incompetence. Here, a rapid, deep y descent from a tall v wave gives the venous pulse a collapsing appearance. A prominent v wave with a rapid y descent may also occur in constrictive pericarditis: differentiation of these two conditions on the basis of the jugular venous pulse is unreliable. In the presence of tricuspid stenosis the y descent is characteristically slow—a sign of good specificity.

The inspiratory increase in venous pulse (Kussmaul sign) occurs in constrictive pericarditis but may also be noted sometimes in right ventricular failure; hence its specificity is low.

In tricuspid regurgitation expansile pulsation of the liver is associated with the abnormalities of the jugular venous pulse described above. Traditionally, hepatic pulsations are considered an important sign of tricuspid regurgitation. Its diagnostic value is greatly exaggerated: the presence of a pulsating liver actually adds little to the information obtained from inspection of the jugular pulse.

EVALUATION OF CARDIAC PHYSICAL FINDINGS

The discussion in Chapter 2 focused upon approaching the diagnosis with specific objectives in mind. At the completion of the physical examination the first phase of the diagnostic workup is at an end. Before any laboratory studies are arranged the clinician should take stock of the yield of the history and physical examination. It is customary to make at this point a preliminary diagnosis, register an "impression." Two principal questions need to be considered:

1. Is the presence of cardiac disease firmly established?

2. If heart disease is present, how far along the pathway to the definitive diagnosis has one reached?

The first question applies to patients without symptoms in whom cardiac disease is suspected and the physical examination inconclusive, or to those whose symptoms may or may not be indicative of cardiac disease but whose examination reveals no abnormalities (e.g., ischemic heart disease). In this type of problem one should be satisfied that physical examination included all methods of examination and that special attention had been paid to subtle signs.

The answer to the second question is based on the preliminary diagnosis, and may show a wide range in terms of its relationship to the final diagnosis:

- An unequivocal diagnosis has been established by the examination irrespective of any other information to be obtained later (e.g., in mitral stenosis).

- A reasonable diagnosis has been established when combining the history and the findings on examination (e.g., history of myocardial infarction followed by the appearance of an apical systolic murmur; the murmur is found to be characteristic of mitral regurgitation; the diagnosis of postinfarctional mitral regurgitation is thus reasonably well established).

- The examination narrowed the diagnostic choices to two or three conditions (e.g., mitral regurgitation vs. ventricular septal defect).

- The examination brought out several diagnostic possibilities that need to be investigated by further studies.

The last two of the above situations account for the majority of cases. Clinical judgment should now dictate the nature and amount of further workup that will be arranged for the patient. It is important, however, to spell out goals and objectives of further examinations. In cases with inconclusive findings laboratory studies need to be selected with preference for those most likely to provide an answer (e.g., in ischemic heart disease a treadmill stress test may take precedence over "routine" blood tests and radiographic studies). In patients in whom the diagnosis is firmly established by physical examination further studies are usually necessary to evaluate the stage or the severity of the disease.

Throughout this chapter physical signs of cardiac disease have been listed with emphasis placed upon their reliability in leading to a correct diagnosis. It cannot be stressed too strongly that the clinical cardiologist performing the examination is the key individual whose judgment directs the diagnostic chain. If not, diagnostic decisions will be delegated to the radiologist, the electrocardiographer, the clinical physiologist, or even a computer — each of them far removed from the patient and his problem.

Bibliography

Aronow WS, Uyeyama RR, Cassidy J, Nebolon J: Resting and postexercise phonocardiogram and electrocardiogram in patients with angina pectoris and in normal subjects. Circulation *43*:273, 1972.

Bethell HGN, Nixon PGF: Understanding the atrial sound. Brit. Heart J. *35*:229, 1973.

Bruns DL: A general theory of the causes of murmurs in the cardiovascular system. Amer. J. Med. *26*:360, 1959.

Craige E, Millward DK: Diastolic and continuous murmurs. Prog. Cardiovasc. Dis. *14*:38, 1972.

Hancock EW: The ejection sound in aortic stenosis. Amer. J. Med. *40*:560, 1966.

Leatham A: Splitting of the first and second heart sounds. Lancet 2:607, 1954.

Leatham A: Auscultation of the heart. Lancet 2:793, 1958.

Mounsey P: The opening snap of mitral stenosis. Brit. Heart J. *15*:135, 1952.

Reddy PS, Shaver JA, Leonard JJ: Cardiac systolic murmurs; Pathophysiology and differential diagnosis. Prog. Cardiovasc. Dis. *14*:1, 1972.

Shaver JA, Nadolny RA, O'Toole JD, Thompson ME, Reddy PS, Leon DF, Curtiss EI: Sound pressure correlates of the second heart sound. Circulation *49*:316, 1974.

Warren JV, Leonard JJ, Weissler AM: Gallop rhythm. Ann. Int. Med. *48*:580, 1958.

Wood P: The arterial pulse. *In* DISEASES OF THE HEART AND CIRCULATION, 3rd Ed. Eyre and Spottiswoode, London, 1968, p. 26.

Wood P: The jugular venous pulse. *Ibid.*, p. 49.

5
Radiology

Radiologic examination of the heart and great vessels involves two principal techniques:

1. Conventional radiography supplemented by fluoroscopic examination,

2. Contrast radiography—angiocardiography.

Inasmuch as angiocardiography has become a part and parcel of the "invasive" examination of the cardiovascular system in conjunction with cardiac catheterization, both of these procedures are discussed conjointly in Chapter 8. This chapter thus deals only with conventional radiography.

In the past radiography was supplemented by auxiliary techniques other than injection of the contrast medium: orthodiagraphy, roentgenkymography, electrokymography and laminography (tomography). These techniques are now seldom used in conjunction with examination of the heart and great vessels—they were made obsolete by contrast techniques.

TECHNICAL CONSIDERATIONS

The standard radiographic examination of the heart involves chest films. As a minimum, anteroposterior and lateral views are needed; preferably two additional oblique views should be taken, supplemented by contrast visualization of the esophagus. These four chest films showing the cardiovascular shadow and the barium-filled esophagus are often referred to as "four cardiac views." Fluoroscopic examination is often added to this examination. Its role is to permit crude observation of cardiac motion and identification of intracardiac calcification.

Fluoroscopic examination may be supplemented by cinefluorography in cases where the motion of the cardiac shadow or of the calcification may need documentation. In the past fluoroscopic examination was used in physicians' offices in lieu of radiographic examination; today there is little justification for this, especially since image intensification (which has superseded conventional fluoroscopy) is seldom available in individual offices.

The standard technique for recording chest radiographs involves a tube-patient distance of 2 meters (or 6 feet) or more. This distance minimizes the parallax of roentgen rays and makes shadows of the various intrathoracic structures appear in relatively correct sizes and relationships. In seriously ill patients a short tube-patient distance may have to be used with a portable radiographic apparatus. Here the size of various structures may be exaggerated, some more than others. The inadequate reproducibility of sizes of cardiovascular structures makes comparison of serial portable films of limited value.

Comparison of the sizes of the heart and related structures in serial films constitutes an important part of diagnostic radiology. The limitation of portable films has already been mentioned. The standard 2 meter film reproduces the respective sizes of structures adequately and is suitable for comparison. However, even this technique has limitations which should be taken into consideration when comparison of films is indicated:

1. Clarity of detail depends upon the exposure of the film: overexposed films accentuate "hard" shadows, losing details of softer tissues; underexposed films accentuate softer shadows, e.g., the pulmonary vascularity. Thus, in comparing pulmonary vascularity, films of identical exposure and penetration are needed.

2. The standard technique requires taking a deep inspiratory film. The degree of voluntary hyperinflation of the lungs varies, hence the position of the diaphragm is a guide as to whether two given chest films offer an adequate basis for comparison of cardiac size. In addition, some patients may perform a Valsalva maneuver, others a Müller maneuver, while holding their breath during exposure; the former reduces and the latter increases cardiac size.

3. The difference between films taken in systole and those taken in diastole may be large enough to imitate cardiac enlargement in the diastolic film when compared with the systolic film, especially in the presence of bradycardia.

4. Mild degrees of rotation—taking films that are not truly posteroanterior but in a mild degree of obliquity—may produce apparent changes in sizes and relationships of various structures. Such changes may not be easy to detect in patients with mild deformities of the spine.

THE OVERALL CARDIAC SIZE

The size of the entire cardiac silhouette can best be estimated in the posteroanterior view, supplemented by the lateral view (Figs. 5–1, 5–2). Elaborate formulas have been designed to express the difference between a normal-sized heart and an enlarged heart. Although the formulas have statistical validity, their diagnostic application is of limited value because of the variability of cardiac size in healthy subjects. In general, most observers agree that if the width of the cardiac shadow exceeds 50 per cent of the width of the thorax, cardiac enlargement is likely to be present.

Estimation of the total cardiac size from the radiograph is reliable at the two extremes of the spectrum: when the heart is at the lower range of the normal size, or when considerable enlargement is present. In between there is a wide overlap between normal and abnormal that no formula can solve. Cardiac size is influenced by the body build, nutrition, the position of the diaphragm, and the degree of inflation of the lungs — to name but a few factors. To these one has to add the factors affecting reproducibility of cardiac size, listed above, to appreciate

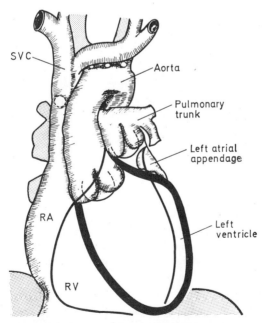

Figure 5–1. Diagram of border-forming structures in the posteroanterior chest film. (From Jefferson, K., and Rees, S.: Clinical Cardiac Radiology, Butterworth & Co., Ltd., London, 1973.)

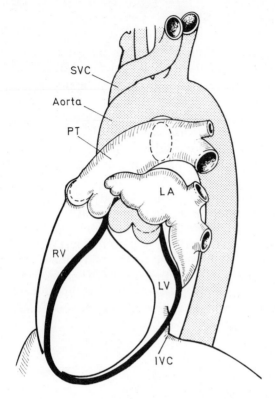

Figure 5-2. Diagram of border-forming structures in the lateral view. (From Jefferson, K., and Rees, S.: Clinical Cardiac Radiology, Butterworth & Co., Ltd., London, 1973.)

the difficulty of an emphatic diagnosis of "cardiomegaly" in patients other than those with at least moderate cardiac enlargement.

CHAMBER SIZE

The importance of recognizing enlargement and hypertrophy of the various cardiac chambers is self-evident. Cardiac radiography offers in this respect a great deal of assistance to the cardiologist. It is important, however, to recognize not only the positive value of chamber analysis but its limitations as well.

Left ventricular enlargement can usually be recognized with little difficulty, since the left ventricle ordinarily forms the apical bulge of the cardiac shadow. Left ventricular hypertrophy without enlargement is usually suspected when that bulge acquires a rounded shape. The

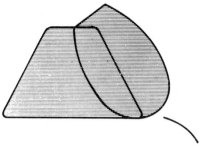

Figure 5-3. Diagram of normal right and left ventricles. (From Jefferson, K., and Rees, S.: Clinical Cardiac Radiology, Butterworth & Co., Ltd., London, 1973.)

specificity of this sign is poor, however. Enlargement of the left ventricle is diagnosed when the apical shadow extends toward the left border of the thorax. The detection of left ventricular enlargement by radiography has a moderate sensitivity and specificity. At present, when the opportunity arises of comparing radiographic films with angiocardiographic delineation of the left ventricular chamber, it can be appreciated how much that chamber can be enlarged with little change in the apical bulge. The specificity of this sign of left ventricular enlargement can be affected by the following potential sources of false-positive diagnoses:

1.   The encroachment of the right ventricle upon the apical bulge may occur in patients with severe right ventricular hypertrophy.

2.   Ventricular aneurysms of the apical regions give similar radiographic readings.

3.   The extracardiac shadow: pericardial fat pad, pericardial effusion, pericardial cysts or tumors, or other extracardiac structures can bring in sources of confusion.

Right ventricular enlargement is less well seen than that of the left

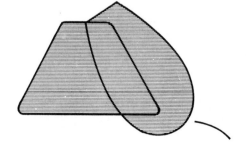

Figure 5-4. Diagram of enlarged left ventricle with a normal right ventricle. (From Jefferson, K., and Rees, S.: Clinical Cardiac Radiology, Butterworth & Co., Ltd., London, 1973.)

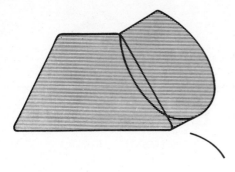

Figure 5-5. Diagram of enlarged right ventricle with a normal left ventricle. (From Jefferson, K., and Rees, S.: Clinical Cardiac Radiology, Butterworth & Co., Ltd., London, 1973.)

ventricle in the radiographic film. Concentric hypertrophy of the right ventricle cannot be recognized at all. Enlargement of that chamber is best shown in the lateral or the left anterior oblique views, since in those the cardiac shadow bulges more anteriorly, approximating the sternum. In the posteroanterior view the enlarged right ventricle often increases the size of the portion of the cardiac shadow to the right of the spine; yet the chamber responsible for most of this part of the shadow is the right atrium, hence this is an indirect sign of right ventricular enlargement. When enlargement involves the outflow tract of the right ventricle, a prominence of the middle arc of the left cardiac border is often found; this, however, overlaps with left atrial enlargement. In severe right ventricular enlargement, seen mostly in some congenital cardiac lesions, the right ventricle may form most of the apical portion of the cardiac shadow (see above). This may be misinterpreted as left ventricular enlargement, or, when the apical arc is elevated, may acquire the appearance of the "coeur en sabot" (like a wooden shoe) traditionally associated with tetralogy of Fallot. In general, right ventricular enlargement is diagnosed radiographically with a low specificity and medium sensitivity.

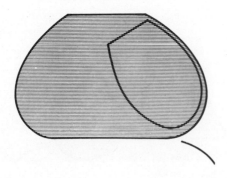

Figure 5-6. Diagram of a grossly enlarged right ventricle with a normal left ventricle. (From Jefferson, K., and Rees, S.: Clinical Cardiac Radiology, Butterworth & Co., Ltd., London, 1973.)

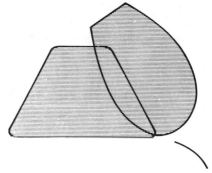

Figure 5-7. Diagram of enlarged right and left ventricles. (From Jefferson, K., and Rees, S.: Clinical Cardiac Radiology, Butterworth & Co., Ltd., London, 1973.)

Left atrial enlargement can be recognized best when that chamber is the only one altered in size. Isolated left atrial enlargement is one of the most characteristic signs of mitral stenosis and represents a valuable radiographic detail supporting such a diagnosis. The left atrium may:

- displace the esophagus posteriorly,

- appear as a prominent left middle arc of the cardiac shadow, just below the pulmonary artery and above the ventricular curve,

- appear as a "double" shadow forming a midportion of the right cardiac border,

- project to the left and posteriorly below the left bronchus and may elevate or compress the bronchus.

With a heart of normal and near-normal size, radiographic diagnosis of left atrial enlargement is of good specificity. Its sensitivity is only fair: angiocardiographic studies occasionally show large size left atria in patients in whom radiographic examination fails to show any atrial enlargement.

In patients with enlargement of more than one chamber, including the left atrium, the specificity of the above guidelines for left atrial enlargement decreases moderately.

Right atrial enlargement can be suspected when the right portion of the cardiac shadow extends rightward in the right lung field. As mentioned, enlargement of the right ventricle alone, enlargement of the right atrium alone, or a combination of both may be responsible for the increase in the size of the cardiac shadow to the right of the spine. Thus, the sensitivity of right atrial enlargement is very low unless it reaches giant proportions.

THE AORTA

Radiographic examination of the aorta should involve inspection of it in all four views. This permits the recognition of the following abnormalities:

- abnormalities of the shape and size of the aorta (dilatation, hypoplasia, tortuosity, aneurysm),

- abnormalities of the aortic arch (right-sided aortic arch, calcifications in it),

- abnormalities of the descending aorta (dilatation, tortuosity, aneurysm, signs of aortic coarctation).

The reliability of the various diagnoses of aortic abnormalities varies a great deal, depending upon the anatomic conditions of other structures, the age and body build of the patient, and other factors. Whenever a critical decision is required regarding aortic abnormalities, contrast visualization is mandatory.

THE PULMONARY ARTERY

Abnormalities of the pulmonary artery play an important diagnostic role in cardiac diseases. This vessel is best seen in the posteroanterior view. The main pulmonary trunk forms the high arc in the left cardiac contour underneath the aortic arch. The right and left pulmonary artery may be seen, when enlarged. Abnormalities of the pulmonary artery include:

1. Its diminished size (usually congenital, associated with some lesions, e.g., tetralogy of Fallot).

2. Enlarged main pulmonary artery—found in conditions associated with increased blood flow to the lungs (usually left-to-right shunts) or with increased pressure in the pulmonary arterial system, or both; also present in valvular pulmonary stenosis (poststenotic dilatation) and in idiopathic dilatation of the pulmonary artery.

The poststenotic or idiopathic dilatation of the pulmonary artery involves primarily the pulmonary trunk but may also extend into the proximal portion of the two arteries. Increased pressures and flows involve the trunk, the two arteries, and their visible principal branches.

The specificity of the pulmonary arterial enlargement is fair. It overlaps with the normal variant, a prominence of the pulmonary arterial shadow found in young individuals, particularly those with thin chests and vertical hearts. It may be confused with extracardiac structures: adenopathy, hilar tumors, and so on. Angiocardiography may show considerable enlargement of the pulmonary trunk and arteries not seen in conventional radiography; hence its sensitivity is only fair.

THE LUNG FIELDS

The lung fields viewed from the cardiovascular standpoint often provide important diagnostic information by permitting an insight into smaller pulmonary vessels as well as an overall estimate of the pulmonary blood volume. The following changes may be considered of diagnostic importance:

1.   Increased pulmonary blood flow is suggested when pulmonary arterial branches are enlarged and the peripheral small branches are dilated, providing a uniform increase in vascularity throughout the lung fields.

2.   Pulmonary hypertension may be suspected when the larger and medium branches of the pulmonary artery are enlarged but the enlargement tapers off abruptly and does not extend into the periphery.

3.   Decreased pulmonary blood flow is implied when the pulmonary arterial branches are smaller than average and the vascular pattern throughout the lungs is reduced. This condition may be present in cyanotic congenital cardiac lesions with pulmonary stenosis associated with large right-to-left shunts. In addition, unilateral or segmental variation in vascularity (i.e., blood flow) can be recognized.

4.   Pulmonary venous congestion usually represents an increase in pulmonary venous pressure and in pulmonary blood volume. Here increase in pulmonary vascular pattern is associated with dilatation of pulmonary veins; pulmonary arterial enlargement may or may not accompany it.

5.   Kerley's B lines represent horizontal shadows located in the lower lung fields, presumed to be related to increased lymphatic drainage due to elevated pulmonary venous pressure or thickened interlobular septa. They are characteristic for mitral stenosis and left ventricular failure.

The information obtained from the survey of the lung fields is of distinct diagnostic value, although the differentiation between the first four conditions listed above may be fuzzy; furthermore, the interpretation is greatly influenced by technical quality of the films. Therefore, the most reliable diagnostic contribution of the changes in the lung fields lies in:

- supporting a clinically considered diagnosis,

- following patients seriatim.

CALCIFICATIONS

Cardiovascular calcifications are among the most valuable yields of radiographic examinations. Some of the calcifications within the cardiovascular shadow are detected by routine radiography; visualization of the smaller calcifications requires special examination by means of fluoroscopy with image intensification. Diagnostically important calcifications include the following:

1. *Valvular calcifications* often acquire crucial importance in evaluation of patients with valvular disease and may become critical issues in certain decisions regarding surgical treatment. Fluoroscopic examination usually permits the separation of the calcification in the mitral valve from those in the aortic valve or in the annulus.

Mitral valvular calcifications:

- may be the simplest way to diagnose mitral valve disease in some atypical cases;

- often point to extensive disease of the mitral cusps, disqualifying the patient from a simple valvotomy;

- may establish the chronicity of mitral involvement in patients with mitral regurgitation, thereby suggesting rheumatic etiology.

Aortic valvular calcifications:

- demonstrate extensive disease of aortic leaflets, suggesting the necessity of valve replacement in surgical candidates;

- demonstrate the location of the outflow obstruction to be at the valve site.

Annular calcifications are of lesser importance than valvular.

2. *Coronary calcifications* are frequently found in routine films or on fluoroscopic examinations. They almost always involve the proximal portions of the principal coronary arterial branches. Although calcifica-

tions indicate atheromatous disease, their presence does not prove serious occlusive disease of these branches. Calcified areas are not necessarily the ones most heavily affected by disease; occasionally coronary calcifications may be found in patients whose coronary arteriograms are normal.

3. *Pericardial calcifications.* These occur commonly in constrictive pericarditis. While there is a wide individual variation in the time needed to develop calcification, they are, as a rule, indicative of chronicity of the pericardial disease. Pericardial calcifications do not always signify significant inflow obstruction, but merely offer a high probability that advanced hemodynamic abnormalities will be found.

4. *Calcifications in the aorta* are very common, particularly in the arch and in its descending portion; there they are of no significance in middle-aged and elderly individuals. Once thought to be specific for luetic aortitis, calcifications of the ascending aorta are now known to occur in other forms of aortitis and even in atherosclerotic disease. Calcifications in the aortic wall frequently provide a good outline of the vessel, thereby permitting occasional differentiation between tortuosity, ectasia, and aneurysm of the various parts of the aorta.

5. *Myocardial calcifications* occur occasionally in ventricular aneurysms. Their diagnostic contribution is small.

6. Other calcifications occasionally found in the cardiac silhouette include calcifications within cardiac tumors (e.g., myxoma), endocardial calcifications in "jet lesions" in valvular regurgitation, calcified thrombi, and unexplained calcifications in the atrial or ventricular myocardium.

FLUOROSCOPY

The role of a fluoroscopic examination is — as stated previously — limited to a supplementary part of the radiographic examination. The principal contributions of the fluoroscopic examination are:

- the opportunity to find and identify small calcifications,
- the ability to view the motion of the heart and great vessels.

The latter involves the following problems:

1. Assessment of cardiac border motion may reveal:

- exaggerated border motion in patients with large stroke output,

- diminished border motion, involving the entire heart or its segments,

- "paradoxical pulsation" of the left atrium (systolic expansion or posterior motion) in mitral regurgitation,

- "paradoxical pulsation" of cardiac aneurysms.

The specificity of these findings is moderate; many of the findings formerly observed by fluoroscopic examination now require angiocardiography for analysis and confirmation, since fluoroscopic examination is considered merely a screening technique. It should be mentioned that differentiation between pericardial effusion and cardiac enlargement is no more reliable on the basis of assessment of border motion than it is on the basis of the alleged difference in shape.

2.   Assessment of the motion of the great arteries may demonstrate the exaggerated pulsation of aortic regurgitation. This, however, is not specific, for it is also found in other conditions with large stroke output (e.g., complete heart block).

Pulsation of the main pulmonary trunk and the principal arteries is commonly increased in congenital heart disease with increased pulmonary flow ("hilar dance"). It may also be seen in lesions with increased pressure and as well in pulmonary valve incompetence; hence it has little discriminating help to offer in the differential diagnosis.

3.   Assessment of the motion of prosthetic cardiac valves is of importance in the examination of postoperative patients. It does sometimes provide early indications of prosthetic valve dysfunction.

INTERPRETATION OF RESULTS

The radiographic examination of the cardiovascular system consists of two parts:

- recording and noting of abnormalities,

- interpretation of their significance.

It is the interpretation that can make the radiographic examination fall flat. Ideally, the interpretation should be made jointly by the radiologist and the clinician who is familiar with the clinical facts. In practice the radiologist fulfills both functions alone, often without the knowledge of the clinical problem involved. The role of the radiologic examination is often misunderstood, both by the clinician and the radiologist. The radiologist is properly concerned with his responsibility of offering most help to the clinician. By noting certain combinations of abnormalities he often suggests certain clinical diagnoses. The clinician, on the other hand, often accepts the radiologic diagnosis as an established fact.

The range of probability that the radiologic diagnosis is correct varies widely. Inexperienced radiologists tend to overread radiologic findings: such diagnoses as "cardiac enlargement," "congenital heart disease," and "rheumatic heart disease" are sometimes suggested when the radiologic examination reveals deviation from the ideal rather than deviation from the normal. Experienced radiologists, particularly those exposed to an adequate volume of angiocardiographic work, are aware of the inadequacies of superficial diagnoses and tend to be more cautious. Yet, it is the clinician who has to weigh the information and apply it to other clinical facts in his possession.

There are very few features that offer anything approximating a firm diagnosis on the basis of radiologic findings alone. One can exemplify this by the following combination of radiographic findings:

- Large left atrium with normal-sized other chambers, associated with calcifications in the mitral valve; the diagnosis of mitral stenosis is highly probable.

- A characteristic notch on the descending aorta combined with scalloping of the ribs; the diagnosis of coarctation of the aorta is almost certain.

Yet, these are exceptions. More often only a lesser level of probability can be achieved. For example:

- The radiologist recognizes increased pulmonary vascularity suggestive of left-to-right shunt; by noting an appropriate chamber enlargement he can suggest further that the shunt is on an atrial level, or on a ventricular level, or on the aortic-pulmonary level. Noting, however, that each component finding has some false-positive and false-negative diagnoses, he recognizes that the probability of being correct in his diagnosis is probably in the 75 per cent range. Many diagnoses have no better probability than 50 per cent.

The importance of viewing the radiologic examination in perspective cannot be overemphasized. When all the findings are reviewed in the light of other clinical data, radiologic study often helps in making dramatic diagnoses. When used in abstract situations or out of context, it is capable of contributing to untold harm in unnecessary restriction of patients, in unneeded cardiac catheterizations, or, conversely, in missing important clues.

Bibliography

Jefferson K, Rees S: CLINICAL CARDIAC RADIOLOGY. Butterworths, London, 1974.
Lester RG: Radiological concepts of the evaluation of heart disease. Mod. Conc. of Cardiovasc. Dis. *37*:113, 1968; *38*:7, 1969.

6

Electrocardiography and Vectorcardiography

Electrocardiography is the most widely used laboratory test in cardiology. While its clinical importance is beyond question, it is noteworthy that the limitations of it are not as widely recognized as its virtues. Consequently one frequently encounters over-reliance upon electrocardiographic findings as well as the failure to recognize the normal variability of the electrocardiogram, with misinterpretation of minor changes. In the following discussion the general principles of electrocardiography will be presented strictly from the standpoint of their relation to the clinical diagnosis of cardiac disease. The discussion will omit reference to the role of electrocardiography in the diagnosis of arrhythmias, to which a separate chapter is devoted.

Vectorcardiography represents an alternate method of presentation of the same electrophysiological events that are displayed in the electrocardiogram. Theoretically, vectorcardiography and electrocardiography should be identical except for loop display vs. scalar display of electrical potential. In practice, vectorcardiography uses a different lead system (in this discussion the most widely accepted Frank lead system will be referred to); hence certain differences between the two are discernible. Some comments regarding the possible superiority of one method over the other will be made at the end of this chapter.

It will be assumed that the reader is acquainted with the basic concepts of electrocardiography and vectorcardiography; hence the customary discussion of the dipole principle will be omitted.

THE NORMAL RANGE

Differentiation between the normal and abnormal has always presented great difficulty in electrocardiography. The general tendency of considering any deviation from the ideal curve a significant abnormality has produced wide abuses in clinical electrocardiography. Examination of large series of normal subjects, such as one surveying 120,000 healthy aviators, showed that many abnormalities may simply be normal variants, as discussed in Chapter 2. Thus, one should always consider "normality" in terms of the Gaussian curve encompassing 96 per cent of the population with an overlap between the remaining 4 per cent of normals and patients who have proven cardiac disease.

It is imperative, therefore, to consider the division between the normal and abnormal electrocardiogram as a broad zone, rather than a sharp line. This overlap between normal and abnormal is particularly difficult to verbalize in conventional electrocardiographic interpretation, since the reader is expected to commit himself to a diagnosis. Minor deviations from the norm are often interpreted as "borderline" findings. However, the fact that a more pronounced electrocardiographic abnormality may represent a normal variant is difficult to transmit to the clinician in a routine reading. It is therefore the responsibility of the clinician who applies the electrocardiographic interpretation to the clinical situation to recognize the limitation of it and to exercise care in diagnosing heart disease based on the electrocardiographic abnormalities, but which is unsupported by other evidence.

ATRIAL ABNORMALITIES (Fig. 6-1)

Depolarization of the atrium inscribes the P waves of the electrocardiogram and the P loop of the vectorcardiogram. Atrial activity is

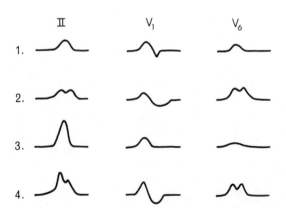

Figure 6-1. Diagram showing the shape of P waves in three electrocardiographic leads: *1*, normal P waves; *2*, P waves in left atrial "hypertrophy"; *3*, P waves in right atrial "hypertrophy"; *4*, P waves in biatrial "hypertrophy."

contained within the rather narrow confines between +30 and +60 degrees in the extremity leads; in the horizontal plane (i.e., chest leads) it is often of low amplitude. In right precordial leads the P wave is frequently diphasic. The duration of atrial activity is between 0.06 and 0.1 secs.; its magnitude in terms of conventional leads is 0.2 mv. or less. The right atrium depolarizes first, the left afterwards: consequently, the first half of the P wave represents predominantly right atrial events, the second half left atrial events.

Abnormalities of atrial depolarization are caused by two principal factors:

- abnormal sequence of atrial depolarization waves produced by ectopic origin of the pacemaker,

- abnormalities induced by anatomic changes (dilatation or hypertrophy) of either or both atria.

Ectopic rhythms produce abnormalities of the P axis; it affects also the shape and duration of the P wave. Such abnormalities are usually, though not always, associated with an abnormal P-R interval.

Left Atrial Abnormality. Also referred to by various electrocardiographic readers as "left atrial enlargement," "left atrial hypertrophy," and "left atrial disease" left atrial abnormality widens the P wave to 0.1 sec. or more. The normally fused two components of the P wave often separate, inscribing bifid P waves in several leads. In right precordial leads the late negative component of the P wave is broader and deeper than normal. Vectorcardiogram shows a larger and more posteriorly directed terminal part of the P loop. It should be noted that the most consistent feature of left atrial abnormality is the prolongation of the P wave and its separation into two components. This same effect can be produced by an interatrial conduction delay, in which the left atrial activation lags behind. Such conduction disturbances produce false-positive "left atrial P waves."

Right Atrial Abnormalities. These produce tall, often single-peaked, "Gothic" P waves, best seen in leads I and II. Right precordial leads often show a predominantly positive (anterior) deflection. Vectorcardiogram shows exaggeration of the anterior portion of the P loop.

Biatrial Abnormalities. They can often be identified when criteria for disease of both atria are present. Because of their sequential rather than simultaneous activation, atrial abnormalities do not cancel each other out.

The interpretation of atrial abnormalities, when considered in a clinical context, can be an important aid in diagnosis. Left atrial abnormalities appear characteristically in mitral stenosis and are also often present in left ventricular failure. If care is exercised not to overread minor deviations from the norm, such P wave changes carry a good specificity, although the sensitivity is only moderate. Right atrial abnormalities are often seen, and may be exaggerated, in congenital cardiac lesions, in some of which they play an important differential role. In acquired cardiac disease they constitute an important clue in chronic cor pulmonale (though not a very sensitive one) and may appear acutely in pulmonary embolism.

The gamut of changes occurring in P waves in connection with ectopic rhythms will be discussed in Chapter 17.

VENTRICULAR HYPERTROPHY

Hypertrophy of either or both ventricles may affect the electrocardiogram in a characteristic manner. These changes rank high in the diagnostic application of electrocardiography.

Left Ventricular Hypertrophy. This produces changes that fall into three categories:

- increased voltage of the QRS complexes,

- abnormalities of repolarization (ST-T changes),

- prolongation of the QRS duration, preferentially affecting the ventricular activation time.

High QRS voltage is the sign most widely present, having the highest potential sensitivity. The widely accepted minimum voltage criteria for the recognition of left ventricular hypertrophy include the following:

- S in lead V_1 + R in lead V_5 or V_6 greater than 3.5 mv.

- S in V_2 + R in V_5 or V_6 greater than 4.5 mv.

- R in V_5 greater than 2.5 mv.

- R in AVL greater than 1.1 mv.

- R in I + S in III greater than 2.5 mv.

As explained in Chapter 2, selection of the diagnostic criteria cannot increase the sensitivity of a test without sacrificing its specificity. The above criteria occupy an intermediate position; when applied, they include a fair number of false-positives and false-negatives — more than 10 per cent of each. The inherent inaccuracy of the voltage criteria for left ventricular hypertrophy is related to the fact that precordial (and to a lesser extent extremity) lead voltage is influenced by the distance between the electrode and the heart. Thus in young subjects, in thin-chested individuals, and in those with thoracic deformities, criteria for increased voltage lose validity. Conversely, in patients with hyperinflation of the thorax, voltages are artifactually reduced.

Abnormalities of the ST-T part of the electrocardiogram include the rotation of the ST-T vector away from the QRS vector. Thus, in leads with tall upright QRS complexes T waves become flattened, then inverted; the S-T segmental depression often develops. The addition of these changes to increased QRS voltage greatly increases specificity of the electrocardiogram in detecting left ventricular hypertrophy. However, it is necessary when applying the criteria to recognize the false-positive ST-T changes produced by digitalis administration, as well as by ischemia, or myocardial damage resulting from it.

Prolongation of the QRS complexes occurs only with a severe degree of left ventricular hypertrophy; thus it has a low sensitivity; its specificity is adversely affected by the overlap with conduction disturbances. Delay in ventricular activation time (prolonged interval from the onset of the QRS complex to the initiation of the last downstroke of the R wave to more than 0.05 secs.) is of more theoretical than practical importance, as these changes are relatively infrequently found in left ventricular hypertrophy without an overall prolongation of the QRS duration.

Changes in the vectorcardiogram produced by left ventricular hypertrophy include the production of a larger, more posteriorly directed and usually counterclockwise inscribed QRS loop. In the axial leads increased QRS voltage is evident. It has been shown by Pipberger's group that the voltage of the R wave in lead X plus that of the R wave in lead Z, when totalling more than 2.7 mv., offers a 95 per cent probability that left ventricular hypertrophy is present.

The recognition of left ventricular hypertrophy is of considerable importance in clinical cardiology. Electrocardiographic changes often appear earlier than other manifestations of left ventricular hypertrophy. Evidence of left ventricular hypertrophy, for example, when present in hypertension offers proof of target organ involvement, thus of its severity and persistence. In aortic stenosis it may serve as a means of separating mild from significant degrees of obstruction. It is clear, however, that the diagnostic challenge lies in the recognition of *early* left ventricular hypertrophy. Yet, the early pattern provides also the highest margin of error, a fact which must be taken into consideration when decisions are made on the basis of the electrocardiographic findings alone.

Right Ventricular Hypertrophy. This occurs physiologically in the neonate and persists for the first few months of life. The postnatal electrocardiogram usually shows the QRS axis in the extremity leads shifted rightward beyond 100 degrees; in the precordial leads there is a predominantly positive QRS complex in lead V_1 and a predominantly negative one in lead V_6, with intermediate leads showing transition between the two—thus presenting complete reversal of the adult precordial electrocardiogram. This is the postnatal dextrocardiogram, as opposed to the adult levocardiogram. The vector loop in the horizontal plane is directed anteriorly and rightward, instead of posteriorly and leftward, as it is in the normal adult vectorcardiogram. In congenital cardiac lesions characterized by right ventricular hypertrophy since birth, the electrocardiogram and the vectorcardiogram may show a persistence of the pattern of the dextrocardiogram or changes intermediate between dextrocardiogram and levocardiogram. Such changes have high specificity. In atrial septal defect (where right-sided overload develops with some delay) the normal evolution of the postnatal electrocardiographic changes may take place, but later the electrocardiogram acquires features of right bundle branch block, which becomes an electrocardiographic expression of right ventricular hypertrophy and dilatation due to volume overload.

Electrocardiographic diagnosis of right ventricular hypertrophy in the childhood age maintains good specificity with a reasonable sensitivity. In contrast, patients who acquire right ventricular hypertrophy as adults present a wide range of electrocardiographic abnormalities that are only mildly specific and sensitive. Only seldom do patients acquire the pattern of fully developed right ventricular hypertrophy resembling the postnatal dextrocardiogram: this may occur with severe degrees of pulmonary hypertension at systemic pressure levels. More often changes develop that show only isolated features resembling the neonatal electrocardiogram. Recognizing that electrocardiographic changes produced by right ventricular hypertrophy are a part of a continuum, one can nevertheless conveniently divide acquired right ventricular hypertrophy into the following varieties:

1. Fully developed, severe right ventricular hypertrophy, resembling the neonatal electrocardiogram.

2. Shift of the extremity lead axis beyond + 90 degrees without significant changes in the precordial lead is often found in milder cases of right ventricular hypertrophy (e.g., mitral stenosis of moderate degree). These changes are particularly significant if proof can be obtained that rightward axis shift is acquired. (False-positive cases would primarily involve patients who had always had vertical axis, related to body build.) A differential point in the axis shift is the development of left posterior fascicular block (see infra), which somewhat reduces the specificity of this change.

3. The development of positive deflections in leads V_1 and V_2: these can take the form of an RS complex, a qR complex or an rsR' complex. This pattern overlaps with incomplete right bundle branch block and posterobasal myocardial infarction.

4. Development of deep S waves in leads V_5 and V_6, often associated with a superior rotation of the extremity lead axis.

5. Appearance of a fully developed right bundle branch block.

Certain trends can be noted linking these electrocardiographic changes with specific diseases. In mitral valve disease, as mentioned, the mere rightward shift of the extremity lead axis often occurs; when it is complicated by increased pulmonary vascular resistance, R waves or rsR' complexes tend to appear in right precordial leads. In chronic lung disease left precordial S waves and superior axis shift may be found or an indeterminate axis of the S_1, S_2, S_3 type. In acute pulmonary embolism sudden development of right bundle branch block may be observed.

Vectorcardiographic equivalents of right ventricular hypertrophy pattern in the scalar electrocardiogram include the horizontal QRS loops that show more anterior forces than usual, those with predominant rightward forces, and a loop directed posteriorly and rightward (instead of leftward); superior and rightward loops may also be encountered, corresponding to the fourth pattern listed above.

In general, right ventricular hypertrophy has a low diagnostic sensitivity. Many patients with clinically and pathologically demonstrated right ventricular hypertrophy nevertheless have electrocardiogram and vectorcardiogram falling into the normal range. Sometimes serial records permit the recognition of subtler changes implying the development of right ventricular hypertrophy, but old electrocardiographic tracings are only occasionally available. The specificity of the electrocardiographic changes indicative of right ventricular hypertrophy is fair to good, especially when supported with clinical correlation.

Biventricular Hypertrophy. This condition can be diagnosed in children with cardiac disease (usually congenital) by showing electrocardiographic or vectorcardiographic features combining the changes produced by hypertrophy of each ventricle. In adults the recognition of biventricular hypertrophy is more difficult, often impossible. Subtler changes produced by right ventricular hypertrophy are frequently masked by those of left ventricular hypertrophy. Occasionally, electrocardiograms showing rightward extremity lead axis shift with changes indicative of left ventricular hypertrophy in the precordial leads are seen in patients with clinically diagnosed biventricular hypertrophy. However, the specificity and sensitivity of this combination of findings is low and its reliability doubtful.

The specificity of electrocardiographic and vectorcardiographic changes suggestive of ventricular hypertrophy can be greatly enhanced if such changes are considered conjointly with atrial abnormalities. Thus, in chronic lung disease lesser changes in the electrocardiogram suggestive of right ventricular hypertrophy — equivocal per se — may become diagnostic if P pulmonale (right atrial P wave) is also present. The combination of rightward axis shift and left atrial abnormality supports strongly the clinical diagnosis of mitral stenosis. Questionable changes suggesting left ventricular hypertrophy acquire more significance when left atrial abnormality is also in evidence.

MYOCARDIAL INFARCTION

Electrocardiographic and vectorcardiographic changes produced by myocardial infarction constitute the widest use — and abuse — of these diagnostic techniques. A wide range of changes is produced by acute myocardial infarction, with many persisting permanently as telltale scars from infarcts. Some changes have a very high specificity, greater than 95 per cent; others may show only subtle abnormalities that can be perceived solely by careful and detailed study of serial tracings.

Electrocardiographic changes resulting from myocardial infarction include two principal categories:

• those affecting the QRS complexes,

• those affecting the ST-T waves.

The former are considered characteristic for transmural myocardial infarction, the latter for partial thickness wall involvement ("nontransmural," "intramural"). There are some theoretical questions as to whether such strict electrocardiographic-anatomic relationship exists in all cases.

Abnormalities of repolarization ST-T changes represent the early alterations of the electrocardiogram and account for the changing pattern. QRS changes may develop with some delay and are often permanent.

S-T segment changes involve the ischemic process and represent "injury current"; they overlap with temporary ischemia, so that only the reversibility or nonreversibility of such changes may decide whether myocardial infarction has taken place. Early changes include exaggerated tall T waves, which become associated with S-T segment elevation. If myocardial infarction develops, then the S-T elevation, involving a positive T wave, persists; after a few hours or days the S-T segment gradually returns to the isoelectric position, while the T waves show late inversion. This stage may persist permanently, or T-waves may return to normal over a period of weeks or months. The duration of the evolution of the ST-T changes (exclusive of the final righting of the T waves) takes from two days to two weeks (Fig. 6–2).

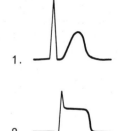

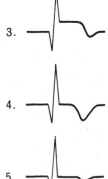

Figure 6-2. Diagram showing the evolution of a typical acute myocardial infarction in the electrocardiographic lead most severely affected by the infarction: *1*, very early stage (seldom "caught"); *2*, early stage; *3*, intermediate stage; *4*, late stage of healing infarction; *5*, chronic residual change.

The entire sequence occurring in conjunction with QRS abnormalities (see below) provides a specificity approaching 100 per cent for the diagnosis of acute myocardial infarction. The sensitivity of these ST-T changes is fairly good but depends upon the location of the infarction. The ST-T sequence without QRS changes is slightly less specific, as some overlap with pericarditis, and possibly with myocarditis, may occur.

Changes in the QRS complexes involve the early activation forces, thus inscribing abnormal Q waves and R waves. Four principal localizations of myocardial infarction are recognized:

- Anterior infarction, inscribing QS waves or QR waves in right and mid precordial leads;

- Lateral myocardial infarction, inscribing abnormal Q waves in leads I, AVL, V_5 and V_6;

- Inferior myocardial infarction, inscribing abnormal Q waves in leads II, III and AVF;

- Posterobasal ("true posterior," "strictly posterior") myocardial infarction, inscribing tall R waves in leads V_1 and V_2.

There is some question whether the division of anterior myocardial infarction into "antero-septal" and "anterior" based on the number of leads involved in the Q wave abnormality is justified. The only certain way of recognizing septal involvement in the infarction is the development of a conduction disturbance.

The specificity of QRS changes produced by myocardial infarction is related to two points:

- the development of significant changes under observation,

- the magnitude of the change.

The sensitivity of the QRS changes is low, inherent in the fact that only full thickness infarcts are likely to produce these changes.

As stated, QRS changes more often than not persist for life. The exact figures as to how many fully developed abnormal Q waves eventually disappear are not available. It is estimated that no more than 20 per cent disappear or change from diagnostic into noncharacteristic abnormalities.

The specificity of the permanent QRS abnormalities produced by myocardial infarction is affected by the following:

1. Normal variants: inferior myocardial infarction overlaps with physiological Q waves. Standards for abnormalities (Q waves greater than 25 per cent of the total QRS voltage, longer than 0.03 secs. in duration) represent criteria with only moderate reliability. Unexplained tall R waves in right precordial leads are occasionally found in healthy individuals, overlapping with posterobasal myocardial infarction.

2. Left ventricular hypertrophy or incomplete left bundle branch block or both may inscribe QS waves in leads V_1 to V_4, thus overlapping with anterior myocardial infarction.

3. Conduction defects, including Wolff-Parkinson-White syndrome, may produce QS waves or deep Q waves in various leads.

4. Right ventricular hypertrophy may produce changes in right precordial leads similar to those of posterobasal myocardial infarction.

5. Certain forms of myocardial disease, including acute myocarditis, chronic cardiomyopathy, and hypertrophic subaortic stenosis, may cause the appearance of Q waves identical with those considered characteristic for myocardial infarction.

Changes in the QRS complexes produced by myocardial infarction are often associated with damage to the peripheral parts of the conducting system, producing right bundle branch block, left anterior or posterior fascicular block, or complete left bundle branch block. Conduction defects other than left bundle branch block do not obscure the presence of myocardial infarction in that the telltale Q waves remain unaffected by the defect. In left bundle branch block abnormal Q waves are obliterated by the conduction defect and the presence of myocardial infarction can no longer be diagnosed on the basis of the QRS complexes.

Vectorcardiographic changes in the QRS loop are similar to those deduced from the scalar electrocardiogram. In general, the early forces are deflected by the infarction and are directed away from the infarcted area. Thus in anterior myocardial infarction there are no anterior forces: this is best noted by inspecting the horizontal plane loop, which may be inscribed in a clockwise direction rather than the normal counterclockwise manner. In the inferior myocardial infarction the early forces are deflected superiorly—the loop remains above the E-point for at least 25 msec. In lateral myocardial infarction early rightward forces are in evidence. In posterobasal myocardial infarction the anterior portion of the QRS loop is exaggerated. The differential diagnosis of myocardial infarction from vectorial loops is similar to that of the scalar 12-lead electrocardiogram; the overlap between infarction, left ventricular hypertrophy, and conduction defect presents diagnostic difficulties. In anterior myocardial infarction this three-way differentiation may be even more difficult than on the basis of the scalar electrocardiogram. Sometimes the vectorcardiogram presents details more clearly visible than the scalar electrocardiogram: defects—"bites" visible in the midportion of the QRS loop—may be better identified as abnormalities than comparable abnormalities in the electrocardiogram.

While the recognition of an old myocardial infarction on the basis of abnormalities of the QRS part of the electrocardiogram and vectorcardiogram presents some difficulties, as discussed above, the interpretation of postinfarctional T waves is even less reliable. Once the evolution of the ST-T portion of the electrocardiogram is completed during the acute stage of infarction, the residual changes overlap with many other conditions affecting repolarization. The great majority of postinfarctional T wave abnormalities fall into the "nondiagnostic T wave changes" group. The only exceptions are the following:

- Late symmetrical, deep T wave inversion is somewhat more likely to be a residual change resulting from infarction than from other causes.

- This type of T wave pattern, preceded by coving (bowing) of the S-T segment, has an even better specificity for old myocardial infarction.

- Persistent S-T segment elevation has a moderate specificity and a fair sensitivity for postinfarctional ventricular aneurysm.

The differentiation of these T waves in relation to the various factors will be discussed in more detail below.

The preceding discussion deals with acute and residual changes produced by acute myocardial infarction in patients who, prior to the attack, had normal electrocardiograms and showed the expected typical changes. Many patients show atypical changes that may present diagnostic difficulties. These include:

1. Atypical evolution of the ST-T changes. This includes delay in the sequential appearance of the changes, reversal of their order, or appearance of only S-T segment depression (signifying subendocardial infarction).

2. Indication of myocardial infarction by minor electrocardiographic changes. Some patients with clear clinical evidence of acute myocardial infarction show only minor T wave changes, perhaps because they involve areas of the myocardium that are poorly accessible to conventional electrocardiographic exploration.

3. Variable Q waves. Occasionally abnormal Q waves pathognomonic of myocardial infarction are recorded but disappear within one or two days.

Some diagnostic difficulties in interpreting the electrocardiogram of acute myocardial infarction stem from the fact that the patient's preinfarction electrocardiogram was already abnormal. The following abnormalities may obscure or minimize electrocardiographic evidence of acute myocardial infarction.

- Left ventricular hypertrophy (from prior hypertension or other cause) affecting the ST-T part of the tracing;

- Old myocardial infarction, especially if associated with ventricular aneurysm;

- Various conduction disturbances (as mentioned above);

- Digitalis effect.

The clinical importance of electrocardiographic diagnosis of myocardial infarction — recent or old — varies greatly. In some cases it represents merely a confirmation of a clinical diagnosis that is already otherwise evident. In other cases it is the crucial bit of evidence for an atypical set of clinical manifestations. Chronic changes may be found in asymptomatic subjects as a surprising discovery with serious implications. It is in the situation in which electrocardiographic diagnosis carries a great deal of clinical weight that the electrocardiographic reader and the clinician should be fully aware of the limitations of the diagnosis. In these cases misinterpretation of diagnostic data can produce avoidable harm to the patient.

INTRAVENTRICULAR CONDUCTION DEFECTS

Diseases of the conducting system as a whole traditionally belong to the section on arrhythmias. However, localized lesions affecting the more peripheral sections of this system do not disrupt the impulse propagation, but merely alter the order of ventricular activation, thereby producing electrocardiographic abnormalities. Intraventricular conduction defects fall into five categories:

- block in the right bundle branch,

- block in the anterosuperior division of the left bundle branch,

- block in the inferoposterior division of the left bundle branch,

- block in the entire left bundle branch,

- other intraventricular conduction defects.

The general principle of conduction disturbance below the bifurcation of the bundle of His involves activation of some portion of the ventricle via a detour, with a delay; hence the shape of the QRS complexes is altered and their duration usually prolonged. Repolarization is also affected by the development of "secondary" T wave changes—directed in the opposite manner to the QRS complexes.

Right Bundle Branch Block. This is arbitrarily divided into a complete and an incomplete form on the basis of the QRS duration (complete = longer than 0.11 sec.; incomplete = 0.10 to 0.11 sec.). Block in the right bundle branch delays activation of the right ventricle and produces late rightward and anterior—occasionally superior—forces that inscribe secondary R waves in leads AVR, V_1, and V_2 and broad S waves in leads I, II, AVL, V_5, and V_6. In the vectorcardiogram the appropriate change in the terminal portion of the loop is directly recorded. The diagnostic significance of right bundle branch block is as follows:

1. It may be found in normal individuals: incomplete form is fairly common; complete form occurs in about one in 500 subjects, Minor delays (small r' in right precordial leads) should be considered normal variant unless other evidence of cardiac disease is found.

2. Right bundle branch block overlaps with right ventricular

hypertrophy (see above) to the extent that they cannot be differentiated by means of the electrocardiogram or vectorcardiogram alone.

3. It may develop acutely and transiently as a result of either increased pressure in the right ventricle (acute cor pulmonale) or direct injury to the right bundle branch (during cardiac catheterization).

4. When produced by organic damage to the right bundle branch it may be caused by ischemic heart disease — acutely in myocardial infarction or chronically without a clinical counterpart — or may be produced by discrete disease of the conducting system. In the latter case, it may be combined with left anterior fascicular block and be a precursor of complete A-V block.

5. It may be a true congenital anomaly (not an expression of right ventricular hypertrophy in some congenital cardiac lesions), related to abnormal course of the conducting system.

The typical right bundle branch block (complete or incomplete) may be looked upon as a center of a spectrum. On one side of it are the various lesser degrees of right-sided conduction delays, often representing normal variants of no clinical significance. On the other side of the center are atypical forms of it, including wide, often bizarre QRS complexes that may be associated with marked right axis shift and broad monophasic QRS complexes in right precordial leads. These changes presumably represent right bundle branch block combined with additional damage to the myocardium or other parts of the conducting system (RBBB + septal myocardial infarction; RBBB + left posterior fascicular block). They also occur in some congenital malformations (e.g., Ebstein's anomaly).

Left Anterior Fascicular Block. This defect is considered likely to be present if the extremity lead axis is shifted superiorly beyond −45°. The QRS complexes may be normal in duration or slightly prolonged, but seldom exceed 0.11 secs. The QRS voltage may be increased, particularly in the extremity leads, overlapping with left ventricular hypertrophy. (Hence the specificity of the pattern of left ventricular hypertrophy is reduced in the presence of superior axis.) Vectorcardiographic equivalent of this conduction defect is provided by a QRS loop that is initiated in the normal direction (contrasting with inferior myocardial infarction), then is directed strongly superiorly.

The concept of a block within the anterosuperior fascicle of the left bundle branch is relatively new; its anatomic and electrophysiologic basis is not yet fully defined. It is not yet known whether such a diagnosis is justified in all patients showing an extremity lead axis of −45° or more. Superior axis produced by inferior myocardial infarction overlaps with this condition to some extent; the differentiation — as stated — rests with the orientation of the initial QRS force; however, the

specificity of this is not yet well defined. A special variety of left anterior fascicular block is found in conjunction with some congenital
malformations of the heart, and is considered characteristic for lesions
caused by maldevelopment of the atrioventricular canal (e.g., septum
primum type of atrial septal defect). The cause of these changes is presumably not an interruption of the fascicle but the anomalous course of
the infra-His portion of the conducting system which causes delayed
activation of the portion of the left ventricle normally activated by the
anterior fascicle.

Left Posterior Fascicular Block. This defect is believed to be
present when the frontal place axis is abnormally shifted to the right —
between +100° and +150°. Inasmuch as right axis shift is also characteristic for certain forms of right ventricular hypertrophy, the specificity of
the diagnosis of left posterior fascicular block is low and the diagnosis
should be entertained only if on clinical grounds right ventricular
hypertrophy appears unlikely.

Left Bundle Branch Block. This represents probably the most
serious disturbance of intraventricular conduction. It is characterized
by prolonged QRS duration of 0.12 or more and by the absence of the
small physiological Q waves present in leads with upright QRS complexes and is usually accompanied by broad notching of QRS complexes. The QRS voltage ranges from abnormally low to very high — the
latter not related to left ventricular hypertrophy. The extremity lead
axis is usually normal. Some patients show a markedly superior axis
shift, which is considered a variant of left bundle branch block. The
vectorcardiographic picture of left bundle branch block is characterized
by a loop inscribed in the horizontal plane in a clockwise manner and
by slowing of the midportion of the loop.

There is some controversy as to whether an incomplete form of
left bundle branch block exists. In a manner analogous to right bundle
branch block this concept postulates generalized slowing in the entire
left bundle without preferential involvement of the two fascicles,
thereby producing an electrocardiographic pattern similar to complete
left bundle branch block but with QRS duration less than 0.12 sec.
Some such cases undoubtedly represent severe left ventricular hypertrophy, which overlaps to some extent with left bundle branch block. In
other cases no specific clinical condition can be identified although
disease in the left ventricular myocardium is frequently present. Until a
better explanation is found, it is not unreasonable to assume that peripheral portions of the left ventricular conduction system (beyond the
fascicular distribution) may show some slowing of lesser degree than
that of complete left bundle branch block. In general, it is noteworthy
that block in either of the two fascicles seldom precedes (if at all) left
bundle branch block, suggesting that the two varieties of conduction
disturbances may be caused by different mechanisms.

Other Conduction Defects. Other forms of intraventricular conduction disturbances are evidenced by a variety of atypical electrocardiographic patterns associated with delay in intraventricular conduction, but without falling in any one of the categories listed above. The spectrum ranges from mere slurring of QRS complexes in otherwise normal electrocardiograms (often overread as I–V conduction disturbance although they almost always represent innocent normal variants), all the way to bizarre unclassifiable broad QRS complexes.

A special place among conduction defects is given to the concept of *"peri-infarction block."* Since this term was first introduced some 20 years ago, there have been many conflicting definitions of it submitted. Many cases of "peri-infarction block" are now clearly examples of fascicular blocks complicating myocardial infarction and should be identified as such. Perhaps this term should be reserved for cases in which the electrocardiogram shows the typical residual QRS changes from an old myocardial infarction with terminal forces directed opposite to the former. The QRS complexes may also be prolonged beyond 0.1 sec.

The clinical significance of conduction defects differs greatly from that of those electrocardiographic findings discussed earlier: both ventricular hypertrophy and myocardial infarction represent electrocardiographic substrates of morphologically demonstrable diseases of the heart. Conduction defects in theory involve damage to the conducting bundles; however, anatomic confirmation of such damage is exceedingly difficult to obtain. Furthermore, its relation to cardiac disease is variable. Thus the finding of a conduction defect calls for the clinical interpretation of its significance, a procedure in which clinical and electrocardiographic findings have to be combined. In interpreting the significance of conduction defect the following points should be considered:

1. The abnormality in question should be identified as a true conduction defect: the overlap between conduction defects and left or right ventricular hypertrophy have been commented upon; the pre-excitation syndrome will be discussed below.

2. Right-sided conduction defects may permit in addition the identification of other electrocardiographic abnormalities: myocardial infarction or left ventricular hypertrophy; this type of association should be noted and possible connection between the demonstrated abnormality and conduction defect considered.

3. Conduction defects as part of congenital cardiac malformations should be considered, particularly if this electrocardiographic abnormality is found in younger individuals (endocardial cushion type of septal defects, Ebstein's anomaly).

4. Milder forms of conduction delay are less likely to be asso-

ciated with serious cardiac disease and often represent normal variants. Minor conduction defects (e.g., notching of QRS complexes) are probably better ignored, unless a specific clinical reason is found to the contrary.

5. Severe, often atypical, conduction defects associated with unusual prolongation of the QRS complexes usually have a serious underlying cause, but it is not necessarily irreversible myocardial damage; electrolyte imbalance and drug toxicity may cause these changes as well. The determination of the permanency of these abnormalities in the search for the underlying cause is imperative.

6. The commonly used association of an etiological label with conduction defects — i.e., the automatic assumption of the presence of ischemic heart disease — is unwarranted.

In discussing conduction defects it is necessary to include a presentation of the problem of the *"pre-excitation syndrome,"* which does not represent delay in intraventricular conduction but resembles it morphologically. A part of the Wolff-Parkinson-White syndrome, this condition involves premature activation of some portion of the ventricles via short-circuiting bypasses. The ventricular complex may represent a fusion of the wave front activating some portion of the ventricle prematurely with that activating the remainder of the ventricle via the natural conducting system. The resulting QRS complexes are prolonged, resemble bundle branch block complexes and are associated with a shortened P-R interval. The most characteristic feature of the QRS complexes is the delta wave, i.e., stepwise notching on the upstroke of the QRS complexes visible in leads with predominantly upright QRS complexes. The two commonest forms of pre-excitation are:

- type A, with precordial leads resembling right ventricular hypertrophy;

- type B, with precordial leads resembling left bundle branch block.

There are many intermediate and atypical forms of pre-excitation. In some, deep Q waves are present, imitating major changes from myocardial infarction. Vectorcardiographic loops in pre-excitation show the predictable changes in the QRS loop, but are characteristically recognized by the slowing of the initial portion of that loop. From the standpoint of the electrocardiographic diagnosis, the following points should be emphasized:

1. While the diagnosis in typical cases is easy, less typical forms may be mistaken for serious abnormalities (left ventricular hypertrophy, myocardial infarction).

2.   The P-R interval is occasionally not shortened but normal, in which case the electrocardiographic diagnosis may be more difficult.

3.   Every effort should be made to provoke a change in the normal complexes (the conducting bypass may become inactivated by various maneuvers: exercise, Valsalva test, drug administration), so that a basic electrocardiogram can be recognized (see also Chapter 20).

The clinical syndrome associated with pre-excitation will be discussed in Chapter 20.

T WAVE ABNORMALITIES (Fig. 6-3)

Few areas of electrocardiography offer more challenge to the electrocardiographic reader than the changes in the T waves. The wide overlap between the factors affecting repolarization of the ventricles, on the one hand, and the normal variability of the ST-T part of the electrocardiogram, on the other hand, make abnormalities of repolarization of low order in specificity.

Electrophysiologically, T wave abnormalities are divided into two main categories:

1.   Those related to abnormal order of depolarization of the ventricles, such as in bundle branch block—secondary T wave abnormalities.

2.   Those unrelated to an altered sequence of depolarization—primary T wave abnormalities.

In the latter category a wide range of changes can be distinguished:

- lower T wave amplitude than that expected for a given lead (in relation to the QRS complex amplitude),
- flat, isoelectric T waves,
- diphasic T waves,
- inverted T waves showing no characteristic morphologic features,
- tall, exaggerated T waves,
- broad, upright T waves fused with U waves,
- upright T waves fused with elevated S-T segments,
- inverted T waves showing specific features:
  - symetrically inverted T waves with isoelectric S-T segments,

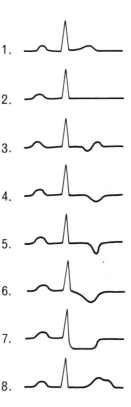

Figure 6-3. Diagram showing various T waves in an electrocardiographic lead: *1*, normal T wave; *2*, flat T wave; *3*, diphasic T wave (− +); *4*, inverted T wave; *5*, symmetrical, late T wave inversion, somewhat more likely to represent an old ischemic injury; *6*, T wave inversion preceded by downward sloping of the S-T segment, often seen after digitalis administration; *7*, inverted T wave fused with a horizontally depressed S-T segment, usually denoting ischemia; *8*, upright T wave fused with a U wave.

- T waves fused with coved (arched) S-T segments,
- T waves fused with sagging S-T segment depression,
- T waves fused with horizontally depressed S-T segments,
- broad inverted T waves with prolonged Q-T interval.

Isolated S-T segment changes include the following:

- temporary S-T segment depression:
  - horizontal,
  - upward slanting,
  - downward slanting,
- permanent S-T segment depression,
- temporary S-T segment elevation,
- permanent S-T segment elevation,

Wide variation of the T waves in healthy subjects have important bearing upon their diagnostic interpretation.

First, permanent T wave inversion in the lead that usually shows upright T waves (e.g., AVL) may be considered normal in certain rotation of the electrocardiographic axis. It is considered acceptable that the spatial angle between the T vector and QRS vector does not exceed 60 per cent (usually the angle is narrower, making the direction of the T wave follow the principal direction of the QRS complexes).

Second, many diurnal physiological factors are known to influence T waves and may cause their variation in shape and duration from day to day or from hour to hour. Among these are: respiratory changes, activities affecting body position, postprandial influences, and hyperventilation.

Third, a variety of noncardiac influences may affect T waves: changes in the state of the autonomic nervous system, electrolyte imbalance, gastrointestinal disorders, noncardiac drugs, and other factors.

Fourth, cardiac drugs are known to affect the T waves of the electrocardiogram seriously and consistently — notably, digitalis and antiarrhythmic agents.

A great many anatomic and physiologic derangements of the heart are capable of producing T wave abnormalities. Yet, many electrocardiographic readers, almost in a reflex manner, associate T wave abnormalities with ischemic heart disease. Even those T wave abnormalities that show certain distinctive morphologic features often have low specificity. Clues derived from T wave changes are helpful only in a most general manner:

- Late, symmetrical T wave inversions are often seen as residual changes from myocardial infarction (Fig. 6–3, 5); their significance is enhanced by the simultaneous presence of residual Q waves. However, they can also be found occasionally in later stages of pericarditis and in cerebrovascular accidents (the latter associated with Q-T prolongation).

- Inverted T waves marked by S-T segment coving have the highest specificity as postmyocardial infarction residuals, but they do have false-positives.

- Inverted T waves preceded by depressed or sagging S-T segments occur after digitalis administration, in ventricular hypertrophy and in subendocardial infarction (Fig. 6–3, 6). As temporary changes they occur in ischemia; their specificity will be discussed below.

A great deal of attention is being paid to serial T wave changes. It is indeed important to be aware that intermittent myocardial ischemia and minor ischemic myocardial damage are frequently manifest by constantly changing shape and direction of the T waves. It is equally important to recognize, however, that some normal subjects have "unstable" T waves because of a number of factors, some listed above, some unidentified, so that T wave changes may occur from day to day without demonstrable cardiac disease.

Abnormalities of the S-T segments also vary in their diagnostic contribution. S-T segment depressions have very low specificity: they have been mentioned in connection with T wave abnormalities with which they are usually associated. The common tendency of reading persistent S-T segment depression as "ischemia" is not only unwarranted but represents a contradiction in terms, since a chronic state of ischemia cannot be present (by definition, ischemia is either reversible or produces cell death). Persistent S-T segment elevation has a fair specificity in indicating fully developed ventricular aneurysm or major areas of dyskinesia. However, this change overlaps with the occasional normal variant of "early repolarization."

STRESS TESTS

Stress tests have been in use for many years as a means of detecting myocardial ischemia. Originally introduced as the two-step test of Master, the older test has now been widely replaced by the more sophisticated treadmill or bicycle test.

The two-step test is simple in terms of the necessary equipment and consumes relatively little of the supervising physician's time. The advantages of the more complex treadmill test include the following:

- The treadmill test gives the patient an opportunity to perform exercise he is more accustomed to engaging in (few patients are used to running up a flight of stairs).

- This procedure permits observation *during* exercise as well as after its termination: the two-step in its original form records abnormalities only in the recovery period.

- The treadmill test establishes the patient's exercise tolerance and allows observation regarding the highest cardiac rate attained during exercise (unless it is advisable to discontinue the test at submaximal heart rates).

The sensitivity of the treadmill test for the detection of ischemia during or after exercise is naturally higher than that of the two-step test. Yet the latter has a surprisingly good overall record.

Criteria for a positive test vary from institution to institution (Fig. 6–4). As in other diagnostic procedures, a more liberal acceptance of abnormalities improves the sensitivity of the test at the expense of lower specificity. Most experts agree upon two points:

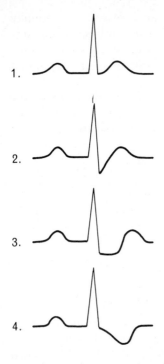

1.

2.

3.

4.

Figure 6–4. Diagram showing the shape of S-T segment changes occurring during and after a stress test: *1*, normal ST-T waves; *2*, junctional S-T segment depression (usually considered a normal response); *3*, segmental S-T depression, found in ischemia; *4*, downward-sloping S-T segment with inversion of the T wave, also considered a "positive" test for ischemia.

1. A horizontal depression of the S-T segment of 1 mm. or more, or one slanting downward, constitutes a positive test for ischemia, when such a pattern is evident during exercise, during recovery from exercise, or both.

2. An upward-slanting depression involving mostly the S-T junction occurs frequently in normal subjects and is of no diagnostic significance.

Points of uncertainty and disagreements include the following:

1. Is an upward-slanting junctional depression with a considerable portion of the S-T segment below the isoelectric line to be considered positive or negative for ischemia?

2. How significant, as an indication of ischemia, is a mere inversion of T waves without S-T segment change during or after exercise?

3. How should one interpret S-T segment depression in patients who have T wave abnormalities in the control pre-exercise electrocardiogram?

4. Can electrocardiographic response to stress testing be quantified? This question involves the speed with which the ischemic changes appear during exercise, as well as their magnitude.

The answers to these questions are not clear and require further investigation. The mere point that these questions are subject to disagreement suggests that their diagnostic contribution is uncertain and their acceptance should be made with considerable caution when applied to individual cases.

Depression of the S-T segments represents the classic evidence for myocardial ischemia and is the principal diagnostic goal for the stress tests. In some cases, however, other electrocardiographic abnormalities may occur:

- S-T segment elevation developing during stress testing is considered evidence for ischemia with more serious implications than S-T segment depression.

- Arrhythmias often appear during or after exercise: atrial arrhythmias are probably of little diagnostic significance. Ventricular arrhythmias — premature contractions, ventricular salvos, tachycardias, even ventricular fibrillation — occur more frequently in ischemic heart disease. Nevertheless the appearance of ventricular arrhythmias as the *sole* abnormalities during or after stress testing is not considered a positive result but rather suspicious and suggestive for ischemia.

- Intraventricular conduction defects appear occasionally during stress testing. These usually represent rate-related conduction defects and need not be indicative of ischemic heart disease.

Stress testing represents an important addition to the diagnostic use of the electrocardiogram. It should be emphasized that the performance of such tests is not without risk to the patient, and both the patient and the person performing the test should be aware of this. Defibrillation facilities are mandatory in any stress-testing laboratory.

Stress tests are widely used as a noninvasive diagnostic means of evaluating patients with chest pain, as well as of surveying the general population. Yet the sensitivity and specificity of these tests are not well defined. It is known that false-positive S-T segment depression identical with that produced by ischemia may be found in patients taking digitalis and in patients with left ventricular hypertrophy and normal T waves. False-positive stress tests have been shown in a disturbingly high proportion in healthy women. Their incidence in healthy men is not known. False-negative stress tests are recognized by the fact that many patients with other demonstrated manifestations of ischemia show negative stress tests. Here the limitation may be the currently used lead system, which is most sensitive to ischemic changes in the anterior and lateral walls of the heart.

The stress test is limited, in addition, by the fact that clear-cut results in the detection of ischemia are possible only in the patient whose resting electrocardiogram is normal—at least in the commonly used leads. Furthermore, poor motivation or physical impediments may prevent patients from attaining the level of exercise necessary to stress the heart sufficiently for the production of ischemia. The most widely accepted goal of treadmill testing is to stress the patient to 80 or 90 per cent of the predicted maximal cardiac rate. In some centers the attainment of maximal heart rate is aimed at. The endpoint—stopping the test earlier on command by the physician—is prompted by positivity of the test at an earlier stage. However, if the patient cannot attain the desired submaximal cardiac rate, the test is inconclusive.

ELECTROCARDIOGRAPHIC INTERPRETATION

Ideally the electrocardiogram should be interpreted by the clinician who examines the patient and who has the capability of reviewing its contribution to the diagnosis. In a sense, the application of the electrocardiogram to the diagnosis on the basis of someone else's interpretation might be considered analogous to the establishment of a diagnosis on the basis of another clinician's physical examination. The concept of strict application of the electrocardiogram to the bedside diagnosis is acknowledged in some institutions, in which uninterpreted electrocardiographic tracings are placed in the patient's chart. However, practical considerations make this goal difficult to attain. Electrocardiography has thus become a diagnostic "test" similar to radiography, in which an expert-consultant reads the electrocardiogram and submits the report to the clinician. Modern technology has produced some further modification of this principle: electrocardiograms are being interpreted by distant "super-experts" who collect tracings from wide areas via telephone transmission. Furthermore, computer interpretation of electrocardiograms is being widely investigated as the "ultimate" in electrocardiography.

Acknowledging the fact that a "formal" interpretation of the electrocardiogram offers a realistic solution to the problem, one cannot help noting the negative aspects of this approach as it is being practiced. Successful clinical application of the electrocardiogram that is interpreted by someone other than the clinician in charge of the patient is contingent upon two conditions:

1. The electrocardiographic reader must be acquainted with the clinical problem that led to the request for an electrocardiographic examination.

2. The clinician should appreciate the fact that the interpretation

does not represent a firm diagnosis but merely a suggested condition with the highest probability to fit the given electrocardiogram.

Neither of these two conditions is as a rule fulfilled. Electrocardiographic readers are seldom acquainted with the clinical situation; they may or may not be given a working diagnosis — frequently the patient's age is the only available information. The clinician receiving the report all too frequently considers the conclusion a firm diagnosis and acts accordingly.

Throughout this chapter comments have been made regarding an estimated specificity and sensitivity of the various electrocardiographic deviations from the norm as related to clinical conditions. Most of these are mere estimates; in only very few instances are actual figures available. Nevertheless, one can guess that the average electrocardiographic diagnosis (even when based on the knowledge of clinical data) carries a probability not higher than 75 per cent of being anatomically or physiologically correct. Only a few electrocardiographic abnormalities have a higher specificity — in the high nineties, some undoubtedly fall into the category of 50 per cent or less.

The failure to appreciate the potential inaccuracy of the electrocardiogram results in its wide abuse and may lead to tragic consequences. Untold harm is being perpetrated by attaching the stigma of heart disease to healthy subjects because of an innocent electrocardiographic imperfection, by hospitalizing patients on the basis of an overdiagnosed reading of "myocardial infarction," or by subjecting patients to coronary arteriography on the basis of unusual normal variants.

If the electrocardiogram is to be fully taken advantage of as a valuable aid in clinical diagnosis, the following conditions might be considered:

- Electrocardiographic readers should become consultants in a manner similar to the radiologist: the clinician submits a request for electrocardiographic examination with pertinent clinical information, preferably stating the reason for ordering it. If necessary the reader can discuss the problem with him and modify the interpretation. This will require subjecting the selection of electrocardiographic readers to the same scrutiny for qualifications as the hospital radiologist or pathologist. Hospitals in smaller communities could be linked by telephone to nearby hospitals with adequate cardiological facilities, with readers still available for phone consultation. Mass-produced reading stations and computer reading should be discouraged, at least in terms of electrocardiograms for acute care hospitals.

- The electrocardiographic reader and the clinician should

both be fully cognizant that the electrocardiograph records the sum of activity generated by action potentials of the heart: any conclusion from it regarding anatomic abnormalities or changes in the physiological state are only inferential, therefore may be inaccurate.

- Both parties should recognize the broad variations in the normal and the overlap between the various conditions producing abnormalities in the electrocardiogram.

DIAGNOSTIC ASPECTS OF ELECTROCARDIOGRAPHY VS. VECTORCARDIOGRAPHY

For many years the question has been asked whether the diagnostic accuracy of the electrocardiogram can be improved by using vectorcardiography. Vectorcardiography has two advantages:

- It uses a corrected lead system, less subject to distortion from unusual body build or other extraneous factors.

- Loop presentation emphasizes certain relationships in the manner that a graph shows some details better than a table.

The disadvantage of loop vectorcardiography is its inability to display the cardiac rate and rhythm; measurement of complexes is thus made more difficult in the vectorcardiogram.

While the advantage of a corrected, orthogonal lead system clearly makes the vectorcardiogram a potentially superior, more consistent technique, this would only be valid if electrocardiography were a deductive science in which electrocardiographic-anatomic relationships could be predicted from models. This is not now the case—electrocardiography still remains an empirical art with its diagnostic contribution based on correlations between the electrocardiograms and the anatomic or clinical findings in a large number of cases. Obviously, electrocardiography has the advantages of much wider experience; its range of normal and abnormal is more widely known than that of the newer and more complex vectorcardiography. Thus, given a diagnosis in which the electrocardiogram and the vectorcardiogram show discordant findings (e.g., in the differential diagnosis between myocardial infarction and left ventricular hypertrophy), one does not have the security to recognize the vectorcardiogram as the more reliable test. Studies comparing the diagnostic accuracy of electrocardiography and vectorcardiography showed that one method seemed better in some problems and the other in other problems (Simonson et al.). Our own experience comparing findings in the two techniques in patients in whom the diagnosis was established by other means confirmed this fact by showing the electrocardiogram more reliable in some cases and the vectorcardiogram in others. When looking for the superiority of one method over the other, one is tempted to call it a draw.

Bibliography

Chou TC: Clinical aspects of vectorcardiography. *In* Cardiac Diagnosis by NO Fowler, Hoeber Med. Div., Harper and Row, New York, 1968.

Constant J.: Learning Electrocardiography. Little, Brown & Co., Boston, 1973.

Grant RP: Clinical Electrocardiography. McGraw-Hill Book Co., New York, 1957.

First SR, Bayley RH, Bedford DR: Peri-infarction block; electrocardiographic abnormality occasionally resembling bundle branch block and local ventricular block of other types. Circulation *2*:31, 1950.

Flower NC, Horan JG: Subtle signs of right ventricular enlargement and their relative importance. In Advances in Electrocardiography, edited by RC Schlant and JW Hurst. Grune and Stratton, New York, 1972. p. 297.

Goldman MJ: Principles of Clinical Electrocardiography, 7th Editon. Lange Medical Publications, Los Altos, California, 1970.

Grant RP: Left axis deviation. An electrocardiographic-pathologic correlation study. Circulation *14*:233, 1956.

Hiss RG, Lamb LE: Electrocardiographic findings in 122,043 individuals. Circulation *25*:947, 1962.

Holt JH, Barnard ACL, Lynn MS: A study of the human heart and a multiple dipole electrical source. II. Diagnosis and quantitation of left ventricular hypertrophy. Circulation *40*:697, 1969.

Horan LG, Flowers NC: Diagnostic power of the Q-wave: Critical assay of its significance in myocardial deficit. *In* Advances in Electrocardiography, edited by RC Schlant and JW Hurst. Grune and Stratton, New York, 1972, p. 321.

McCaughan D, Littman D, Pipberger HV: Computer analysis of the orthogonal electrocardiogram and vectorcardiogram in 939 cases with hypertensive cardiovascular disease. Amer. Heart J. *85*:467, 1973.

Morris JJ, Estes EH, Whalen RE, Thompson HK, McIntosh HD: P-wave analysis in valvular heart disease. Circulation *29*:242, 1964.

Romhilt DW, Bove KE, Norris RJ, Conyers E. Conradi S, Rowlands DT, Scott RC: A critical appraisal of electrocardiographic criteria for the diagnosis of left ventricular hypertrophy. Circulation *40*:185, 1969.

Rosenbaum MB, Elizari MV, Lazzari JO, Nau GJ, Levi RJ, Halpern MS: Intraventricular trifascicular blocks. Review of literature and classification. Amer. Heart J. *78*:450, 1969.

_____ The differential electrocardiographic manifestations of hemiblocks, bilateral bundle branch block, and trifascicular blocks. *In* Advances in Electrocardiography, edited by RC Schlant and JW Hurst. Grune and Stratton, New York, 1972, p. 145.

Selzer A, Ebnother CL, Packard P, Stone AO, Quinn JE: Reliability of electrocardiographic diagnosis of left ventricular hypertrophy. Circulation *17*:255, 1958.

Selzer A, Naruse DY, York E, Kahn KA, Mathews HB: Electrocardiographic findings and concentric and eccentric ventricular hypertrophy. Amer. Heart J. *63*:320, 1962.

Selzer A, York E, Naruse DY, Pierce CH: Electrocardiographic findings in 500 cases with hypertrophy of cardiac ventricles, Amer. J. Med. Sci. *240*:543, 1960.

Simonson E: Differentiation Between Normal and Abnormal in Electrocardiography. C. V. Mosby Co., St. Louis, 1961.

Simonson E.: Electrocardiography stress tolerance tests. Prog. Cardiovasc. Dis. *13*:269, 1970.

Simonson E, Tuna N, Okamoto N, Toshima H: Diagnostic accuracy of the vectorcardiogram and electrocardiogram. A cooperative study. Amer. J. Card. *17*:829, 1966.

Surawicz B: The pathogenesis and clinical significance of primary T-wave abnormalities. *In* Advances in Electrocardiography, edited by RC Schlant and JW Hurst. Grune and Stratton, New York, 1972, p. 321.

7

Other Noninvasive
Diagnostic Methods

PHONOCARDIOGRAPHY

Phonocardiography has been used for decades; first used as a means of graphic registration of the vibrations associated with cardiac sounds and murmurs, it had been widened to display simultaneously several physiological events within the cardiac cycle. As such it has provided means of obtaining important information not only concerning audible events, but cardiac function as well. The introduction of intracardiac phonocardiography further widened the field. Yet, intracardiac phonocardiography can be performed only during invasive procedures; its complexity makes it suitable only as a research tool.

Conventional phonocardiography is virtually limited to multichannel recording of physiological events. The recording of heart sounds alone or in conjunction only with the electrocardiogram does not offer sufficient diagnostic information to make it worthwhile.

Minimal equipment used in phonocardiography consists of a 4-channel physiological recorder; more channels are often preferred. The most frequently used combination consists of two sound channels, the electrocardiogram, and a pressure recording device that should be used to display external carotid arterial pulse curve, external jugular venous pulse, or the apexcardiogram. An additional channel recording respiratory phases may be useful; sometimes more than one pressure event needs to be shown—hence the preference for more than four channels in some institutions.

Presently available equipment provides the opportunity to record cardiac sounds and murmurs with preferential amplification of certain frequency bands, a procedure which greatly facilitates sound analysis. The technique of phonocardiography is difficult and time-consuming,

110

if the recording is obtained at a level of quality high enough to ensure accurate interpretation. Only too often phonocardiography is abandoned as useless to the clinician because poor equipment or poor technique provided inferior records. Because of the cost of good equipment and the investment in the necessary manpower to provide good phonocardiographic records, a phonocardiographic unit probably should not be started outside a busy cardiac center.

Phonocardiographic records display many normal and abnormal heart sounds with greater sensitivity than murmurs. Most audible sounds can be recorded; furthermore, inaudible vibrations are occasionally displayed in the phonocardiographic records as well:

- Low amplitude pulmonary valve closure in pulmonary stenosis can be recorded.

- In some cases low-frequency sounds, such as those of S3 and S4, may produce recordable and palpable vibrations, but be inaudible on auscultation.

Cardiac murmurs are recorded, provided they are easily audible. (Grade I murmurs are almost never displayed on the phonocardiogram.) Often a lengthy search for appropriate sound filters is needed, particularly for murmurs of high frequency. Considering the fact that murmurs are less well recorded by phonocardiography than perceived by auscultation, phonocardiography cannot be used as means of determining whether or not a murmur is present.

The clinical importance of phonocardiography lies less in the capability of providing a record of auscultatory findings than in permitting exact timing of certain auscultatory findings, thereby helping in the differential diagnosis. Among the diagnostic uses are the following:

1. The timing of murmurs in relation to sounds or other events identifying parts of the cardiac cycles. Differentiation between ejection systolic murmurs and regurgitant murmurs is often made and is especially important if murmurs appear in atypical form. Late systolic murmurs occasionally are confused with early diastolic murmurs; the differentiation can easily be accomplished by phonocardiography.

2. Identification and differentiation of heart sounds and other acoustical phenomena: S3 and S4 gallop sounds can be timed and identified; mitral opening snap can be diagnosed and differentiated from late pulmonary valve closure or from an S3 gallop sound. Ejection sounds and midsystolic clicks can be displayed and timed. Unusual sounds, such as pericardial knock or tumor "plop," can be demonstrated.

Carotid pulse tracing serves as a means of demonstrating abnormalities of the arterial pulse, which usually are perceived by palpatory examination. As a rule, the carotid arterial pulse curve approximates the central aortic pressure curve, thus the rate of rise of the upstroke, the anacrotic notch or the bisferiens type pulse are well shown in the appropriately recorded carotid pulse curve. The carotid pulse also provides timing landmarks:

- the onset of the left-sided ejection, shown by the beginning of the carotid upstroke;

- the aortic valve closure, shown by the incisural notch.

Both these events are recorded with a delay of about 20 msec. (hence the second sound is not simultaneously recorded with dicrotic notch).

The apexcardiogram records the motion of the apical impulse. The normal apexcardiogram consists of the following components:

- the atrial component — the *a* notch on the upstroke of the outward motion of the apex,

- the systolic peak, or the E point, representing the maximum excursion of the outward motion,

- the descent in midsystole, often interrupted by a plateau, then continuing to the nadir of the tracing — the O point,

- the rapid-filling wave,

- the slow-filling wave,

- further outward motion leading to the *a* notch.

When properly recorded, the apexcardiogram reflects left-sided physiological events of the cardiac cycle (Fig. 7–1). Its value in clinical diagnosis includes the following points:

- The O point is a reliable timing device for the opening of the mitral valve.

- The apex of the angle between the rapid-filling phase and the slow-filling phase times the third heart sound.

- Qualitative changes with clinical implications are as follows:

  a. An exaggerated *a* notch (becoming an *a* wave) has the same significance as a loud S4 gallop sound.

  b. Diastolic upstroke — rapid-filling phase — reflects the speed of left ventricular inflow; in mitral stenosis the slope is reduced.

  c. Exaggerated diastolic motion may produce a wave at

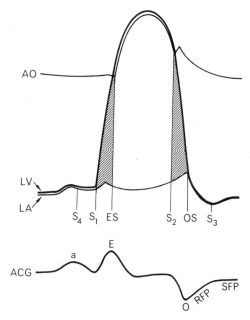

Figure 7-1. Diagram showing left ventricular pressure events with simultaneously recorded apexcardiogram. (See text for description.)

AO

LV

LA

S_4 S_1 ES S_2 OS S_3

E

a

ACG

O RFP SFP

the end of the rapid-filling phase coinciding with an S3 gallop sound.

    d. A sustained apical impulse can be recorded in the presence of left ventricular hypertrophy.

Venous pulse tracings record the jugular pulse wave. All abnormalities of the venous pulse discussed in Chapter 4 can be displayed, yet the venous pulse record serves only as a qualitative display without the quantitative aspects of the carotid and apical pulse tracing. Once an important part of the "polygraph" used for the analysis of arrhythmias, this aspect is now of only historical importance. The principal reason that the venous pulse is less useful in timing is that it relates to *right-sided* cardiac events, whereas the other phenomena relate to the left ventricle.

    As mentioned, *systolic events* of the left ventricle can be timed and measured with reasonably good fidelity noninvasively by a combined phonocardiographic-electrocardiographic-sphygmographic record (Fig. 7-2). The various measurements are based on the following intervals:

- *Total electromechanical systole* — from the Q wave of the electrocardiogram to the aortic component of the second sound;

- *Left ventricular ejection time* — from the beginning upstroke to

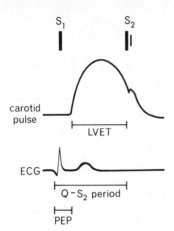

S_1

S_2

carotid pulse

LVET

ECG

$Q-S_2$ period

PEP

Figure 7-2. Diagram showing simultaneously recorded phonocardiographic tracings of heart sounds, the carotid pulse curve, and the electrocardiogram — used for the measurement of systolic time intervals. (See text.)

the trough of the incisura or dicrotic notch of the carotid pulse curve;

• *Pre-ejection period* — derived by substracting the left ventricular ejection time from the total electromechanical systole.

These three measurements have been used widely as part of the various indices of left ventricular function. In addition, it is possible to measure or calculate other events within the cardiac cycle, such as the electromechanical delay, the isovolumetric contraction period, the isovolumetric relaxation period, the rapid-inflow phase, the diastasis, and the atrial asystole.

The functional significance of the above measurement is based on the observation that, with reduced performance of the left ventricle, the pre-ejection period (PEP) may be prolonged, the ejection time shortened (LVET), with the total electromechanical systole remaining constant. The ratio of the two — PEP/LVET — has been used as one index of impairment of left ventricular function that can be obtained by a noninvasive method.

Phonocardiography and the auxiliary recording methods require great technical accuracy and precision. This is especially true for the use of this technique as noninvasive evaluation of cardiac function. While the validity of these measurements, when carefully performed, is without question, their application as a diagnostic method for the evaluation of a given patient has yet to be tested in terms of specificity and sensitivity. It is virtually certain that wide overlap exists between the normal and the impaired left ventricle. It will require a large number of patients, of different ages, with a variety of cardiac diseases to establish an abnormal zone with moderate reliability. At present, such measurements are used to display differences between groups of cases and to follow some patients longitudinally, as has been shown in studies of the effect of digitalis.

ECHOCARDIOGRAPHY

This is a relatively new technique applied to cardiology. Within a very few years it has established itself as one of the most important and valuable diagnostic methods. New applications of this technique are being constantly suggested and its total potential use has not yet been defined. It appears equally valuable as a research tool and as a routine diagnostic method of study.

The principle of echocardiography is based on the reflection of ultrasonic waves by media of different acoustical densities. Sound waves are sent from the surface of the body toward the heart and are reflected by its various structures. These reflected sound waves, sensed by a transducer at the body surface, are recorded on photographic paper, either alone or in conjunction with other physiological and electrical events (Fig. 7–3). Not all structures reflect ultrasonic waves back to the transducer—only those that are perpendicular to the ultrasonic beam. The structures that reflect ultrasonic waves can be explored in relation to their thickness and their relationship to other structures as well as their motion. The most important uses of echocardiography are:

1. The diagnosis of pericardial effusion. This method permits a reliable estimation of the presence and amount of pericardial fluid in areas within the "view" of the beam. They are highly sensitive in generalized pericardial effusion, but localized effusions "out of sight" of the ultrasonic beam or partly formed effusions can be missed.

2. Study of the mitral valve. Motion of mitral cusps, their relationship to each other, their thickness, and their position during the cardiac cycle can be reliably recorded. Thus, the diagnosis of mitral stenosis can be established along with a rough estimate of its severity. Mitral valve calcifications as well as calcifications of the mitral annulus can be demonstrated. Mitral regurgitation can usually be shown, especially its rheumatic variety, that due to rupture of chordae tendineae, and that caused by late systolic prolapse of a leaflet. The specificity of these diagnoses is fairly good and their sensitivity fair.

3. Study of the aortic valve. Reduced motion of the aortic leaflet and increased echoes from the aortic root permit the diagnosis of aortic stenosis with reasonable reliability. Aortic regurgitation can be recognized indirectly, by a fluttering motion of the mitral valve within the stream of regurgitant blood.

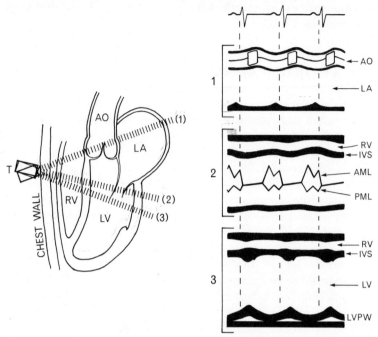

Figure 7-3. Diagram showing normal echocardiographic tracings. The left part of the diagram presents the three standard directions in which the transducer (T) sends ultrasonic beams. The right side of the diagram presents an electrocardiographic lead on the top (as timing reference) and three echocardiograms corresponding to the directions of the transducer on the right. Abbreviations: AO—aorta; LA—left atrium; RV—right ventricle; IVS—interventricular septum; AML—anterior mitral leaflet; PML—posterior mitral leaflet; LVPW—posterior wall of the left ventricle.

4.   In valvular heart disease, echocardiography plays an important diagnostic role in patients with multivalvular involvement by permitting an assessment of the condition of the valve other than the most obvious one (e.g., mitral valve involvement in patients with overt aortic regurgitation).

5.   In patients with suspected infective endocarditis, valvular vegetations can often be recognized by abnormal echoes.

6.   The size of cardiac cavities can be assessed; all four chambers can be brought within the "view" of the ultrasonic beam and one dimension of each measured. The sensitivity of the assessment of chamber enlargement is good. This method is also invaluable in permitting longitudinal observations of progression of cardiac disease by

serial studies. From the systolic and diastolic sizes of the left ventricular chamber, the ejection fraction can be calculated with acceptable results for clinical purposes.

7. Motion of the ventricular septum and the posterior wall of the left ventricle can be recorded. This permits the detection of akinesia or dyskinesia of the portion of the myocardium examined by the ultrasonic beam. Generalized decrease in cardiac contractility as well as abnormalities in calculated left ventricular ejection fraction help confirm the clinical diagnosis of cardiomyopathy. In atrial septal defect a paradoxical septal motion is recorded, which is very helpful for screening patients with suspected atrial septal defect. (False-positive findings occur in patients with gross cardiac disease, such as aneurysm of the ventricular septum, left bundle branch block, and tricuspid regurgitation.)

8. The diagnosis of hypertrophic subaortic stenosis is suggested by a disproportionately thickened interventricular septum (in relation to the posterior wall of the left ventricle) and by an abnormal motion of the mitral valve toward the septum in systole.

9. The presence of space-occupying structures of moderate or large sizes can be recorded and diagnosed: intracavitary tumors and large atrial or ventricular thrombi.

10. In the field of congenital heart disease there are a growing number of malformations in which the relationship of the various structures to each other can be clarified. Among the more important lesions are the following: transposition of the great arteries, tetralogy of Fallot, truncus arteriosus, single ventricle, and "double-outlet" right ventricle.

Echocardiography requires good equipment and a great deal of time to explore adequately the various regions of the heart. As in electrocardiography and other diagnostic cardiac techniques, the echocardiographer should be acquainted with the clinical problem and be able to focus upon specific questions. However, the time invested in obtaining good echocardiographic records is well rewarded by the greater reliability of this noninvasive method than that of most of the others. Inasmuch as echocardiography explores directly anatomic structures within the heart, its specificity is in principle higher than that of such indirect techniques as electrocardiography or vectorcardiography. Its limitation lies primarily in the inaccessibility to direct exploration of many areas of the heart.

It should be emphasized that echocardiography requires considerable training. Only wide experience and constant practice will prevent the echocardiographer from falling into the many pitfalls of misintrepretation of the various structures. The danger of overreading echocardiograms is as acute as that discussed in connection with cardiovascular radiology and electrocardiography.

PULMONARY FUNCTION TESTS

The close interrelation between the circulation and the respiration causes disorders of one system almost always to affect those of the other. It is therefore justifiable to include in an evaluation of a cardiac patient with significant disability pulmonary screening tests, and to have a complete pulmonary function panel in all those who are severely dyspneic. We include a pulmonary function panel even in asymptomatic patients if cardiac surgery is contemplated.

The usual evaluation of the respiratory functions consists of three parts:

1. Ventilatory function tests,

2. Determination of pulmonary diffusing capacity,

3. Blood gas analysis.

Other, more elaborate tests are performed in response to specific indications.

The yield of a pulmonary function panel to the overall diagnostic evaluation of the patient with cardiac disease is as follows:

- determination as to whether the respiratory function is normal or abnormal;

- a determination as to whether dyspnea is produced by a restrictive factor (frequently secondary to cardiac failure) or by broncho-obstructive disease;

- an estimation of the severity of obstructive lung disease, if present;

- an analysis of hypoxia, if present.

OTHER PROCEDURES

In addition to the procedures described above, other tests applicable to the cardiac patient deserve a brief discussion.

Isotope scanning has recently been introduced as a procedure demonstrating circulatory pathways in a manner similar to angiocardiography, but using an infinitely simpler procedure. While the principle of contrast visualization of cardiac chambers and vascular structures is the same in both procedures, isotope scanning provides only a fraction of the detail that becomes available as a result of angiocardiography. Consequently, this technique can be used only as a screening method. If the very expensive equipment necessary to scanning is available, screening may be of assistance in selected problems; the use of scanning in cardiology at present does not justify the acquisition of the equipment for that purpose alone.

Circulation time and venous pressure have been traditional bedside tests of cardiac function at the time when direct physiological methods were not available. They are still in use in some institutions. The poor reproducibility of these tests and the many potential sources of error make it wise to dispatch them into oblivion. They do not appear to be worth the time spent, nor the slight risk to the patient of an untoward reaction from the injected detector substance.

Ballistocardiography has been around in one form or other for more than three decades. A worthwhile principle — recording pulsations reflecting the recoil of blood ejected into the great vessels — seems to have become bogged down in a variety of technical difficulties. Thus, while in theory it might be possible to obtain an index of left ventricular contractibility by means of this noninvasive technique, practical considerations of poor reproducibility make it too unreliable to carry diagnostic weight.

Bibliography

Bass H: Pulmonary function studies: aid to diagnosis. Prog. Cardiovasc. Dis. *14*:621, 1972.

Feigenbaum H: Clinical application of echocardiography. Prog. Cardiovasc. Dis. *14*:531, 1972.

Selzer A, Dunlap RW, Wray HW, Russell J: A critical appraisal of the circulation time test. Arch. Int. Med. *86*:491, 1968.

Selzer A: Circulation time and venous pressure: routine tests. Amer. Heart J. *80*:142, 1970.

Weissler AM, Harris WS, Schoenfeld CD: Systolic time intervals in heart failure in man. Circulation *37*:149, 1968.

8

Cardiac Catheterization and Angiocardiography

Cardiac catheterization and angiocardiography deserve probably the major credit for the dramatic advances in diagnostic cardiology in the last two decades. As a research tool and as a diagnostic procedure both are indispensable. These two tests do introduce, however, a new and important factor into cardiovascular diagnosis—the element of *risk* to the patient, which puts them into an entirely different category as "invasive" diagnostic tests. Furthermore, these tests are associated with a major financial investment, both on the part of the institution in which they are performed and on the part of the patient. Therefore, whenever cardiac catheterization and angiocardiography are being contemplated, two questions should be considered by the clinician before the decision is made as to whether or not such procedures are indicated:

1. Is the risk of the procedure justified by the potential benefit to the patient from the information to be derived from the test?

2. Are the available facilities good enough, so that the information gained from the procedure is likely to be the most complete and reliable possible?

Each of the two procedures consists of a technical part and of the interpretation of the findings. Expertise and technical excellence are essential: a technically unsatisfactory electrocardiogram can be repeated at a minor inconvenience to the patient, but an unsatisfactory set of data obtained on catheterization or a technically poor angiocardiogram may mean subjecting the patient to a repeat procedure, thereby doubling the risk and the expense. The importance of the interpretation lies in the fact that there can be no rigid "routine" in the

120

performance of the tests: each part of the procedure has to have a specific goal. Decisions regarding the next step to be undertaken frequently depend on the interpretation of the findings obtained from the preceding step, hence they have to be made on the spot. Consequently, the test is only as good as the captain of the team performing it. Two of the most important prerequisites of good quality hemodynamic and angiocardiographic studies are an adequate caseload and long and steady experience with the tests by the team performing them. However, the quality of work falls off on both ends of the spectrum; inadequate caseload on one end, "assembly line" work of too large a caseload on the other end.

Cardiac catheterization and angiocardiography complement each other. The former involves hemodynamic measurement providing insight into pathophysiology of the disease; inferential information can thus be obtained regarding anatomic relationships. The latter displays directly the anatomic relationships and demonstrates the pathways and sequences of blood flow, thus providing inferential information regarding anatomic-pathophysiologic relationships. In simple problems one of the two procedures may suffice; more often the two are combined.

FACILITIES

A cardiac catheterization laboratory should be of adequate size to accommodate all necessary equipment without crowding. Temperature control and the arrangement of the table should facilitate the attainment of "basal state" (if it is possible) in the patient.

The basic equipment consists of the fluoroscopic-radiographic facilities and the physiological recorder. Image intensification with television viewing is essential. The mobility of the table and x-ray tube should make it possible to perform fluoroscopy and angiocardiography in the various positions and rotations with the least discomfort to the patient. The physiological recorder usually contains eight channels; photographic recording that permits multiple pressure events to be recorded from a single baseline is preferable to direct writing equipment. Oxygen analysis can be performed by a variety of methods (manometry, oximetry, spectrophotometry, etc.). It is essential that results be available during the procedure (even if only preliminary screening results). Angiocardiographic equipment includes a rapid film changer with biplane facilities for large films as well as a single plane cinecamera or two cameras for biplane work. Videotape recorders for instant playback of the cineangiographic image are widely used and are becoming a standard piece of equipment.

The technical members of the team should be familiar with the various steps. Two major objectives must dominate the efforts of the entire team:

- the safety of the patient at all times,
- the attainment of the best possible technical results.

Patient safety is contingent upon the knowledge of all possible complications and hazards of the procedure and on their anticipation and prevention. Continuous monitoring of the rhythm is of course a prerequisite of such procedures. Speed in certain parts of the procedure (e.g., manipulation within the left side of the heart) is important.

Technical excellence depends largely upon the experience of the professional and technical personnel, working together as a team. Only broad experience and continuous work in this area can produce the alertness for all possible sources of error as well as expertise in their avoidance.

CARDIAC CATHETERIZATION

Catheterization of the heart and related structures involves three principal routes of entry:

1. Venous catheterization of the right side of the heart,

2. Retrograde arterial catheterization of the left side of the heart and the principal arteries,

3. Transseptal catheterization of the left heart chambers.

Auxiliary procedures include the following:

- recording of arterial pressure via an arterial needle,
- the use of indicator dilution techniques,
- the use of modifiers of the patient's basal state, such as exercise, drug administration, intracardiac pacing,
- recording of intracardiac action potential.

The technique of catheterization of the right side of the heart is well known. The cardiac catheter is introduced through one of the veins in the cubital fossa via a cutdown, or percutaneously into a femoral vein, and guided under fluoroscopic control into the right-sided cardiac chambers and the pulmonary arterial system. The pulmonary arterial "wedge" pressure permits the recording of pressures in the pulmonary venous system; a catheter wedged firmly into a branch of the pulmonary artery separates the distal part of the artery from the pulmonary arterial system; that artery then acts as an extension of the catheter, thus providing a connecting channel with the capillary system. After the pulmonary "wedge" pressure is recorded, the catheter is placed in the main pulmonary artery, an arterial needle inserted, and necessary measurements of flows and pressures taken. Using the Fick principle for the determination of cardiac output, oxygen consumption should be measured simultaneously when arterial and venous samples are drawn. During right-sided cardiac catheterization serial blood samples are taken sequentially from the various chambers as the catheter tip passes through them, in order to explore the possibility of left-to-right shunts. Measurements are recorded during the performance of exercise (usually moving the ergometer pedals in recumbency); all measurements should be taken at least two minutes after the onset of exercise. If left-sided cardiac catheterization is to be performed, certain portions of the study have to be done with two catheters in place at the same time. Simultaneously recorded pressures are preferable to those taken consecutively ("withdrawal curves") for calculations of pressure gradients, if this is possible. Strain gauges or other pressure measuring devices should be frequently rechecked regarding their standardization and the position of the reference baseline.

Catheterization of the right side of the heart provides the opportunity to obtain the following diagnostic information:

1. The diagnosis and localization of left-to-right shunts by means of serial determination of oxygen samples from the various chambers. The following conditions are suggested if oxygen content of blood samples shows a significant increase in a given chamber and in chambers downstream from it:

- atrial septal defect — increased oxygen content in the right atrium (against caval samples), in the right ventricle, and in the pulmonary artery;

- ventricular septal defect — increased oxygen in the right ventricle and in the pulmonary artery;

- aorticopulmonary communication — increase in the pulmonary artery.

2. Pressure measurements yield the following potential information:

- the diagnosis of pulmonary hypertension,

- an analysis of the type of pulmonary hypertension,

- the diagnosis of inflow or outflow obstruction within the right ventricle,

- the diagnosis of right ventricular diastolic hypertension and right atrial hypertension,

- observation regarding changes in contour of pressure curves.

3. With the aid of some auxiliary procedures the following information can be added:

- right-to-left shunts,

- arterial hypoxemia,

- measurements of cardiac output,

- responses of pressures and flows to exercise,

- determination of pressure and collection of samples from special venous systems: coronary, hepatic, renal.

4. During catheterization of the right side of the heart, selective angiocardiography can be performed as the means of visualization of the following areas:

- the venous system,

- the right heart chambers,

- right-to-left shunts,

- anomalous pulmonary venous connections,

- left heart chambers, including cineangiographic study of the left ventricle (less satisfactory than by means of left ventricular or left atrial injection but adequate for many purposes),

- evaluation of the various complex malformations of the heart.

Catheterization of the *left side of the heart* is considered a supplementary procedure to right-sided studies. Since the entry to the arterial system and the left side of the heart carries a higher risk than that of the right side, left heart catheterization must have well-defined goals that cannot be fulfilled by other, simpler procedures. It should be noted that, except for the presence of valvular abnormalities in the left ventricle, measurements of pressures and collection of samples can be obtained without catheterization of the arterial system: The systolic pressure in the left ventricle is close to that obtained from a systemic artery through an arterial needle. The diastolic pressure and the left atrial pressures can be obtained through pulmonary arterial wedging. Left-sided arterial samples are obtained from the systemic artery. Catheterization of the left side of the heart is required for the following purposes:

1. To measure pressure in the left ventricle in the presence of inflow or outflow obstruction in that chamber;

2. To provide an opportunity for performing selective angiocardiographic studies of the left side of the circulation, which includes the following:

> - left ventriculography, to assess left ventricular contractility, to demonstrate mitral regurgitation, and to demonstrate details of the mitral valve;
>
> - visualization of the aortic root, to demonstrate aortic abnormalities, aortic regurgitation, and aorticopulmonary and aorticocardiac communications;
>
> - visualization of the coronary arterial circulation.

The choice of entry in the left side of the circulation varies from institution to institution. Preference is often based upon experience and familiarity with techniques. Entry into the aorta and the coronary circulation requires retrograde arterial study; the choice here lies between brachial arterial cutdown and percutaneous femoral catheterization. Entry into the left heart chambers can be accomplished in a retrograde manner via the arterial system, or via the transseptal route.

Transseptal left heart catheterization carries a somewhat higher risk than retrograde arterial catheterization. Its use offers certain advantages over the retrograde technique, and these advantages often justify the higher risk:

> - In patients with severe aortic stenosis, when the crossing of the valve orifice is difficult and time-consuming;
>
> - Angiocardiographic studies with injection into the left atrium may be needed in some conditions;
>
> - If aortic valve prosthesis is present, exploration of the left side of the heart has to be done via the transseptal route;
>
> - In hypertrophic subaortic stenosis transseptal catheterization offers some advantages, e.g., avoidance of catheter "trapping" in the apical portion of the left ventricle.

Transseptal catheterization of the left side of the heart should be avoided in patients in whom the presence of atrial thrombi or tumors is suspected.

Interpretation of Catheterization Findings

The first step in the process of interpretation of the results of cardiac catheterization has to start *during* the procedure by the process already mentioned, namely a critical review of each finding as it is displayed or recorded in order to detect possible errors that could invalidate these and some of the subsequent findings. During the performance of the test the operator should ask himself these questions:

1. Is each location of the catheter correct? It is necessary to double-check catheter location by means of fluoroscopic inspection and by the pressure recording from the given point. In some conditions, e.g., in congenital heart disease, even such double-check may not be enough, for abnormal chamber relationship and unusual connections may be present, obliterating the ordinary criteria. An injection of angiographic contrast substance is often used to reinforce this information.

2. Is there reasonable probability that the patient is in a "basal state" throughout the procedure? Many measurements, such as the cardiac output and the left atrial pressures can show misleading values if undue apprehension, pain, or excitement is present during the critical points of the study.

3. Is enough attention paid to the details of each measurement? For example, it is essential to be meticulously careful in collecting expired air for the determination of oxygen consumption, to collect the appropriate blood samples simultaneously, and so on.

4. Is each pressure tracing properly recorded? A variety of artifacts can distort pressure curves, such as inadequate damping, leaks in the connection between the catheter and the recording apparatus, faulty standardizations, incorrect establishment of the 0 reference point. Whenever pressure gradients are recorded by using two channels, it is imperative that the two recording transducers have identical sensitivity.

The second step in the interpretation of results involves a critical review of the final data obtained at cardiac catheterization. The limitations of each result should be considered. One of the important points is the reproducibility of the findings and the decision as to whether or not they are abnormal.

Cardiac output is most frequently determined by means of the Fick formula:

$$\text{Cardiac output} \atop \text{(L./min.)} = \frac{\text{oxygen consumption (ml./min.)}}{\text{arteriovenous oxygen difference (ml./L)}}$$

$$\text{Cardiac index} \atop \text{(L./min./M}^2\text{)} = \frac{\text{cardiac output (L./min.)}}{\text{body surface area (M}^2\text{)}}$$

Measurement of oxygen consumption is the weaker and more poorly reproducible part of this equation. The arteriovenous oxygen difference alone expresses reliably whether or not the resting cardiac output is normal, if the arteriovenous oxygen difference lies between 3.5 and 4.5 ml. of oxygen per 100 ml. of blood (35 to 45 ml. per liter). An arteriovenous oxygen difference of 5.0 ml./100 ml. or higher is definitely abnormal. This usually corresponds to a cardiac output (index) of 2.5 L./min./M² or less. Measurements of the adequacy of the increase of cardiac output in response to exercise are more difficult to evaluate. The usual increase in healthy individuals averages 600 ml. of cardiac output for each 100 ml./min. increment in oxygen consumption. An alternate way of evaluation defines normal exercise response: the arteriovenous oxygen difference increases no more than 2.0 ml./100 ml. when oxygen consumption rises to twice the resting level. It is seen that both standards require measurement of oxygen consumption at rest as well as during the exercise test. The reproducibility of measurement of oxygen consumption, which is only moderate at rest, may be even worse during exercise when the patient hyperventilates (the commonest potential error of measurement is the inability to collect all the expired air because of perioral leaks). In general, the assessment of the "exercise factor" should be considered as an approximation rather than an exact measurement.

Measurement of the pulmonary arterial pressure is less likely to be subject to error than that of cardiac output. The variation of pressure in the lesser circulation that occurs in the nonbasal state is only minor, so that the reproducibility of that measurement is good.

Pulmonary resistances are calculated from the well-known formulae, which, however, oversimplify relationships, hence do not represent exact values. Nevertheless, resistances within the lesser circulation play an important role in the diagnosis of various cardiac diseases and show a reasonable reproducibility:

$$\text{Total pulmonary resistance} = \frac{\text{mean pulm. arterial pressure (mm.Hg)}}{\text{cardiac output (L./min.)}}$$
(mm.Hg/L./min.)

$$\text{Pulmonary vascular (arteriolar)} = \frac{\text{pressure gradient: P.A. } \overline{m} - \text{L.A. } \overline{m}}{\text{cardiac output (L./min.)}}$$
resistance (mm.Hg/L./min.)

P.A. $\overline{m}$ = mean pulmonary arterial pressure.
L.A. $\overline{m}$ = mean left atrial pressure.

Example: normal average level:

$$\frac{12 \text{ mm.Hg}}{6 \text{ L/min.}} = \text{TPR} = 2 \text{ mm.Hg/L/min.} = 160 \text{ dynes sec./cm.}^5$$

$$\frac{6 \text{ mm.Hg}}{6 \text{ L/min.}} = \text{PVR} = 1 \text{ mm.Hg/L/min.} = 80 \text{ dynes sec./cm.}^5$$

These values are often expressed in the other, widely used units of dynes sec./cm.[5]. Above values can be converted into the latter units by multiplying them by 80.

Atrial and ventricular diastolic pressures are important indices of ventricular function, although these measurements have to be taken within the contexts of the stroke output they "kick off." Elevation of ventricular diastolic pressure (with the corresponding increase in the *a* wave of the atrial pressure) occurs not only in ventricular failure, but also with increased stiffness (lower compliance) of this chamber. This occurs in ventricular hypertrophy and in ischemic heart disease before heart failure sets in (see Chapter 14). Elevation of the *mean* atrial or ventricular diastolic pressure is, as a rule, a better index of impending or actual cardiac failure. Upper limits of mean atrial (or ventricular diastolic) pressure in normal individuals are 5 mm. Hg on the right side and 10 mm. Hg on the left side of the circulation.

Qualitative changes in the *atrial pressure contours* often convey diagnostic information. The absence of *a* waves occurs not only in atrial fibrillation but may be observed with ineffective atrial contraction (such as frequently occurs immediately after restoration of sinus rhythm by electric shock). Tall *v* waves with a rapid *y* descent are most often found when the atrioventricular valves on the appropriate side are incompetent, but cardiac failure of that ventricle without significant valvular regurgitation may produce the same change. The slope of the *y* descent represents a rough guide of atrioventricular filling: a slow *y* descent in the left atrial trace supports the clinical diagnosis of mitral stenosis; rapid *y* descent is against its presence. However, this sign (which has been subject to some elaborate formulae) is influenced by other factors and has only a moderate sensitivity and specificity. In constrictive pericarditis the right atrial pressure presents an "M"-shaped pattern.

The contour of *ventricular and arterial pressure* also is of diagnostic value. In pericardial constriction the early diastolic "dip" with a late diastolic plateau (square root sign) are frequently present in one or both ventricular curves; they are not specific for this condition, as they also occur occasionally in certain forms of cardiac failure. In hypertrophic subaortic stenosis the left ventricular and systemic arterial pressure curves show a bifid pressure peak, with an early systolic percussion wave separated from the main pressure peak by a "dip." In pulmonary valve incompetence the pulmonary arterial and the right ventricular pressure curves may be identical. Changes in aortic stenosis and aortic regurgitation are well known. The slope of the upstroke of the ventricular or the central aortic pressure curve is often measured as an index of left ventricular contractility (dp/dt); such measurements are less reliable when recorded by conventional means than when produced by an intracardiac miniaturized pressure transducer, in which the distortions due to the transmission of the pressure through a long column of fluid in the catheter are avoided.

Measurements of *valve area* have been found useful and relatively accurate, considering the number of assumptions going into the equation and the limitations inherent in the performance of the component measurements. The formula is as follows:

$$\text{Valve area} = \frac{\text{flow through the valve in ml./sec.}}{K \times \sqrt{\text{pressure gradient across that valve (mm.Hg)}}}$$

It is noteworthy that the valve area is directly related to the flow, and inversely related to the *square root* of the pressure gradient; three points of caution should be applied because of this relationship:

- Small variations in cardiac output produce larger variations in the pressure gradient;

- Calculations of valve area become very inaccurate with small pressure gradient (hence when the cardiac output is low);

- The widespread custom of using pressure gradient alone as an index of the severity of valve stenosis may be greatly misleading, unless it is specifically stated that the cardiac output is normal.

Calculations of *shunts* have to be done with caution. They are the least reliable of all measurements performed during cardiac catheterization. It is important, therefore, to appreciate the fact that the results represent in reality only crude approximations rather than exact measurements. The basis for the diagnosis of intracardiac shunts is the presence of "step up" in oxygen content in serial samplings from the various portions of the heart. In unidirectional shunts their approximate quantification can be done with the use of a modification of the Fick formula, as follows:

$$\text{Pulmonary blood flow} = \frac{\text{oxygen consumption}}{\text{arteriovenous oxygen difference across the lungs}}$$

$$\text{Systemic blood flow} = \frac{\text{oxygen consumption}}{\text{systemic arteriovenous oxygen difference}}$$

The arteriovenous oxygen difference across the lungs is represented by the subtraction of the oxygen content of pulmonary venous blood from that of pulmonary arterial samples; the systemic arteriovenous oxygen difference is obtained by subtracting the oxygen content of caval blood from that of systemic arterial blood.

In pure left-to-right shunts the pulmonary flow is larger than the systemic flow; by subtracting the latter from the former the magnitude of shunt can be estimated. In right-to-left shunts the pulmonary flow is subtracted from the systemic flow. Bidirectional shunts require the use of complex formulae; the accuracy is even lower than that of the unidirectional shunts.

Inasmuch as the absolute magnitude of shunts is less important than the relationship of the pulmonary to systemic flow, a simplified version of presenting intracardiac shunt is to show the ratio of pulmonary to systemic flows. By dividing the systemic arteriovenous oxygen difference into the pulmonary arteriovenous oxygen difference a ratio of the outputs of the two ventricles is established. Thus, left-to-right shunts are usually presented as 2 to 1, 3 to 1, and so on; right-to-left shunts are presented as 1 to 1.5, 1 to 2, and so on.

The quantification of the shunts — particularly left-to-right — and the determination of flow ratios is fraught with errors because of the difficulty of obtaining samples of blood that are really representative of caval blood or of pulmonary arterial blood. In atrial septal defect "caval" blood is collected from the superior vena cava, or, occasionally, from superior and inferior venae cavae. In neither case are such samples truly representative of all the well-mixed blood returning to the right side of the heart. Streamlining of bloods with different oxygen contents produces variability and poor reproducibility of oxygen content in the samples. In patent ductus arteriosus the pulmonary arterial blood does not contain a homogeneous mixture of blood arriving from the right ventricle and that returning from the aorta via the ductus: samples show variable oxygen content depending on what distance from the ductal orifice they were collected. Thus, the lack of homogeneity of the oxygen content of blood samples in left-to-right shunts reduces the accuracy of the Fick formula, which in subjects without intracardiac shunts shows excellent reproducibility.

In addition to the detection of intracardiac shunts by the differences of oxygen content from various areas of the heart, the location of shunts — hence the implied presence of defects — can be diagnosed on the basis of most proximal location of the oxygen step-up in the right side of the heart. A reliable detector of left-to-right shunts is the hydrogen inhalation test, which is very sensitive and specific for the presence of shunts — no matter how small — but which cannot quantify shunts. This test consists of inhalation of hydrogen while a platinum electrode attached to the tip of the catheter acts as a detector. Hydrogen appearance, signaled by deflection of a galvanometer, occurs normally in the right heart chambers within 10 to 15 seconds; left-to-right shunts produce premature arrival of hydrogen, reducing the time to 2 to 3 seconds. When the catheter tip is advanced from the caval system to the right atrium, the right ventricle, and the pulmonary artery, the first area in which the hydrogen test is positive suggests the entry of the shunt. An analogous test for the detection of right-to-left shunts uses dye dilution techniques: the dye is injected in the right side of the heart and the dilution curve recorded on the arterial side. Premature arrival of the dye is visualized by a hump upon the ascending limb of the curve. The location of the shunt is determined by the *last* chamber in which dye injection produces the hump (e.g., in ventricular septal defect injection of the dye into the right ventricle produces a hump, but an injection into the pulmonary artery does not).

The *interpretation* of the findings of cardiac catheterization should always be made in the light of the probable clinical diagnosis. In a purely diagnostic study in which the physiological measurements confirm the tentative clinical diagnosis, the interpretation becomes perfunctory. If the clinical impression and physiological findings are discordant, then a critical survey of every step of the procedure and of every measurement must be made, for the clinician will have to weigh the yield of the catheterization study against the information obtained by other means: cardiac catheterization data will stand or fall in its reliability and critical interpretation. Thus it is necessary to be aware of and to look out constantly for sources of error in the procedure and in the results.

The *sources of error* in cardiac catheterization are many — more than can be discussed in this chapter. The awareness of all factors that can lead to error is probably the most important single feature of a good cardiac catheterization team. The common sources of error during cardiac catheterization include the following:

1. Misinterpretation of the location of the catheter tip. The location of the tip of the catheter is determined primarily by fluoroscopic examination, and secondarily by the nature of pressure tracing recorded through the catheter and the type of blood samples drawn from it. Both can be misleading. Fluoroscopic image can be observed in only one plane; inasmuch as two or more chambers overlap in casting a shadow upon the screen, location of the catheter tip in an area where it is not customarily seen can mislead the operator. Thus, the catheter may enter the left ventricle through the foramen ovale and the left atrium but appear to the operator to be in the right ventricle; catheters advanced through the coronary sinus into the coronary venous system often appear to be in the right ventricle.

2. Errors in collection of blood samples. The potential sources of error include the misinterpretation of the chamber from which the sample is drawn, obtaining samples when the patient is not in a basal state, drawing pulmonary arterial samples from a distant branch of the pulmonary artery, thus producing a contamination of pulmonary capillary blood, and many others.

3. Errors in the recording and interpretation of pressure curves. Even if special care is exercised in appropriate calibration of the recording system and in assuring good transmission of the pressure to

the strain gauges, many errors may be present owing to inadequate damping of the system, misinterpretation of motion artifact due to wide swing of the catheter tip, misinterpretation of the area from which the curve is taken, and others.

4.   Errors in the collection of inspired air for the determination of cardiac output have already been mentioned.

A critical examination and re-examination of every step should be done routinely: An overall supercritical approach is particularly important when the principal reason for cardiac catheterization is the assessment of cardiac function, the performance of longitudinal studies, or a comparison of preoperative and postoperative findings.

It is important to differentiate those conclusions obtained from the results of cardiac catheterization that *prove* a certain point from those that *suggest* (indirectly) certain conclusions. Thus,

- A pressure gradient proves obstruction in the path of circulation between the two points of measurement (contingent only on the authenticity of the appropriate measurements), but stenosis of a valve located between the two points is merely implied.

- Varieties of pulmonary hypertension (passive, hyperkinetic, pulmonary arteriolar) are *demonstrated;* their underlying causes implied.

- Valve incompetence can only be implied, not demonstrated by abnormalities of pressure contour (*v* waves in atrial tracings, low diastolic pressure in arterial tracings).

ANGIOCARDIOGRAPHY

Once used as a method of contrast visualization of the entire circulatory system by intravenous injection, angiocardiography is today virtually 100 per cent selective, i.e., the radiopaque medium is introduced via a catheter and injected into only that part of the circulatory system to be visualized. The flow of opacified blood is recorded by means of either a series of large films exposed sequentially, using a rapid film changer, or by cinematography. The former is superior whenever details need to be studied, the latter when fluid dynamics and cardiac motion are to be reviewed. The uses of angiocardiography are too numerous to be listed here; only the more important categories will be mentioned in this brief discussion:

1.   In congenital heart disease angiocardiography is used as a means of "exploring" the cardiovascular system: demonstrating abnormal communications and structures, the relationships of the various

parts of the cardiovascular system to each other, and so on. Here the experience and ingenuity of the operator is at a premium, since decisions regarding the number of injections of the contrast medium, the location of such injections, as well as the appropriate positioning of the patient often have to be made on the spot, with a clear grasp of the overall problem as well as the results obtained, before the next decision is made. In older children and in adults, where the probability is higher that simpler lesions are present rather than multiple cardiac lesions, specific plans are made in advance, especially in patients in whom a clinical diagnosis can be established with a reasonable probability.

2. In valvular heart disease angiocardiography can separate valvar from subvalvar or supravalvar stenosis and from other lesions simulating stenosis: cardiac tumors, cor triatriatum, and so on. Valvular regurgitation can be demonstrated by injection of the contrast medium downstream to the incompetent valve. The degree of regurgitation can be roughly estimated and is often expressed on a scale from + to ++++. The type of valve lesions that produce regurgitation can frequently be identified.

3. Left ventriculography has become an important adjunct to cardiac catheterization plus angiocardiographic studies in all patients who display clinical evidence of cardiac failure or even of reduced effort tolerance. Ventriculography can be used quantitatively as a means of calculating the end-systolic and end-diastolic volumes and the ejection fraction. More often it is used in a qualitative manner to distinguish poorly contracting ventricles from those that contract well. In patients with coronary artery disease left ventriculography provides means of recognizing and localizing abnormal focal areas of contraction: aneurysms, akinetic, hypokinetic, and dyskinetic segments.

4. Aortography is used to explore the possibility of simple or dissecting aneurysms, to demonstrate aortic regurgitation, aortitis, abnormal communications arising from the aorta, and coarctation of the aorta.

5. Coronary arteriography has now become one of the most frequently performed angiographic procedures. The technique of coronary arteriography now universally used consists of repeated selective injections of small amounts of contrast medium into either of the two coronary arteries and recording views in multiple body positions by cinematography (less often by cut films).

Interpretation of Findings

It might appear at first glance that angiocardiographic films — whether cut films or cinematographic — represent the ultimate in demonstration of anatomic detail of structures, contingent only on the technical excellence of the films, so that the interpretation of such films could be considered perfunctory. The truth is that clear-cut answers to questions posed prior to the study are not always available. In a substantial proportion of cases the interpretation is difficult, requiring thorough knowledge of the subject, experience in the procedure, and time to study and restudy the pictures. This can best be illustrated by defining a few areas of difficulty in interpretation:

1. In many cases of congenital heart disease, particularly in those with multiple and complex lesions, the unraveling of the path of the circulation and the identification of each structure may be exceedingly difficult.

2. Evaluation and estimation of the severity of valve incompetence is fraught with difficulties. The degree of the opacification of the chamber receiving the regurgitant stream and the speed with which it opacifies—the usual indices of the severity of regurgitation—are related not only to the volume of regurgitant blood but also to the size of the receiving chamber in which the nonopacified and the opacified blood mix. Artifactual valve incompetence has to be taken into consideration as well; e.g., aortic regurgitation develops in normally competent valves with certain positions of the injecting catheter tip; the mitral valve becomes incompetent physiologically during a premature contraction.

3. Coronary arteriography is subject to a great many pitfalls, even though it is generally considered to be the final yardstick in deciding whether or not ischemic heart disease is present.

First, stenotic lesions in the coronary branches may be deceptive even if a sufficient number of views are taken. The degree of obstruction cannot be actually measured, only estimated. The distinction between a 60 per cent obstruction, which is usually physiologically "silent," and a 70 per cent lesion, which may be significant in terms of interfering with the flow beyond the obstruction, is thus impossible to make with any degree of accuracy.

Second, streamlining of opacified blood can occasionally show artifacts that have the appearance of obstructing lesions.

Third, subtotal or total occlusions can easily be overlooked altogether if they are located at the point of origin of the branch.

Thus, both the interpreter of the films and the clinician must be fully aware of the limitations of angiocardiography. This can be expressed by applying a more modest language to the interpretation than is the current custom, as well as using caution in drawing clinical conclusions from the results.

RISKS OF CARDIAC CATHETERIZATION AND ANGIOCARDIOGRAPHY

As stated previously, the risk of all invasive procedures is related to the experience and skill of the team performing the study. The incidence of death and complications from these procedures varies in a manner similar to the incidence from various noncardiac operations performed by surgeons possessing different levels of skill and experience. Available figures indicate a wide range in the mortality and morbidity from invasive procedures between institutions; in part such differences are related to the size of the respective caseloads.

Fatal and nonfatal complications are influenced by several factors:

- Age—the risk of catheterization and angiocardiography is highest in infants.

- Type of procedure—catheterization of the right side of the heart carries the lowest risk, transseptal left heart catheterization and coronary arteriography the highest.

- Condition of the patient—seriously ill patients are obviously at higher risk than those in satisfactory clinical condition.

- Specific lesions—some lesions are believed to offer higher likelihood of mishaps. Among these are aortic stenosis, severe pulmonary hypertension, and Ebstein's anomaly of the tricuspid valve. Aortic stenosis is widely recognized as a disease in which the risk of the procedure is increased; not enough data are available to judge the extent of such increased danger in the other conditions.

The following complications may occur in the course of cardiac catheterization and angiocardiography:

1. *Arrhythmias.* These occur physiologically as a result of catheter stimulation of the ventricular endocardium. Various tachyarrhythmias occur frequently. Ventricular fibrillation occurs occasionally but as a rule presents no major hazard because the patient can be instantly defibrillated: often the procedure is continued afterward. Bradyarrhythmias are more serious unless they represent a simple vasovagal reaction. Fatal arrhythmias are very rare.

2. *Perforation of a cardiac chamber or the aorta.* Right atrial perforation may be of no consequence; that of other chambers may or may not lead to *cardiac tamponade.* The safety of the patient often depends upon the operator's alertness in recognizing this complication, especially since such cardiac tamponade may have atypical features. The most

serious and treacherous form of cardiac tamponade due to hemopericardium is seen as a complication of transseptal cardiac catheterization.

3. *Hypotensive episodes.* These occur more often in individuals who are seriously ill (except for vasovagal syncope). They represent a potentially serious complication in patients with aortic stenosis.

4. *Ischemic episodes* occur in patients who are undergoing coronary arteriography as well as in those in whom other diagnostic procedures are being performed. Some evolve into *myocardial infarction.* During coronary arteriography some myocardial infarcts have been traced to a dissection of the coronary artery initiated by the manipulation of the coronary catheter.

5. *Embolic complications.* These occur during catheterization of the left side of the heart or, in congenital heart disease, with right-to-left shunts, during right-sided catheterization. Hemiplegia and coronary embolism represent the most serious of such complications; they occur at a rate between 0.1 and 1.0 per cent of coronary arteriographies. Pulmonary emboli are very rare.

6. *Hemorrhages* may occur after retrograde arterial catheterization and can range from subcutaneous hematomas to major arterial bleedings. Most occur upon termination of percutaneous arterial catheterization; occasionally delayed bleeding may occur, as late as 24 hours after the procedure.

7. *Infections* occur infrequently and involve mostly the skin at the point of incision. Serious infections are rare. It is surprising to note the extreme rarity of infective endocarditis following cardiac catheterization procedures, considering that the population undergoing such studies presents the highest risk of such infection.

8. *Arterial thrombosis* may occur at the site of the introduction of the catheter or distally to it, both in percutaneous catheterization and after arterial cutdown. Vigilance regarding such complications is well rewarded, since most of them are successfully treated surgically. Rarely, serious peripheral ischemic disease of an extremity may develop after the procedure.

9. *Reactions to the contrast medium* after angiocardiography are rare now, since major improvement has been made in lowering toxicity of the solutions to a negligible level. Rarely, hypersensitivity reactions may occur. It is to be remembered, furthermore, that the contrast material is a hypertonic solution, and that there is a limitation to how much of it can be injected.

In general, considering the fact that seriously ill, occasionally moribund patients have to undergo lengthy studies prior to life-saving operations, and that during such diagnostic studies manipulations within the heart and the great vessels are performed and foreign substance injected, the procedures are amazingly well tolerated. In many laboratories with well-coordinated active teams, emergency procedures are being performed in patients who are in the early stages of acute myocardial infarction, in those in cardiogenic shock, as well as in deeply cyanotic moribund neonates, and yet such procedures have shown good diagnostic yields and acceptable risks. Nevertheless, the risk of the procedure is highly individual; thus recommendations for such studies should be made only after the risk is considered for the particular laboratory in which the study is to be performed.

INDICATIONS FOR INVASIVE CARDIAC STUDIES

The risk of invasive diagnostic tests must be equated and balanced against benefits derived from the information that is to be gained by the procedure. At the present stage of medical and surgical cardiology, indications for invasive procedures are related more to the nature of the problems than to the type of cardiac disease, for in almost every condition a situation can arise wherein such diagnostic study would be indicated. It is therefore impossible to provide a complete list of indications, but rather to submit the common problem in which studies need to be considered.

1. When congenital heart disease is clinically apparent or suspected, a diagnostic study may be indicated. The goals would be:

- the establishment with certainty as to whether or not organic cardiac disease, no matter how mild, is present in a child or young adult;

- the selection of patients for surgical treatment;

- the establishment of preoperative baseline data (e.g., regarding the presence or degree of pulmonary hypertension) for future reference.

The benefits of a diagnosis in nonsurgical cases include helpful points in the future management of the patient, e.g., regulation of activities, and more accurate knowledge of the patient's prognosis, often offering valuable reassurance to overanxious parents. The "luxury" of performing invasive studies in patients who are not serious surgical candidates is justifiable by the fact that the invasive investigation of cardiac murmurs suspected of representing congenital heart disease requires, as a rule, only the performance of catheterization of the right side of the heart, with its negligible risk.

2. In valvular heart disease all patients in whom surgical treatment is being considered should benefit from an invasive diagnostic study, even if a firm diagnosis can be established by simpler means. While this opinion is not universally accepted—in some centers many patients are sent to open heart surgery without diagnostic catheterization—it is based on two reasons:

- Clinical symptoms do not always reflect the severity of valvular disease, nor can clinical means assess its severity sufficiently to eliminate the risk that operation may be performed in the presence of mild disease.

- Since valve surgery is not curative, patients run the risk of recurrence of symptoms, the interpretation of which may hinge upon the knowledge of preoperative dynamics.

These reasons also justify the performance of postoperative studies in patients who obtained satisfactory results, to be used as a reference point later, should disability recur.

In addition, in some asymptomatic patients a simple "function study" (e.g., right-sided cardiac catheterization with exercise test) may provide a reference point for longitudinal follow-up. This is particularly helpful in mitral stenosis to determine whether the lesion is or is not progressive.

3. In ischemic heart disease a complete hemodynamic-angiographic study is indicated when patients show indication of disturbed cardiac function, such as may develop after acute myocardial infarction.

4. Severely symptomatic patients in whom the diagnosis cannot be clarified by clinical means may be subjected to an invasive study as means of exploring rare or atypical forms of surgically treatable cardiac diseases.

5. Selective coronary arteriography is now widely used and most certainly overused in some quarters. The prime candidates for such studies are patients in whom revascularization procedure is contemplated, and, occasionally, candidates for certain other cardiac operations (e.g., aortic stenosis presenting angina-like chest pain). As a purely diagnostic procedure it is occasionally indicated in young individuals with atypical chest pain to whom the stigma of serious heart disease is attached and in whom uncertain diagnosis might interfere with livelihood or mental health.

It should be re-emphasized that it is less important to place patients in specific diagnostic categories in which invasive procedures are justifiable than to review each individual case from the standpoint of the risk and benefit.

Bibliography

Adams DF, Fraser DB, Abrams HL: The complications of coronary arteriography. Circulation *48*:609, 1973.

Braunwald E, Swan HJC: Cooperative study on cardiac catheterization. Circulation 37–38 (Suppl. III), 1968.

James TN: Angina without coronary disease (sic). Circulation *42*:189, 1970.

Report of Intersociety Commission for Heart Disease Resources: The optimal catheterization and angiocardiographic laboratory. Circulation *43*:A 138, 1971.

Selzer A, Willett FM, McCaughey DJ, Feichtmeir TV: Uses of cardiac catheterization in acquired heart disease. New Engl. J. Med. *257*:66, 121, 1957.

Selzer A, Sudrann RB: Reliability of the determination of cardiac output in man by means of the Fick principle. Circ. Res. *6*:485, 1958.

Selzer A, Popper RW, Lau FYK, Morgan JJ, Anderson WL: Present status of diagnostic cardiac catheterization. New Engl. J. Med. *268*:589, 654, 1963.

Sones FM, Shirey EK: Cine coronary arteriography. Mod. Concepts Cardiovasc. Dis. *31*:735, 1962.

9

Diagnostic Synthesis

Throughout preceding chapters the diagnostic process was presented as a sequential chain of decision-making steps, in which each bit of information is reviewed in the light of the final goal and each test has a specific objective. This process provides the clinician with opportunity to be selective, to withhold certain methods of examination if their contribution to the diagnosis is anticipated to be of little importance. This approach is likely to provide the best diagnostic yield at a reasonable or justifiable risk to the patient with some control over the expense of the evaluation.

Unfortunately, a more widely practiced approach to diagnostic evaluation of a patient with suspected or known cardiac disease is that of ordering a battery of tests at once, collecting all the results of the tests, and then attempting to put together the information into a final diagnosis. The negative aspects of this approach are self-evident. Some examples are presented in Chapter 2.

In discussing the avenues of reaching the final diagnosis, it is necessary to discuss the end-product and to attempt its precise definition.

The term "final diagnosis" as used in the common connotation and in the legal sense is in reality rather misleading. When a patient enters a hospital, the attending physician can record a tentative, provisional diagnosis. However, rules require the writing of a final diagnosis when the patient is signed out upon discharge from the hospital, regardless of whether or not a firm clinical diagnosis has been made. Similarly, death certificates, disability certificates, insurance forms—all require a final diagnosis. Perhaps it would be justified—and more honest—if the clinician were permitted to indicate upon the chart or the certificate how *firm* his diagnosis is. One might consider the following classification:

Class I. Diagnosis certain. This category would include cases in which the diagnosis is established beyond reasonable doubt—i.e., those patients in whom all clinical and laboratory findings clearly concur into a single disease entity, and those in whom invasive laboratory procedures led to an unequivocal diagnosis.

Class II. Diagnosis probable. This category would include conditions in which most of the clinical and laboratory signs support a diagnosis, but some atypical features, or absence of certain expected signs, makes the diagnosis fall short of certainty.

Class III. Diagnosis reasonable. This category would contain cases with discordant findings, in whom the majority of signs or tests — weighted in their respective importance — suggest the diagnosis.

Class IV. Diagnosis questionable. Here one would include patients whose findings do not fit well into any single diagnostic category; however, one diagnosis seems more probable than others.

Translating this hypothetical classification into a specific clinical example, one can select acute myocardial infarction. The range of diagnosis would then be from Class I in which classic findings are present in all respects, to Class IV in which atypical chest pain was present, minor electrocardiographic changes and borderline enzyme elevation were found, yet good medical judgment may require that the patient be treated as a mild myocardial infarction.

This classification would provide the clinician with a range of probabilities with which he can estimate the chance of his diagnosis being correct. Class I diagnosis would offer a 95 per cent or better probability, the other classes appropriately lower probabilities. Class IV may be associated with a probability of correctness of only 30 per cent, but this figure would still be higher than alternative possibilities.

It is unlikely that the proposed diagnostic classification would ever receive official sanction. It is nevertheless a helpful aid in the mental process of diagnostic synthesis. The clinician could consider the diagnosis from the standpoint of the various categories and ask the questions:

- Is a better diagnostic category attainable in a given case by further studies?

- If it is, are its advantages to the patient sufficiently clear to justify the undertaking of further studies?

Throughout this section it has been repeatedly pointed out that each clinical finding and each diagnostic test has some limitations and pitfalls. Thus, one could extend the above diagnostic classification, applying it to the various component parts of the diagnostic evaluation. The process of evaluating the probability of each finding or of each test and then arriving at an overall probability of the final diagnosis would be ideally suited for computer analysis, if data were available to express the sensitivity and specificity of each sign and each test in meaningful numbers. Since such data are not available, the probability and accuracy of each test have to be estimated or guessed by the clinician—largely on the basis of his own experience—a process totally unsuitable for computer programming.

The process of diagnostic synthesis can be exemplified by some clinical situations that are commonly encountered:

1.   If findings on examination and results of the various laboratory studies concur in pointing to a certain condition, the diagnosis becomes easy and reliable.

2.   The clinician may face the situation in which most of the findings support a certain condition, but one or two are inconsistent with such a diagnosis. If this occurs, he has to decide whether the majority of concurrent findings or the discordant finding carries more weight. To exemplify such a situation, imagine a patient who has all the clinical, radiographic, and electrocardiographic findings of aortic stenosis; however, two discordant findings develop: (1) the classic murmur of grade IV intensity was reported as being absent one year earlier; and (2) no gradient across the aortic valve is found on cardiac catheterization. The synthesis suggests two possibilities: either the observation regarding the previous absence of the murmur was faulty and an error occurred during measurement of the left ventricular and aortic pressures, or the diagnosis of aortic stenosis is incorrect. Both possibilities are realistic, but the second is more probable (mitral regurgitation due to rupture of chordae tendineae to the posterior cusp may masquerade clinically as aortic stenosis).

3.   Findings are contradictory—each points in a different direction. Such cases require the full ingenuity of an experienced clinician, who will have to weigh each finding separately and select the ones that carry most weight.

In general, the clinician faces three types of problems in the differential diagnosis:

- The establishment of a diagnosis in patients who, beyond reasonable doubt, have heart disease;

- The differential diagnosis between cardiac disease and diseases of other organs or systems;

- The question of the presence or absence of heart disease in an otherwise healthy individual.

This last problem is an especially difficult and challenging one, which only too often is solved automatically in favor of the presence of cardiac disease (given an abnormal finding, the heart is considered guilty until proven innocent).

The differentiation between the normal and abnormal is admittedly difficult and in many areas it is impossible to go beyond probabilities because of the overlap between the two. It has already been mentioned that the definition of the norm is based on a Gaussian curve and that, in a given test, by the usual standards 4 per cent of the healthy population show findings that are generally considered abnormal. A common situation arises when a single abnormal finding is discovered in an individual who has no symptoms and no previous knowledge of cardiac disease. Such a finding may be an abnormal electrocardiogram, an enlarged heart in the roentgenogram, or a cardiac murmur. A similar situation also occurs when a single suspicious symptom is present: e.g., dyspnea or chest pain.

The diagnostic synthesis in such cases should start with a critical review of the possibility of a technical error (even considering the possibility of mistaken identity) in laboratory abnormalities. When satisfied that the abnormality is authentic, the possibility of an alternate explanation for the test, the sign, or the symptom should be looked for (normal variant, innocent or less serious abnormalities than the clue suggests). When the conclusion seems inescapable that the clue is a correct one, the clinician faces two decisions:

- Should the diagnosis be pursued to obtain a higher probability?
- Should the patient be fully informed of suspicion or discovery of cardiac disease?

Both questions rank high among difficult problems in clinical cardiology. Should every youngster with a suspicious cardiac murmur undergo cardiac catheterization? Should every person with atypical chest pain have coronary arteriography? Such problems can only be solved individually. A teenager, who, because of a murmur has been kept away from sports, and whose parents are anxious regarding his heart, would benefit from having the authoritative answer as to whether or not organic cardiac disease is present. Another similar patient, who had no previous knowledge of a murmur, can be handled on the basis of clinical probability: murmurs more likely to be innocent can be clinically discarded; those with likelihood of congenital heart disease, investigated. The question of the selection of patients for coronary arteriography is more difficult because of the higher risk in this diagnostic procedure. In general, the benefit of the doubt should be resolved, if possible, without subjecting the patient to invasive studies, unless specific benefit to the patient can be identified.

The problem of informing the patient about cardiac abnormalities requires a good deal of clinical wisdom. There is very little doubt that there are as many cardiac cripples around who have no disabling cardiac disease but who suffer from irreversible cardiac neurosis as a result of a wrong diagnosis or careless statement about their hearts as there are true cardiac invalids. A young individual with a small ventricular septal defect may have an outlook for the future no different than if he had a normal heart. These patients should undoubtedly be told of their murmurs, because they would be found by other examiners, but a proper explanation should be given so that they can be made to comprehend the problem and not only accept it without ill effects but also be protected against future physician-alarmists.

The process of diagnostic evaluation of a cardiac patient involves other steps besides the identification of the disease: the assessment of where the patient fits within the natural history and course of the disease. This assessment includes:

- The functional classification of disease (cardiac status);
- Assessment of the severity of the lesion;
- Review of etiological and hereditary factors.

Functional classification of cardiac disease has been based for half a century on four classes designed by the New York Heart Association, and adopted as the "official" diagnostic terminology by most insurance companies, governmental agencies, and hospitals. The functional classification is based upon the patient's ability to perform his customary activities. This is supplemented by a companion therapeutic classification which recommends how active the patient should be. The functional classification is as follows:

Class I – No limitation of physical activity;

Class II – Slight limitation of activity (ordinary activity produces symptoms);

Class III – Marked limitation of activity (less than ordinary activity produces symptoms);

Class IV – Inability to carry out any activity without symptoms; symptoms may be present at rest.

The limitation of this classification is obvious, in view of how often factors other than activity may evoke serious cardiac symptoms. Recently a revision of the functional classification has been proposed by the Criteria Committee of the New York Heart Association, which submits a broader basis for an overall assessment of the stage of a cardiac disease. The new classification is as follows:

Cardiac status
1. Uncompromised
2. Slightly compromised
3. Moderately compromised
4. Severely compromised

Prognosis
1. Good
2. Good with therapy
3. Fair with therapy
4. Guarded despite therapy

Some time will undoubtedly elapse before the new classification will acquire official sanction and the old one is abandoned. Nevertheless, the clinician should find it easier to fit his patients into the new categories and the reproducibility of classification from physician to physician and from institution to institution will probably be improved.

The assessment of the severity of lesions applies to most chronic forms of cardiac disease. A patient with classic signs of mitral stenosis may have no symptoms or may have minor, nonprogressive symptoms over long periods of time. His mitral stenosis may during this time progress from trivial to moderately severe obstruction of the mitral orifice. Patients with congenital heart disease may develop severe pulmonary hypertension without showing progressive symptomatology. Obviously, such factors have important bearing upon medical or surgical therapy and their recognition is as important as the basic diagnosis.

The etiology of cardiac disease no longer plays the important role it did two or three decades ago, mostly because of the shift of emphasis upon the physiological rather than the anatomic basis of cardiac disease. Nevertheless, etiological factors are part of the diagnosis and should be followed, particularly whenever epidemiological, familial, and hereditary influences play an important role and may have some bearing upon preventive aspects of the disease.

As a final recapitulation, it is necessary to look upon the mental process of cardiac diagnosis as involving two separate parts:

- The diagnosis per se, i.e., the act of recognizing whether or not cardiac disease is present, and its identification.

- The consequence of the diagnosis: How will the knowledge of this fact influence the health and the life of the patient?

The second aspect should always take precedence over the first, otherwise academic curiosity might lead to the performance of some procedures that may not be in the best interest of the patient.

Bibliography

Major changes made by Criteria Committee of the New York Heart Association (Editorial). Circulation *49*:390, 1974.

Selzer A, Cohn K: Functional classification of cardiac disease: A critique. Amer. J. Card. *30*:306, 1972.

10

Approach to Treatment

Within one generation cardiac therapy underwent a fundamental change, from the ritualistic art of handing the patient a prescription for an inert substance to a semiscientific use of powerful drugs, and then to other effective methods of treatment and to spectacular cardiac operations. The qualification "semiscientific" is necessary to emphasize the fact that scientific methods of evaluation of the therapeutic results are only beginning to make inroads in everyday cardiological practice.

The use of effective forms of therapy has its price: the great majority of therapeutic agents (in a broad sense, i.e., including operations) carry with them a risk to the patient. The risk, involving morbidity and mortality, necessitates careful forethought regarding the need for the therapy as well as an evaluation as to what would happen to the patient if no treatment were to be offered to him. Thus it is important to emphasize the foremost principle of therapy: *The risk of the treatment has to be at least balanced and preferably outweighed by its benefit to the patient.*

In general terms, therapy involves two principal forms:

- *Remedial therapy*—treatment of a manifestation of disease;

- *Prophylactic therapy*—treatment aimed at the prevention of the development of cardiac disease, the prevention of a complication or of a later stage of existing disease.

Remedial therapy involves risk to all patients subjected to it, with benefits presumably accrued in all. Prophylactic therapy involves risk to all individuals subjected to it, but benefit is accrued only to a fraction of those. Obviously in balancing risk against benefit of a therapeutic step this distinction has to be sharply defined.

Cardiac therapy has to be thought of in broadest terms. In various acute diseases, e.g., myocardial infarction, infective endocarditis, therapy involves a finite period of time after which it may be terminated. In chronic diseases, which include the majority of cardiac problems, therapy includes decisions not only involving the traditional forms of treatments (medical, physical, surgical) but the planning of the patient's daily life, including his vocation, his recreational activities, his place of work and of residence, and his travels. It should also be appreciated that "letting loose" a patient with cardiac disease without any therapy is a decision that has to be considered as carefully as any other form of treatment.

Defining cardiac therapy in the above terms, and recognizing its broad implications upon a patient's life, it is important that each decision be considered in the light of specific objectives, exemplified by the following questions:

1. Does the patient need active therapy?

2. Is it possible to make a reasonable assessment of the risk of the contemplated therapy?

3. Can the benefit of the contemplated therapy be assessed?

4. Could the therapy alter the psychological makeup of the patient?

5. Could therapy impose financial hardship on the patient or his family?

THE RISK

In considering the therapeutic equation (risk vs. benefit) it is necessary to consider both parts of the equation in broader terms than they are often defined. Risk in its narrow sense is thought of in terms of an untoward reaction to a drug, or death or a complication resulting from treatment; the risk of surgical therapy is most often considered from the standpoint of the immediate surgical mortality, with only peripheral consideration given to late complications and deaths.

The risk of therapy should include all the consequences to the patient and his family resulting directly or indirectly from a given therapeutic step. A youngster may be advised to give up his favorite sport or to select a vocation not to his liking. How will this recommendation affect his life? Patients are often advised to take off a few months from work, to change their job to one of lesser responsibility than they deserve or have earned, to change their place of residence. Will such steps disrupt the patient's family life, lead to a state of depression, or cause financial ruin? Even the initiation of therapy—the act of informing the patient that he has a "murmur" or an abnormal electrocardiogram which necessitates certain restrictions—may produce far-reaching consequences in the form of crippling cardiac neuroses. The tragedy is that only too often therapeutic restrictions with all such negative consequences are made on the basis of incomplete or even outright wrong diagnoses!

THE BENEFIT

As in the case of the risk, the benefit of therapy must be considered in the broad sense and must be critically evaluated. It is obvious that the range of benefits from cardiac therapy is very wide, from a well-defined, immediately measurable therapeutic effect, to a nebulous beneficial effect dreamed up by armchair strategists on the basis of theoretical speculation and animal experiments. Many controversies concerning the various therapeutic approaches to some forms of cardiac disease arise because benefits are based on arguments which include a little black magic from past generations, irrelevant animal experiments, poorly designed and uncontrolled clinical trials.

In trying to assess the benefits of therapy one should first consider whether or not its effectiveness can be directly measured. In advocating chronic therapy one can further consider the benefits from the standpoint of how well the therapy can be monitored.

Measurements of therapeutic effectiveness vary with the therapeutic goals. In general, therapy directed against objective effects or endpoints is easier to evaluate than that for subjective symptoms. In measuring *objective* effects of therapy one can distinguish the following:

- Immediate effects, e.g., restoration of sinus rhythm by electroshock;

- Intermediate effects, e.g., response to initiation of diuretic therapy in patients with fluid retention;

- Long-range effects, e.g., cure of infective endocarditis;

- Effects of continuous therapy, e.g., digitalis control of atrial fibrillation, therapy of hypertension.

Among *subjective* effects of cardiac therapy one can exemplify the immediate effects by the relief of an anginal attack after sublingual administration of nitroglycerin, and its long-range effects by the elimination of anginal attacks after an aorto-coronary bypass operation.

The effectiveness of therapy should be appraised if possible by appropriate monitoring. This can be done by a variety of methods:

1.   Direct measurement of the desired effect, e.g., the recording of blood pressure reduction in response to therapy for hypertension.

2.   Observing objective indices directly related to the desired ef-

fect, e.g., weight reduction in response to diuretic effect; decrease of blood cholesterol level in response to lipid-reducing therapy.

3. Observing objective indices related indirectly to the desired effect, e.g., level of prothrombin activity during anticoagulant treatment, or level of quinidine in the blood.

4. The patient's observation of the subjective effects, e.g., the recording of the number of anginal attacks after initiation of anti-anginal therapy.

In relatively few forms of therapy is the above exemplified monitoring available or assessment of the benefit clearly possible. In most, it is necessary to approach each form of therapy by asking the question: How well is the therapeutic effectiveness of an agent demonstrated? This question cannot often be answered for each case in which therapy is applied; rather, it may be necessary to rely on the demonstration of the effectiveness by results of formal studies. Thus, the great majority of therapeutic endeavors involve situations in which individual judgment is difficult. The great biological variability of symptoms of disease, as well as the variability of objective signs against which therapy is directed, makes the cause-effect relationship between therapy and clinical improvement difficult to prove. Other factors—psychological influences, suggestion—play a role in influencing results of therapy that may outweigh the effect of the therapeutic agent. Modern pharmacology relies more and more on controlled clinical studies, the purpose of which is the elimination of all other factors than the drug in question upon the manifestation of the disease or symptoms. The design of such studies is difficult and results often inconclusive; consequently good studies are not yet available for many drugs used in cardiology.

When dealing with long-range therapy of chronic disease, its benefit can be expressed in terms of the effect of the treatment upon the natural history of the disease. This method, in theory, permits quantification of the benefit, hence is highly desirable. However, only exceptionally is the natural history of a disease sufficiently well known to constitute a basis for comparison. As an example one can mention the results of the Veterans Administration Cooperative Study of anti-hypertensive therapy (Fig. 10–1). Here the "yardstick" is the occurrence of morbid events and two curves—those of patients receiving antihypertensive therapy and those untreated—are compared. The effectiveness of the therapy is clearly demonstrated by the difference between the two curves and its benefit thus adequately established.

In comparing effects of cardiac surgery upon the natural history of cardiac disease attempts are usually made to use the mortality as the basis of comparison. Figure 10–2 shows a curve depicting the effect of aortic valve operation upon the natural history of aortic stenosis. It is

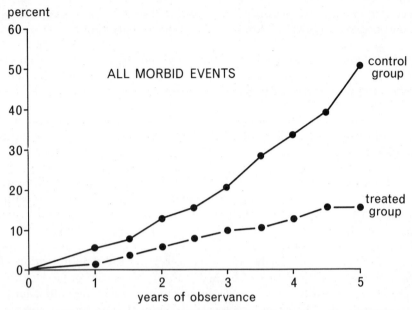

Figure 10-1. Comparison between patients with hypertension on antihypertensive therapy with control patients showing the incidence of morbid events. (Redrawn from the Veterans Administration Cooperative Study of Antihypertensive Therapy. By permission, copyright American Medical Association.)

seen that in asymptomatic patients the curve slopes down gently, only slightly lower than the actuarial curve of the general population. When symptoms develop, a sharp increase in mortality occurs. Operation temporarily accentuates the mortality by an immediate loss owing to a 10 per cent risk of the operation, but shows a satisfactory straightening of the line in survivors, indicating the net benefit. However, in a hypothetical case, assuming early surgery in patients without symptoms (advocated by some), surgical treatment might be associated with a net setback of the natural history: several years may elapse before the curve of treated patients crosses that of untreated patients, thus affecting unfavorably—though temporarily—the natural history of aortic stenosis.

It should be pointed out that curves of mortality with and without surgical therapy are as a rule based on uncontrolled studies, often not pertaining to comparable populations. Their validity is sometimes doubtful. This is particularly true in the various statistics quoted in support of the success of aorto-coronary bypass operations performed for treatment of ischemic heart disease; all too frequently survival curves in surgically treated patients are matched with the worst available "medical" series. It is for this reason that several authorities strongly urged the organization of a randomized controlled study which would have some statistical validity. (Such a study is now being conducted by the Veterans Administration Hospital group.)

PROPHYLACTIC THERAPY

For reasons stated above, it is necessary to take a particularly cautious approach to prophylactic therapy, especially if it is associated with a risk, however small.

By definition, prophylactic therapy involves treatment of subjects who are merely thought to be susceptible to a disease, to a manifestation of a known disease that is not yet in evidence, or to the development of a complication of a known disease. This means that *all* subjects are treated at a time when the treatment is not yet needed; many are treated for a condition they will never develop—with or without therapy. Obviously the risk-benefit ratio has to be scrutinized even more skeptically in this situation than in conventional remedial therapy. One should approach prophylactic therapy by asking the following questions:

- Are the goals of the therapy well defined?

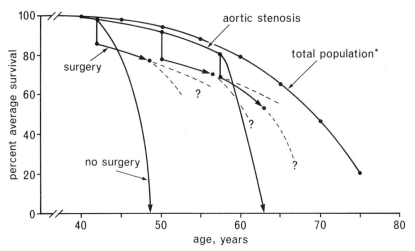

*U.S. vital statistics, males, 1963

Figure 10-2. Curve showing average survival in the male population after the age of 40, comparing the normal population with that with aortic stenosis. See text for detailed discussion. (Modified from Ross and Braunwald, by permission of the authors and the American Heart Association, Inc.)

- How often does the condition against which prophylactic therapy is aimed occur naturally?

- How well is the protective action of the contemplated therapy demonstrated?

- Can the risk-benefit ratio be reliably estimated for this therapy?

Some established forms of therapy can serve as excellent examples of the relativity of the risk-benefit ratio. Given a method of treatment that is virtually devoid of risk, or in which the risk is minimal, there might be justification for its use even if the benefits are poorly defined or their magnitude unknown. In this category one can place the recommendation to discontinue cigarette smoking or to undertake a low-fat and low-cholesterol diet for the prevention of ischemic heart disease (given well motivated subjects); similarly, antibiotic therapy in connection with dental manipulations may be administered prophylactically for the prevention of endocarditis in susceptible subjects. On the other end of the spectrum, anticoagulant therapy for chronic ischemic heart disease has been largely and properly abandoned (except for a few diehard enthusiasts) because of the high risk and unproved benefits.

In the following three chapters the common methods of therapy used in patients with cardiac disease are discussed. An attempt is made to present the subject critically, separating points that have been reasonably well established from those based on tradition, speculation, and inadequately controlled clinical studies.

Bibliography

Dykes NHM: Uncritical thinking in medicine. The confusion between hypothesis and knowledge. J.A.M.A. *227*:1275, 1974.

Ross J, Braunwald E: Aortic stenosis. Circulation *38*(suppl. V, 61), 1968.

Veterans Administration Cooperative Study Group on Antihypertensive Agents: Effects of treatment on morbidity in hypertension. J.A.M.A. *213*:1143, 1970.

11
Drug Therapy

GENERAL PRINCIPLES

The clinician taking care of a patient with heart disease may be called upon to use every type of drug therapy, inasmuch as most such patients have a lifelong affliction and may be stricken with various intercurrent and unrelated illnesses in addition to their cardiac disease. In this section drug therapy most directly related to heart disease will be discussed as well as some principles of drug treatment in general.

The clinician has today at his disposal a number of powerful drugs that may help patients with cardiac disease but may also harm them and even kill them. The critical, even skeptical approach, presented in the preceding chapter is fully justified when dealing with drugs that have a high toxic potential. Furthermore, the correct use of drugs requires a thorough understanding of drug kinetics, drug actions and drug interactions, far beyond that usually supplied by the drug manufacturer in the usual release or printed in the *Physicians' Desk Reference.*

Drug Kinetics

Cardiac drugs are as a rule not used topically; the usual mode of administration consists of oral, sublingual, subcutaneous, intramuscular, or intravenous administration. Rectal drug administration is now rarely used. In order to reach its target-organs the drug has to be absorbed and transported. Drug action thus is first dependent upon the absorption of the drug. Such absorption may be fast or slow, complete or incomplete, consistent or changeable (related to various secondary factors). As soon as the drug enters the body, factors begin to develop that rid the body of the foreign substance: the drug is excreted, secreted, or metabolized. The relationship between the absorption and elimination of the drug determines the mode of drug administration and the dosage. The pharmacologist, borrowing a term from the radioisotopes, estimates the *half-life* of the drug, i.e., the time necessary to lower the concentration of a drug in the body fluid to one half of its peak.

The administration of a drug with a short half-life is different from that of one with long action. Given a drug in the former category, such as quinidine, its peak serum concentration is reached within one or two hours; the fall-off of the concentration curve is intercepted by the effect of the next dose—4 or 6 hours later—producing a new increase in concentration. A gentle wavy concentration curve is thus maintained, presumably keeping the drug concentration at all times within the effective zone. On the other hand when using drugs with a long half-life (in the past often referred to as "cumulative"), such as digitalis or coumarin derivatives, a stable drug concentration can be attained with drug administration at intervals of a day or even less frequently (Fig. 11–1).

A major step to better understanding of drug administration was the demonstration of the fact that drug elimination does not take place in absolute terms of destruction or excretion of a certain amount of the drug per unit of time, but rather is a function of the concentration of the drug. Its elimination is thus a fraction of the amount of the drug in the body. By means of this mechanism a drug concentration in the body reaches a plateau. In drugs with a short half-life the plateau is reached promptly, in long-acting drugs slowly. From the practical standpoint it is now clear that digitalis and coumarin drugs can be brought up to an effective level by administration of daily "maintenance" dosages without initial loading. However, the plateau is not reached until several days after the initiation of the therapy. Thus the purpose of the drug loading technique in long-acting drugs is to reach the effective zone at once, rather than after a long delay.

Drug Effectiveness

Whereas drug kinetics determine the concentration of the drug in the body at any given time, its effect upon the target organ is further related to two factors:

- The threshold of effective drug action (the lowest concentration of the drug at which its effect is measurable);

- The dose-effect relationship.

A third factor, to be discussed later, is the threshold of drug toxicity.

There is a great variation in these factors with different drugs. For example, quinidine used for the suppression of premature contractions is often effective at a very low serum concentration. It shows a good dose-effect relationship in the sense that stronger anti-arrhythmic action follows higher drug concentration. On the other hand, the two long-acting drugs already mentioned — digitalis and coumarin derivatives — have a high threshold of effectiveness. Both drugs also have a low threshold of toxicity, making them effective, without harm to the patient, only within a narrow therapeutic zone.

The general principles of evaluating the effectiveness of drugs have already been mentioned in Chapter 10 in terms of therapy in general. Drugs used most effectively and reliably are those in which the effect is directly measurable and can be continuously monitored. As an example, one can mention the action of diuretics in patients in chronic cardiac failure, where body weight permits accurate monitoring, or the use of digitalis in controlling ventricular rate in atrial fibrillation. In such cases individual dosage schedules can be provided for a patient, titrating the drug as needed. The majority of cardiac drugs do not possess such a reliable demonstration of therapeutic efficacy; therefore, evidence for their effectiveness has to rest with critically evaluated results of controlled studies. Modern pharmacology has provided techniques that are capable of assessing drugs adequately with a minimum of bias. The most widely used method of study is the double-blind technique that eliminates suggestion and bias on the part of the patient and

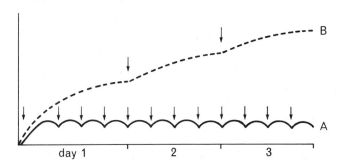

Figure 11-1. Diagram showing the concentration of two hypothetical drugs (ordinate) administered at points indicated by arrows. Drug A, with a short half-life, permits maintenance of a steady level, attained at once, when administered four times a day. Drug B, with a long half-life, accumulates slowly: after three days its final level has not yet been attained.

the physician alike. Valuable as this method of study is, it can occasionally lead the investigator astray, especially when dealing with end-effects which are potentially influenced by psychogenic factors that can make the placebo effective. Studies that purported to show that nitroglycerin is ineffective for anginal attacks (objective evidence clearly demonstrates its effectiveness) may serve as an example of a "false negative" result of a double-blind study.

Drug Toxicity

Almost all effective drugs are toxic; differences between them lie only in the type of toxicity and the magnitude of the risk involved in the drug administration. Toxicity is used here in its widest connotation, that is, to include all undesirable effects of drug administration.

Such undesirable effects fall in various categories:

- Side-effects, related to the pharmacologic action of the drug on areas other than the target organ (e.g., diarrhea after quinidine, headache after nitroglycerin).

- Idiosyncratic reaction to a drug that can range from general anaphylactic reaction to involvement of one or more organs or systems (e.g., blood dyscrasia, skin eruption).

- Dose-related toxicity, which may be produced by administration of higher than usual dosage, by vagaries of drug kinetics, or by individual sensitivity to a drug (shifting both the therapeutic and the toxic threshold to a lower drug concentration).

- Toxicity produced by drug interaction (e.g., potentiation of coumarin drugs by salicylates.

It is obvious that the major objective of drug therapy is to obtain the maximum possible benefit from a drug without subjecting the patient to its toxicity. Thus, the prevention of toxicity and anticipation of various factors that would enhance toxicity are important goals of rational drug therapy. Among definable factors that should always be assessed when drug therapy is being initiated are:

- *The age of the patient;* as a rule sensitivity to a drug increases with age, so that it is prudent to consider using, if possible, lower dosages in older patients.

- *The size of the patient:* many drugs are administered in terms of dosages per kg. of body weight. This aspect is not always sufficiently emphasized. While dose-effect relationship is not always sufficiently clear to go through such calculation for each drug, one should at least categorize patients into three or four groups regarding size when deciding upon dosages.

- *Renal function.* Since the kidney is the major organ for drug excretion, impairment of renal function plays the expected major role in altering drug kinetics. The importance of using smaller doses for drugs primarily excreted through the kidney (e.g., digoxin) whenever renal function is impaired, cannot be overemphasized.

- *Hepatic function.* Many drugs are metabolized in the liver; impairment of hepatic function requires the appropriate caution in administration of such drugs (e.g., coumarin drugs).

- *Gastrointestinal function.* The absorption of drugs administered orally is obviously related to gastrointestinal function. Inquiry into a possibility of gastrointestinal disturbances is an important step in initiation of drug therapy. The use of alternate routes of drug administration may occasionally be indicated when serious uncertainty regarding gastrointestinal function exists.

- *Peripheral circulation.* Drugs administered parenterally other than intravenously are, as a rule, absorbed better than those administered orally. However, patients in shock may be so vasoconstricted that no effective absorption takes place from hypodermic or intramuscular depots. In such patients only the intravenous route is effective.

While in general the avoidance of toxicity is the prime prerequisite of proper drug therapy, there are situations in which drugs may have to be administered in spite of side effects or even serious toxic effect. Setting priorities when dealing with life-saving situations would justify the use of quinidine in spite of diarrhea, the use of toxic antibiotics (e.g., those with serious nephrotoxic effects) for treatment of infective endocarditis, or even the use of penicillin and related drugs in the presence of known hypersensitivity to these antibiotics (under the protection of corticosteroids) in life-threatening infections specifically responsive to these drugs.

Drug Interactions

When more than one drug is administered to a patient, each drug can exert its independent action without relationship to the other; more often, however, there is some interaction between the drugs which may profoundly influence the therapy. The basic directions of such interactions are:

- Synergism — potentiation of the action of a drug by the other drug (either unidirectional or bidirectional);

- Antagonism — a drug's diminishing the effectiveness of the other drug.

The knowledge of drug interaction is of great importance in therapy. Anticipation of such interaction may alter therapeutic plans of action; it may be necessary to be more vigilant for side effects of toxicity; it may be important to regulate the use of casual drugs in patients who are maintained on a chronic drug therapy. A few specific examples may clarify such relationships:

- Combinations of antiarrhythmic drugs may offer some advantages over the use of single drugs, by lesser toxic potential or by better effectiveness of combined therapy.

- Drug toxicity may develop in patients on well-tolerated maintenance drug therapy as a result of the action of another drug or the *effects* of the other drug's actions (e.g., digitalis toxicity may appear after the effects of the administration of diuretics have taken place).

- The casual use of aspirin for a headache may lead to a serious hemorrhage in a patient on a coumarin drug because of aspirin potentiation of the anticoagulant potency.

CARDIAC AND RELATED DRUGS

Digitalis

Digitalis is the oldest cardiac drug, one which has perhaps been more thoroughly studied than any other therapeutic agent. Paradoxically, it is also a drug about which there are more unanswered questions than those applicable to other drugs.

The actions of digitalis have been thoroughly evaluated from the standpoint of animal pharmacology, biochemistry, electrophysiology, and cellular ultrastructure. Human studies have been rather sketchy, with a paucity of well-controlled investigations. An important step in better understanding of pharmacodynamics has been accomplished by the development of reliable digitalis blood assays.

Of the many actions of digitalis, the following net effects upon the heart and circulation constitute the basis of its clinical use:

1. It slows the rate of propagation of the depolarization wave through the various parts of the cardiac conducting system.

2. It strengthens the mode and the force of cardiac contraction.

Some of the other actions that may influence the clinical effects of digitalis include:

3. Mild pressor effect upon the arterial system;

4. Mild negative chronotropic effect;

5. Mild venopressor effect;

6. Enhancement of latent pacemaker cells (in large doses).

Clinical uses of digitalis fall into three categories:

- Its effect upon atrioventricular nodal transmission, permitting effective control of ventricular rate in atrial fibrillation and other atrial tachyarrhythmias;

- Its antiarrhythmic action, primarily the prevention of recurrent supraventricular tachyarrhythmias (also termination of some rapid ectopic rhythms);

- Its inotropic effect, improving cardiac performance in heart failure.

In discussing the use of digitalis in these three categories one should sharply separate the first two indications for digitalis use from the third one. Both the control of ventricular rate in atrial fibrillation and its action of converting or preventing ectopic atrial rhythms are the results of its dromotropic action (slowing conductivity). In atrial fibrillation ventricular slowing is accomplished by better triage of impulses traversing the AV node owing to increased refractoriness of the node. The other antiarrhythmic actions may be related to the interruption (or the prevention) of re-entry rhythms. It should be emphasized that all these actions of digitalis have a *measurable endpoint*. In control of atrial fibrillation the ventricular rate provides an easy method of monitoring the effectiveness as well as the dose needs of this drug. The interruption of an ectopic tachyarrhythmia provides a finite endpoint for a short-term intervention. The preventive use of digitalis against tachyarrhythmias is applied most commonly in patients whose attacks occur frequently enough to provide some basis for measurement of its effectiveness, although its efficacy for this purpose is not as great as in its other uses.

In sharp contrast, the use of digitalis for its inotropic effect in cardiac failure provides little or no opportunity for either assessing its immediate effectiveness or for monitoring its chronic use. Tradition calls for the use of digitalis "until the desired effects have been accomplished." In practice it is very seldom that this can be done. The reasons for this are as follows:

- Clinical criteria for the quantification of cardiac failure are very poor (see Chapter 13). The reliability and reproducibility of symptoms and signs of cardiac failure, even of some of the laboratory findings, are too poor, and the action of digitalis not dramatic enough to recognize a clear-cut beneficial effect that can be attributable to digitalis alone.

- Given a patient in cardiac failure in whom digitalis treatment is initiated, it is exceptional to use digitalis as the *sole* therapeutic agent. As a rule, bed rest, low sodium diet, diuretics, and other therapeutic agents are instituted at the same time, yet the credit for improvement is often given to digitalis.

Reviewing critically the clinically demonstrated evidence on which digitalis therapy in patients with cardiac failure who are in sinus rhythm is based, one comes up with the following observations:

1. In acute hemodynamic studies digitalis is capable of improving cardiac performance (as expressed by pressures and flows) in a substantial number of patients in failure (66 to 75 per cent), but such improvement is *not* forthcoming in those with normal hemodynamics (regardless of whether such patients have normal hearts or well-compensated heart disease).

2. Measured contractility of the cardiac muscle (assessed directly during cardiac operations) is enhanced acutely in normal and in hypertrophied hearts. Yet the importance of this finding in terms of overall cardiac performance is not known.

3. Indices of the mode of cardiac contractility (dp/dt, systolic ejection intervals) improve acutely after digitalis administration both in normals and in patients in cardiac failure. Here, too, clinical relevance is questionable.

On the other hand some obvious questions are at present unanswered:

1. What are the reliable figures regarding the consistency and the magnitude of hemodynamic improvement following digitalis administration? (Available figures are based on small series.)

2. Is there a dose-effect relationship, or is digitalis effect upon cardiac performance an "all-or-none" type of result?

3. Is the measurable improvement after digitalis maintained and,

if so, for how long? Is the maintenance therapy important, or even necessary?

4. Is there a qualitative or quantitative difference in the responses to digitalis administration in the various types of cardiac failure (acute failure vs. chronic failure; decompensation of chronically hypertrophied heart vs. failure due to myocardial disease)?

The answers to these and other questions regarding digitalis inotropism are urgently needed if we are to place digitalis therapy on a rational basis. Until they are available this aspect of digitalis use resembles more the crude empiricism of Withering's time than modern scientifically based drug use. One can submit the following hypotheses regarding digitalis inotropism without finding any conclusive information as to which of them is correct:

- Digitalis is a dependable drug improving cardiac performance in the majority of patients in cardiac failure and such improvement is well maintained by continuous digitalis therapy.

- Digitalis has an inotropic effect that improves cardiac performance when first administered. Such improvement (by reduction of cardiac size and shift of cardiac performance to a more efficient function curve) is maintained regardless of whether or not digitalis therapy is continued.

- Digitalis may improve cardiac performance in an acute study, but this effect is transient with prompt return of circulatory dynamics to its original state; therefore the benefit to the patient is insignificant.

- Digitalis is an inconsistently acting, weak inotropic agent and should not be used for its inotropic effect alone.

Our present approach is based on the first hypothesis. Whether the speculations and extrapolations upon which this hypothesis rests can be supported by more direct evidence remains to be seen. At the present time the therapeutic equation has to be based on comparing relatively high risk with uncertain benefits.

Digitalis Toxicity. The serious problem created by digitalis toxicity has been emphasized and re-emphasized from time to time, only to be promptly forgotten in the light of new information on the cellular action of digitalis or a few enticing, if indirect, clinical studies. It has been shown that digitalis toxicity is a principal reason for the hospitalization of an appreciable percentage of patients admitted in cardiac failure. The exact number of fatal digitalis intoxications is difficult to determine accurately, but it is estimated to represent a significant fraction of patients taking digitalis (Beller et al.).

Toxic effects and side effects of digitalis administration include those affecting the heart and those involving other organs.

Cardiac toxicity of digitalis represents the serious aspect of it and is largely responsible for the digitalis fatalities. The cardiac manifestations of digitalis toxicity include the following:

1. Ventricular arrhythmias in increasing order of seriousness: occasional ventricular ectopic beats, ventricular ectopic beats appearing as bigeminal rhythm, multifocal ventricular premature beats, ventricular tachycardia, ventricular fibrillation.

2. Supraventricular arrhythmias including the following: atrial or AV junctional tachycardias with 1 to 1 or 2 to 1 response; AV junctional tachycardias with atrioventricular dissociation, AV junctional tachycardias with alternating intraventricular conduction ("bidirectional tachycardias"), accelerated AV junctional rhythm with retrograde atrial activation or AV dissociation.

3. Conduction disturbances, including simple prolongation of AV conduction, higher degree of heart block (Wenckebach phenomenon, complete heart block).

4. Bradyarrhythmias, including slow idionodal or idioventricular rhythms, regular bradycardia appearing in patients with atrial fibrillation, sinus bradycardia.

It is perhaps no exaggeration to say that no arrhythmia exists that could not be induced by digitalis overdose. It is noteworthy, however, that two common arrhythmias—atrial flutter and atrial fibrillation—are very seldom traceable to digitalis intoxication.

Extracardiac digitalis toxicity includes gastrointestinal disturbances (nausea, vomiting, rarely diarrhea), visual disturbances (yellow vision, blurring of vision), headaches, confusion, drowsiness, psychoses, gynecomastia, paresthesias, and other, rare manifestations. Digitalis, among commonly used drugs, is one of the rarest in causing allergic manifestations, although skin eruptions and thrombocytopenia have been reported.

Digitalis toxicity can be brought about in several ways:

- Larger than usual doses are used either for initial administration or for maintenance therapy.

- Individual sensitivity making ordinary doses of digitalis toxic for a given patient.

- The appearance of an interacting additional factor for digitalis toxicity, one that sensitizes the patient to digitalis. Such factors include hypopotassemia, hypoxia, renal failure, drug interaction (diuretics, calcium, catecholamines), and electroshock for conversion of arrhythmias.

Management of digitalis toxicity involves three steps:

1. Anticipation and prevention of potential toxicity,

2. Discontinuation of the drug,

3. Active therapy.

Obviously, prevention of digitalis toxicity is the safest approach. Two principles are important in the prevention of digitalis toxicity: the use of conservative dosages, and a thorough understanding by the physician and the patient of the various precipitating factors. Thus, a patient tolerating well digitalis maintenance doses may develop a gastrointestinal upset that could lower the potassium level and render a therapeutic dose toxic; similarly, an upper respiratory infection may produce hypoxia with similar effect.

In patients who show digitalis toxicity that is not life-threatening, discontinuation of the drug is the safest form of action. Since it is a drug with a long half-life, signs of digitalis toxicity may persist for days, even for a week or two, during which time careful supervision of the patient is the only care needed.

Active therapy is primarily directed against repetitive ventricular arrhythmias and alternating tachycardias. The action of the various antiarrhythmic agents in advanced digitalis toxicity is the subject of controversy. According to some, diphenylhydantoin is more effective than quinidine, lidocaine, or procainamide; according to others propranolol is the drug of choice. Data supporting such recommendations are far from convincing; it is more likely that each antiarrhythmic agent may on occasion work when another fails. The choices of such drugs may well rest with individual preferences rather than a proven superiority of any agent. Because of the synergism between electroshock therapy and digitalis, the termination of digitalis-induced tachycardias by DC shock is highly hazardous, and can be suggested only in patients in whom all other means have failed and whose life is in danger. This maneuver then becomes a calculated high-risk procedure.

Active therapy for digitalis-induced bradycardias is seldom needed. Yet patients who cannot tolerate slow cardiac rates because of increasing cardiac failure or disturbances of sensorium may have to be treated by pacing. The decision as to whether temporary pacing or permanent placement of a pacemaker should be performed has to be made in each case individually, after weighing all factors involved.

Digitalis Administration. Digitalis is used orally or parenterally. Oral administration includes digitalis leaf and purified digitalis glycosides (digoxin, digitoxin, gitalin). Parenteral digitalis preparations and equivalent drugs include ouabain, deslanoside, lanatoside C, digoxin, and digitoxin.

The principal route of digitalis administration is oral. Intravenous digitalis may be used in urgent situations. Other forms of parenteral digitalis are seldom used, the principal indication for them being inability (or inadvisability) of taking food by mouth.

Digitalis leaf is seldom used at present. While the principal reason for its abandonment is the fact that biological assaying of such a crude drug makes wide variation of potency likely, recent experience has shown that even the pure glycoside, digoxin, may show variation of bioavailability of sufficient magnitude to be of concern to the therapist. The oral drugs show wide difference in pharmacokinetics: ouabain and deslanoside have short half-lives; the estimated half-life of digoxin is 1.5 to 2 days; that of digitoxin 7 to 9 days. The oral preparations could be used without initial loading (as already indicated), but their effect, evidenced by the plateau of drug concentration, would take about a week in the first case and 4 to 5 weeks in the second case. Consequently, it is the usual practice to load the patients initially by administering 5 to 10 times the maintenance dosage over the first 24 to 48 hours, thereafter placing the patient on the maintenance schedule.

The use of digitalis in patients with atrial fibrillation and rapid ventricular response is best done by monitoring the effect of each dose by means of the ventricular rate. It is from the experience with patients who are in atrial fibrillation that most relevant clinical information has been extracted regarding dose schedule, individual sensitivity, and other aspects of digitalis administration. Such observations also led to the widely held view that digitalis is ineffective until the patient receives the full loading dose, hence its narrow therapeutic range requiring "juggling" between the ineffective zone and the toxic zone, which are close to each other. These views have been extrapolated to the use of digitalis for its inotropic action. The problem of the dose-effect relationship has not been fully reinvestigated with the use of modern techniques. Even in atrial fibrillation it is not known whether the high threshold of effectiveness of digitalis is a fact or a myth.

Recently two observations have been put forth relevant to this subject: first, experimental data indicated a possible dissociation between the inotropic action and the dromotropic effect of digitalis. This, if confirmed in man, might indicate that extrapolation of data on digitalis administration from patients in atrial fibrillation to those treated for its inotropic action may be invalid and the dose-effect relationship different for the two actions of digitalis. Second, indirect evidence, based on indices of ventricular contractility, shows that there may be lesser effect of small doses of digitalis and more pronounced effect following administration of larger doses—thus a more conventional dose-effect relationship than is generally accepted. If confirmed by more direct studies of cardiac performance in man, these "straws in the wind" may justify a reconsideration of current concepts of digitalis administration.

The usual dosage of digitalis for an average-sized patient, put in terms of digoxin — by far the most widely used digitalis preparation — is 0.325 mg. as the maintenance dose with a range (derived by monitoring patients in atrial fibrillation) from 0.125 to 0.5 mg. The loading dose ranges from 1.0 to 2.5 mg., usually spaced during the initial 24 to 36 hours. The wide individual variation of sensitivity to digitalis administration is shown by patients who develop toxicity at 0.1 mg. maintenance level and require 0.05 mg. or less, and by some who can be controlled only by 1.0 mg. per day or more. In sinus rhythm, such observations cannot be made except in situations of unusual sensitivity shown by toxicity at a low level. In general an average dose schedule has to be followed, usually consisting of 1.0 to 2.0 mg. loading dose and 0.25 mg. maintenance dose.

Digitalis Assay. Recent years have witnessed an important advance in digitalis therapy, namely, a quantification of the amount of digitalis in the serum of patients taking this drug. Biological, chemical, isotope labeling, and other methods have been used; the most practical method that can be made available in the average hospital is the radioimmunoassay technique. Available for digoxin, digitoxin, and ouabain, this method is most often used to assay digoxin as the most widely used digitalis glycoside. Digitalis assay has been responsible for the better understanding of the pharmacodynamics of this drug.

The important question for the clinician is: To what extent is digitalis assay helpful in the management of an individual patient who is taking digitalis or is being considered for digitalis therapy? At present the assay technique permits the separation of three groups of patients:

1. Patients with a grossly ineffective level of digoxin,

2. Patients within the therapeutic range,

3. Patients within the toxic range.

Investigators who study large numbers of patients indicate that there is a wide overlap between the three zones of digitalization. Thus it is only occasionally possible to draw definitive conclusions from the knowledge of which category the patient is in. Given an individual who has arrhythmias compatible with digitalis toxicity, if digitalis assay shows him to be in the ineffective zone, the probability is high that the arrhythmias are produced by factors other than digitalis. If such a patient is in the toxic range, arrhythmias can reasonably be considered evidence of digitalis toxicity. Assays in the broad range between the two extremes do not provide usable clues.

Prophylactic Digitalization. The use of digitalis for preventing anticipated manifestations of cardiac disease has been widely recommended. The use of digitalis for the control of repetitive or paroxysmal arrhythmias has already been discussed. Here, in order to justify the risk of digitalis administration, one should consider that such therapy is indicated in patients in whom arrhythmias occur with considerable frequency, or in patients with arrhythmias that have a definitely demonstrated deleterious effect upon the circulation.

More recently some enthusiasm has been generated in using digitalis for the prevention of cardiac failure. Such prophylactic therapy has been advocated in patients with cardiac disease prior to major operations (cardiac or noncardiac), during acute myocardial infarction, or in any other condition in which heart failure might occur. The need for a specific knowledge of the risk-benefit ratio in prophylactic therapy has been emphasized earlier. The risk of digitalis is moderately high; its potential benefit under such circumstances is totally unknown. (The supporting evidence for such use of digitalis has been entirely extrapolated from animal studies!) In view of the reservations and the many unanswered questions regarding *therapeutic* use of digitalis for its inotropic effect, its *prophylactic* use for that purpose appears unwarranted.

Diuretics

Diuretic therapy ranks high among effective methods of control of cardiac failure. Diuretic drugs differ from many other cardiac drugs:

- They are administered to perform a specific task, hence there is no need to maintain an effective level of the drug.

- Their effect can be directly measured.

The goal of diuretic therapy is to eliminate the excess fluid in the body. The great majority of diuretics exert their action only if excess fluid is actually present. However, the newer, more powerful diuretic agents are capable of acting in subjects without fluid retention, thereby introducing the risk of dehydration.

Diuretics vary greatly in the mode of their dehydrating action. These drugs are customarily grouped into agents with similar chemical structure or with similar action of both. The most important groups are:

1. *Thiazides*. This group of drugs was the first used effectively by oral administration. Mild to moderate in potency, thiazides interfere with water and sodium excretion in the distal tubule. They enhance potassium excretion and often lead to hypokalemia, unless potassium supplementation, in the diet or as potassium salts, is administered. Thiazides also may produce hyperuricemia. Thiazides are the fa-

vorite "starting" diuretics in patients with mild or moderate degree of fluid retention.

2. *Ethacrynic acid and furosemide.* These two drugs, chemically unrelated to each other, are the most powerful diuretic agents available. Their introduction (both were made available about the same time) has signaled an important advance in diuretic therapy, for they act when all other diuretics, singly or in combination, are no longer effective. Administered both orally and intravenously, these drugs exert their action upon the salt and water absorption in the proximal tubule and the ascending limb of the loop of Henle. They are fast-acting (orally within one half hour, intravenously within minutes), but their effect is of short duration. The use of these diuretics also may lead to potassium depletion and uric acid retention.

3. *Aldosterone antagonists.* Spironolactone, the principal representative of this type of diuretic, blocks competitively the action of aldosterone upon the cells in the distal tubule. Of considerable theoretical interest, this drug is poorly absorbed, slow-acting, and is rarely used alone. It does, however, potentiate the use of other diuretics and its principal use is in cases where diuretic combinations are indicated.

4. *Triamterene* blocks the distal tubular cells in the manner of spironolactone, but independently of aldosterone action. It also is slow-acting, often requiring two or three days of continuous therapy before its effects are apparent; its use, therefore, is also preferred as an adjunct rather than as the principal diuretic agent. It is a potassium-sparing diuretic.

5. *Organic mercury compounds.* Once the most widely used diuretics, mercurial salts have been largely replaced by newer drugs. Their major disadvantage is that they are effective only by parenteral administration. They affect the water and sodium reabsorption in the distal tubule and act more reliably in acid urine. In many institutions mercurial diuretics are no longer in use.

Other drugs, now seldom used unless specific reasons exist, include the following:

- Carbonic anhydrase inhibitors (e.g., Diamox),

- Osmotic diuretics (mannitol, glucose),

- Acid-forming salts (ammonium chloride).

Toxicity of Diuretics. Untoward effects of diuretic therapy can be categorized as follows:

- By-product of the normal diuretic action,

- Effect of excessive diuresis,

- True toxic effects.

The commonest by-products of diuresis are hypokalemia and hyperuricemia. The extent of such changes in the composition of the serum depends upon the diet and the individual sensitivity of patients. The effect of excessive diuresis is dehydration, constriction of circulating blood volume, and eventually shock.

Toxic effects vary from drug to drug. Ethacrynic acid and furosemide may produce deafness, hepatic coma, and glucose intolerance. Thiazides have been reported as producing agranulocytosis, cutaneous vasculitis, and thrombocytopenia.

The most important principle in the use of diuretics is to administer the smallest dose that is effective and—if possible—to use these drugs intermittently.

Administration of Diuretics. Diuretic therapy is the most effective means of controlling cardiac failure. In acute heart failure or in patients in previously untreated chronic failure, diuretics produce prompt relief from symptoms. In many patients who have recovered from the initial bout of failure, continuous diuretic therapy may insure good control of failure and permit the patient to lead an asymptomatic existence. These benefits are unmistakable, clear-cut, and can be directly measured. One goal of prudent therapy is to reduce the risk of diuretic therapy to a minimum. This can be done by the following steps:

- The assessment of the function of organs potentially affected by diuretic therapy: renal function, hepatic function, glucose tolerance.

- Potentiation of diuretic therapy by dietary sodium restriction, thereby reducing demand for diuretic therapy.

- Selection of a diuretic or a combination of diuretics least likely to produce side effects or toxicity.

- Use of smallest effective dose with preference to the intermittent administration of the drug. Self-monitoring by the patient by keeping weight charts is a prerequisite for effective therapy.

Antiarrhythmic Agents

The principal antiarrhythmic drugs include the following: quinidine, procainamide, lidocaine, diphenylhydantoin, and propranolol. Table 11–1 shows some of the characteristics of these drugs. While their actions overlap in some respects, each should be discussed separately from the standpoint of risk and benefits.

TABLE 11-1. ANTIARRHYTHMIC DRUGS*

Drug	Effects on ECG	Half-life	Dose and Interval	Route	Adverse Effects	Therapeutic Plasma Levels
Diphenylhydantoin (Dilantin; and others)	Shortens QT	24-36 hrs	1 Gm loading dose then 300-400 mg/day 50 mg q5min to 250 mg (can be repeated after 2 hrs) then 300-400 mg/day	PO IV	Ataxia, nystagmus, drowsiness, coma. Hematological effects. Cardiac toxicity with rapid IV injection.	10-20 µg/ml
Lidocaine (Xylocaine; and others)	Shortens QT	1.5-2 hrs	50-100 mg then 1-4 mg/min	IV	Drowsiness or agitation, disorientation, coma, seizures, paresthesias, cardiac depression, cardiac arrhythmias.	1-5 µg/ml
Procainamide (Pronestyl; and others)	Prolongs QRS, QT and PR (±)	3-4 hrs	500 mg-1 Gm then 2-8 Gm daily 250-500 mg q3-4h No more than 100-200 mg q5min to 1 Gm 1-3 mg/min maintenance	PO IM IV	Lupus-like syndrome common, GI symptoms, rash, hypotension, arrhythmias, heart block.	3-8 µg/ml
Propranolol (Inderal)	Prolongs PR (±) No change QRS Shortens QT	2-4 hrs PO 2 hrs IV	10-40 mg q6h 1-5 mg in 1 mg increments	PO IV	Heart block, heart failure, asthma, hypotension.	50-100 ng/ml
Quinidine (many brands)	Same as procainamide	6 hrs	100-600 mg q4-6h	PO or IM	GI symptoms, cinchonism, rashes, thrombocytopenia, hypotension, heart block or tachyarrhythmias.	3-7 µg/ml

*From The Medical Letter, Vol. 26, No. 25, 1974.

Quinidine

The oldest antiarrhythmic drug in use, quinidine is still the most effective, often referred to as a "broad-spectrum antiarrhythmic agent." The recognition of its high toxic potential has limited some of its uses, but it remains an indispensable agent for some types of arrhythmia.

Quinidine is a short-acting drug; its half-life is estimated at about 4 hours after oral administration. A sustained effective level of quinidine is relatively easy to attain by administration of quinidine every 4 to 6 hours. It is also a drug with a good dose-effect relationship in that low levels of quinidine may have effective suppressive action upon some milder forms of arrhythmia, while high levels may be necessary to terminate or suppress arrhythmias more resistant to therapy.

The action of quinidine consists of slowing of the conduction through the heart and depressing automaticity of ectopic pacemaker cells. These two principal actions of quinidine make this drug effective in most tachyarrhythmias, and in the suppression of ectopic beats. Both supraventricular and ventricular varieties respond to quinidine. The principal uses of quinidine include the following:

- Termination of paroxysmal atrial arrhythmias (tachycardia, flutter, fibrillation),
- Termination of chronic atrial fibrillation or flutter,
- Prevention of recurrences of such arrhythmias,
- Termination and prevention of junctional tachyarrhythmias,
- Prevention or suppression of ventricular premature contractions,
- Termination and prevention of ventricular tachycardia,
- Prevention of ventricular fibrillation.

Quinidine toxicity falls into three categories:

1. Side effects of the expected quinidine antiarrhythmic action,

2. Dose-related toxic effects at high quinidine levels,

3. Idiosyncratic reactions to quinidine.

Toxic effects and side effects of quinidine include cardiac and noncardiac manifestations. Toxic cardiac manifestations represent the principal risk of quinidine administration and are characterized by their sudden appearance, occasionally leading to unheralded disasters.

Among side effects most consistently accompanying quinidine administration are gastrointestinal disturbances, namely diarrhea, occasionally accompanied by nausea and vomiting. The effect of quinidine upon the gastrointestinal tract in such disturbances must be considered "the price to pay" for quinidine's beneficial effect; only in extreme cases do such side effects constitute a cause for discontinuation of quinidine. Other side effects include manifestations of cinchonism (tinnitus, dizziness, weakness, drowsiness, headaches). An important cardiac side effect is the negative inotropic effect of quinidine (depressing cardiac performance). This, however, seldom plays a significant *clinical* role in quinidine therapy, unless serious myocardial disease is present.

Dose-related toxic manifestations of quinidine action include severe gastrointestinal disturbances and cinchonism, in which cases reduction of the quinidine dose could make quinidine administration tolerable to the patient. The serious and unpredictable quinidine toxicity relates to the heart: it includes a variety of ventricular arrhythmias: single ventricular premature contraction, multifocal premature beats, ventricular "salvos," bouts of ventricular tachycardia and ventricular fibrillation. Cardiac toxicity is usually, but not always, associated (not necessarily preceded) by electrocardiographic abnormalities: prolongation of the Q-T-U interval, increased duration of the QRS complex. While in the majority of patients ventricular arrhythmias develop in response to quinidine toxicity in a sequential manner, i.e., from the simpler to the most serious ones, this may not be the case. At times, the sequence develops too fast to discontinue quinidine treatment, or even to institute remedial therapy. Paroxysmal ventricular fibrillation ("quinidine syncope") unquestionably is responsible for most quinidine deaths; it may occur with little or no warning.

Idiosyncratic reactions include true allergic manifestations of quinidine intolerance: skin rash, asthma, collapse, serum-sickness-like manifestations. Hypersensitivity reactions associated with quinidine administration include thrombocytopenic purpura and drug fever. However, the most serious manifestation of quinidine hypersensitivity — being life-threatening — is the development of cardiotoxicity, including quinidine syncope, at a normal or even low quinidine concentration.

Administration of Quinidine. Quinidine is a drug with a potentially high risk, in this respect being second only to digitalis. Even though documentary evidence is not available on the frequency of sudden death in cardiac patients caused by quinidine-induced ventricular fibrillation, it is the impression in some cardiology centers that such deaths are not uncommon, and in fact may account for a significant fraction of unexpected sudden deaths in cardiac patients. Thus quinidine therapy has to be considered a calculated risk; the benefits of quinidine therapy are, however, much more clearly defined and measurable than those of digitalis therapy for cardiac failure. The following guidelines should be considered before starting quinidine therapy:

- Alternate, less toxic methods of antiarrhythmic therapy should be undertaken, if effective.

- Short-term quinidine therapy or the initiation of maintenance therapy is preferably to be carried out in the hospital with proper monitoring facilities.

- In patients maintained on quinidine therapy, monitoring by means of electrocardiography and quinidine blood level is indicated at reasonable intervals.

- Patients should be carefully instructed about drug interactions affecting quinidine, about factors possibly sensitizing them to quinidine, and about warning signs of impending quinidine toxicity (e.g., unexplained attacks of dizziness — see below).

Quinidine administration is limited at present to the oral route. Parenteral quinidine is considered too hazardous — the need for such form of therapy has to be filled by alternate drugs. Quinidine sulfate is the universally used form of this drug; quinidine gluconate (Quinaglute) and quinidine polygalacturonate (Cardioquin) are recommended as long-acting drugs requiring less frequent administration. Their superiority to quinidine sulfate has not, however, been definitely established.

As stated, an effective quinidine concentration can be maintained by the administration of the drug orally every 6 hours. The dose ranges from 0.2 to 0.4 gm. per administration. Larger doses with more frequent administration had been used in the past for a rapid build-up of the drug for the purpose of converting atrial fibrillation to sinus rhythm. This method has been abandoned in favor of electroshock therapy. As a short-acting drug, quinidine does not require loading: its proper therapeutic concentration is reached within one to two hours and is sustained with relatively little variation as long as the therapy is continued. Serum quinidine concentration, determined usually 2 to 3 hours after the last dose, ranges between 2 and 6 mcg./ml. Higher concentration is to be avoided because of the risk of toxic doses. (There is some overlap between therapeutic and toxic doses, but definite toxicity is likely to be present at levels above 10 mcg./ml.) There is also a wide overlap between ineffective and effective blood concentration at the lower end of the scale. As with digoxin, serum quinidine levels are guidelines to therapy rather than exact measurements.

While factors potentiating quinidine effect are not as readily identified as those in digitalis, it is probable that impaired renal function, hypoxia, and electrolyte imbalances are likely to increase chances of adverse reaction to quinidine; careful dose adjustment in the presence of such abnormalities is advisable. Quinidine is often administered together with a digitalis preparation; there is an impression, as yet undocumented, that serious cardiotoxic reaction, such as quinidine syncope, may be developing more often in patients on combined drug schedules rather than in those taking quinidine only. Quinidine is known to interact with reserpine, which increases the potency of quinidine. Combinations of antiarrhythmic drugs are recommended by some: quinidine with procainamide or quinidine with propranolol. A synergistic effect of such combination with a lessening probability of toxicity is thought to exist; adequate proof of such advantages is not available, since such recommendations are based on uncontrolled studies.

Treatment of quinidine toxicity is seldom necessary: as a drug with a short half-life, discontinuation of it produces a prompt fall in quinidine concentration, hence cessation of toxicity. The only exception is in quinidine syncope. In this, the most serious manifestation of quinidine toxicity, alertness for the occurrence of ventricular arrhythmias is essential. Quinidine syncope may be preceded by electrocardiographic evidence of quinidine effect (changes in depolarization and repolarization). In patients on quinidine maintenance therapy serious attacks are frequently preceded by brief episodes of dizziness (thought to represent bouts of less serious arrhythmias). Alertness of the patient and his family in prompt reporting of such episodes is important. Quinidine syncope may occur repetitively over a period of hours, even a day or two; ventricular fibrillation may be spontaneously terminated, or may be converted by electroshock. Isoproterenol infusion has been recommended as an antidote for cardiotoxicity of quinidine; the evidence of its effectiveness is only conjectural.

Procainamide

From the electrophysiological standpoint the action of procainamide is identical with that of quinidine. Clinically, however, it has been suggested that its effect upon atrial arrhythmias is weaker than that of quinidine, while in ventricular arrhythmias it exerts comparable antiarrhythmic action. There is, however, an important difference between these two drugs: procainamide has a much wider safety margin, which permits its use in high dosages as well as intravenous administration. Theoretically, cardiotoxicity of procainamide is comparable to that of quinidine; in practice serious arrhythmias are very rare, and occur almost exclusively after intravenous administration. As in quinidine, this drug has a negative inotropic cardiac effect, which is of insufficient magnitude to be of clinical importance. Procainamide exerts, however, an important hypotensive action, and its administration in patients in cardiac failure or after myocardial infarction requires monitoring of arterial pressure. Undesirable effects of this drug are fewer than with quinidine: gastrointestinal upsets are rare; cinchona effects are not evoked by it. The principal risk of procainamide consists of the following:

- Hypersensitivity reactions (skin eruptions, blood dyscrasias);

- Systemic lupus erythematosus-like disease, which develops only after long-term procainamide therapy. The high frequency of this reaction in patients on prolonged procainamide therapy suggests that it represents a direct effect of the drug rather than an abnormal response in sensitive individuals. Fortunately this disease is promptly reversed upon termination of therapy.

The dosage of procainamide varies from 0.5 to 1.0 gm. per dose, administered orally every 3 to 4 hours. With a short half-life and a kinetic pattern similar to that of quinidine, this mode of administration may assure continuous effective concentration of the drug, although some advocate its administration every three hours. Higher dosages up to 10 gm. per day have also been suggested, but their advantages have not been demonstrated. Intravenous procainamide has been used in the past extensively for the termination of serious ventricular arrhythmias; its use has been largely replaced by lidocaine or electroshock therapy.

Lidocaine

Lidocaine is probably the most widely used antiarrhythmic agent in hospitalized patients at the present time. A short-acting drug, with poor absorption from the gastrointestinal tract, it is unsuitable for oral administration and is best used by continuous intravenous infusion.

The electrophysiological basis of the action of lidocaine includes a suppressive effect upon ectopic pacemaker cells (in common with quinidine and procainamide). However, lidocaine does not exert the action of slowing the conductivity, differing in this respect from the two other drugs. Its effectiveness is primarily targeted upon ventricular ectopic rhythms. The biological half-life of lidocaine is estimated to be 2 to 3 hours; however, ordinary dosages maintain an effective antiarrhythmic blood concentration for only one half hour or less. Lidocaine is largely metabolized in the liver, hence its concentration is not related to renal function. However, hepatic congestion secondary to cardiac failure produces slowing of lidocaine metabolism and may bring about an undesirably cumulative concentration of this drug in response to the usual therapeutic dosages.

As with the other antiarrhythmic agents, cardiotoxicity of lidocaine is occasionally observed; however, its undesirable effects involve preferentially the central nervous system. Confusion, drowsiness, paresthesias, and convulsions may develop during lidocaine administration. Such toxic effects are not especially rare, since lidocaine infusions are often given in increasing dosages for therapy-resistant ventricular arrhythmias, in the hope that higher doses might accomplish what lesser ones failed to do.

The administration of lidocaine most commonly includes an intravenous bolus of 50 to 100 mg. for sustained arrhythmias, or continuous intravenous drip delivering 100 mg. per hour, used for repetitive arrhythmias or for arrhythmia prophylaxis. Sometimes both methods are used. An intramuscular bolus of 200 mg. has been recommended as prophylactic therapy (e.g., early in the course of myocardial infarction). The effectiveness of this treatment has not yet been demonstrated by well-controlled studies.

Diphenylhydantoin (Phenytoin)

An anticonvulsant drug used extensively for treatment of epilepsy, diphenylhydantoin (Dilantin) has been used as an antiarrhythmic agent for many years. It has not reached wide popularity, but merely occupies the place of a second or third-choice drug for many arrhythmias. It has important differences from the other antiarrhythmic agents:

- Its electrophysiological basis is different from the other antiarrhythmic drugs in that it *shortens* the action potential and the refractory phase and enhances AV nodal conduction.

- From the standpoint of pharmacokinetics, it is a long-acting agent with a half-life of at least 24 hours.

Because of its mode of action diphenylhydantoin might be expected to be especially suitable for reentrant arrhythmias and for those evoked by digitalis toxicity. In practice, superiority of this agent over other antiarrhythmic drugs remains to be demonstrated.

As a long-acting drug, diphenylhydantoin requires initial loading followed by maintenance by means of smaller doses. It is metabolized in the liver. Diphenylhydantoin toxicity affects the heart and the central nervous system. Serious ventricular tachyarrhythmias as well as bradycardias and conduction disturbances have been described after administration of diphenylhydantoin, but almost always such complications involve rapid intravenous administration and are avoidable by more cautious administration.

Diphenylhydantoin toxicity other than that causing arrhythmias includes effects upon the central nervous system (nystagmus, seizures), and also aplastic anemia.

Diphenylhydantoin loading may be accomplished by the oral or intravenous route. The oral route is preferred for the prevention of repetitive arrhythmias, the intravenous one for treatment of existing arrhythmias. Intravenous administration involves repeated injection (slow) of 100 mg. doses up to 1,000 mg., unless the arrhythmia is terminated sooner. Oral loading also is managed by the administration of 1 gm. of this drug. Maintenance dose is 200 to 400 mg. per day.

Propranolol

A newer antiarrhythmic agent, propranolol exerts two principal actions:

- Blockade of beta-adrenergic receptors,

- Direct cardiac effect similar to that of quinidine.

Both actions contribute to the antiarrhythmic effect of this drug: the beta-adrenergic blockade affects arrhythmias initiated or perpetuated by catecholamine stimulation (involving beta-adrenergic enhancement); the quinidine-like effect provides a further base for the broad effectiveness of propranolol.

Both the pharmacokinetics and the full range of clinical usefulness of propranolol are less well known than those of the other antiarrhythmic agents. This drug appears to have a short half-life (3 hours), does not require initial loading, and maintains its effect when administered every 6 hours. It has certain distinctive antiarrhythmic features:

- It is the only drug that consistently slows SA nodal discharge, hence is effective in controlling sinus tachycardia.

- It blocks transmission of impulses through the AV node, effectively slowing ventricular rate in atrial fibrillation and in other atrial tachyarrhythmias; this action is more consistent and dependable than that of digitalis.

In addition, propranolol exerts a "broad-spectrum" antiarrhythmic effect similar to that of quinidine, being perhaps preferentially more effective against atrial than ventricular arrhythmias.

It has two serious by-products of its cardiac actions:

1. It depresses myocardial performance, thereby producing or accentuating cardiac failure. This effect is much more pronounced than that of quinidine and procainamide and may lead to serious consequences.

2. It may produce excessive slowing of the SA node or various lower pacemakers, leading to undesirable bradyarrhythmias.

With proper monitoring propranolol is a drug with a considerable safety margin. Large doses have been used for its effect in reducing anginal attacks without major ill effects. Toxic manifestation, such as gastrointestinal disturbances, somnolence, depression of renal function, and thrombocytopenia, have only rarely been observed. Its beta-adrenergic blocking effect makes the administration of this drug contraindicated in patients susceptible to bronchospasm, and it should be applied with caution in diabetics.

Propranolol may be administered intravenously in increments of 0.5 to 1.0 mg. for the termination of arrhythmias. Larger doses than 5 mg. are seldom used. The usual mode of administration is via the oral route, the dose ranging from 40 to 360 mg. in 24 hours in four divided doses.

Antianginal Drugs

The evaluation of drugs used for the control of attacks of angina pectoris is exceedingly difficult for several reasons:

- Angina is a subjective manifestation of disease, hence unsuitable for independent evaluation.

- Most anginal attacks are of short duration and subside spontaneously, whether or not a drug is being administered.

- Since angina is most frequently provoked by exercise, patients usually stop exercise *and* take a drug, making it difficult to separate the effects of the two therapeutic interventions.

- There is great variability in the development of anginal attacks; psychogenic and neurogenic factors play an important role in their provocation.

The history of drug therapy for angina pectoris includes many examples of drugs enthusiastically recommended but later abandoned as useless. It is important to note that some such agents were actually tested by well-designed studies, even by the double-blind technique, with results seemingly indicative of drug effectiveness but later disproved. The difficulty in evaluation of antianginal drugs lies in the fact that placebo agents frequently show a definite antianginal effectivness, owing to suggestion and psychogenic action.

Nitroglycerin (Glyceryl Trinitrate). This is the oldest and still the most effective drug used on a short-term basis for the abortion of an anginal attack or for the prevention of an anticipated attack.

The best demonstrated effective route of administration of nitroglycerin is sublingual. As a drug that deteriorates rapidly, a fresh supply (six months old or less) of the drug should be assured. Nitroglycerin has a very rapid and transient action, making it suitable only for an existing or anticipated attack. The drug can be used repeatedly with no cumulation or ill effect. Tachyphylactic reduction of effectiveness does not ordinarily occur, though prolonged use of nitrates may induce dependence, as demonstrated by nitroglycerin factory workers.

The action of this drug can be demonstrated objectively in patients who happen to have anginal attacks (or in whom such attacks are provoked) while hemodynamic measurements are being made. A prompt return of abnormally elevated left atrial and left ventricular diastolic pressure is consistently found within 30 seconds to 3 minutes after sublingual administration of nitroglycerin. Its action has been postulated as involving two mechanisms:

- A coronary dilating action producing a redistribution of coronary flow with better perfusion of ischemic areas;

- A reduction of cardiac workload, hence myocardial oxygen demand, by its effect of lowering peripheral resistance and reducing venous return.

The second mechanism probably has more support in its favor.

Nitroglycerin exerts no toxicity in its ordinary sense. An unpleasant side effect frequently accompanying its use is headache and a throbbing sensation. In some cases nitrogylcerin has been blamed for having precipitated hypotension and shock when administered during the initial attack of pain accompanying acute myocardial infarction. It is impossible to establish a cause-effect relationship between nitroglycerin administration and hypotension in a condition with so many factors affecting the circulation.

The dose of nitroglycerin ranges from 0.2 to 0.6 mg.; the dosage should be titrated by the patient.

Long-acting Nitrates. The nitroglycerin-like effect is also present in other nitrates, which have been tried for many years as a means of preventing anginal attacks on a sustained basis rather than for individual attacks. They include erythrityl tetranitrate (Cardilate), pentaerithrityl tetranitrate (Peritrate), isosorbide dinitrate (Isordil), and sustained action nitroglycerin preparations.

These preparations are available in two forms: sublingual pellets and oral tablets. The evaluation of the effectiveness of long-acting nitrates is difficult for reasons explained above. To date no convincing evidence has been submitted that oral administration of any of such drugs produces a significant action upon reducing the frequency of anginal attacks or improving effort tolerance. Sublingual use of such agents is similar to that of nitroglycerin, but there is reasonable evidence that a sustained effect over a period of one to two hours after administration may persist. Such drugs, particularly when combined with propranolol, appear to offer a medical regimen that controls angina in many patients beyond the expected placebo effect. However, further, large-scale studies are needed to provide the conclusive proof of such effect.

Nitrates have few side effects (nitroglycerin-like headache) and low toxicity (rare hypersensitivity reactions are reported, e.g., skin eruptions). They do however lead to a development of tolerance, which may cross over to other similar drugs; e.g., they may make nitroglycerin less effective in terminating attacks.

Propranolol.   This drug, already discussed for its antiarrhythmic action, has been used successfully for angina. Its mode of action is not entirely clarified; several actions seem to be involved:

- Beta-adrenergic blockade eliminates the triggering of anginal attacks of catecholamine release.

- Cardiac depressant effect as well as beta blockade reduces myocardial oxygen demands.

- Exercise may be performed at lower cardiac rates, hence may be more economical.

- Its hypotensive effects add to the reduction of cardiac workload.

Propranolol is used orally in increasing doses. High doses are frequently used and are often effective when lower doses fail. Such doses are higher than those necessary for the beta-adrenergic blocking effect, suggesting a combined action of autonomic and direct cardiac contribution.

Antihypertensive Drugs

These agents will be discussed in conjunction with the treatment of hypertension in Chapter 39.

Antithrombotic Therapy

While not strictly cardiac drugs, agents affecting intravascular thrombosis play an important role in cardiology. They involve three groups of drugs:

1. Anticoagulant drugs (preventing formation of fibrin clots);

2.   Antiplatelet drugs (preventing platelet aggregation);

3.   Thrombolytic drugs (dissolving existing intravascular thrombi).

Except for thrombolytic agents, drugs in this category are used in prophylactic therapy. Therefore, a strict definition of the risk-benefit ratio needs to be made in setting rational guidelines for such therapy. There is little doubt that intravascular thrombosis may produce serious morbidity, permanent disability, and death. The high stakes in the prevention of such sequelae represent a justified calculated risk. The question as yet undetermined, except for few specific instances, is whether or not such drugs are really capable of effectively preventing intravascular clotting, and to what extent.

Intravascular thrombosis against which therapy is aimed involves the following areas:

1.   Venous thrombosis (thrombophlebitis, deep venous thrombosis);

2.   Intracardiac thrombosis (mural thrombosis in the atrium in atrial fibrillation, in the ventricle after myocardial infarction, in ventricular aneurysm);

3.   Thrombosis in or around prosthetic devices (artificial valves, patches, grafts);

4.   Arterial thrombosis (primarily coronary and cerebral).

Recent advances in the knowledge of blood coagulation and intra vitam thrombosis point to a basic difference between thrombi forming within the arterial system and those in the venous system. Arterial thrombi are initiated by platelet aggregation with secondary fibrin deposits ("white clots"); intravenous thrombosis consists primarily of fibrin clots ("red clots"). As a consequence, rational therapy calls for the use of appropriate specific agents for the two types of thrombosis.

Antithrombotic therapy has to have a definable objective in terms of its duration:

- It may aim at acute protection from thrombosis, e.g., during open heart operation, during cardiac catheterization.

- It may aim at protection over a finite period, e.g., temporary anticoagulation during acute myocardial infarction, treatment of thrombophlebitis and phlebothrombosis.

- It may aim at permanent protection, by indefinite anticoagulant or antithrombotic therapy.

- Thrombolytic therapy at present involves only short-term treatment of a known thrombotic process.

In terms of risk, there is a fundamental difference between anticoagulant drugs and those aimed at platelet aggregation. Anticoagulant drugs tamper with the physiological clotting mechanism: an effective anticoagulant action of a drug automatically produces a danger of hemorrhage; the patient's only protection is an intact vascular system. Drugs aimed at platelet aggregation carry no basic risk other than that the individual drug may impose.

In terms of the benefits of anticoagulant therapy the definition of the protection attained by the therapy is very difficult to assess. Certain observations can be accepted as reasonable:

- Acute heparinization effectively protects from intravascular thrombosis.

- Intermittent heparinization over a period of days or weeks offers reasonable protection from intravascular clotting.

- Long-term or intermediate-term oral anticoagulation offers only partial protection from thrombosis, and does not eliminate it.

Thus, with the risk of anticoagulant therapy high and benefits difficult to measure, such therapy can be justified only by the very high stakes of the possibility of saving the patient from death or disability. As expected, the interpretation of the therapeutic equation varies widely.

Heparin is the oldest and the most widely used anticoagulant drug; it can be used only parenterally, hence it is mostly suited for short-term anticoagulation and is usually administered to hospitalized patients.

The index of heparin effectiveness is the prolongation of clotting time. Heparin has a short half-life, but in contrast to many other drugs its half-life is dose-dependent. The most effective sustained action of heparin is attained by frequent intravenous administration of the drug (usually every 4 hours). The usual dose is 5,000 to 10,000 units per dose. Larger doses (e.g., 40,000 units) provide a very high initial level and a longer sustained therapeutic level when given every 6 to 12 hours; this regimen, however, is less dependable than more frequent injections, although it is not known whether short "bursts" of anticoagulant effect may not suffice to keep blood from clotting. Depot heparin administered intramuscularly and the administration of concentrated heparin intradermally or hypodermically were popular in the past, but are less so at present because of the still less dependable anticoagulant effect by this technique, as well as the frequency of local hemorrhages at the site of injections. A new method for the use of heparin is being tested as prophylaxis against postoperative phlebothrombosis. It consists of low, safe doses of heparin (5000 mm. subcutaneously every 12 hours). Initial results are very promising.

The principal risk of heparin therapy is that of hemorrhage. As a protein it is capable, rarely, to elicit anaphylactic reaction or allergic reaction (skin eruptions, asthma, etc.). The antidote to heparin in bleeding patients is protamine. Long-range use of heparin may cause osteoporosis.

Coumarin drugs are the only group of oral anticoagulants used in this country; the two most frequently used agents are warfarin (Coumadin, Panwarfin) and bishydroxycoumarin (Dicumarol).

These drugs act on the liver and antagonize vitamin K; their effect on the clotting process is thus indirect and requires several days until available vitamin K (used for the synthesis of factors II, VII, IX and X) is exhausted. Its action can be monitored by prothrombin time determination. The effective level of anticoagulation by means of this method is a prothrombin time 1¾ to 2½ times that of a control individual, or, in terms of prothrombin concentration, 20 to 30 per cent of normal. It should be noted that with the onset of anticoagulant therapy prothrombin time readings do not reflect therapeutic effectiveness, since prothrombin time lengthens and falls into the required therapeutic range several days before the full anticoagulant activity takes place.

Warfarin, the most widely used oral anticoagulant today, is a long-acting drug with a half-life of about two days. By initial loading the therapeutic level is reached earlier, although it is possible to reach the desired effect by starting a patient on regular maintenance. Some authorities recommend the slower method of not using initial loading, especially if elective, long-term anticoagulation is being initiated. The daily dose varies widely from 2 to 15 mg. of warfarin (bishydroxycoumarin requires 5 to 10 times larger dosage). Loading is usually done by using 3 to 10 times the maintenance dose.

There are several unique features of oral anticoagulant therapy that make this method fraught with difficulties beyond that of other drugs. They include the following:

- Prothrombin time test—an indirect one—has only moderate reliability as a means of monitoring the proper level of anticoagulant activity. Technically it is not always well reproducible, depending upon the freshness of the reagents and the experience of the technician.

- The therapeutic range between a totally ineffective level offering no protection against thrombosis and that threatening serious hemorrhagic complications is very narrow. The maintenance of the patient in this zone requires often tricky "juggling" of the dosages.

- Some individuals show wide swings and variations in the prothrombin time on a maintenance of the same dosage; this may sometimes be related to hepatic disease but often cannot be traced to any factor. The impracticality of performing such tests more often than at weekly intervals in patients on long-term anticoagulation often produces dilemmas and calls for compromises.

- Coumarins are among drugs most sensitive to interaction with other drugs. Long lists of drugs potentiating or reducing the potency of anticoagulant action are available and should be made known to each patient. Among those are aspirin and phenylbutazone, which increase the potency, and barbiturates, which decrease the potency.

With so many factors influencing the action of oral anticoagulants, it is not surprising that patients often are outside the recommended therapeutic zone. Some are in the ineffective zone, a circumstance which may have no immediate bearing in prophylactic therapy, but others may be over the danger level. This therapy thus carries a high risk of hemorrhages, some of which may be fatal.

The antidote to coumarin bleeding or to a very high prothrombin time is the administration of vitamin K_1. In emergencies blood transfusions may be necessary. Coumarins have few dangers other than that of hemorrhage. Rarely allergic reactions occur; some gastrointestinal irritation may be present; allopecia has been described.

Platelet antiaggregants are drugs which on a good theoretical basis can be considered as effective against thrombosis within the arterial system, but which have as yet not undergone extensive enough clinical trials to test such effect in man with arterial disease. Among the several drugs with potential effects of this nature are aspirin, dipyridamole (Persantine), and sulfinpyrazone (Anturane).

A wide gap separates these drugs from anticoagulants. They have no action interfering with the normal clotting mechanism and therefore carry little risk of hemorrhage. These drugs have very low toxicity, consisting of occasional gastrointestinal irritation and rare allergic reactions. In dealing with drugs with a minimal risk, especially aspirin, in which long experience has shown that long-term use carries a minimal risk, the uncertain potential benefit may well balance the small risk and make the drug acceptable for use even without final evidence of its effectiveness. Yet, the high cost of Persantine and Anturane has to be taken into consideration.

Thrombolysins are represented by a group of enzymes that are capable of dissolving intravascular thrombi. The theoretical reasoning behind such therapy is sound, but so far it has been bogged down by practical difficulties. The two enzymes that have undergone clinical trials are streptokinase and urokinase.

Streptokinase is a highly antigenic substance; released for use in this country for a short time, it produced so many undesirable reactions that it was withdrawn. Further purification may overcome some of these serious drawbacks in the future (trials in Europe with new preparations have been more successful).

Urokinase has the advantage over streptokinase of not being antigenic. It is, however, very difficult to obtain and will be very expensive when released for use. Current investigative trials have been quite successful.

The potential use of such agents holds the highest promise in the dissolution of pulmonary arterial thrombi. They would, of course, also be useful in other forms of venous thrombosis; pulmonary embolism has been selected for clinical trial as the most serious manifestation of venous thrombosis (see Chapter 40). Their use in arterial thrombosis is uncertain. The theoretical promise for the use of thrombolytic therapy in acute myocardial infarction has been greatly weakened by recent evidence suggesting that coronary thrombosis plays a lesser part in the pathogenesis of acute myocardial infarction than was believed in the past.

Bibliography

Aronow WS: The medical treatment of angina pectoris. Amer. Heart J. *84*:273, 445, 567, 706, 834.

Beller, GA, Smith TW, Abelmann WH, Haber E, Hood WBJ: Digitalis intoxication. A prospective clinical study with serum level correlations. New Engl. J. Med. *284*:989, 1971.

Bigger JT, Heissenbuttel RH: The use of procainamide and lidocaine in the treatment of cardiac arrhythmias. Prog. Cardiovasc. Dis. *11*:515, 1969.

Bourne HR: Unrecognized therapeutic measures including placebo. *In* CLINICAL PHARMACOLOGY, by KL Melmon and HF Morelli. The Macmillan Co., New York, 1972, p. 549.

Braunwald E: Studies on the cardiocirculatory actions of digitalis. Medicine *44*:233, 1965.

Collaborative analysis of long-term anticoagulant administration after myocardial infarction. Lancet *1*:203, 1970.

Damato AN: Diphenylhydantoin. Pharmacological and clinical use. Prog. Cardiovasc. Dis. *12*:1, 1969.

Doherty JE: Digitalis glycosides. Pharmacokinetics and their clinical implications. Ann. Int. Med. *79*:229, 1973.

Gettes LS: The electrophysiological effects of antiarrhythmic drugs. Amer. J. Card. *28*:526, 1971.

Gianelly R, von der Groeben JO, Spivack AP, Harrison DC: Effects of lidocaine in ventricular arrhythmias in patients with coronary heart disease. New Engl. J. Med. *277*:1215, 1967.

Koch-Weser J., Klein SW: Procainamide dosage schedules, plasma concentration and clinical effects. J.A.M.A. *216*:1454, 1971.

Lucchesi BR, Whitsett LS: The pharmacology of beta adrenergic blocking agents. Prog. Cardiovasc. Dis. *11*:410, 1969.

Lyon AF, De Graff AC: Antiarrhythmic drugs: I. Mechanism of quinidine action. II. Clinical use of quinidine. Amer. Heart J. *69*:713, 834, 1965.

Melmon KL: Drug reactions. *In* CLINICAL PHARMACOLOGY, by KL Melmon and HF Morelli. The Macmillan Co., 1972, p. 568.

Morelli HF: Drug interactions. *Ibid.*, p. 585.

Rowland M.: Drug administration and regimens. *Ibid.*, p. 21.

Selzer A, Hultgren HN, Ebnother CL, Bradley HW, Stone AO: Effect of digoxin on the circulation in normal man. Brit. Heart J. *21*:335, 1959.

Selzer A, Kelly J Jr: Action of digitalis upon the nonfailing heart. A critical review. Prog. Cardiovasc. Dis. *7*:273, 1964.

Selzer A, Malmborg RO: Hemodynamic effects of digoxin in latent cardiac failure. Circulation *25*:695, 1962.

Selzer A, Wray HW: Quinidine syncope: paroxysmal ventricular fibrillation occurring during treatment of chronic atrial arrhythmias. Circulation *30*:17, 1964.

Selzer A, Walter RM: Adequacy of preoperative digitalis therapy controlling ventricular rate in postoperative atrial fibrillation. Circulation *34*:129, 1966.

Selzer A, Cohn KE: Production, recognition and treatment of digitalis intoxication, Calif. Med. *113*:1 (Oct.), 1970.

Smith TW, Butler VP, Haber E: Determination of therapeutic and toxic serum digoxin concentrations by radioimmunoassay. New Engl. J. Med. *181*:1212, 1969.

Smith TW: Contribution of quantitative assay techniques to the understanding of clinical pharmacology of digitalis. Circulation *46*:188, 1972.

Thomson PD, Melmon KL, Richardson JA, Cohn KE, Steinbrunn W., Cudihee R, Rowland M: Lidocaine pharmacokinetics in advanced heart failure, liver disease and renal failure in humans. Ann. Int. Med. *78*:499, 1973.

Urokinase pulmonary embolism trial. Phase I results. A cooperative study. J.A.M.A. *214*:2163, 1970.

12

Other Forms of Medical Therapy

REGULATION OF EXTERNAL WORKLOAD

Cardiac workload consists of two components:

1.   That necessary to supply the basic metabolic demands of the body;

2.   The sum total of all the voluntary and involuntary increments produced by factors increasing circulatory demands.

In the course of treatment of various forms of cardiac disease it may become necessary or advisable to regulate the voluntary activities or to control the involuntary factors increasing cardiac workload. The regulation of workload may proceed in both directions: restricting it or recommending its augmentation.

Rest is the most restrictive step in cardiac therapy and obviously can be applied only on a temporary basis. The concept of rest has undergone major changes: two or three decades ago it was not unusual to have a cardiac patient lie flat and motionless for long periods of time; today such extreme measures are considered unnecessary, even harmful, and only a modified form of rest (including bed and chair rest) is applied for limited periods of time.

Rest, along with all other therapeutic measures, has to be reviewed from the standpoint of risk vs. benefit.

The negative aspects of rest include the following:

1.   Metabolic changes produced by inactivity and the loss of conditioning;

2. The risk of deep venous thrombosis and its sequel—pulmonary embolism.

3. The psychological impact of the rest and of its implication to the patient that it signifies serious disease.

The benefits of rest are purely conjectural. It is virtually impossible to design properly controlled studies that would prove that rest is beneficial in conditions in which it is applied. Certain speculative ideas as well as actual observations are pertinent to the problem of therapeutic rest:

1. In acute diseases involving the myocardium it might be advisable to keep external workload at a minimum in order to conserve cardiac reserve, even if the patient has an unimpaired effort tolerance. This principle serves as the justification for rest therapy in acute myocardial infarction and in acute rheumatic carditis. While no one can argue with the logic of this reasoning, there are sufficient examples of patients who refuse to cooperate, or who had clinically unrecognized attacks of infarction or carditis, to indicate that immediate harm does not necessarily result if normal activities are pursued during these illnesses.

2. Patients in severe cardiac failure are often treated with rest, in addition to other measures (drugs, oxygen, etc.). One frequently gets the impression, though not the proof, that rest makes an important contribution to the overall success of the regimen. In some cardiac surgical centers intensive medical therapy including a period of rest is given to patients prior to cardiac operations if cardiac failure is present. Here again, such a course is justified by the impression that this regimen reduces the risk of operations.

3. Long periods of bed rest have been credited with spectacular improvement in patients with chronic myocardial disease. The impracticability of enforcing this regimen (in terms of months of complete rest), and its expense make it difficult to gather sufficient data to provide convincing evidence of benefits.

Thus, at the present time the benefit of rest therapy *may* outweigh its risk in the following conditions:

- In acute myocardial infarction—for a period not to exceed three weeks in uncomplicated cases;

- In acute carditis (including nonrheumatic myocarditis), provided the diagnosis is established beyond doubt and the time period not excessive;

- In patients in severe cardiac failure, as an adjunct to other forms of therapy.

Restriction of activities constitutes the next step in therapy regulating external workload. This involves recommendations to patients to eliminate certain physical activities which are within their effort tolerance, such as the following:

1. Recommendations regarding the occupational activities:

   • vocational guidance in young patients,

   • restrictions regarding more strenuous aspects of regular work,

   • decisions regarding disability and retirement.

2. Regulation of recreational activities:

   • elimination of recreational sports,

   • restriction regarding vacations,

   • restriction on travel.

In considering the pros and cons of restriction of activities beyond the point permitted by the patient's symptoms, there are virtually no hard data to support either side of the argument about exercise. Sudden death during exercise is known to occur in patients with aortic stenosis (particularly in juveniles with congenital aortic stenosis), in hypertrophic subaortic stenosis, and in patients with ischemic heart disease. Such accidents, however, constitute only an infinitesimal fraction of patients with chronic heart disease. Furthermore, it is not known whether sudden death would not have occurred during lesser, everyday activities in these cases. On the other hand, it is necessary to consider the serious psychological impact upon some patients and the detrimental financial aspects of various restrictions which balance or even overbalance their ill-defined benefits.

At the present state of knowledge restriction of activities other than bed rest should be based on some definable objective and on common sense. The frequently encountered excess caution is to be deplored, as is the tendency to use inflexible rules. Only too often one finds school children deprived of participation in physical education programs and in games because of the mere fact that a cardiac murmur had been noted. Similarly, it is common to find physicians requesting automatically 3 to 6 months' sick leave or disability period for patients with acute myocardial infarction, regardless of how benign the course was or how firmly the diagnosis established. Also, permanent disability or early retirement is often recommended for patients with nondisabling angina or with other forms of cardiac disease, even though effort tolerance is fair and symptomatology nonprogressive. This only compounds the already serious problem of individuals not being able to find employment the moment any mention of "heart disease" is made.

On the other hand, it is common sense for one to advise a young-ster with compensated serious heart disease against choosing pro-fessional athletics as a career, or to recommend retirement or change of occupation to a 60-year-old longshoreman who continuously per-forms strenuous physical work in spite of advanced ischemic heart disease.

Thus, restriction of activities in any form should be recommended with full consideration of all the factors involved, medical as well as nonmedical. In the great majority of cases activities can best be regu-lated by the patient's symptoms rather than restricted by the physician's advice.

Exercise therapy represents the reverse to the previously discussed aspects of regulation of external workload. It involves two modes of approach:

1. Graded exercise as a means of rehabilitation of patients recov-ering from acute cardiac diseases;

2. Regular reconditioning therapy, now used extensively in the treatment of ischemic heart disease.

The transition from rest to full activity has to take place gradually, if for no other reason, as a result of the patient's limited tolerance of exercise. It is felt that this transition can be facilitated by guidance from trained physiotherapists. Whether the expense of physiotherapy is jus-tified by specific advantages is not always certain. Other than the ex-pense, there can be no objection to physiotherapy if it is available.

Exercise therapy is based on observation that patients with ische-mic heart disease and chronic angina often improve in response to such therapy. While some suggestions have been made that exercise therapy may favorably affect the natural history of ischemic heart disease, it is more likely that exercise therapy exerts a nonspecific effect upon the patients:

- Better conditioning is associated with a sense of well-being;

- There is objective evidence that exercise can be performed more economically (from the metabolic standpoint) by trained, well-conditioned subjects.

No critically appraised information is available on how much exer-cise is needed as a minimum to exert a beneficial effect, whether such effect is quantitatively related to the amount of exercise, and whether or not it is necessary to reach a submaximal level (in terms of heart rate) of exercise in order to obtain a benefit (as is claimed by some workers in the field). The apparent success of supervised "exercise classes" now widely organized in many localities may be related to the psychological impact of the interaction of patients and to a greater probability that patients will follow a program.

Pregnancy constitutes an involuntary increase in cardiac workload. While the increment of cardiac work is not as great as strenuous exercise, it imposes the load continuously, hence it affects the circulation profoundly. The specific risks of pregnancy involve the following:

1. Appearance of cardiac failure,

2. Appearance of peri-partum cardiomyopathy,

3. Development of pulmonary hypertension,

4. Development of infection, including infective endocarditis,

5. Problems with anticoagulation in patients with prosthetic valves,

6. Development of hypertension,

7. Aortic dissection in coarctation of the aorta.

The principal risk to most women with cardiac disease who become pregnant is the precipitation of cardiac failure, which may be temporary or responsive to therapy, may be sudden and cause death, or may be partly reversible but may bring the patient one step down on the course of a chronic disease.

The physician has the following means of controlling the untoward effects of pregnancy upon the heart in women with cardiac disease:

- Unqualified opposition to pregnancy, with sterilization,

- Recommendation against pregnancy,

- Recommendation to terminate early pregnancy,

- Recommendation for the performance of surgical correction of the cardiac lesion during pregnancy,

- Medical management during pregnancy,

- Cardiological supervision during labor and delivery.

While the effect of pregnancy on women with cardiac disease is admittedly unpredictable, it is now generally believed that its risk is probably smaller than it was considered in the past. It is probable that a patient with cardiac disease who can perform ordinary activities without symptoms (Class I) undertakes a risk in carrying a child that is only very slightly higher than that of a normal woman. Thus the usual diseases of childbearing age—rheumatic and congenital heart disease—are characterized by long periods of asymptomatic state, in which the risk of pregnancy is acceptable. Since the attitudes of women toward pregnancy vary widely, it may be best to inform the patient of the higher risk to her and permit her to make the choice whether or not such pregnancy should be undertaken or completed. As in the case of restriction of activities, physicians frequently tend to take the attitude of undue caution toward pregnancy, erring on the side of recommending against pregnancy in cardiac patients. Only the most careful individual consideration of the risk of pregnancy and a frank discussion of the problem with the patient involved will provide a fair approach to this difficult problem.

REGULATION OF ENVIRONMENTAL FACTORS

A patient with cardiac disease may find himself in an environment which might adversely affect the disease, or which could make him more symptomatic. The regulation of such environmental factors, if feasible, should be undertaken with the same consideration of pros and cons as other therapeutic approaches.

Stress

Superimposed upon the minimum daily stresses of ordinary existence are the stresses of competitive work or play. Such stresses have been blamed as contributory risk factors for the development of ischemic heart disease and hypertension, as well as a variety of noncardiac diseases. No one can deny that stresses of meeting deadlines, of competing with peers, and of trying to please superiors exert a visible influence upon the psychological makeup of an individual and may produce some subjective effects that are eliminated by rest or vacation. It is not certain, however, whether the circulatory effects of stressful situations fall within the normal reserve of the heart or exceed it; therefore the potential harm is unknown. This difficulty is compounded by the fact that measurement of stress cannot be done with any degree of accuracy, with the sole exception of its effect upon the arterial pressure. The reliability of the fluctuation of blood pressure as an overall index of stress is not known.

The attitude of physicians in regard to stress has been similar to that toward restriction of activities; that is, the advocacy of undue caution. One cannot discard the possibility that in some individuals a medical recommendation forcing someone to take a position of lesser responsibility than he deserves, or to retire, may in itself magnify the stress rather than reduce it. In this field of nonscientific guesswork one has to "play it by ear" in regard to management of patient responsibilities.

Altitude

Altitude of 5,000 feet or more introduces an element of arterial hypoxia which may affect normal individuals as well as cardiac patients. There is no evidence that high altitude per se has a consistently deleterious effect upon the course of cardiac disease. Inhabitants of high altitude (up to 14,000 feet) suffer from cardiac disease to a comparable extent to those at sea level. The only specific effect of high altitude hypoxia is the production and aggravation of pulmonary hypertension. It has been shown that children with congenital heart disease have a higher incidence of pulmonary hypertensive complications; it is probable that failure of postnatal closure of the ductus arteriosus may be increased by altitude. Thus, in terms of specific contraindications, patients with clinical conditions predisposing to pulmonary hypertension should, if possible, avoid high altitude.

Inasmuch as hypoxia is directly proportional to altitude, the effects of altitude are more likely to develop above 9,000 feet than in the 5,000 to 9,000 range. In terms of complications, it is also important to know whether a patient who goes to a high altitude area for rest and recreation will take enough leisure time to spend the first day or two resting, thereby permitting acclimatization, or whether he will commence a strenuous pack trip immediately upon arrival at that area. In general, ischemic heart disease may be more prone to become aggravated by high altitude in terms of symptomatology than other forms of cardiac disease. Occasionally, first symptoms of cardiac disease (often previously unknown) develop while in high altitude. Thus, as in other forms of regulation of the patient's mode of living, individual decisions have to be made as to whether a patient is to be permitted to go to such areas or not, balancing the importance of a particular trip (or permanent move) against the likelihood of evoking difficulty.

A common question pertaining to altitude is the need for restriction of cardiac patients from commercial aviation. At present, when altitude pressurization is routine, and the pressure in the cabin is equivalent to 2,000 to 5,000 feet, there appears to be no need to withhold plane travel from any but class 4 patients, and even those often undertake such trips without problems.

Climate

Patients with cardiac disease do not differ from the general population in their being more comfortable in the moderate ranges of temperature and humidity. Whether hot and humid environment can actually harm patients is difficult to decide. Subjects have been studied in such unfavorable surroundings and found to have some impairment of cardiac performance. Abnormalities thus recorded do not indicate serious derangement of cardiac function, and their significance is not known. Restrictions regarding climate fall into the category of more pleasant options rather than necessities for cardiac patients.

TOBACCO AND ALCOHOL

Within the area of management of patients with cardiac disease, the reduction of the various risk factors plays a variably important role. The two common poisons taken by the patients voluntarily, tobacco and alcohol, undoubtedly play a role in the production and aggravation of cardiac disease. Statistics regarding higher incidence of coronary atherosclerosis in smokers are reasonably convincing and tobacco is a recognized risk factor in ischemic heart disease. When recommending that the patient abandon the use of tobacco, one cannot find the same socioeconomic ill effects that have been mentioned in connection with other restrictions, although admittedly some patients would consider the quality of life less desirable if they were to give up smoking. Two compelling reasons may cause patients to continue this habit: inadequate will power to stop smoking and the substitution of smoking for another undesirable factor, obesity.

The role of alcohol is in a somewhat different category, in that the heart is relatively insensitive to alcohol damage, so that the excessive drinker is more likely to suffer other consequences than heart disease. It is only the entity of "alcoholic cardiomyopathy" that is tentatively traced to alcohol damage, and in this entity — as will be pointed out — it is not yet definitely established as to whether alcohol plays the principal etiological role or is mainly a contributory factor.

DIETARY THERAPY

There are only two special diets that are widely used in patients with cardiac disease and are relevant to cardiac therapy:

- Low sodium diet,

- Low fat and low cholesterol diet.

Low sodium diet plays a smaller role in the therapy of cardiac disease today than it did a decade or two ago. Once popular, extreme restrictions of sodium to 100 mg. or less per 24 hours are now seldom recommended. The reason for such change is twofold:

- The awareness of potential harm to the patient in the form of iatrogenic electrolyte imbalance,

- The availability of more powerful diuretics.

It is now generally recognized that diuretic therapy, sodium restriction, and rest can all accomplish the same end. The respective contribution of each of these factors can be adjusted in patients who follow a chronic regimen controlling cardiac failure, so that they become least disruptive to the patient's habits.

It is prudent to advise patients with lesions that are likely to produce cardiac failure to begin mild dietary adjustment of the sodium intake early, at the stage when they are fully compensated. A gradual elimination of sodium is less traumatic to patients than the abrupt change from a regular diet to one severely restricted. This is particularly true for patients with certain dietary habits or of certain ethnic cultures in which high sodium intake is customary. The average "low sodium diet" in patients hospitalized is usually that of 2.0 gm. of salt (= 0.8 gm. of sodium) per 24 hours. Patients are often instructed to continue such diets at home when discharged from the hospital; in practice they seldom adhere to such restrictions; most prefer the use of diuretics. Inasmuch as aggravation of failure, or even attacks of frank pulmonary edema may follow a single dietary indiscretion, it is wise to instruct patients to take additional diuretics if they are to indulge in an unusually salty meal.

Low fat and cholesterol diet is still a matter of controversy in regard to its role in ischemic heart disease. The controversy revolves around two questions:

- The role of high fat, high cholesterol diet in the etiology of coronary atherosclerosis,

- The role of dietary restriction of cholesterol and saturated fatty acids in the treatment of existing ischemic heart disease.

Evidence for an etiological role of high content of saturated fatty acids and cholesterol in ischemic heart disease is based on mass epidemiological observations: There is irrefutable evidence that some ethnic groups, nations, or inhabitants of geographical areas whose dietary habits include a small contribution of the presumed offenders and whose serum cholesterol has significantly lower mean values have a lower incidence of ischemic heart disease than comparable groups with high fat intake. It has been pointed out that in our culture infants are born with a low serum cholesterol level, but that level gradually increases, presumably in response to our customary diet. While there are still some skeptics who question even this relationship, the evidence seems reasonably convincing. As a corollary to accepting this relationship, a change of dietary habits in most Western countries appears desirable; furthermore, the principal effort needs to be aimed at infants and children, for it is probably easier to maintain the low cholesterol level present in infancy throughout life than to aim at lowering it later, once "hypercholesteremia" for this standard becomes established.

The question of reversibility of ischemic heart disease in response to dietary therapy (or cholesterol-lowering agents) is more difficult to answer. Whether or not the atherosclerotic process, one advanced sufficiently to produce the symptomatic stage, can be arrested or reversed remains to be demonstrated. Several studies have been conducted in regard to this problem, none as yet yielding significant information. Until authoritative information is available to answer this question, one can recommend such dietary restrictions to patients with ischemic disease on the basis that, while potential benefits are uncertain, no direct risk is involved. However, one should consider the negative aspects of such a diet, namely the objections of some patients to the loss of favorite meals, the technical difficulty of attaining such diets in places other than the home, and the additional cost of such a diet. Well-motivated patients are often willing to make such sacrifices, even on the basis of only the conjectural possibility that their disease may thereby be less apt to progress.

PSYCHOTHERAPY

It should be recognized that there is a psychotherapeutic angle in every contact between the physician and the patient. It is often overlooked by the physician that almost every layman recognizes that the heart is the most important organ in the body: heart disease is probably the most dreaded of all illnesses and the one with the most serious connotations. Careful handling of a patient may make the difference between success and disaster. A considerate approach to a patient with heart disease may lead to his cheerful acceptance of his fate and the opportunity to lead a tolerable and even pleasant life in spite of the handicap. A careless and brutal approach may have a disastrous effect on a patient with trivial heart disease who could become a hopeless cripple from iatrogenic cardiac neurosis. It is, of course, true that the psychological makeup of the patient is a contributory factor if cardiac neurosis develops, but there is a considerable leeway, and the skill of handling often determines the result.

Psychotherapy should not be approached solely from the standpoint of situations requiring expert care by a psychiatrist. Only a very small fraction of cases fall into this category. Rather, it is the mode of handling the psychological component that accompanies every problem related to the heart — not only cardiac disease but also suspicion of cardiac disease. The clinician taking care of the patient has to assume the principal responsibility for handling this component. Psychotherapeutic considerations color all dealings with patients but are of particular importance in patients who have recovered from an acute cardiac disease (e.g., myocardial infarction) or who suffer from non-disabling or only mildly disabling cardiac lesions. Here the question as to how well the patient is rehabilitated often depends upon the management of aspects other than the physical treatment of disease. The responsibility for neurotic disability often can be placed squarely upon the shoulders of the clinician who neglects to consider the psychological component of the illness.

It is often necessary to weigh the psychological component of cardiac disease upon the therapeutic scale as an important risk factor that may require certain compromises in therapy. The importance of communication with the patient regarding the diagnosis of heart disease has already been stressed. The need for elaborate diagnostic tests should always be considered in the light of the possible conclusions the patient may draw from the mere performance of such studies. The frequency of follow-up visits in asymptomatic patients needs to be considered carefully in this light, as well as the desirability of recommending continuous drug therapy. The experienced cardiologist often assumes the calculated risk of providing less than ideal care or making less elaborate diagnostic evaluation for the benefit of sparing the patient the psychological trauma.

VARIOUS SHORT-TERM FORMS OF THERAPY

Inhalation therapy. The past decade saw a change from empirically administered oxygen to patients with myocardial infarction or in cardiac failure to a rational, scientifically controlled inhalation therapy. The traditional oxygen tent that accomplished little, except perhaps to provide cool surroundings for the patient in a non-air-conditioned room, is no longer in use. Modern inhalation therapy has two principal objectives:

- To correct impaired gas exchange,

- To relieve the overload of increased work of breathing.

It is generally recognized that the prime indication for the administration of oxygen is arterial hypoxia. Cyanosis is a poor index of impaired respiratory gas exchange because of the following reasons:

1. Peripheral cyanosis from stasis and low cardiac output occurs more commonly than central cyanosis due to arterial hypoxemia.

2. Central cyanosis, when easily detectable, indicates severe degree of arterial hypoxemia; early treatment is indicated, before visible cyanosis is present.

Simple arterial hypoxemia occurs in cardiac patients as a result of a variety of mechanisms:

- Hypoventilation, often resulting from drugs,
- Pulmonary atelectasis,
- Other forms of ventilation-perfusion imbalance,
- Diffusion difficulties.

Administration of oxygen corrects hypoxemia entirely or partially, depending on the extent of intrapulmonary shunting. It is now generally considered correct to start oxygen in a low concentration of 40 per cent or less, in order to avoid CO_2 retention; in simple cases, not associated with dyspnea, a face mask of the venturi type is most often used. If ineffective, or if respiratory distress is present, respiratory assist devices are indicated.

Respirators are generally available using either of two principles:

- Delivery of inspired gases under measured positive pressure,
- Delivery of a predetermined volume of inspiratory gases.

Pressure respirators can be used by means of a tight-fitting face mask; delivery of the gas may be triggered by the patient's inspiration. The pressure of delivery is predetermined by prior adjustment or may be automatically cycled. Such respirators are also frequently used via an endotracheal tube in the postoperative period and under other special conditions.

Volume respirators can be used only through an endotracheal tube and are fully automatic. They effectively take over the work of breathing and occasionally have dramatically beneficial effects in severely dyspneic patients.

Phlebotomy, once a frequently used procedure for the relief of severe cardiac dyspnea and pulmonary edema, is now used very seldom. The principle of phlebotomy has not been challenged, and its hemodynamic effects upon left ventricular failure are still considered beneficial; however, easier and more effective methods of accomplishing similar ends are now available:

- Intravenous diuretics can effectively reduce blood volume within minutes;
- Respiratory assistance may control severe dyspnea more effectively.

It is nevertheless well to remember that phlebotomy may be indicated under some circumstances, for example, in plethoric patients or in areas where respiratory care is not available.

Electroshock therapy has become one of the most important advances in cardiac therapy. Used for a long time for open chest reversal of ventricular fibrillation, electroshock acquired its present importance in response to two major advances:

- The development of external resuscitation (1960),

- The development of a timed delivery of direct-current shock as a safe means of conversion of tachyarrhythmias other than ventricular fibrillation (1962).

Today's equipment consists of a capacitor capable of delivery of up to 400 watt-seconds (joules) of direct current by means of paddles applied to the patient's skin. The delivery is triggered by the R waves of the electrocardiogram so that it falls outside the vulnerable phase of repolarization.

Electroshock therapy is used in three forms:

1. As an emergency during cardiac arrest (ventricular fibrillation);

2. On a semi-emergent basis for conversion of tachyarrhythmias in patients who are in acute cardiac distress or in shock;

3. As an elective procedure.

In addition to its use in emergency defibrillation of ventricles, electroshock therapy is used to terminate all forms of tachyarrhythmias. Since it is a procedure that carries a definite risk, the indications have to be well spelled out in terms of potential benefits. Specific situations in which electroshock therapy is not indicated include the following:

- Repetitive tachyarrhythmias, i.e., short bursts of tachyarrhythmias interrupted by periods of sinus rhythm;

- Arrhythmias suspected of being substitute rhythms or escape rhythms or where evidence exists that the physiological pacemaking mechanism is malfunctioning;

- Tachyarrhythmias suspected of being caused by digitalis toxicity (this is a relative contraindication—in life-threatening situations electroshock may be necessary as a calculated risk).

Indications for electroshock therapy include the following:

- Chronic atrial fibrillation in patients with a reasonable prospect of maintenance of sinus rhythm;

- Chronic atrial flutter;

- Tachycardias of atrial, junctional, or ventricular origin that do not respond to other forms of medical therapy and are poorly tolerated by the patient.

Electroshock administration is very painful and requires either general anesthesia or the administration of tranquilizers (hydroxyzine — Vistaril) in sufficient doses to produce amnesia. The risks of the procedure include the following:

- Risk of anesthesia in general;

- Depression of the SA pacemaker with serious bradyarrhythmias;

- Uncontrollable tachyarrhythmias (multifocal ventricular ectopic beats, ventricular tachycardias, ventricular fibrillation);

- Potentiation of digitalis toxicity with the production of digitalis arrhythmias;

- Possibility of systemic embolism from fibrillating atria (remote).

The development of rhythm disturbances as a complication of electroshock therapy most often takes place immediately after the administration of the shock, but may also be delayed and occur minutes, even hours, after the conversion. The safety of the procedure may be enhanced if the patient's rhythm is monitored for 1 to 6 hours after shock administration.

The conversion of tachyarrhythmias if they are short-term or paroxysmal is handled differently from those established for a long time. The former, as a rule, require a weaker shock (25 to 100 watt-seconds) and are seldom treated with drugs before or after the shock; the latter are usually treated with quinidine or procainamide (second choice) for 24 to 48 hours prior to the procedure, and for a time afterward, varying from one or two weeks to permanent administration of such drugs. Atrial fibrillation usually requires higher wattage (100 to 400 watt-seconds). Inasmuch as there is a possibility that the magnitude of the shock is related to potential damage to the myocardium, it is customary to start the patient with administration of lower wattage and then to administer higher doses until conversion is accomplished, or until a 400 watt-second shock is shown to be ineffective. If secondary arrhythmias are triggered by shock administration which does not accomplish conversion, it may be safer to abandon the procedure.

The success rate of electroshock therapy in restoring sinus rhythm is about 85 per cent; figures differ in the various categories, as will be pointed out in the discussion of arrhythmias. Often sinus rhythm does not appear at once but after an intermediate period of a junctional bradycardia.

Electroshock therapy has revolutionized the treatment of arrhythmias. It is nevertheless a procedure fraught with considerable difficulties regarding indications, details of administration, and the handling of problems arising from its use. It has a significant incidence of morbidity and mortality and should always be considered a calculated risk; potential benefits should clearly outweigh the risks. This procedure should be kept in the hands of the experienced cardiologist or other clinicians familiar with all ramifications. Casual or occasional use of it may unnecessarily magnify its risk, perhaps to the point of outweighing *all* potential benefits except in dire emergencies.

PACEMAKERS

Along with electroshock therapy, the introduction of pacemakers has signaled a major advance in the therapy of cardiac disease. First used in complete heart block with syncopal attacks, it has been applied to a wide variety of disturbances of cardiac rhythm. Pacemaking is used in two general forms:

- As a temporary procedure, using the pulse generator outside the body;

- As permanent therapy, using an implanted pulse generator.

Currently used pacemakers include the following:

1. Fixed rate pacemaker, firing at a constant rate at all times.

2. Demand pacemaker, triggered by the R wave of the patient's heart beat. Here the stimulus is applied at a fixed interval from the last R wave. The pacemaker thus is inactive whenever a spontaneous beat occurs earlier in relation to the last R wave than the present interval, thereby being inhibited except when spontaneous rate falls below that of the pacemaker.

3. Demand pacemaker inhibited by the R wave of the patient's heart beat. Similar effect operates in this type to the previous one, but utilizing a different mechanism of inhibition when adequate cardiac action takes place.

4. P-triggered pacemaker. Here the sensing lead in the atrium recognizes atrial activity and generates a ventricular stimulation after an interval equivalent to the normal P-R time. This pacemaker, more physiological than others (because of the capability to follow changes of SA rate) has the drawback of its complexity.

Pacemakers are now almost exclusively placed transvenously, both for temporary as well as for permanent use; as a consequence pacemaker stimulation is as a rule endocardial. Only rarely epicardial stimulation is used, mostly when thoracotomy is performed for another reason. Therapeutic pacing is used in the great majority of cases by ventricular stimulation. Occasionally, when AV conduction is intact, atrial pacing may be indicated.

The risk of pacemakers includes the following:

- Serious or even fatal arrhythmias during its placement. This is rare during elective pacemaker insertion but represents a hazard in seriously ill patients, e.g., during acute myocardial infarction.

- Perforation of the right ventricle. This complication varies in its consequences, at times producing no significant sequels.

- Stimulation of the diaphragm. Not a life-threatening complication, this nevertheless may be very bothersome for the patient, who may refuse to tolerate it.

- Various forms of pacemaker malfunction. These include premature failure of the batteries, interruption of wiring, and loss of myocardial contact due to fibrosis of the endocardium around the electrode. As a result of such failures of the pacemaker function the original condition for which the pacemaker was inserted may become operative again or, rarely, pacemaker-induced serious arrhythmias may develop.

- Rarely, pulmonary emboli from mural thrombosis, or damage to the tricuspid valve may develop.

While the pacemaker has been used successfully in a great many cardiac conditions, the principal goals of pacemaker therapy can be summarized as follows:

1. Treatment of bradyarrhythmias serious enough to become a hazard to the patient's life.

2. Prevention of cardiac (or ventricular) standstill, whenever the risk of it has been established.

3. Prevention of tachyarrhythmias that are initiated by excessive slowing of cardiac rate.

4. Overdrive suppression of certain tachyarrhythmias.

In considering these goals, the selection of cases for pacemaker therapy requires careful consideration of all factors within the framework of the therapeutic equation (risk vs. benefit).

Bibliography

DeSanctis RW: Diagnostic and therapeutic uses of atrial pacing. Circulation *43*:748, 1971.

Escher, DJW, Furman S: Pacemaker therapy in chronic rhythm disorders. Prog. Cardiovasc. Dis. *14*:459, 1972.

Fox SM III, Naughton JP, Gorman PA: Physical activity and cardiovascular health. Mod. Concept. Cardiovasc. Dis. *41*:17, 21, 25, 1972.

Furman S, Escher DJW: The pacemaker follow-up clinic. Prog. Cardiovasc. Dis. *14*:545, 1972.

Kosowsky BD, Barr I: Complications and malfunctions of electrical cardiac pacemakers. Prog. Cardiovasc. Dis. *14*:501, 1972.

Lown B: Electrical reversion of cardiac arrhythmias. Brit. Heart J. *29*:469, 1967.

Proceedings of the International Symposium on Physical Activity and Cardiovascular Health. Canad. Med. Assoc. J. *96*:695, 1967.

Resnekov L: Present status of electroversion in management of cardiac arrhythmias. Circulation *47*:1356, 1973.

Resnekov L, Lipp H: Pacemaking in acute myocardial infarction. Prog. Cardiovasc. Dis. *14*:475, 1972.

Resnekov L, McDonald L: Complications in 200 patients with cardiac dysrhythmias treated by phased direct current shock and indications for electroversion. Brit. Heart J. *24*:926, 1967.

Selzer A, Kelly JJ Jr., Johnson RB, Kerth WJ: Immediate and long-term results of electrical conversion of arrhythmias. Prog. Cardiovasc. Dis. *9*:90, 1966.

13
Surgical Therapy

Cardiac surgery in general and open heart surgery in particular are recognized as major breakthroughs in medicine in this century. The dramatic impact of operations performed upon the heart has generated an enthusiasm among the medical profession as well as among the lay public that has at times blurred the guidelines of prudent therapeutic approaches. Thus, the usual two modes of approach to treatment—the conservative and the aggressive approach—have in certain aspects given place to a rational approach and an irrational approach. An example of irrationality is cardiac transplantation; initiated with a minimum of preparation and a maximum of publicity, cardiac transplantation has spread rapidly to the four corners of the world and has been publicized to an extent unprecedented in medical history, only to be retired to one or two institutions in which the basic research is being performed—where it should have been initiated and remained in the first place!

The physicians' enthusiasm for the drama of open heart surgery coupled with the public's clamor for quick cures of serious heart diseases generated an atmosphere in which operations were often performed for the sole reason that they were available, without respect to their merit in terms of long-range effects upon the course of the disease. Risk has been considered solely on the basis of the immediate effects of the operation. It is thus necessary to outline a careful analysis of surgical treatment, looking at it from an appropriately unbiased perspective.

The problem of surgical treatment involves three general types of operations:

1. Curative operations (e.g., atrial septal defect);

2. Corrective operations (most valve operations);

3. Palliative operations (e.g., Blalock anastomosis).

Related to cardiac operations is the problem of noncardiac operations that are indicated in patients with chronic cardiac disease. Each type of cardiac or noncardiac operation may be elective, urgent, or may represent an emergency.

Surgical treatment of cardiac disease needs the same balancing of the two therapeutic factors—risk vs. benefit—as all other forms of treatment. It is important, however, that these factors be appropriately defined and be considered in a broad sense rather than with a simplistic narrow approach.

DEFINITION OF RISK

Under the concept of risk one should include every consequence or complication related to the operation directly or indirectly. These include:

- Operative death;

- Late death related to the operation or its consequences;

- Excess morbidity after the operation (unusual complications, postoperative syndromes, infections, etc.);

- Poor surgical results (e.g., persistence of cardiac defect, production of valvular regurgitation, unsuccessful relief of valvular stenosis or repair of valvular regurgitation, periprosthetic leaks);

- Failure of the patient to improve clinically (predominance of "myocardial factors" rather than mechanical load prior to the operation: the play of other factors interfering with the corrective aspects of the operation);

- Damage to the patient at the time of the operation (cerebral damage, myocardial damage, other "accidents");

- Disabling late complications related to the operation (e.g., thromboembolism from thrombi formed around prosthetic material, hemolytic anemias);

- Increased risk of further operations upon the heart;

- The expense of the operation and of the time-loss from work.

DEFINITION OF BENEFITS

Surgical benefits require the consideration of two overall aspects:

1. Prolongation of the life of the patient;

2. Improvement of clinical symptomatology—the "quality of life."

In order to determine whether life would be prolonged, it is necessary to have a reasonable knowledge of the natural history of the given disease, as well as to recognize the prognostic guidelines of the various signs, symptoms, or measurements of the severity of the lesion. The major deficiency in setting proper guidelines for surgical therapy is the inadequate, often fragmentary knowledge of the natural history of disease (see also Chapter 10). In congenital heart disease — the first group of diseases to be tackled surgically — mean survival figures were based on autopsy studies and were highly biased, providing an unduly pessimistic picture. Inasmuch as the "natural" history of such lesions no longer exists, since it would be improper in symptomatic individuals to withhold surgical treatment, attempts are being made now to estimate indirectly the prognosis of such lesions. Similar considerations are given to all other forms of cardiac disease that are now amenable to surgical therapy.

The evaluation of symptomatic improvement appears to be easier than the determination of the overall prognosis, inasmuch as the patient serves as his own control, comparing symptoms before and after the operation. Yet, such evaluation, when based on subjective manifestations of disease, is fraught with pitfalls.

First, the patient's symptoms prior to the operation may not have been caused by the cardiac lesion that is to be repaired. (Dyspnea due to pulmonary disease, noncardiac chest pain, or other symptoms may have been present.)

Second, subjective improvement may be related to the long period of rest.

Third, suggestion plays an important role in the symptomatology. A great many patients claiming dramatic improvement after open heart operations have been shown by objective studies (hemodynamic evaluation, coronary arteriography) to be no better than prior to the operation.

Because of such pitfalls it is advisable to look for objective indices of improvement. Routine cardiac catheterization prior to cardiac operations is an important part of preoperative evaluation of the cardiac patient. Even in patients whose diagnosis is established beyond reasonable doubt by noninvasive techniques, hemodynamic data represent an important background material against which it may become necessary to measure future studies in patients who did not receive the expected benefit from the operation. Having such data, there is merit in performing repeat studies even in patients who profess to have shown considerable symptomatic improvement following the operation. It is not surprising that cardiac centers in which clinical evaluation alone determines surgical results are more optimistic in regard to surgical results than those in which there is reliance on more objective measurements of surgical success!

SELECTION OF PATIENTS FOR SURGERY

The process of selection of patients for surgical treatment is obviously related to the underlying disease; it will be discussed in Part II of this book. However, certain basic principles may be worth stating here in an effort to establish general guidelines for the case selection.

Cardiac operations involve a broad range of conditions as well as a wide spectrum of symptomatology. On one end of the spectrum are patients who are well, asymptomatic, in whom the operation is entirely prophylactic; on the other end are those who are moribund, in whom a high-risk operation is performed as a desperate last step, comparable to some forms of radical surgery for the treatment of cancer.

Prophylactic operations may be based on the principle that although the majority of patients with a certain lesion may suffer no grave consequences from it, some may acquire a serious disease, the risk of which is higher than that of the operation. An example of such a lesion is patent ductus arteriosus too small to produce a significant dynamic overload, but which represents a vulnerable point for the development of infective endocarditis.

A situation intermediate between a prophylactic operation and a corrective operation is represented by the atrial septal defect: here the majority of patients at the time of operation are asymptomatic; the goals of the operation are (1) to protect the patient from pulmonary hypertension (the probability is about 15 per cent), and (2) to prevent the development of cardiac failure late in life (probability of about 75 per cent).

The performance of such prophylactic, or "semiprophylactic" operations as exemplified above, looked upon from the standpoint of risk vs. benefit, is justified under three conditions:

1. The operation is curative, or comes close to it;

2. The risk of the operation is very small;

3. The incidence of sequels or complications which are to be prevented is known and overbalances the risk of the operation.

Analyzing from this standpoint operations for closure of the duct and correction of the atrial septal defect*, one can make a much stronger case for the atrial septal defect. Here, in highly regarded cardiac surgical units the mortality is under 2 per cent, and the likelihood of any late sequelae from the operation itself other than the immediate operative risk is remote; on the other hand, the benefits are clear-cut

---

*In this discussion remarks referring to closure of atrial septal defect apply to operations performed in childhood or adolescence. Closure of adult atrial septal defect is often no longer "curative."

and important. In patent ductus arteriosus the risk of the operation is still lower (probably 0.1 to 0.3 per cent). The heart is never entered, no body perfusion is used — yet the incidence of endocarditis is not known, so the equation cannot properly be completed. It is probable that closure of even small ducts is justifiable, but one can base such a recommendation only on a general clinical impression, not on scientific evidence.

The two conditions discussed above are among the very few that can be "cured" by an operation. Most other operations merely correct a lesion to a lesser or greater extent. The operation may anatomically approach a "cure" (e.g., total repair of tetralogy of Fallot) but still leave the patient with some potential or actual cardiac handicaps; the operation may merely improve the situation mildly, leaving the major disease untouched (e.g., resection of cardiac aneurysm). Most surgical lesions lie in between such extremes. The surgical decisions have to be based on equating the probability of the degree of correction that can be attained with the anticipated difficulties.

Palliative operations may have dramatic effects, e.g., upon cyanosis, but are nevertheless of the lower order in terms of surgical priorities. By definition they do not affect the disease itself but merely correct some of its consequences. Here the benefits must be well defined, the disease manifestation against which the operation is designed of large order of magnitude and of serious consequences to justify this type of operation.

GENERAL SURGERY IN CARDIAC PATIENTS

From experience with cardiac surgery we have learned that seriously ill cardiac patients can undergo long and elaborate operations with relative safety, given the appropriate team facilities. Similarly, in general surgery, it appears that the additional risk of operating upon patients with chronic cardiac disease is small on the average, ranging from no increment in risk in patients with well-compensated cardiac disease to a moderate increase but not a prohibitive one in patients in cardiac failure. Such additional risk can be minimized if the same care is exercised in connection with general surgery as is given to patients who undergo cardiac surgery in regard to preparation, anesthesia, and postoperative care. It is important that cardiac patients in whom a surgical procedure is contemplated be reviewed by a cardiologist or internist and that the decision be not solely a surgical one.

There are a few guidelines and special situations that deserve mention:

• A decision regarding continuation of cardiac drugs should

be carefully reviewed (digitalis, diuretics, antihypertensive drugs, etc.).

- In patients with ischemic heart disease special care should be exercised to avoid wide variation of blood pressure, or hypoxia.

- Patients with valve disease undergoing urological surgery should be viewed as potential candidates for infective endocarditis.

- Patients on a chronic anticoagulant regimen require special consideration concerning the interruption of this program.

THE CARDIOLOGIST'S CONTRIBUTION TO OPEN-HEART SURGERY

The participation of the cardiologist in the care of patients who undergo open-heart surgery varies from department to department. In general, care during the procedure is given to the patients mostly by the anesthesiologists and other members of the surgical team; frequently, however, the preoperative preparation of the patient as well as the postoperative care are undertaken with the active participation of the cardiologist.

Preparation of Patients for Surgery

After the diagnostic evaluation has established a valid indication for cardiac surgery, the medical and surgical members of the team jointly decide on the timing of the operation. The preparation ranges from a routine evaluation of the patient's condition to an elaborate treatment aimed at the reduction of the surgical risk.

The preoperative evaluation should be performed on all patients immediately prior to the operation. If diagnostic studies determining operability had been performed shortly before the operation, they should incorporate the various tests to be listed below. If time has elapsed between the diagnostic study and the surgical operation, certain tests need to be repeated even if this interval is no longer than one week. Such tests include:

1. A 12-lead electrocardiogram,

2. A chest roentgenogram,

3. Routine blood studies.

The following studies are recommended as routine prior to open heart surgery, but need not be performed immediately before the operation:

1. Study of respiratory function,

2. Study of renal function,

3. Study of hepatic function,

4. Serum electrolyte measurements,

5. Blood clotting panel,

6. Search for infections (including dental care),

7. Review of cerebral function.

In view of the fact that most patients require assisted respiration in the immediate postoperative period, it is helpful to the patient if he has the opportunity to acquaint himself with the respirator, to have its action explained to him prior to the operation, and to try its use in advance of the operation.

Special problems requiring more elaborate handling occur in very ill patients, particularly those who are in cardiac failure. They include the following:

1. Patients in severe cardiac failure often benefit from a period of intensive hospital treatment, consisting of rest, low sodium diet, and drug therapy. The duration of the therapy varies in relation to the seriousness of the patient's condition. It is important that a stable state be attained 2 or 3 days prior to the operation, so as to prevent the possibility of excessive fluid loss and electrolyte imbalance that occasionally is produced by massive diuresis. In treating seriously ill patients in congestive cardiac failure it is occasionally necessary to weigh carefully the advantages of preoperative treatment that may reduce the operative risk against the possibility of further deterioration or death before the operation can be performed. An individual survey has to be made in each case to guide the choice of optimal time of the operation; the following points need to be considered, among others:

- The natural history of the underlying disease (e.g., aortic stenosis with overt cardiac failure carries a very poor prognosis; it is often better to operate immediately, even if optimal medical treatment has not been instituted).

- The question as to whether or not a precipitating factor is responsible for cardiac failure (abrupt development of cardiac failure may sometimes be traced to a complication: a bout of arrhythmia, pulmonary embolism; a decision regarding whether to operate before the complication is eliminated, or vice versa, needs to be made).

• The extent of previous therapy and the patient's response to it should be carefully reviewed.

2. Patients who are on chronic drug therapy require planning regarding their drug administration:

• Digitalis is a subject of considerable controversy concerning its role in surgery in general, and in open heart surgery in particular. In the author's opinion, the risk of digitalis administration does outweigh its potential benefits unless poorly controlled atrial fibrillation is present. Thus, there is good justification to discontinue digitalis 2 or 3 days prior to the operation (as in electroshock therapy); several unavoidable factors often develop after the operation (hypoxia, electrolyte imbalance, acidosis) that may potentiate digitalis effect, bringing into the open latent toxicity.

• Diuretics should not be used during the last 2 or 3 days prior to the operation, in order to avoid electrolyte imbalance and hypovolemia.

• Anticoagulants have to be stopped in time to restore clotting mechanism to its normal function.

• Drugs affecting catecholamine release or influencing the autonomic nervous system (reserpine, propranolol) should be stopped at least 48 hours in advance of the operation.

• Patients on chronic corticosteroid therapy require special care regarding their adrenal function.

• Antibiotics are not used prophylactically; however, active infections should be treated in advance of the operation.

3. Patients with metabolic disease (diabetes, gout, etc.) should be appropriately controlled prior to the operation.

Postoperative Management

Routine care includes the monitoring and periodic checking of the following:

• arterial pressure

• central venous pressure

• urinary output

- blood balance (blood loss through chest tubes and its replacement)
- sensorium
- respiratory status (including blood gases)
- cardiac rhythm
- hematocrit
- acid-base balance
- chest roentgenogram (2 to 4 times in the first 24 hours)
- 12-lead electrocardiogram (at least once in the first 24 hours)
- electroencephalogram, if clinically indicated.

Frequent physical examinations are performed, with special reference to evidences of cardiac failure, pulmonary abnormalities, and neurological abnormalities. In uncomplicated cases the patient wakes up promptly and usually requires a minimum of intervention except for analgesic drugs and intravenous fluid infusion. Assisted respiration is usually needed via the endotracheal tube at first, then a T-piece, and then a mask. Physiotherapy (breathing exercises) starts at once and the patient is encouraged to cough; the proper tracheobronchial "toilet" is important.

Early Postoperative Complications. These are most commonly related directly to the operation. They include:

1. *Excessive bleeding.* The range of blood loss varies greatly from patient to patient. Excessive bleeding requires surgical judgment regarding at which point it may be necessary to reopen the thorax in order to find the source of bleeding.

2. *Neurological damage.* Late regaining of consciousness, confusion, restlessness, and agitation occur frequently in older patients, and are almost always totally reversible. Prolonged coma and focal neurological damage usually is more serious, signifying brain damage due to embolism or cerebral ischemia.

3. *Cardiac failure.* Whenever clinical evidence of cardiac failure appears in the immediate postoperative period, it is imperative that a careful analysis of the various possible factors responsible for it be made. Such factors range from the insignificant and readily correctable to the very serious. They include:

- Hypervolemic overload due to too much or too rapid blood replacement;
- Ectopic tachyarrhythmias;

- Tamponade — pericardial or peri-cardiac hematoma;
- Myocardial damage — either pre-existing before the operation or surgically induced;
- Unsuccessful operation (reopening of a defect, poor valve repair, leaky valve prosthesis, etc.)

4. *Oliguria and anuria* may occur in patients who were in cardiac failure prior to the operation, in which case it is caused by sodium and water retention. It often responds well to the administration of diuretics. When associated with hypotension, it may be more serious, since it may be caused by failing cardiac function or by renal tubular necrosis.

5. *Hypotension* is most commonly a simple manifestation of hypovolemia. More serious causes include failing cardiac function (preshock state) and the "shock-lung" syndrome.

6. *Tachycardia,* ranging between 120 and 160, is frequently observed. A differentiation between sinus mechanism and ectopic tachycardias must be made, for treatment is different for each. Sinus tachycardia most frequently relates to hypovolemia or fever; occasionally the cause of it is not apparent. Ectopic tachycardias, including atrial flutter or fibrillation, should be treated conservatively; in patients who were on digitalis prior to the operation this drug should not be used to control such tachycardia, for the arrhythmias may be due to the operation's unmasking of latent digitalis toxicity. Many patients tolerate the rate of 150 without too much discomfort; should, however, cardiac failure or hypotension develop and it is thought to be related to the rapid rate, electroshock therapy may be necessary to terminate the ectopic rhythm. (Such intervention requires the ectopic origin of the tachycardia to be actually *proven.*) Intolerance of rapid rates may occur in prosthetic valves.

7. *Other forms of arrhythmias* — ventricular ectopic beats, salvos, tachycardias — may occur in response to hypoxia, acid base or electrolyte imbalance, or myocardial damage. Correction of the initiating cause, if such can be identified and is correctable, is a more appropriate approach than the use of antiarrhythmic drugs. If active antiarrhythmic therapy is needed, lidocaine is the drug of choice.

8. *Bradyarrhythmias* occur less frequently than rapid rhythms. The commonest is junctional bradycardia with an atrial standstill (or retrograde atrial activation); postoperative complete heart block occurs occasionally. Even though a temporary use of the pacemaker may be indicated by the patient's intolerance of slow rates, most such slow rhythms are self-limited and require no long-range therapy.

9. *Hypoxia* is controlled by assisted respiration and the use of oxy-

gen. The persistence of hypoxia in spite of intensive ventilatory assistance is usually a sign of a serious problem, signifying a pulmonary complication (atelectasis or embolism) or severe cardiac failure.

10. *Icterus* occurs occasionally in the early postoperative period and is usually caused by excessive hemolysis, particularly in patients who prior to the operation were in chronic right ventricular failure.

11. *Excessive febrile reaction* occurs in some individuals without identifiable cause; it is necessary, nevertheless, to investigate the possibility of an infection and institute therapy based, whenever possible, on the identification of the infecting organism. Shotgun antibiotic therapy is to be discouraged.

Delayed (Intermediate) Complications. The complications just described include those that are characteristic of the immediate postsurgical period, although some of them could develop days or weeks thereafter. The following comments apply to complications primarily developing after the immediate postoperative period:

1. *Pulmonary complications;* these include atelectasis, pneumonitis, pleural effusion, and intrathoracic hematomas. These complications may necessitate prolonged use of assisted respiration and are frequent sources of a febrile postoperative course. Pulmonary complications occur more frequently in patients who exhibited prior to the operation obstructive pulmonary disease or who had severe elevation of pulmonary vascular resistance.

2. *Cardiac arrhythmias.* Ventricular ectopy and tachyarrhythmias occur characteristically during the immediate postoperative period. Atrial arrhythmias, on the other hand, are frequently delayed. Of the tachyarrhythmias, atrial flutter and fibrillation tend to appear later in the postoperative course than supraventricular tachycardias. Atrial arrhythmias, in general and atrial flutter or fibrillation in particular appear commonly in patients in whom the surgical procedure included manipulation or repair in the atria. Thus, atrial septal repair which traumatizes the right atrium and mitral valve surgery producing trauma to the left atrium show an incidence of postoperative atrial arrhythmias six times higher than ventricular septal repair or aortic valve surgery (in which areas other than the atria are the target of surgical manipulation). Atrial arrhythmias occur with a frequency ranging from 10 to 50 per cent in patients with atrial septal surgery or mitral valve surgery; the incidence increases sharply with age. The time of onset of such arrhythmias varies between 2 and 14 days after the operation, with only an occasional occurrence of arrhythmias beyond the second week. In the great majority of cases these arrhythmias revert to sinus rhythm either spontaneously or in response to quinidine treatment; occasionally electroshock therapy may be necessary. These

arrhythmias tend to be recurrent, but the tendency to arrhythmias subsides within a month or two after the operation.

3. *Psychotic episodes* and periods of confusion may occur with some delay; the more serious forms of neurological damage have already been mentioned as immediate sequelae. Confused periods and psychotic episodes occur frequently in elderly patients 2 to 10 days after the operation; their duration is variable, but in most cases such episodes clear within two to three weeks.

4. *Icterus* occurring early is, as stated, the result of hemolysis in the great majority of cases. It may develop at once, or after a few days' delay. Its duration varies, but it seldom lasts longer than three weeks. Late icterus due to hepatitis will be discussed below.

5. *Cardiac failure.* Sudden delayed appearance of cardiac failure requires immediate evaluation in order to determine its underlying mechanism. Simpler tests, such as electrocardiography, roentgenography, and echocardiography, often aid the carefully performed physical examination; in case of inconclusive findings, cardiac catheterization and angiocardiographic studies should be performed.

6. *Febrile episodes* that develop as a recrudescence after the temperature has returned to normal require a comprehensive search for the cause. Infective endocarditis, the most serious of all possibilities, is fortunately a rare postoperative complication. While blood cultures should be a part of the investigation, careful examination of the urinary tract, the respiratory apparatus, and the incision site should be made.

Late Complications and Sequelae of the Operation. Complications that develop after the patient has been discharged from the hospital include the following:

1. *Failure to improve* after the operation. When the patient after open heart surgery returns to reasonable activities he is expected to perform better than prior to the operation. This general rule does not apply, of course, to patients who are operated upon while asymptomatic or with minimal symptoms. Yet an evaluation of the effects of the operation may not be easy, for many patients are limited by incisional pain, incomplete clearing of pulmonary sequelae of the operation, or simply by physical deconditioning. In some patients it may take several months before the full benefit of the operation becomes apparent. Nevertheless, undue reduction of effort tolerance requires a thorough search for factors that may be responsible for it. These include:

• Unsatisfactory surgical repair,

• Misjudgment of the mechanical factor (correctable factor) as responsible for the patient's disability, when myocardial disease may have been its cause,

- Intraoperative myocardial damage,

- Postcardiotomy syndrome,

- Anemia,

- Hepatitis.

2. *Hepatitis* is estimated to develop in 1 to 5 per cent of patients who undergo open heart surgery. Its onset varies from a few weeks to six months after the operation. The severity of hepatitis varies from a subclinical illness, often discovered by laboratory studies taken in response to minor complaints, to serious and even fatal cases.

3. *Hemolytic anemia.* In addition to immediate postoperative hemolysis related to the massive blood transfusions at the time of the operation, some patients with prosthetic valves develop chronic hemolytic anemias as a result of continuous mechanical damage to the erythrocytes. This damage is almost always related to periprosthetic leaks. Mild and moderate hemolysis may not require therapy, but severe anemia often necessitates reoperation and replacement of the prosthesis.

4. *Systemic embolism* occurs most frequently, though not exclusively, in connection with prosthetic cardiac valves. The question as to whether the incidence of emboli is reduced by anticoagulant or platelet-antiaggregant therapy has not yet been resolved since no controlled studies have been reported. The introduction of newer models of prosthetic valves and the use of homograft and heterograft valves have materially reduced, though not completely eliminated, the incidence of embolic complications.

5. *Complications related to anticoagulant therapy.* As stated earlier, continuous oral anticoagulant therapy carries a considerable risk; whenever used in patients with prosthetic valves, occasional hemorrhagic complications of varying seriousness can be expected. Patients on anticoagulant regimens should be supervised regarding (a) the proper monitoring of prothrombin time, and (b) the presence or the development of contraindications to the continuation of such therapy (e.g., peptic ulcer).

6. *"Postpericardiotomy syndrome"* is a term applied to a variety of complications appearing with some delay after the operation. Although some defy efforts at classification, two sets of symptom-complexes are specific enough to be singled out:

- *A febrile illness* presumed to be due to an abnormal immune reaction; its symptoms and signs include chest pain, arthralgias, malaise, pleural and pericardial effusions, and occasionally cardiac failure.

• *Lymphocytic splenomegaly* — presumed to be a viral disease — can also be associated with fever and malaise; characteristically abnormal lymphocytes or monocytes appear in the blood smear and hepatosplenomegaly is often present; palpable lymph nodes may be found.

Both these complications are in the great majority of cases benign; their duration varies from a few days to two or three weeks, and they require no specific medication. Occasionally patients are quite ill, in which case steroid therapy has been applied successfully to produce remission. The rheumatic-like postpericardiotomy syndrome may take a cyclic course, recurring every few weeks or months for three to six remissions.

Bibliography

DeCesare W, Rath C, Hufnagel C: Hemolytic anemia of mechanical origin in aortic valve prosthesis. New Engl. J. Med. *272*:1045, 1965.

Humphries JO, Gott VL, Benson SW: Care of the patient undergoing valvular heart surgery. Prog. Cardiovasc. Dis. *15*:449, 1973.

Intersociety Commission for Heart Disease Resources: Optimal resources for cardiac surgery. Circulation *44*:A 221, 1971.

Kirklin JW, Rastelli GC: Low cardiac output after intracardiac operations. Prog. Cardiovasc. Dis. *10*:117, 1967.

Kornfeld DS, Zimberg S, Malm JR: Psychiatric complications of open-heart surgery. New Engl. J. Med. *273*:287, 1965.

Mundth ED, Austen WG: Postoperative intensive care in cardiac surgical patients. Prog. Cardiovasc. Dis. *11*:228, 1965.

Osborn JJ, Popper RW, Kerth WJ, Gerbode F: Respiratory insufficiency following open-heart surgery. Ann. Surg. *156*:638, 1962.

Popper RW, Knott JMS, Selzer A, Gerbode F: Arrhythmias in open heart surgery. I. Atrial septal defect. Amer. Heart J. *64*:455, 1962.

Popper RW, Selzer A, Osborn JJ, Kerth WJ, Robinson SJ, Gerbode F: Arrhythmias after cardiac surgery, II Cyanotic tetralogy of Fallot with comment regarding ventricular septal defect. Amer. Heart J. *68*:32, 1964.

Sanderson RG, Ellison JH, Benson JA, Starr A: Jaundice following open heart operations. Ann. Surg. *165*:217, 1967.

Seaman AJ, Starr A: A febrile postcardiotomy lymphocytic splenomegaly: new entity. Ann. Surg. *156*:956, 1962.

Selzer A, Popper RW, Gerbode F: Incidence and causes of arrhythmias following open heart surgery. Memorias del IV Congreso Mundial de Cardiologia, Mexico. *2*:145, 1963.

Selzer A, Kelly JJ Jr, Gerbode F, Kerth WJ, Osborn JJ, Popper RW: Case against routine use of digitalis in patients undergoing cardiac surgery. J.A.M.A. *195*:549, 1966.

Uricchio JF: The postcommissurotomy (post-pericardiotomy) syndrome. Amer. J. Cardiol. *12*:436, 1963.

Williams JF, Morrow AG, Braunwald E: The management of "medical" complications following cardiac operations. Circulation *32*:608, 1965.

14

Causes and Mechanisms of Cardiac Failure

Definitions. "Heart failure" is a term that is both too broad and too vague to have an adequate definition, especially in view of its literal connotation. Several definitions have been suggested, none of which is suitable without many qualifications and explanations. The best and most widely used definition states that "heart failure exists when the heart as a pump is incapable of meeting all metabolic demands of the body." Using this definition as a baseline, one can proceed with discussion of the problem in its broad sense.

The term "cardiac failure" is applied to a set of clinical signs and symptoms, therefore denoting *clinical* rather than physiological evidence of inadequacy of cardiac function. It is customarily used to describe evidence of functional abnormality of the heart at rest: the reduction of exercise tolerance caused by heart disease — a condition in which the pump obviously cannot meet the excess metabolic needs of tissues — is, in the usual connotation, not considered evidence of cardiac failure.

Causes of cardiac failure in its clinical context involve three general mechanisms. Only the first two strictly qualify for the term cardiac failure as the primary process; the third involves secondary effects upon the heart.

1. Pump failure produced by *increase* in cardiac workload that taxes the myocardial reserve beyond its capability.

2. Pump failure caused by anatomic or functional alteration of the myocardium that makes the weakened ventricle incapable of carrying out adequately the *normal* load.

3. Conditions that interfere with the pumping action of the heart but do not directly involve myocardial function.

The first mechanism includes potentially all conditions in which the workload of the heart is increased. The heart may fail acutely in response to a sudden intolerable overload, such as is exemplified by a perforation of a valve in infective endocarditis or, more often, chronically by exhausting the reserve capability of the ventricle that has developed compensatory hypertrophy.

The second mechanism operates in conditions that involve various forms of myocardial disease or focal damage to the myocardium produced by ischemic insults. Here, too, acute failure may ensue (e.g., acute myocardial infarction), or the heart may fail gradually, chronically.

The third mechanism involves various processes in which there is interference with the movement of blood, usually by reduction of inflow to the heart. It includes the following conditions:

- Reduced blood volume and venous return—noncardiac shock;

- Interference with the diastolic filling of the heart by excessive tachycardia;

- Pericardial tamponade and pericardial constriction;

- Stenosis of atrioventricular valves interfering with ventricular filling;

- Mechanical obstacles: tumors, large thrombi;

- Extreme bradycardia.

These conditions, as stated, are not included in the concept of cardiac failure, although their clinical consequences overlap with those of heart failure.

DEVELOPMENT OF CARDIAC FAILURE

Cardiac Reserve. Under ordinary conditions the resting workload of the heart constitutes only a small part of its top capabilities. The metabolic needs of strenuous exercises may be as much as 20 times its resting demands. However the cardiac workload does not rise in proportion to the increase in demands, thanks to the normal oxygen reserve in the arterial blood. The arterial blood is 95 per cent saturated with oxygen; the venous blood returning to the heart is ordinarily 75 per cent saturated with oxygen; consequently only 20 per cent of the oxygen supply is extracted by the tissues. Thus, if oxygen demands during heavy work increase 20-fold, they can be met by extracting four times more oxygen from arterial blood and, in addition, by increasing the cardiac output five times, thereby offering five times more oxygenated blood. Inasmuch as there is a slight increase in arterial pressure during exercise, the cardiac workload upon each ventricle (roughly, the product of pressure and cardiac output) during maximum exercise rises to between five and six times its basal level. There is evidence to show that the weight of the heart is related to the amount of work performed by an individual; thus a physiological work hypertrophy occurs in an analogous fashion to hypertrophy of exercising skeletal muscles. In general, the voluntary increase in cardiac load is well tolerated. There is no evidence that heart failure can develop as a result of strenuous exercise in the absence of some pathological process.

In contrast to voluntary workload and its consequence, namely the physiological hypertrophy of the cardiac ventricles, cardiac disease may impose an involuntary cardiac overload. Such increase in cardiac workload differs from that of the voluntary workload in the fact it operates continuously rather than intermittently. It constitutes a stimulus for pathological hypertrophy. It is probable that the physiological cardiac hypertrophy and mild degree of pathological cardiac hypertrophy overlap and are identical. However, pathological hypertrophy, by the time it becomes clinically recognizable, has already surpassed the degree of hypertrophy that voluntary exercise can produce.

Hypertrophy. Increased size of a cardiac ventricle is basically a compensatory phenomenon. Increase in cardiac workload is the principal, though not the only, stimulus for the growth of myocardial fibers. Work hypertrophy occurs typically in hypertension of either circuit, in valvular heart disease, and in some congenital cardiac lesions. A related type of cardiac hypertrophy develops in ischemic heart disease in which replacement of cardiac fibers by fibrosis reduces their number to a point that the normal cardiac workload becomes excessive for the number of available fibers. Cardiac failure — presumably the process of chronic dilatation and stretch of a cardiac chamber — also may lead to hypertrophy of the affected ventricle. Finally certain humoral stimuli (catecholamines ?) are believed to produce myocardial hypertrophy without increase in cardiac workload. This mechanism may be operative in "idiopathic" types of cardiac hypertrophy which occur in some forms of cardiomyopathy.

There are inherent disadvantages related to the function of a hypertrophied myocardial fiber as compared with a normal fiber. Even though clinically hypertrophied hearts may seem to perform normally, even supernormally, refined tests of cardiac function often show some impairment of their performance. Thus, once an abnormal workload develops and provides the stimulus for compensatory cardiac hypertrophy, an abnormal process is initiated which constitutes a continuum, with fully compensated hypertrophy on one end and cardiac failure (decompensation) on the other.

Theoretically, the process of work hypertrophy is reversible: if the stimulus ceases to exist hypertrophy regresses. This, however, does not always occur in cardiac disease. Medical or surgical treatment of conditions overloading the heart leads to regression of clinical signs of cardiac hypertrophy. Yet, in many instances the cardiac ventricle remains hypertrophied and its function stays abnormal. It is as if there was a "point of no return" in the process of hypertrophy. It has long been believed, even though the evidence is not conclusive, that hypertrophied fibers may have impaired oxygen delivery, thus show relative ischemia (in spite of adequate coronary blood supply). Large hearts often show subendocardial fibrosis similar to that found in ischemic heart disease. Thus, the change from latent to overt malfunction of a hypertrophied ventricle represents the onset of "decompensation."

There are two basic types of external workload:

- Preload—i.e., the handling of venous return;

- Afterload—i.e., working against peripheral resistance.

Pathological increase in cardiac workload is thus produced either by increased preload ("volume overload", "diastolic overload") or by increased afterload ("pressure overload", "systolic overload").

Responses of the ventricle to increased workload of each type are not identical. In volume overload hypertrophy is associated with dilatation; in pressure overload the size of the chamber (its end-systolic volume) remains normal, leading to "concentric" cardiac hypertrophy. In the latter case ventricular dilatation appears late, only when overt cardiac failure makes its appearance.

The process of compensatory hypertrophy and of decompensation shows a great individual variability. Some patients develop a pronounced degree of hypertrophy in response to a certain excess workload, whereas others might develop only mild hypertrophy with a similar workload. Similarly, hearts may fail weighing 500 gm. in some patients, while in others under seemingly similar circumstances the heart can grow to a weight of 1,200 gm.

The two cardiac ventricles act as two independent pumps, each subject to its own workload. Thus abnormal increase in workload affects each ventricle separately; furthermore, each ventricle can decompensate without affecting the function of the other.

As mentioned above, decompensation of a hypertrophied cardiac ventricle is one of two mechanisms producing primary pump failure. The other factor is *damage to the myocardium.* A variety of conditions may affect adversely the myocardium; they include inflammatory, metabolic, and ischemic factors. Myocardial disease may involve the entire ventricle—even the entire heart—may be scattered throughout a ventricle, or may affect circumscribed areas of the myocardium. In many such cases secondary hypertrophy develops, as explained above, which may produce an overlap with the first mechanism.

It should be pointed out that in most cases of chronic cardiac failure cardiac hypertrophy and myocardial damage coexist and operate jointly in maintaining impaired cardiac function; primary myocardial disease produces secondary hypertrophy; cardiac hypertrophy leads to myocardial damage. However, in acute forms of cardiac failure (e.g., acute myocarditis, acute valvular regurgitation) the two principal mechanisms producing cardiac failure act separately.

Nonmyocardial causes of circulatory failure are listed above; they involve neither increased workload nor the myocardium. The principal mechanism of producing clinical manifestations similar to those of cardiac failure is the reduction of venous return, which in turn reduces cardiac output and results in the elevation of atrial pressures. Some of these interfere with the overall cardiac performance acutely and temporarily, such as in pericardial tamponade or tachycardia; in others a chronic obstruction to flow is maintained (e.g., mitral stenosis). The importance of this group lies in the fact that basically functional abnormalities are reversible by means other than treatment of cardiac failure.

In the foregoing discussion cardiac failure is presented as the endpoint to the capability of the myocardium to carry a given workload with physiological responses. Frequently, however, the development of cardiac failure occurs earlier than the exhaustion of compensatory powers of the myocardium, namely in response to various extraneous precipitating factors. Among such factors are the following:

- Arrhythmias: extremes of cardiac rate, loss of atrial transport function, loss of energy due to ineffective contraction (bigeminy, atrial fibrillation);

- Infections increasing metabolic demands upon the circulation (the commonest—respiratory infection);

- Additional increase in workload: voluntary (excessive exercise) or involuntary (pregnancy);

- Intercurrent or additional disease (hypertension, ischemic insults, pulmonary disease, renal disease);

- Excessive salt loading.

The importance of the precipitating factors lies in their potential reversibility, hence cardiac failure occurring in response to one of these causes carries a better outlook than that occurring spontaneously.

CAUSES OF CARDIAC FAILURE

The various conditions that can produce cardiac failure can be divided into those producing failure of the left ventricle, of the right ventricle, and of both ventricles. Failure may develop acutely or chronically.

Conditions primarily overloading the left ventricle include the following:

1. Acute

    a. Sudden development of incompetence of the aortic or mitral valve (valve perforation, rupture of chordae tendineae, rupture of head of papillary muscle)

    b. Hypertensive crisis

2. Chronic

    a. Aortic stenosis

    b. Aortic regurgitation

    c. Hypertension

    d. Patent ductus arteriosus

Conditions primarily overloading the right ventricle:

1. Acute

    a. Massive pulmonary embolism

2. Chronic

    a. Pulmonary stenosis

    b. Atrial septal defect

    c. Pulmonary hypertension

Conditions affecting both ventricles:

1. Acute

    a. Perforation of ventricular septum

    b. Acute arteriovenous fistula

2. Chronic

    a. Mitral regurgitation

   b. Ventricular septal defect

   c. Various high output states

   d. Various combined valve lesions

Conditions affecting primarily the myocardium:

1. Acute

   a. Temporary ischemia (anginal attacks)

   b. Acute myocardial infarction

   c. Acute myocarditis

2. Chronic

   a. Chronic myocardial disease

   b. Late stage of ischemic heart disease

   c. Late stage of cardiac hypertrophy

HIGH OUTPUT STATES

During the past two decades, when physiological measurements in man became commonplace, many patients were found to have cardiac output higher than normal. It was also observed that clinical evidence of cardiac failure could be found in patients who had higher than normal cardiac output. The concepts of "high output state" and "high output failure" were introduced. More recently some doubt has been expressed as to whether the term "high output failure" is really justifiable; if it is, it may be a rare condition, given out-of-proportion importance in many books and articles.

The causes of higher-than-average cardiac output are manifold. The difficulty in approaching this condition critically lies in the fact that apprehension on the part of the patient who undergoes physiological studies manifests itself by a high oxygen consumption, hence producing temporarily high output related to an unsteady physiological state. Thus only repeated determinations of cardiac output with reasonable evidence that the patient approaches a basal condition should be accepted in assessing the "high output state."

The generally recognized conditions that sometimes, but not always, may be associated with elevated resting cardiac output include the following (see also Chapter 42):

1. Increase in metabolic needs of tissues (hyperthyroidism, occasionally pheochromocytoma);

2. Early stages of essential (idiopathic) hypertension;

3. Obligatory connections between high and low pressure areas in the circulation: intracardiac shunts, aortopulmonary or aortocardiac shunt, arteriovenous shunts and fistulas;

4. Idiopathic high output state (probably a very rare condition).

Circulatory interconnections listed above include conditions in which high cardiac output is limited to only one side of the circulation (intracardiac shunts) and those with a hypercirculatory state within both circuits (arteriovenous fistula).

Theoretically, high output failure includes patients with well-documented clinical signs and symptoms of cardiac failure in whom an abnormally elevated resting cardiac output is found. One could well imagine that if a 20 L./min. flow through the heart is produced by a peripheral arteriovenous fistula, an overloaded, failing heart may still eject 10 L./min. while in failure. It is, however, difficult to locate many authenticated cases exhibiting such findings.

PHYSIOLOGICAL CONSEQUENCES OF CARDIAC FAILURE

Inasmuch as the principal function of the heart is the delivery of oxygen to the tissues, impaired function of the pump results first of all in inadequate oxygen delivery at times when the demand is elevated. Thus, even though *clinical* criteria for cardiac failure require some evidence of cardiac malfunction at rest, its *physiological* manifestations are first evident during exercise. Yet such malfunction merely produces earlier termination of the voluntary effort; upon cessation of exercise abnormalities may disappear and adequate oxygen delivery may be re-established.

Left ventricular failure constitutes the principal form of cardiac failure. Ventricular function in general is customarily expressed in terms of the relationship between ventricular filling pressure and the cardiac output. Function curves depict this relationship by indicating the quantity of blood ejected for each increment of filling pressure (Fig. 14–1). Thus significant impairment of cardiac function occurs when higher pressures are needed to eject equivalent quantities of blood compared with the prefailure function. When abnormal cardiac function is present under resting conditions, circulatory derangement may take place in one of two ways:

1. Normal cardiac output is ejected with abnormally high filling pressure;

2. Abnormally low cardiac output is ejected with a normal filling pressure.

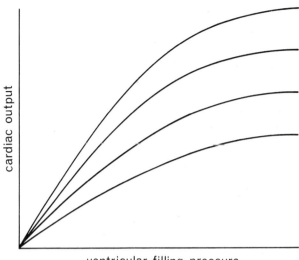

cardiac output

ventricular filling pressure

Figure 14-1. A "family" of ventricular function curves showing the relationship between (left) ventricular filling pressure and cardiac output. The two lower curves exemplify depressed ventricular function; the upper curves, normal function.

It is only in advanced forms of cardiac failure—usually its chronic form—that *both* low cardiac output and elevated filling pressure is found. The diagrammatic presentation of events leading to cardiac failure is depicted in Figure 14–2.

When the ventricular *filling pressure* is abnormally elevated, the presence of cardiac failure is implied but not definitely demonstrated. Such finding requires differentiation between cardiac failure and an altered ventricular function curve due to decreased compliance of the ventricle. It has been demonstrated that a hypertrophied ventricle or a ventricle affected by ischemia or fibrosis is less compliant than normal ventricles, and therefore requires higher filling pressure to eject a comparable amount of blood to those under normal conditions. While during resting state low compliance and early heart failure overlap, responses to exercise are more normal in patients with noncompliant ventricles than in those in cardiac failure.

The immediate consequences of cardiac failure are more pronounced in patients who show a predominant elevation of filling pressure than in those with lowered cardiac output. High ventricular filling pressure—elevated left atrial pressure—raises the pressure gradient across the lungs, hence increases pulmonary capillary pressure and pulmonary arterial pressures. When the right ventricle responds normally to the increased load of pulmonary hypertension, a temporary discrepancy between outputs of the two ventricles may develop, producing an

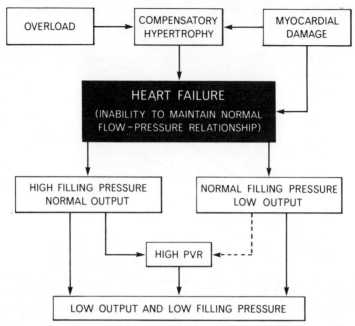

Figure 14-2. Diagrammatic presentation of factors leading to cardiac failure and their physiological consequences. (PVR — pulmonary vascular resistance).

increase in the central (i.e., intrapulmonary) blood volume. The combination of high pulmonary capillary pressure and increase in central blood volume often alters pulmonary mechanics, producing shortness of breath. Sudden increase in pulmonary capillary pressure in patients who never had the opportunity to develop adaptive mechanisms may produce pulmonary edema. Finally, in some patients — pulmonary vascular hyperreactors (about 15 to 20 per cent of the population) — pulmonary arteriolar spasm may develop via a reflex initiated by left atrial hypertension, producing severe pulmonary hypertension and increased load upon the right ventricle.

The development of lowered cardiac output at rest has relatively little immediate effect upon the circulation unless the reduction is extreme. The intricate regulatory mechanism adjusting regional flows reduces some of the more wasteful circuits, directing more blood to the essential organs. Furthermore, tissues can extract more oxygen from the ample reserve in the blood. However, at a certain point the limitation of regional flow initiates a process of retention of sodium and water (partly from fall in renal perfusion, partly from hormonal imbalance), which eventually produces one of the major problems accompanying cardiac failure — edema and fluid retention. This may be aggravated by increased hydrostatic pressure in the capillaries, which occurs in right ventricular failure, if present.

A sudden severe fall in cardiac output involves some of the *acute* emergencies that develop as a result of acute cardiac failure. The most extreme form is cardiac arrest — a total cessation of the pumping action produced by ventricular standstill, by ventricular fibrillation, or by critical tachyarrhythmias so rapid that no effective ejection of blood is possible. Cardiac arrest produces instant hypoxic cessation of cerebral function. Reversibility of brain function represents the critical point at issue, regardless of whether or not cardiac function can be re-established.

Serious impairment of cardiac function produced by an abrupt fall in cardiac output may lead to the clinical syndrome of *shock.* The clinical spectrum involving syncope, collapse, and shock has a common physiological basis — inadequate (or absent) perfusion of the brain and other essential regions of the body. Hypoperfusion of organs may be caused by a wide variety of mechanism within or without the heart. Such mechanisms include the following:

- Inability to maintain adequate perfusion pressure due to failure of the pressor-regulating mechanism. This includes postural faints, vasovagal syncope, and related functional disturbances.

- Reduction of blood volume with resulting decrease of venous return to the heart: included here are various peripheral forms of shock, such as hemorrhagic and septic.

- Cardiogenic shock produced by pump failure: acute myocardial infarction, acute development of overload (perforation of a valve, perforation of the ventricular septum, rupture of a papillary muscle, massive pulmonary embolism, etc.).

- Cardiogenic shock produced by nonmyocardial factors (pericardial tamponade, excessive, but not critical, tachy- or bradyarrhythmias).

The essence of shock syndromes is thus the sudden fall in cardiac output from a variety of causes. The filling pressures vary — their level is of relatively little importance in the physiological consequences of shock. In cardiogenic forms of shock (myocardial and nonmyocardial alike) filling pressures are elevated; pulmonary edema is rare but may develop in association with shock. However, high diastolic pressures may be present only during the initial stage. Once the vicious circle of shock sets in, the effective circulating blood volume may be reduced, the venous return may fall, and diastolic pressure in the ventricle may return to normal. The essential determinant of shock is the individual adaptation to the sudden fall in cardiac output. Some patients develop severe vasoconstriction; the arterial pressure may be maintained through this mechanism, yet organ perfusion may be seriously impaired. Some patients develop excessive fall in arterial pressure owing to inadequate adaptation of the pressure-regulating mechanism. In these, organ perfusion may also be impaired by low perfusion pressure. Thus, it should be realized that the level of arterial pressure is a poor index of the adequacy of circulatory adaptation to shock. It is likely that the center band of the spectrum — patients who neither develop excessive arterial hypotension nor excessive vasoconstriction — represent those with a good physiological adaptation, who may not go into shock in spite of severe reduction of cardiac output.

The serious consequences of reduction of cardiac output develop only in acute stages of cardiac failure. Chronic cardiac failure characterized by a low cardiac output produces no characteristic clinical manifestations comparable to those secondary to high filling pressures. Only when very low cardiac output persists over long periods of time may it affect the overall metabolic activity of the body and produce cardiac cachexia. An inconstant clinical counterpart of low cardiac output is fatigability that may limit the patient's activity; more typically, shortness of breath is the limiting factor.

Failure of the *right ventricle* is, as stated, much less common than left ventricular failure. The right ventricle, its workload being only a fraction of that of the left, may play a satellite role and fail secondarily to left ventricular failure. The old clinical truism stating that the commonest cause of right ventricular failure is failure of the left ventricle holds true and has a sound physiological basis. Elevation of pulmonary arterial pressure secondary to high left ventricular filling pressure increases right ventricular workload. This is occasionally magnified by the pulmonary arteriolar constriction that develops in some patients in cardiac failure. The right ventricle may tolerate the additional load adequately or may fail in response to it. Primary failure of the right ventricle caused by right-sided cardiac lesions elevates right ventricular filling pressures and often renders the tricuspid valve incompetent. Yet the clinical manifestations of this are less pronounced than left-sided pressure rises. Producing few symptoms, right-sided failure presents no difficulty in its clinical recognition, since hypertension in the caval system is subject to direct recognition by inspection.

REVERSIBILITY OF CARDIAC FAILURE

One of the crucial points concerning the subject of heart failure is whether or not cardiac function can be significantly improved and whether entirely normal circulatory functions can be re-established in patients who are in cardiac failure. This point, briefly touched upon earlier, requires further amplification.

The theoretical possibilities concerning improvement in cardiac function are:

1. Cardiac failure may be eliminated by removal of its causes.

2. Cardiac failure may be eliminated by effective cardiac therapy aiming at improvement of cardiac function.

It should be obvious that the elimination of clinical signs and symptoms associated with cardiac failure is simplest in conditions in which the heart itself is not involved in the process. Thus, elimination of arrhythmias, correction of pericardial tamponade or constriction, removal of tumors, and correction of atrioventricular valve stenosis all produce restoration of the normal or near-normal circulatory dynamics to the extent such complete elimination of the causative factors is possible.

In the group of patients who develop cardiac failure after a long period of cardiac overload, reversibility is less well understood. As mentioned, compensatory hypertrophy may regress when the overload is eliminated. Among the examples of such regression — in addition to those in animal studies — are the physiological disappearance of right ventricular hypertrophy of the postnatal period, indirect evidence of regression of ventricular hypertrophy after successful pulmonary valvotomy for pulmonic stenosis, and regression after effective anti-hypertensive therapy in severe hypertension. Patients with successfully treated valvular disease in the older age group (e.g., aortic valve disease) may fail to show significant regression of ventricular hypertrophy. Nevertheless, even if no reversal of hypertrophy is accomplished, cardiac failure can often be effectively eliminated by the reduction of the cardiac workload, which permits improvement in function even if normalization is not produced.

Cardiac failure produced by myocardial disease is, as a rule, not amenable to the elimination of its cause; the exception can be found in the rare cases of focal myocardial disease — e.g., aneurysms — with serious hemodynamic consequences, in which surgical resection of the defect may significantly improve circulatory dynamics.

The elimination of cardiac failure by means of medical therapy aimed at improving cardiac function is disappointing, when looked upon from the hemodynamic standpoint. Regardless of how dramatic results of therapy may appear clinically, patients who were in chronic cardiac failure seldom show significant hemodynamic normalization in response to therapy. One is thus justified in considering medical therapy of cardiac failure as a means of *controlling* rather than *eliminating* cardiac failure.

It should be emphasized that the above remarks apply to patients with chronic cardiac failure. Many acute forms of heart failure affect circulatory functions only temporarily, and the functions revert to normal either spontaneously or in response to simple medical measures. As examples one can mention here ischemic attacks producing immediately reversible cardiac failure, heart failure that may develop in uncomplicated attacks of acute myocardial infarction, or cardiac failure in the course of acute myocarditis, e.g., in rheumatic fever.

Bibliography

Badeer HS: Metabolic bases of cardiac hypertrophy. Prog. Cardiovasc. Dis. *11*:53, 1968.

Braunwald E, Ross J Jr, Sonnenblick EH: Mechanisms of contraction of the normal and failing heart. New Engl. J. Med. *277*:794, 853, 910, 1012, 1967.

Dodge HT, Baxley WA: Hemodynamic aspects of heart failure. Amer. J. Cardiol. *22*:24, 1968.

Fishman AP: Pulmonary edema—The water exchanging function of the lungs. Circulation *46*:390, 1972.

Friedberg CK: Edema and pulmonary edema. Pathological physiology and differential diagnosis. Prog. Cardiovasc. Dis. *13*:546, 1971.

Genest J, Granger P, DeChamplain J, Boucher R: Endocrine factors in congestive heart failure. Amer. J. Cardiol. *22*:35, 1968.

Robin ED, Cross CE, Zelis R: Pulmonary edema. New Engl. J. Med. *288*:239, 292, 1973.

Shillingford J, Thomas M: Hemodynamic effects of acute myocardial infarction in man. Prog. Cardiovasc. Dis. *9*:570, 1967.

Selzer A, McCaughey DJ: Hemodynamic patterns in chronic cardiac failure. Amer. J. Med. *28*:337, 1960.

Selzer A: Hemodynamic sequelae of sustained elevation of left atrial pressure. Circulation *20*:243, 1959.

Spodick DH: Acute tamponade. Diagnosis and management. Progress Cardiovasc. Dis. *10*:64, 1967.

Swan HJC, Forrester JS, Diamond G, Chatterjee K, Parmley WW: Hemodynamic spectrum of myocardial infarction and cardiogenic shock. A conceptual model. Circulation *45*:197, 1972.

Thal AP, Kinney JM: On the definite classification of shock. Prog. Cardiovasc. Dis. *9*:527, 1967.

Wright RE Jr, McIntosh HD: Syncope: A review of pathophysiological mechanisms; Prog. Cardiovasc. Dis. *23*:580, 1971.

15

Recognition and Evaluation of Cardiac Failure

The clinical spectrum of cardiac failure encompasses a broad range of severity. In mild heart failure the diagnosis may be difficult; in severe failure it is often apparent at a glance. A clinician approaching the problem of a patient suspected of being in cardiac failure has to concentrate upon several questions:

- Are the symptoms and signs under consideration actually caused by cardiac failure?

- Is there an acute or a chronic process?

- Is the nature of the underlying process known?

- Is there a precipitating factor responsible for this bout of failure and, if so, is it reversible?

- How severe is cardiac failure?

- Is there a possibility of directing therapeutic efforts toward the *cause* of cardiac failure, or only toward its *manifestations*?

Many times the answers to some of these questions are self-evident. However, the problem may be one of considerable perplexity, as the discussion that follows will show.

HISTORY

When taking a history of a patient who may be in cardiac failure, some areas have to be explored in depth:

1. The effort tolerance and its limitation by dyspnea;

2.   The presence or absence of other forms of dyspnea: paroxysmal nocturnal dyspnea, orthopnea, Cheyne-Stokes respiration, nocturnal attacks of coughing;

3.   Wide variations of body weight and details of urinary output—both as manifestations of fluid retention;

4.   The possibility of fatigability as a manifestation of cardiac failure;

5.   Background details that may suggest the presence of chronic cardiac disease responsible for heart failure: rheumatic fever, knowledge of cardiac disease in the past, hypertension, etc.;

6.   Background details that may offer an alternative explanation for signs and symptoms: chronic pulmonary disease, anemia, renal disease, endocrine imbalance.

Each detail of the history has to be critically examined and evaluated along the lines suggested in Chapter 3. Of particular importance is the appraisal of dyspnea, which constitutes the cardinal symptom of impending or existing left ventricular failure. For example, one has to avoid the pitfalls of considering dyspnea due to poor physical conditioning as evidence of impaired left ventricular function, or of accepting hyperventilation as paroxysmal dyspnea. In differentiation between dyspnea due to cardiac disease from that produced by respiratory disease, it should be noted that dyspnea in chronic obstructive lung disease is usually slowly and gradually progressive except in the presence of obvious respiratory infections; in cardiac dyspnea wide fluctuations of the effort tolerance and of its paroxysmal forms are common.

In evaluating evidences of fluid retention, particular attention should be paid to premenopausal women who occasionally show an exaggeration of perimenstrual fluid retention. Such patients are occasionally misdiagnosed as presenting cardiac failure.

Points elicited from the history need to be examined from the negative standpoint as well. As an example of a false-positive background history one may cite patients with known valvular heart disease whose dyspnea is caused by coexisting obstructive lung disease with no direct cardiac participation in the origin of their disability.

PHYSICAL EXAMINATION

Physical findings vary widely with the extent of cardiac failure, with its duration, and with the involvement of one or both ventricles. Under the overall term of cardiac failure are included some special forms of acute heart failure, as defined in the preceding chapter.

Cardiac arrest and syncope represent the extreme forms of acute cardiac failure in which there is sudden cessation of an effective pumping action. The two mechanisms — ventricular standstill and ventricular fibrillation — may persist until corrected or until death ensues, or may be self-limited, temporary, or paroxysmal.

When examining a patient in collapse, the critical issue is to determine the following:

- Whether or not there is effective cardiac action;

- The rhythm (standstill, ventricular fibrillation, extreme tachycardia or bradycardia);

- The state of cerebration (patient totally or partially unresponsive, convulsive seizures).

While resuscitative procedures are being conducted, further information can be obtained from the family.

Shock represents the next portion of the continuum with a considerable overlap with syncope. The critical issues in the physical examination include the following:

- color (flushing vs. pallor),

- sensorium (responsiveness, restlessness),

- cardiac rate and rhythm,

- quality of peripheral pulses,

- evidence of vasoconstriction, skin temperature, perspiration,

- estimation of venous pressure,

- signs of pulmonary congestion,

- level of arterial pressure.

These points may provide information helpful in the differential diagnosis of shock, specifically in separating cardiogenic shock from simple vasomotor collapse (including vasovagal attack) or noncardiac shock.

Positive signs pointing to cardiac origin of shock include evidence of myocardial infarction (by history, electrocardiography), presence of elevated venous pressure, and presence of pulmonary vascular congestion. On the negative side, evidence for involvement of other organs or systems, bleeding, presence of serious infection, and a history of diabetes all point to mechanisms other than the heart. Excessive bradycardia or tachycardia, if present, increase the probability of cardiac mechanism of shock.

Acute pulmonary edema is the most common manifestation of acute left ventricular failure. The characteristic picture of a patient, dyspneic and anxious, coughing and expectorating frothy pink sputum, is well enough known and needs no further elaboration. Occasionally differential diagnostic difficulties may arise in the following areas:

- Associated bronchospasm may cause the pulmonary edema of left ventricular failure to be confused with bronchial asthma;

- Pulmonary edema — as demonstrated by radiography — may have only minimal physical signs (in patients with emphysema).

- Pulmonary edema due to other mechanisms (high altitude, heroin) resembles left ventricular failure.

Physical findings supporting the diagnosis of pulmonary edema due to left ventricular failure include the following:

- evidence of left ventricular hypertrophy,

- gallop sounds,

- increased venous pressure,

- evidence pointing to acute myocardial infarction.

Acute right ventricular failure is a characteristic finding in massive pulmonary embolism and will be discussed in Chapter 40.

Chronic cardiac failure presents itself with the conventional clinical signs; it may involve failure of the left ventricle, of the right ventricle, or of both ventricles. Physical examination of patients in chronic cardiac failure involves signs affecting the heart, the arterial system, the venous system, and various peripheral signs.

In inspecting a patient several important points can be observed:

Cyanosis is commonly found in patients in cardiac failure. It may be produced by a central or peripheral mechanism. Central cyanosis — that associated with lowered arterial oxygen saturation — is most commonly related to impaired pulmonary oxygen exchange; rarely reversed shunting through a patent foramen ovale may produce hypoxemia. Peripheral cyanosis is an indication of low cardiac output and often is associated with signs of vasoconstriction.

Icterus may be present in patients with chronic right ventricular failure, particularly when chronic tricuspid valve incompetence is present. The mixture of cyanosis and jaundice often gives such patients a characteristic appearance.

Malar flush — red color of cheeks associated with a slightly cyanotic hue — is also evidence of low cardiac output. It is most commonly found in patients with mitral stenosis with pulmonary hypertension.

Other details perceived upon inspection include signs of dyspnea—obvious respiratory distress during talking or moving about the room; ascites, occasionally presenting itself as a very prominent clinical feature; and cardiac cachexia, which may be encountered in patients with long-standing cardiac failure.

Given a patient with *pure left ventricular failure,* physical findings are subtle. The principal sign is an S3 gallop sound, which may be palpated and auscultated. The evaluation of an S3 gallop should be done with caution, especially in younger individuals. In some patients with increased flow through the mitral valve an S3 gallop sound may be present without cardiac failure, as explained in Chapter 3.

Given a patient with cardiac disease affecting the left ventricle, the presence of an S3 gallop sound does not automatically mean chronic cardiac failure. This sign may appear temporarily during and after exercise, or during anginal attacks. A permanent S3 gallop occasionally precedes other evidence of cardiac failure by months or even years. Nevertheless, with the exceptions noted here, it is a highly specific sign of left ventricular functional abnormality, signifying pressure abnormalities in the left atrium and left ventricle during the *early* diastolic period.

The presence of an S4 gallop sound in cardiac failure is common in patients who are in sinus rhythm (its validity as an abnormal sign is contingent upon a normal P-R interval). It is, as indicated earlier, a sign of low specificity, since it is related to altered left ventricular compliance as well as to left ventricular failure. Therefore, it is often present in left ventricular hypertrophy without any impairment of function. It is also present in many normal individuals over the age of 50. Its value as a sign of cardiac failure lies in its occasional prominent appearance in patients followed longitudinally.

Pulmonary rales constitute the traditional sign of pulmonary congestion secondary to left ventricular failure. They are a clinical finding of low reliability. Medium or coarse rales of pulmonary edema are good evidence of pulmonary "congestion". However, fine basal rales may be produced by factors other than left ventricular failure. Conversely, pulmonary rales are absent in left ventricular failure often enough so that clear lungs on auscultation are of little diagnostic aid.

Elevated venous pressure is the cardinal sign of right ventricular failure. Inspection of the venous pulse above the clavicles and of the deep jugular pulse permits easy detection of systemic venous hypertension. The pulse contour is also usually altered: in right ventricular failure a rapid *y*-descent is usually present. When the *v*-wave appears exaggerated, the presence of tricuspid regurgitation is likely to be found. It should be emphasized that right ventricular failure secondary to left ventricular failure is often found only initially. Treatment—often merely putting the patient to bed—promptly reverses right ventricular failure, even if signs of tricuspid valve incompetence were present.

Fluid retention is a feature of both left ventricular failure and right ventricular failure. It is well recognized that as much as 3 to 5 kg. of fluid may be retained without any clinical evidence. When fluid retention is clinically evident, hydrothorax and ankle edema are usually the early signs; extensive anasarca and ascites are apt to be present with long-standing, neglected cardiac failure. In the differential diagnosis one should look with suspicion at unilateral hydrothorax or unilateral ankle edema as possibly caused by noncardiac factors. Other causes of fluid retention, in general, should be adequately weighted in the differential diagnosis.

Pulsus alternans is a clinical sign that is moderately specific for left ventricular failure. The finding of pulsus alternans is detected by careful examination (disappearance of alternate arterial sounds upon inflation of the blood pressure cuff to a point of 10 to 20 mm. Hg below the systolic level in patients with regular sinus rhythm).

Physical examination in patients suspected of presenting cardiac failure includes, of course, a search for the presence of heart disease that may represent the basis for cardiac failure. Of particular importance are evidences of hypertrophy of either or both ventricles. The presence of valvular heart disease, congenital lesions, hypertension, or ischemic heart disease may represent the background upon which heart failure develops. Equally important as the presenting signs in the physical examination is a search for a precipitating factor, as explained in Chapter 14.

RADIOGRAPHY

Radiography plays an important role in the diagnosis of cardiac failure. While its role in general has been discussed earlier, two specific points are relevant to the recognition and the differential diagnosis of cardiac failure:

1. The presence of cardiac enlargement,

2. The presence of pulmonary vascular congestion.

Cardiac enlargement is not an obligatory finding in patients in cardiac failure. It is, nevertheless, unusual for patients to develop heart failure with a normal-sized heart. Thus, the presence of a normal-sized heart (particularly one in the lower range of normalcy) should cause one to give priority to a diagnosis other than cardiac failure as an explanation of suspicious clinical findings.

"Pulmonary vascular congestion" is a rather ill-defined combination of accentuated vascular shadows with prominence of the larger pulmonary veins, especially upper zone vessel dilatation. It overlaps with the normal film, with increased bronchial markings in bronchitis, and even with left-to-right shunts of congenital heart disease. Nevertheless, pulmonary vascular congestion, especially when combined with small amounts of pleural fluid in both costrophrenic angles, represents an important confirmatory sign of cardiac failure. It is particularly important as a means of following the progress of the patient: serial tracings permit the patient to act as his own control in the evaluation of the pulmonary vascular changes. It is important that meticulous technique be used to make films comparable with each other. The extreme form of pulmonary vascular congestion radiographically is the picture of acute pulmonary edema with its characteristic "butterfly" or "snowstorm" appearance.

ELECTROCARDIOGRAPHY

Electrocardiography is basically unrelated to cardiac function, so that the change from a compensated state to severe cardiac failure is not as a rule associated with any electrocardiographic alterations. Nevertheless, some diagnostic information can often be obtained from an electrocardiographic tracing:

- The presence of left or right ventricular hypertrophy may help determine the nature of the disease causing failure;

- The presence of a normal electrocardiogram should suggest the possibility that the signs and symptoms considered to represent cardiac failure may be caused by some other condition;

- The development of left atrial abnormality often precedes or coincides with the onset of cardiac failure;

- Administration of digitalis for cardiac failure may induce electrocardiographic abnormalities, which may later be misinterpreted as signifying serious cardiac disease; caution should be applied to electrocardiographic interpretation in patients receiving digitalis.

OTHER LABORATORY PROCEDURES

Phonocardiography offers means of confirming auscultatory and palpatory findings during physical examination. Recording an S3 gallop sound may permit a more refined differential diagnosis if the nature of the diastolic sound is not entirely clear. This can be done by timing of the sound and a simultaneously taken apexcardiogram. The latter also may record abnormal diastolic chest wall motion. Recording the venous pulse curve permits a better analysis of the venous pulse waves than inspection alone.

Pulmonary function tests play an important role in the differential diagnosis of cardiac vs. pulmonary dyspnea.

Stress tests. While the treadmill stress test is primarily used for the detection of ischemia, it is occasionally useful in testing the patient's effort tolerance and thus providing objective evidence to confirm or to contradict a history of disability.

Echocardiography is increasingly useful as a multifaceted diagnostic tool. In patients evaluated for cardiac failure an echocardiogram may provide the following useful information:

- It can confirm the presence of cardiac enlargement by direct demonstration of increased size of the ventricular cavity;

- It may show decreased contractility of the posterior wall of the left ventricle, such as may be present in cardiomyopathy or in ischemic heart disease;

- It may provide means of estimating the ejection fraction by noninvasive technique.

HEMODYNAMICS

As an invasive technique requiring hospitalization and associated with a considerable expense to the patient, hemodynamic and angiocardiographic evaluation is obviously not a routine method of diagnosis of cardiac failure. In specific instances it does provide, however, critical information that cannot be obtained by simpler means. Indications for the performance of cardiac catheterization and angiocardiographic studies include the following (related specifically to cardiac failure):

1. Patients in cardiac failure of uncertain origin, where the possibility of a surgically correctable lesion is considered;

2. Patients with valvular or congenital heart disease in whom the extent and the presence of failure is not clear, and whose surgical correction may be contingent upon hemodynamic studies;

3. Patients with ischemic heart disease in whom any form of cardiac surgery is being considered (revascularization, aneurysmectomy, etc.);

4. Patients who develop clinical findings suggestive of cardiac failure after cardiac operations;

5. Selected cases with chronic cardiac failure in which the progress of therapy is being objectively monitored.

When approaching a hemodynamic study of a patient in cardiac failure, certain guidelines have to be carefully noted:

- Cardiac failure is a "fluid" state with hemodynamic findings influenced by previous activity, steady state, and other factors.

- Diuretic therapy may exert a profound effect upon hemodynamics; The state of hydration of the patient has to be taken into consideration in the interpretation of the data.

- Other drug therapy, e.g., digitalis, may also influence hemodynamics.

When cardiac failure is fully developed, hemodynamic abnormalities are clear-cut and their interpretation presents no difficulty. In early cardiac failure the overlap between the normal variants and heart failure may make firm diagnoses hazardous. As explained in the preceding chapter, physiological abnormalities produced by the failing cardiac ventricle fall into three categories:

1. Abnormalities of atrial and ventricular diastolic pressures,

2. Abnormalities of cardiac output,

3. Combined abnormalities of both pressures and flows.

Such abnormalities may be present during the resting study, or may only be provoked by exercise.

In an arbitrary manner, recognizing that hemodynamic abnormalities in cardiac failure represent a continuum, one can divide such abnormalities into the following patterns:

1. Normal findings at rest; during recumbent exercise, abnormalities of pressure or flow or both become apparent (e.g., left atrial mean pressure rises to 30 mm. Hg; cardiac output does not rise in proportion to the increase in oxygen consumption).

2. Left ventricular failure is apparent at rest with predominant pressure abnormality (e.g., resting mean left atrial pressure is 25 mm. Hg; further rise occurs with exercise; cardiac output is at the lower range of normal; its increase with exercise is subnormal).

3. Left ventricular failure is apparent at rest with predominant flow limitation (e.g., left atrial resting pressure is 15 mm. Hg. and rises to 20 with exercise; resting cardiac output is 2.0 L./min./M^2; it fails to increase during exercise.

4. Left ventricular failure is evident with combined pressure and flow abnormalities (e.g., left atrial mean resting pressure is 30 mm. Hg; cardiac output is 1.6 L./min./M^2; left atrial pressure rises to 35 with exercise; cardiac output increases to 2.0 L./min./M^2).

5. Right ventricular dynamics are likely to remain normal in pattern 1; in pattern 3 abnormalities may become apparent during exercise; in patterns 2 and 4 systolic pulmonary hypertension of varying degree occurs; elevation of right atrial pressure may or may not be present. Some patients show reactive pulmonary hypertension, namely elevated pulmonary arteriolar resistance in excess of 3 mm. Hg/L./min. or 240 dynes sec. cm^{-5}; in such cases significant elevation of right atrial pressure is the rule and right atrial pressure curves suggesting tricuspid regurgitation are common.

6. Pure right ventricular failure presents itself as a consequence of pulmonary hypertension. Right ventricular diastolic pressures and right atrial hypertension are present and tricuspid regurgitation is common. Left-sided dynamics are normal or mildly abnormal; cardiac output may be normal or subnormal; all abnormalities are accentuated by exercise.

Angiocardiography fulfills a specific role in the evaluation of a patient in cardiac failure, which is to permit observations concerning cardiac contractions. This involves the following situations:

- Qualitative estimation of the overall contractility of the left ventricle by cineangiographic study of the left ventricle;

- Study of segmental motion of the cardiac border by left ventriculography in ischemic heart disease with focal myocardial scarring;

- Qualitative estimation of the ejection fraction, the end-systolic and the end-diastolic volume.

EVALUATION OF CARDIAC FUNCTION

The preceding section dealt with the recognition of cardiac failure. In patients who have chronic cardiac disease, particularly in those who fall into the category of chronic ventricular overload, the terms "compensation" and "decompensation" can be used only in the crudest clinical terms. While it is true that patients with clinical evidence of severe cardiac hypertrophy may perform normally and be unequivocally in functional class I, it is nevertheless certain, as already explained, that a hypertrophied heart is a diseased heart with its function to some extent compromised. Early disturbance of ventricular function can only be surmised, or sometimes may be detected by complex tests. Thus from the very inception of the process of compensatory hypertrophy in response to chronic overload there is a gradual transition to the appearance of overt cardiac failure with the stage of failure being merely an arbitrary late portion of a spectrum. Thus it becomes important at times to evaluate cardiac function and to be able to place the patient's position upon the functional spectrum. Function tests play an important role in investigative work dealing with the course of cardiac disease and with the effects of therapy. In routine clinical work functional evaluation becomes of importance in surgical problems, particularly in decisions as to whether or not a patient is operable (e.g., in ischemic heart disease, mitral regurgitation), and at which point operations should be performed.

Clinical evaluation of cardiac function is of limited value because of the wide overlap between normal and abnormal and the dependence on the patient's physical conditioning. Stress testing by means of treadmill or bicycle ergometer tests is of value only in longitudinal follow-up studies, when the patient's performance can be compared with his own performance in the past.

In evaluation of cardiac function, invasive methods have been widely applied. Cardiac catheterization provides the means of performing the crucial hemodynamic measurements and, by repeating such measurements during exercise, of evaluating the patient's responses to increase of workload. Such studies require only catheterization of the right side of the heart and therefore carry an acceptably low risk.

Among more elaborate function tests measuring the contractility of the myocardial fibers are measurement of the initial slope of the ventricular or aortic pressure curve (dp/dt). The theoretical validity of such measurement is well established; however, technical considerations make such measurements fully reliable only when the curve is recorded by a manometer in situ (micromanometer), for pressure transmitted by means of a column of fluid in the catheter may distort it, thereby lessening its reliability.

Another index that has been widely used is the maximal contractile element velocity (V_{max}), which is derived from pressure measurements performed during cardiac catheterization. Although theoretically representing an important index of cardiac contractility, the feasibility of obtaining a reliable measurement of this index has been questioned.

The most widely used functional index of cardiac performance is obtained by angiocardiography. As already mentioned, end-systolic and end-diastolic volumes can be measured from angiographic tracing, and the ejection fraction thus calculated. Ideally, such measurements should be performed by the biplane technique and by means of the rapid film changer. However, an acceptable shortcut of using a cine-angiographic single-plane technique is available, and such measurements show reasonably sensitive values as a crude function index, though probably not precise enough for research purposes.

In Chapter 7 a brief discussion of systolic time intervals measured by means of phonocardiographic and sphygmographic recording was included. Such noninvasive indices of ventricular function tests have been receiving increasing attention. The validity of the concept is well established and the accuracy of the measurement appears reasonable. However, the overlap between the normal and abnormal is wide and the influence of various extraneous factors makes reproducibility only fair. Thus, their value as a single determination in patients with cardiac disease has considerable limitations. The use of echocardiography, as another noninvasive function test, was mentioned earlier. This method is gaining wide acceptance as a moderately reliable way of estimating the ejection and following the progress of the disease longitudinally.

SIGNIFICANCE OF CARDIAC FAILURE

As emphasized in this chapter as well as in the preceding one, cardiac failure represents a fluid phase in the natural history of cardiac disease; its recognition and evaluation has to be considered from a perspective that examines the duration of cardiac failure, its permanency, its severity, and its potential reversibility.

The relationship between the extent of cardiac failure and the severity of the underlying disease, on the one hand, and the patient's disability, on the other hand, is rather crude. Severe cardiac disease with cardiomegaly—whether in valvular heart disease or in cardiomyopathy—may be associated with relatively little clinical disability. Patients, especially those with sedentary work habits and occupations, may be comfortable, have few symptoms, and remain unchanged for months or years. Some such patients show severe hemodynamic abnormalities with evidence for both left and right ventricular failure. Others may have only modest hemodynamic abnormalities. In ischemic heart disease associated with serious myocardial damage, such as in large ventricular aneurysms, clinical manifestations and hemodynamic abnormalities also show a wide range—from intractable clinical and serious hemodynamic evidence of cardiac failure to a virtual asymptomatic state with only minimal hemodynamic abnormalities.

Thus, from the standpoint of the prognosis and as an indication for the various forms of treatment, it is necessary to refine all observations and to view them in the light of the patient's overall clinical condition. For example, aortic regurgitation is known to produce severe degrees of cardiac hypertrophy; there is very little doubt that the hypertrophied left ventricle is functionally seriously impaired and the indices of myocardial contractility are expected to be grossly abnormal. Yet, many such patients, especially those under the age of 40, remain not only free from symptoms but capable of performing strenuous exercise, occasionally outperforming healthy individuals of comparable ages. The problem of cardiac failure is especially challenging to the clinician. Good judgment and experience are needed to proceed with proper evaluation of it, to know how far to go in arranging invasive and elaborate tests, and to be able to interpret the results adequately. The stereotyped approach to cardiac failure of two decades ago, advocating "digitalis, diuretics, and low-sodium diet," no longer has a place in today's cardiology.

Bibliography

Friedberg CK: Edema and pulmonary edema. Pathologic physiology and differential diagnosis. Prog. Cardiovasc. Dis. *13*:546, 1971.

Mason DT, Spann JF Jr, Zelis R, Amsterdam ER: Alterations in hemodynamics and myocardial mechanism in patients with congestive heart failure. Prog. Cardiovasc. Dis. *12*:507, 1970.

Selzer A, Popper RW, Lau FYK, Morgan JJ, Anderson WL: Present status of diagnostic cardiac catheterization. New Engl. J. Med. *286*:589, 654, 1963.

Spodick DH: Acute cardiac tamponade. Diagnosis and management. Prog. Cardiovasc. Dis. *10*:64, 1967.

Sonnenblick EH, Parmley WW, Urschel CW, Brutsaert DL: Ventricular function: evaluation of myocardial contractility in health and disease. Prog. Cardiovasc. Dis. *12*:449, 1970.

Wood P. Heart Failure: *In* Diseases of the Heart and Circulation, 3rd Ed. Eyre and Spottiswoode, London, 1968, p. 291.

16

Management of Cardiac Failure

The management of a patient in cardiac failure has to be approached from a broad standpoint. Only when the evaluation of the patient is completed should therapy be started, save for dire emergencies, A careful analysis of the problem then permits one to take one of the several options pertaining to treatment:

1. No therapy directed specifically toward cardiac failure is needed. As an example of this approach one can cite some cases of acute myocardial infarction or of acute rheumatic fever, in which mild cardiac failure develops temporarily.

2. Therapy is directed toward the factor which has precipitated a bout of cardiac failure. Example: restoration of sinus rhythm in patients in whom cardiac failure developed with the onset of atrial fibrillation.

3. Therapy is directed toward alleviation or elimination of the underlying disease that caused cardiac failure. Example of medical therapy: control of hypertension, cure of infective endocarditis; surgical correction of a valve lesion or its replacement; correction of a congenital defect.

4. Therapy is directed toward alleviation of cardiac failure and its consequences.

ACUTE FORMS OF CARDIAC FAILURE: CARDIAC EMERGENCIES

Sudden development of cardiac failure often produces medical or surgical *emergencies*. In general such acute forms of cardiac failure fall into three categories:

• acute pulmonary edema,

244

- shock,

- acute congestive failure (not specifically involving either of the above syndromes).

Acute Pulmonary Edema

Acute pulmonary edema ranges from a self-limited, temporary condition to rapidly fatal forms. When a patient is found to be in pulmonary edema, immediate therapy has to be initiated, while at the same time the situation is analyzed in order to determine the cause and mechanism of such an attack.

Pulmonary edema is most frequently a manifestation of acute left ventricular failure. Other forms of pulmonary edema (high altitude, heroin-induced) are noncardiac and need not be discussed here. Failure of the left ventricle may be unprovoked, but a precipitating factor can often be identified. Pulmonary edema involves a vicious circle: high capillary pulmonary pressure produces alveolar transudation and pulmonary congestion. As a result of this, increased respiratory effort ensues, and arterial hypoxia may develop. Both of these consequences may further impair left ventricular function. In addition, apprehension often induces hypertension, which may add to left ventricular load. Thus, the objectives of the treatment of acute pulmonary edema involve the following:

1. Elimination of the precipitating factor, if possible,

2. Improvement of left ventricular function,

3. Correction of deficiency in oxygenation.

The order in which the necessary therapeutic steps are taken has to be decided individually. Priorities depend upon the urgency of the situation and the judgment as to which of the objectives is attainable the fastest way.

Among the precipitating factors, one stands out as potentially immediately reversible, namely tachyarrhythmias. Appropriate treatment — intravenous drug administration or electroshock therapy — may in many cases slow the ventricular rate or re-establish normal rhythm rapidly enough so that it may be the only treatment necessary.

Treatment aimed at improvement of ventricular function includes the following approaches:

- Direct inotropy by means of digitalis. The uncertainty regarding the use of this drug for its inotropic action was discussed in Chapter 11. Its effect and reliability in such emergencies as acute pulmonary edema is unproved, except in the case of uncontrolled atrial fibrillation.

• Reduction of preload as means of "decompression" of the pulmonary circulation and improvement of left ventricular performance is a logical approach in pulmonary edema. This may include:

1. Phlebotomy;

2. Use of rotating tourniquets;

3. Reduction of blood volume by means of rapid-acting diuretic drugs administered intravenously.

The use of powerful new diuretics (ethacrynic acid, furosemide) has stirred considerable enthusiasm in treatment of pulmonary edema. Even though dramatic effects are frequently observed, some controlled studies have thrown doubt upon consistency of their effectiveness. It appears probable that diuretics would be most effective in cases where there is an appreciable increase in circulating blood volume.

• Reduction of ventricular load and interruption of the vicious circle by administration of morphine. Its general sedative effect as well as its specific effect reducing the work of breathing often has a dramatic impact in terminating attacks of pulmonary edema.

• Oxygen administration. The use of simpler means, such as a venturi mask, may correct hypoxia and its consequences. If this is ineffective, use of respiratory assistance should be considered, first using positive pressure respirators, then, in resistant cases, intubating the patient for the use of automatic breathing.

Shock

Shock represents a clinical syndrome produced by many causes. Only "cardiogenic" shock represents a form of cardiac failure in its proper connotation. This form of shock is most frequently found in acute myocardial infarction; other causes include massive pulmonary embolism and sudden ventricular overload (such as occurs in acute valvular incompetence).

The principal defect occurring in shock is the inadequate perfusion of vital organs. This may be due to inadequate perfusion pressure—hypotension—and reduced cardiac output (see Chapter 14).

The goal of therapy for cardiogenic shock is to improve the perfusion of the cerebral, cardiac, and renal circulations and to maintain sufficient flow of blood to supply minimal needs of other tissues. Low cardiac output and hypotension are related to each other but independently variable. As already explained, very low cardiac output may be present with normal or even slightly elevated arterial pressure owing to compensatory vasoconstriction. Conversely, severe hypotension does not automatically mean a critically reduced cardiac output. The use of pressor agents is a subject of controversy in cardiogenic shock: the possibility that maximum vasoconstriction is already present and elevation of pressure throws an unnecessary load upon the left ventricle while having no effect upon organ perfusion undoubtedly is correct in some cases. Yet, in others—when the pressure-regulating mechanism is defective—they may be helpful. On the other hand, alpha-adrenergic blocking agents and related drugs have a hypotensive effect (therefore reduce afterload) and may improve organ perfusion in shock, in patients with excessive vasoconstriction.

Thus the drug of choice in the therapy of cardiogenic shock cannot be decided upon unless both arterial pressure and cardiac output are known, and even then the use of such agents is merely inferential. The approach to a patient in shock involves first of all a rapid assessment of the overall situation. As the first step the diagnosis of *cardiogenic* shock has to be confirmed and its probable cause determined.

Pericardial tamponade due to hemopericardium constitutes an example of reversible shock in which a correct diagnosis is often lifesaving. Shock due to acute massive pulmonary embolization often presents a surgical emergency: failure to respond to initial therapy points strongly toward a decision in favor of emergency embolectomy.

Cardiogenic shock occurring in the course of acute myocardial infarction carries a very high mortality (about 80 per cent), which has shown very little improvement in response to the many forms of therapy introduced from time to time. It is reasonably well established that the underlying cause of such shock is extensive damage to the myocardium, probably beyond the capability of maintaining the circulation under any circumstances. Only borderline cases may be salvageable. Supportive therapy includes a choice of drugs discussed above. Inotropy is disappointing—digitalis appears to do more harm than good. Isoproterenol, which is an effective inotropic drug, has been recommended by some, but is discouraged by others because of its effect in increasing myocardial oxygen demands, an effect thought to outweigh its myocardial stimulating action.

The use of circulatory assist devices is still in an early developmental stage. Intra-aortic balloon pumping and other forms of pumps introduced into the arterial system have been shown to increase both arterial pressure and cardiac output. It is apparent that such devices are capable of correcting the basic deficiency responsible for shock; however, it has not been demonstrated with what frequency, if at all, such temporary assistance alters the final outcome. Thus far the most promising use, although still far from satisfactory, has been in patients who can be supported with the aid of such devices in preparation for a surgical procedure – a small proportion of cases.

Acute Congestive Failure

Acute congestive failure spans an entire range of severity, from mild episodes occurring in the course of some cardiac diseases to severe forms constituting emergencies, equaling in seriousness pulmonary edema and shock.

Acute congestive failure differs in two ways from chronic cardiac failure:

1.   It may be a temporary, reversible disturbance of cardiac function.

2.   It is usually characterized by sudden onset.

Milder forms of reversible acute cardiac failure include bouts in the course of acute myocardial infarction, acute myocarditis, and acute rheumatic fever; they include also episodes in the course of chronic cardiac disease in which the onset of failure is clearly related to an extraneous factor. Thus in order to diagnose "acute" forms of cardiac failure it is necessary to recognize its cause and mechanism. It should be noted that the reversibility of acute forms of cardiac failure can be accomplished in many but not all cases. In some, acute cardiac failure is merely a stage that establishes itself in a chronic form.

Vigorous therapy of acute cardiac failure is indicated only in its most serious, emergent forms. Otherwise, therapy ranges from none at all to the conventional therapy, described in connection with chronic cardiac failure, on the following page.

In dealing with acute congestive cardiac failure of appreciable severity, the first objective is to determine its cause. Abrupt development of severe cardiac failure is unlikely to take place without a specific cause, often a serious one. The patient's life may depend upon identification of such a cause. The most treacherous causes are atypical forms of valvular disease. Some patients with aortic stenosis or, less often, mitral stenosis may decompensate suddenly and, when first seen in cardiac failure, do not show the typical clinical features of the valve disease. Yet, in some such cases immediate operation is not only lifesaving but may render such a patient totally asymptomatic. Other emergencies include acute forms of valvular regurgitation: aortic regurgitation produced by valve perforation or by dissecting aneurysm and mitral regurgitation produced by rupture of chordae tendineae or by rupture of a head of a papillary muscle. Arrhythmias causing sudden severe cardiac failure have already been discussed; their recognition usually presents no difficulty; correction is often simple.

TREATMENT OF CHRONIC CARDIAC FAILURE

Most patients in the category of chronic cardiac failure suffer from a long-standing cardiac disease which at a given point in its natural history enters the stage of cardiac failure. Treatment of chronic cardiac failure should be undertaken with a prime guiding principle in mind: maximum possible control of failure with minimum possible therapy.

As explained in connection with acute cardiac failure, the initial step in the therapy requires an investigation and correction or elimination where possible of precipitating causes. Some such causes are self-limited; if the patient's condition permits, therapy may be postponed, and it may become altogether unnecessary when effects of such factors are gone. Precipitation of cardiac failure by single insults include the following:

- overexertion,
- salt intake in excess of the usual habits,
- overhydration (often iatrogenic),
- increase in blood volume (e.g., blood transfusion rapidly administered).

Temporary conditions, not falling into the category of "single insult," include:

- infection,
- arrhythmias,
- pulmonary infarcts,
- hypertensive crises,
- hypoxia.

When such precipitating factors in the production of heart failure have been ruled out, the next priority concerns the possibility of finding a treatable cause of cardiac malfunction. Once such a factor is identified, one can consider the feasibility and the risk in its elimination or alleviation.

Some cases of cardiac failure involve acute diseases of the heart. In most such cases normal cardiac function may be restored after the acute process is terminated; in some permanent damage to the myocardium is produced and residual chronic cardiac failure ensues. These include the following:

- acute myocardial infarction,
- rheumatic fever,
- acute myocarditis,
- infective endocarditis.

Cardiac failure represents the potential late results of all forms of cardiac disease. Treatable forms of cardiac disease include hypertension (systemic and pulmonary) and the various forms of surgically correctable cardiac conditions, including valvular heart disease, congenital malformation, and some forms of ischemic heart disease.

After the first two steps—consideration of precipitating factors and treatable causes of cardiac failure—one should initiate plans for the therapy of cardiac failure per se. Such therapy has three principal goals:

1. Elimination and control of aggravating factors,

2. Improvement of ventricular function,

3. Control and prevention of fluid retention.

Among aggravating factors, the control of which may favorably influence cardiac failure are the following:

- Excessive activity; restriction of activities ranges from a brief period of rest at home or at the hospital for severe failure to the elimination of recreational activities and limitation of occupational activities in milder cases.

- Excess body weight; weight reduction may be an important therapeutic objective in overweight patients.

- Control of cardiac rate and rhythm; while extreme ranges of cardiac rate may produce cardiac emergencies (see above), lesser degrees of arrhythmias often act as aggravating factors; treatment includes the control of ventricular rate in atrial fibrillation, elimination of ectopic rhythms, pacing in excessive bradycardias.

- Elimination of risk factors: tobacco, control of diabetes.

- Elimination of infections.

Improvement of ventricular function is thought to be accomplished by the inotropic use of digitalis. The limitation and uncertainty of the continuing effectiveness of this drug has been discussed in Chapter 11. This drug is used traditionally for its inotropic effects as a mainstay in the treatment of cardiac failure. In addition, indirect influence upon cardiac performance is exerted by several of the other methods, including elimination of some of the aggravating factors (particularly arrhythmias, regulation of activities) and the regulation of fluid balance.

The elimination and prevention of fluid retention constitutes probably the most effective means of controlling cardiac failure; certainly the new era of management of cardiac patients was initiated by the introduction of effective diuretic agents. The clinician has at his disposal a wide span of interventions in the management of fluid control:

- Simple restriction of sodium intake in the diet may suffice in milder cases. This may vary from a mere elimination of excess salt in food to moderately restricted dietary sodium.

- The occasional use of diuretics, guided by variation in body weight.

- Regular use of diuretics. Here the gradation involves milder diuretics (e.g., thiazides), the powerful newer diuretics (ethacrynic acid and furosemide), the adjustment of their dosages, and, finally, the use of diuretic combinations.

Therapy of cardiac failure involves three steps:

1. Initiation of the treatment according to a plan arrived at after the appraisal of all the factors involved in a given case.

2. Adjustment of therapy after the results of the initial therapy become apparent.

3. Maintenance therapy, adjusted periodically according to the patient's responses and needs.

There are cases in which maintenance therapy is unnecessary: the initial therapy may restore compensation with the patient remaining out of failure for indefinite time periods. Such a course is the rule in cardiac failure initiated by an obvious precipitating factor but may also occur in patients without any recognizable factor present prior to the onset of failure. However, in the majority of patients, once overt cardiac failure develops, some form of therapy needs to be continued permanently.

The effects of therapy should be monitored and supervised. The object of monitoring includes the following:

- symptoms,

- chart of daily body weight,

- periodic rechecks, including physical examination, chest roentgenograms, electrocardiograms,

• search for evidence of intolerance for drugs or their untoward effects: arrhythmias, serum electrolyte disturbances, hyperuricemia, nitrogen retention.

As stated, treatment of cardiac failure should be initiated and continued on the premise that the minimum amount of treatment represents the best policy. This approach calls for cautious initiation of treatment as well as for periodic attempts to reduce or discontinue the various components of therapy. Thus, digitalis and dietary restriction, sometimes reinforced by a single dose of a diuretic agent, carries many patients in a controllable state for long periods of time. Diuretic therapy needs constant adjustment. Inasmuch as variation in body weight provides a reasonably good means of evaluating the effectiveness of diuretics as well as the need for their administration, a thoughtful trial of drugs, dosages, and frequency of their use should be given in each patient. Only by discontinuing the use of diuretics can one discover that the patient may not need diuretic therapy at all.

"INTRACTABLE" CARDIAC FAILURE

The term intractable cardiac failure is often applied loosely, denoting patients who do not respond to a certain "routine" treatment. Some patients referred to a cardiology service as in "intractable" cardiac failure respond promptly to changes in management. There is, however, a group of patients who remain in cardiac failure, or deteriorate in spite of intensive, well-instituted therapy. They are composed of three types of patients:

1. Those with heart damage beyond repair, not salvageable by any means, truly refractory to any form of therapy.

2. Those with overt or occult lesions amenable to surgical attack, where an operation — even at the cost of very high risk — is often lifesaving.

3. Those that can be brought out of failure by means of expert therapy.

Confronted with a patient purported to be in intractable cardiac failure the first priority is an evaluation. This should include first a clinical study aimed at identification of any factors that may have been overlooked; afterward, hemodynamic and angiocardiographic evaluation are in order, unless specifically contraindicated or shown to be superfluous.

Conditions that may contribute to refractoriness of cardiac failure to therapy include the following:

• clinically "silent" myocardial infarction,

- occult infection,

- pulmonary infarction.

The prognosis for a patient may be brighter if such a condition is detected, inasmuch as some are amenable to therapy or clear spontaneously. Furthermore, refractoriness to treatment may have its source in the untoward effects of earlier treatment:

- digitalis intoxication,

- hypokalemia,

- hyperkalemia,

- hyponatremia,

- hypochloremic acidosis,

- hypochloremic alkalosis.

Cardiac catheterization and angiographic studies are performed in order to consider the following possibilities:

- detection and quantification of valvular lesions,

- detection of congenital lesions (usually atypical),

- detection of resectable cardiac aneurysms,

- detection of unusual forms of cardiac disease (e.g., tumors),

- evaluation of myocardial contractility in patients with valvular heart disease,

- screening of patients with advanced, non-bypassable coronary artery disease.

After the process of diagnostic evaluation is complete, the basic decision is made as to whether surgical therapy comes into consideration at all. If this form of treatment appears in principle feasible, the following points need thorough consideration:

1. Is the mechanical (i.e., removable) factor sufficiently prominent to offer a reasonable possibility for postoperative improvement of the circulatory status?

2. Can one afford the time to proceed with medical therapy before the operation in order to reduce operative risk in the patient?

The answer to these two questions cannot be considered in any quantitative manner; they are subject to "educated guesses" on the part of the combined medical-surgical team. The more experienced the team, the more likely such estimates will be correct.

When the decision is made to subject the patient to medical therapy, the plan for treatment should include the following steps:

- Management of any identifiable factor listed above;

- Correction of any possible consequence of prior treatment: discontinuation of digitalis in suspected intoxication with this drug, correction of electrolyte and acid-base imbalance;

- Intensification of therapy if no untoward effects are present;

- Additional approaches to therapy.

Experience has shown that patients who are refractory to intensive medical therapy on an outpatient basis frequently respond well to treatment in a hospital even though the same regimen is used. The reason for this is not clear: possibly rest and hospital discipline add something to the therapy; possibly patients do not follow prescribed regimens as well as they claim they do. It is nevertheless often worthwhile to try a period of hospital treatment in such refractory patients. In addition to the already mentioned intangible benefit of the hospitalization some other options may be offered to a hospitalized patient:

1. A better trial and adjustment of diuretic therapy by means of monitoring daily weight, fluid intake and output, and serial serum electrolyte determinations.

2. Control of respiration: some patients with markedly increased work of breathing may be brought out of refractoriness by a period of assisted respiration.

3. Mechanical removal of some of the effects of cardiac failure that may perpetuate it: thoracentesis, removal of ascites.

4. Hemodialysis for unresponsive massive edema.

Cardiac failure presents one of the most challenging problems to the clinician. In milder cases, the balance between undertreating and overtreating a patient requires good judgment; in severe cases, experience is at a premium. Here an effective cardiology service may salvage many patients incorrectly considered "intractable."

Bibliography

Brest AN: Management of refractory heart failure. Prog. Cardiovasc. Dis. *12*:493, 1970.

Cairns KB, Porter GA, Kloster FE, Bristow JD, Griswold HE: Clinical and hemodynamic results of peritoneal dialysis for severe cardiac failure. Amer. Heart. J. *76*:227, 1968.

Fowler NO: Management of refractory heart failure. Prog. Cardiovasc. Dis. *12*:493, 1970.

MacCannell KE, Moran NL: Pharmacological basis for the use of adrenergic agonists and antagonists in cardiogenic shock. Prog. Cardiovasc. Dis. *10*:55, 1967.

Selzer A, Popper RW, Gerbode F, Kerth WJ: Effect of surgical relief of cardiac overload upon intractable heart failure. Amer. J. Med. Sci. *251*:283, 1966.

Robin ED, Cross CE, Zelis R: Pulmonary edema. New Engl. J. Med. *288*:239, 292, 1973.

17

Mechanisms of Arrhythmias and Their Recognition

The term "arrhythmia" is used traditionally to denote all deviations from the norm in the sequence and origin of heart action, regardless of whether the rhythm of the heart beat is regular or irregular, slow or rapid. The objections raised in regard to the inadequacy of this term are well taken, and the suggested substitute term "dysrhythmia" seems more satisfactory; nevertheless, the traditional ties of the clinician to the term "arrhythmia" may be too strong to overcome. Since it is likely that the term "arrhythmia" will continue to be widely used, it is important that its proper definition be understood.

The subject of arrhythmias has undergone drastic conceptual changes during the last decade. The knowledge of electrophysiology has "exploded" and its clinical application is firmly demonstrated. Furthermore, the wide use of cardiac monitoring has brought the subject of arrhythmias into the common use of virtually every clinician and many nurses. Whereas it is beyond the scope of this book to provide a detailed discussion of the subject, it may nevertheless be useful for the reader to note a few basic definitions of terms that will be used in the next four chapters.

BASIC DEFINITIONS

Impulse formation. The automaticity of cardiac action is contingent upon periodic depolarization of myocardial fibers, a mechanism which initiates cardiac contraction. The cardiac muscle is composed of two types of myocardial cells: most myocardial fibers exhibit no changes in

255

potential during the diastolic phase. Some cells, however, namely those comprising most of the components of the conducting system, have the property of spontaneous diastolic depolarization (sloping phase 4) and these constitute the *pacemaker cells* (Fig. 17–1); the rate of the depolarization — of impulse formation — determines how active the pacemaker is. It has been demonstrated that under abnormal conditions — ischemia, myocardial disease, toxic effects of certain agents — ordinary myocardial cells may develop diastolic depolarization and become pacemaker cells.

Both ordinary myocardial cells and pacemaker cells respond to stimuli — either propagated from other cells or extraneous — in a manner dependent upon the phase of the cardiac cycle. Immediately after its depolarization the cell is totally unresponsive to any stimulation *(absolute refractory phase);* thereafter — still during systole — the cell responds only to stimuli of higher than normal intensity *(relative refractory phase).* During most of diastole the cell responds normally to stimuli. However, following the relative refractory phase there are two brief periods, the vulnerable phase and the supernormal phase, about which there is a controversy as to whether they are always present or occur only under special circumstances. Both of these periods are located

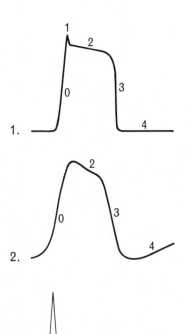

Figure 17–1. Drawing contrasting the electrical potential obtained from single cells (*1* and *2*) with a simultaneous conventional electrocardiogram (*3*). Curve *1* shows potential of an ordinary myocardial cell; curve *2*, of a pacemaker cell. (Phases 0 to 4 are indicated on the two upper curves.)

toward the end of the systolic phase and the beginning of the diastolic phase. During *the vulnerable phase*, stimulation may initiate chaotic rhythm (fibrillation), and during the *supernormal phase*, cells respond to subliminal stimuli.

NORMAL MECHANISMS

The physiological pacemaker is located in the sinoatrial node (SA node), hence the normal cardiac rhythm is termed sinoatrial or sinus rhythm. The impulse originating there is propagated through the atria by way of three internodal tracts leading to the AV node. At the same time, the impulse traveling through these tracts depolarizes the atria, producing their systole. The atrioventricular (AV) node has a slow conduction time; the impulse traversing it takes enough time to ensure an adequate interval between the atrial and ventricular depolarization, one essential for the most effective coordination of the cardiac pump. Emerging from the AV node, the impulse spreads rapidly through the remainder of the conducting system — the bundle of His, the bundle branches and their ramification, and the Purkinje fiber system that eventually comes in contact with ventricular myocardium, inducing its depolarization.

As indicated, not only the SA node but most of the conducting system is formed of pacemaker cells; the only difference is that cells of its other parts have a slower rising phase 4 slope than the SA node cells, thereby exhibiting a slower rate of impulse formation. The only part of the conducting system that has very few pacemaker cells is the AV node; its role is that of a relay station. Its delaying action of the impulse traversing it has already been discussed. In addition, the AV node sifts through impulses, blocking some weaker and undesirable ones.

In health the SA node is the only active pacemaker of the heart. Other areas of the conducting system represent merely potential pacemakers that become activated solely in case of emergency. Such pacemakers play a standby role, taking over impulse formation if the impulse from the SA node fails to arrive. In this capacity their role is sequential. The next highest concentration of pacemaker cells after the SA node is located at the junction of the AV node and the initial portion of the bundle of His. It represents the secondary pacemaker ready to discharge at a rate of some 10 to 20 beats slower than that of the SA node. Single beats or rhythms originating there are termed "AV junctional" or "AV" beats or rhythms. The old term "nodal" rhythm has been dropped after the demonstration that the AV node is not an active pacemaker. Portions of the conducting system below the AV nodal junction are characterized by gradually slower inherent rates of impulse formation down to about 30 beats per minute for peripheral portions of the conducting system originating "idioventricular rhythms."

The first line of defense against failure of impulses to arrive at the AV nodal junction on time represents the secondary center; more peripheral portions generating still slower rates are referred to as tertiary centers. The mechanism of impulse formation at the lower centers by default, i.e., produced by failure of the proper impulse to arrive from above, is referred to as the *escape mechanism.* Thus *escape beats* occur when one impulse is delayed, *escape rhythm* when impulses stop arriving for a long enough time to permit the lower center to initiate its own, slower rhythm.

The normal pacemaker is under the continuous "monitoring" influence of the autonomic nervous system; its rate is constantly adjusted according to needs by autonomic impulses, primarily those mediated by sympathetic control. The normal sinus rate in adults varies between 60 and 80 beats per minute, with an outside range of rare normal variations of from 40 to 100. In children the normal sinus rate ranges from 150 in an average infant to 90 in a 3-year-old. The rhythm is basically regular except for mild respiratory variation in cycle length. In some normal subjects, particularly in those with inherently slow basal rates, considerable variation may develop, presumably owing to an increase in vagal tone. This is especially pronounced in some children, in whom the sinus arrhythmia may cause the AV junction to throw in an occasional escape beat to fill some unusually long pauses. The heart rate is normally accelerated by sympathetic influence as a part of cardiac regulation. The maximum acceleration reaches the 180 to 200 beat per minute range during strenuous exercise (somewhat lower maximal rates develop in older individuals). Physiological changes and responses of the heart rate via the autonomic nervous system–SA node mechanism include the following:

- rate acceleration during exercise,

- rate acceleration with excitement,

- responses to Valsalva maneuver,

- bradycardia of athletes (often brought about by intensive physical conditioning),

- increased vagal activity producing slowing (e.g., nausea).

Influences of certain abnormal states, extracardiac in nature, may also produce changes in cardiac rate:

- fever,

- hyperthyroidism or other hypermetabolic states,

- conditions associated with abnormal vagal or sympathetic activity.

In contrast to the responsiveness of the SA nodal pacemaker to autonomic control, lower pacemaking centers show little response to nervous regulation. The AV junction shows minor variation in response to sympathetic impulses. For example, individuals who have permanent AV junctional rhythm (either congenital or acquired) show very little, if any, acceleration of the cardiac rate during exercise. However, vagal impulse may affect the conduction through the AV node. Tertiary centers show no evidence of autonomic rate control.

ABNORMAL MECHANISMS

Under abnormal conditions — not necessarily produced by organic disease of the heart — the orderly process of impulse formation and its distribution through the heart may be altered, inducing a variety of disturbances of cardiac rhythm and rate. The basic abnormalities affecting this process fall generally into two major categories:

1. Disturbances of impulse formation,

2. Disturbances of impulse conduction and propagation.

Abnormalities of impulse formation involve the dominance of pacemakers other than the SA node. All such pacemakers are referred to as *ectopic*. Their only physiological role is, as stated, a passive one, namely to stand by, ready to discharge only if a higher impulse fails to arrive. This role is fulfilled when an ectopic pacemaker discharges at its inherent rate of impulse formation.

Whenever an ectopic pacemaker assumes an abnormal role, i.e., discharges at a rate higher than its usual automaticity, one of the following situations may arise:

1. It may assume the control of the entire heart, suppressing the SA nodal function.

2. It may assume the control of the atria, but the rate may be too rapid to find components of the conduction system ready to transmit impulses because of the refractory phase. The ventricle would then respond only to every second, third, or fourth impulse, or to an irregular number of impulses (as in atrial fibrillation).

3. It may assume control of the ventricles only, the atria being protected by retrograde block and activated antegrade from the physiological SA nodal pacemaker (a form of atrioventricular dissociation).

4. It may compete with the SA node for the control of the heart, each pacemaker capable of activating the heart when it finds the conducting system out of refractory phase (parasystole, atrioventricular dissociation with capture).

5.   It may encounter a refractory state of the adjacent tissues that interferes with its propagation ("exit block"), and therefore be able to activate the heart only under special circumstances, intermittently (a variety of parasystole).

Disturbances of conduction and propagation of the impulse include a wide and varied range of conditions and account for a number of clinical arrhythmias. The normal conducting system has been briefly described above. Physiologically the propagation of impulses proceeds from the SA node to the Purkinje fibers. However, the conducting system in addition has the potential capability to conduct impulses in the reverse direction as well. Loss or reduction of conductivity in either direction may play an important role in the pathogenesis of some arrhythmias.

The more important disturbances of conduction include the following mechanisms:

1.   The inability to conduct impulses caused by the normal or pathologically prolonged refractory period. This functional disorder of conduction may affect the entire conducting system or any part thereof, since recovery of conductivity occurs at different speeds in its segments.

2.   An organic interruption of the conducting pathways. Cardiac rhythm is disturbed principally if the bundle of His or all peripheral connections between the AV node and the ventricles are severed.

3.   Organic or functional mechanisms delaying conduction into the periphery but not entirely disconnecting it, thereby producing temporary, intermittent, or incomplete AV blocks.

4.   Premature activation of some portions of the ventricles due to short circuits between the atria and the ventricles, such as are present in Wolff-Parkinson-White syndrome.

5.   Disturbances of conduction in focal areas. The most important of these is the re-entry phenomenon, which involves a focal delay within the conducting system, combined with retrograde (unidirectional) block. The impulse is delayed by the coexistence of these two conditions in an area until cells distal to it have recovered from the refractory phase and can respond to stimuli. Such an impulse then may form either a continuing wave or a single return beat ("echo"). This mechanism is thought to be involved in coupled ectopic beats, in some forms of supraventricular and ventricular tachycardias, in atrial flutter, and in the tachyarrhythmias of the W-P-W syndrome.

6.   Retrograde block occurring in some ectopic tachycardias originating in the AV junction or below prevents the impulse from

reaching the atria and produces AV dissociation in that the atria still follow the normal sinus mechanism.

7.   AV dissociation represents a term used in a variety of disturbances of conduction. Often misused as a synonym for complete AV block, the term atrioventricular dissociation applies merely to the independence of a ventricular complex from the appropriate atrial complex. Thus any mechanism that can cause the atria and the ventricles to beat independently from each other — be it for a single beat or permanently — qualifies for this term. Complete heart block, which represents a specific form of atrioventricular dissociation, has a well-defined connotation: interrupted connection between the atria and the ventricles with the former following the sinus automaticity and the latter an independent *escape* rhythm. When such a situation arises, the broader term of atrioventricular dissociation should be avoided in favor of the more specific term of heart block.

CAUSES OF ARRHYTHMIAS

Arrhythmias range from physiological events to life-threatening emergencies, from single abnormal beats to permanent disturbance of cardiac rhythm. Not all forms of arrhythmias require treatment. However, the importance of establishing or at least suspecting the cause of a given arrhythmia cannot be overemphasized, since such information may materially affect the approach to the case, its interpretation, its prognosis and its therapy. The more important causes of arrhythmias are listed below:

1.   Organic causes

   a.   Congenital: congenital AV block, W-P-W syndrome;

   b.   Acquired damage to the conducting system due to fibrotic disease of the conducting system or its vicinity, to ischemic heart disease, or to surgical interruption of conducting pathways:

   c.   Diseases of the atria: atrial arrhythmias occurring in mitral valve disease and in atrial septal defects, and many other diseases;

   d.   Diseases of the ventricles: myocarditis, acute myocardial infarction, cardiac aneurysm, etc.

2.   Nonorganic causes involving pathophysiological factors

   a.   Hypoxia;

   b.   Disturbance of the acid-base balance;

   c. Electrolyte imbalance (particularly of potassium);

   d. Drugs, toxins, and other noxious agents;

   e. Mechanical stimulation (e.g., cardiac catheterization, pacemaker insertion).

The clinician faced with a problem of arrhythmias in a patient is obligated to go beyond the mere labeling of the arrhythmia. The proper analysis of such a case involves the consideration of the following problems that are related to the causes of arrhythmias:

- Is there known underlying heart disease in the patient with arrhythmia? If so, is the arrhythmia presumed to be related to cardiac disease?

- Could the arrhythmia be the first manifestation of previously unknown cardiac disease? There are ample examples of arrhythmias representing the first evidence of ischemic heart disease, of myocarditis; atrial fibrillation occasionally draws attention to previously unrecognized diseases of the mitral valve.

- What is the significance of the arrhythmia? Is treatment indicated? If so, should arrhythmia or the underlying factor receive first therapeutic priority?

RECOGNITION OF ARRHYTHMIAS

The astuteness with which in the past clinicians were able to diagnose and identify correctly many arrhythmias from a bedside examination or by means of polygraphic tracings is worthy of admiration. Even today, experienced clinicians can frequently recognize certain arrhythmias at bedside. Nevertheless, it is now required that disturbances of rhythm be documented by a permanent record; hence, electrocardiographic diagnosis is mandatory. It is often unnecessary to take a complete 12-lead tracing if the goal of the electrocardiographic examination is merely the diagnosis of the arrhythmia. Examination of the cardiac rhythm can be performed adequately by means of leads II, V_1 and V_6 in the great majority of cases. The crucial part of the electrocardiographic examination is identification and analysis of the P wave. In a small proportion of records the atrial activity is not well demonstrated and needs reinforcement by means of special techniques. Such special electrocardiographic examinations include the following methods intended for better demonstration of P waves:

- Amplification of the P waves by means of special precordial leads taken at higher than standard sensitivity of the machine (leads taken on the right sternal border below the V_1 position, often connected with an indifferent electrode attached to the right arm instead of the V terminal);

• Esophageal leads;

• Right atrial electrograms: this technique is most reliable but should be used only if adequate team facilities for cardiac catheterization are readily available;

• Certain forms of arrhythmias, such as conduction defects (but not exclusively so), can be clarified by recording of the signal from the region of the bundle of His. Other special methods of examination include observations of responses to special procedures, such as carotid sinus stimulation, Valsalva maneuver, use of drugs, and even intracardiac pacing.

It should be made clear that special methods of examination are necessary only in rare instances, since conventional electrocardiography provides enough information for the expert to diagnose the vast majority of arrhythmias. Should special methods of diagnosis become necessary, the complex, invasive techniques are indicated in patients where the exact identification of the arrhythmia carries far-reaching practical significance directly affecting the patient's management. Academic purism is not a sufficient reason to subject a patient to such studies, unless invasive methods are being used for other purposes.

The activities of the principal pacemakers cannot be directly demonstrated in the conventional electrocardiogram. The primary pacemaker — the SA node — is not amenable to any method of recording; any conclusion regarding the function of the SA node is only inferential. The activity of the AV nodal junction is now accessible to direct recording by obtaining the His signal which is generated in that general area. However, as pointed out, the technique of recording this signal is too complex for routine application. The conventional electrocardiogram records depolarization (and repolarization) of the *atria* and the *ventricles;* the diagnosis of arrhythmias depends upon the proper interpretation of the relationship between the two signals from the two sets of chambers.

Analysis of cardiac arrhythmias is facilitated in many cases by the following:

1. Availability of long strips of tracings recording some crucial leads (II and V_1); this permits adequate measurements of various intervals and observation regarding repetitive nature of certain sequences of beats;

2. Availability of old records for comparison of the morphology of P waves and QRS complexes taken prior to the onset of arrhythmias;

3. Use of higher sensitivity and faster speed of recording, whenever indicated;

4. Simultaneous recording of several leads.

In approaching the diagnosis of an arrhythmia, it is helpful to follow a plan, an outline that would permit some simplification of a complex task. Such a plan may be divided into four steps:

1. A scanning of the tracing to determine whether the arrhythmia consists of sporadic interruption of a basically normal rhythm, whether the entire record shows a uniform arrhythmia, whether arrhythmia occurs in groups of beats, or whether an overall repetitive pattern of the abnormality can be detected;

2. Identification of P waves: this step should include determination of whether atrial activity is uniform and whether it is regular;

3. Recognition of QRS complexes: their morphological appearance, uniformity, and regularity;

4. An analysis of the relationship between P waves and QRS complexes.

The *atrial complex*, the P wave, may provide information concerning the origin of the impulse which depolarizes the atria. It is important to differentiate abnormally-appearing P waves produced by anatomic atrial abnormalities, described in Chapter 6, from those caused by abnormalities of its depolarization due to ectopic origin of the rhythm:

- Broad and bifid P waves characteristic of left atrial abnormality may also be produced by disturbances of interatrial conduction, delaying the activation of the left atrium;

- Peaked and tall P waves (P pulmonale) may occasionally be observed without clinical evidence of disease of the right atrium; they may appear and disappear without apparent cause, presumably representing some form of ectopy and/or intra-atrial conduction disturbance;

- Unusually shaped P waves consisting of a gentle initial wave and a sharp terminal spike ("dome and dart P waves") have been reported in some complex congenital cardiac lesions, but can also be found in ectopic impulse formation. This was once thought to represent evidence for the origin of the ectopic rhythm in the left atrium; however, the specificity of this relationship has been disproven; they merely represent a form of ectopy with abnormal depolarization of the atria.

These three varieties of abnormal P waves, in which abnormal impulse formation and the effects of atrial disease overlap, cannot be differentiated on the basis of their appearance alone. When present with a normal rhythm and normal P-R interval, clinical association with cardiac disease may throw the weight of probability toward atrial disease; in the presence of arrhythmias, ectopy is more probable.

The *direction* of the P waves and *change* in their shape when compared with P waves in the same patient taken on another occasion have a higher specificity of indicating ectopic rhythm. The following general guidelines may aid in the analysis of arrhythmias:

1. Normal P waves (in relation to control tracings) present strong evidence (though not proof) that the impulse formation occurs physiologically in the SA node.

2. P waves showing the same direction as control complexes but differing in shape indicate ectopic rhythm with an antegrade activation of the atria. It is now recognized that impulses originating in the AV junction or below it may travel rapidly retrograde along the internodal tracts and activate the atria antegrade; consequently, upright P waves no longer are considered characteristic of "atrial" rhythms but may reflect any form of ectopy. Nevertheless, it is more likely that upright P waves represent ectopy originating in the pacemaker cells scattered in the atrial endocardium.

3. P waves showing superior orientation (i.e., inverted in leads II, III, and AVF, or all three standard leads) represent strong evidence in favor of retrograde activation of the atria, hence of ectopy originating in the AV junction or below.

4. The F waves of atrial flutter are characterized by regular, symmetrical waves inscribed at a rate of 230 to 320/min. They show, in their typical form, a continuous "sawtooth" appearance in leads II, III, and AVF.

5. The f waves of atrial fibrillation resemble those of atrial flutter but are faster (rates above 350/min.), smaller, and less regular. In atrial fibrillation of long standing f waves may become minuscule or even invisible in the standard electrocardiographic tracing.

6. Absent P waves suggest one of three possibilities:

    • Atrial activity is present but the electrical potential generated is of such low amplitude that only special leads (amplified precordial leads, esophageal leads, or atrial electrograms) can demonstrate their presence;

    • Atrial fibrillation of long standing may be present (see above); this is suggested if the rhythm of the ventricular complexes is totally irregular;

- Atrial standstill may be diagnosed if no evidence of atrial activity is discovered by any method, particularly if QRS complexes are equidistant.

Ventricular complexes viewed from the standpoint of arrhythmias appear in one of three forms:

1. Narrow complexes identical with those recorded prior to the onset of an arrhythmia indicate a physiological activation of the ventricles. They may be the result of an impulse originating in the SA node, or an ectopic pacemaker located anyplace *above* the bifurcation of the bundle of His. They are termed "supraventricular" complexes.

2. Broad QRS complexes with various configurations indicative of bundle branch block or other intraventricular conduction defects can be caused by any of the following mechanisms:

- Permanent disease of the lower part of the conduction system (in which case a control tracing also shows wide complexes);

- *Aberration*—a condition in which the impulse traveling from above the bifurcation of the bundle of His finds a part of the lower conducting system still in a refractory phase;

- Response to an ectopic pacemaker located below the bifurcation of the bundle of His.

3. Complexes showing intermediate shapes between (1) and (2) are termed *fusion beats.* The fusion phenomenon indicates that the ventricles are activated by two competing wave-fronts: that arriving from the SA node via the normal channels and that arriving from a "ventricular" ectopic pacemaker. Depending on the temporal relationship between these two pacemakers, either of them can activate the early part of the QRS complex, with the other one accounting for the remainder of the complex. A special form of fusion is the Wolff-Parkinson-White type of complex in which the normal impulse originating in the SA node divides into two pathways reaching portions of the ventricle at different times.

Morphological appearance of QRS complexes, described above, has obvious limitations in its contribution to the diagnosis of arrhythmias:

- Supraventricular complexes demonstrate "high" origin of impulse formation but cannot discriminate between physiological and ectopic rhythm; only occasionally minor aberration may be noted which suggests ectopy over SA rhythm.

- Broad complexes (with conduction defects) can be produced

by any of the above mentioned three mechanisms; their differentiation is difficult. In general, right bundle branch block complexes (particularly those with an rSR' configuration) suggest aberration rather than ventricular ectopy because the right bundle branch has a physiologically longer refractory period than the left. However, in patients with cardiac disease this rule often fails.

Reviewing the relationship between the P waves and the QRS complexes, attention should be paid to the consistency of the relationship:

1. Normal P waves may precede the supraventricular QRS complex by intervals other than the usual range of 0.13 to 0.20. A longer interval usually indicates an AV conduction delay — first degree heart block. A shorter interval may be due to one of the following:

- A normal variant;

- Lown-Ganong-Levine syndrome (diagnosed only if tendency to ectopic tachycardias is demonstrated);

- Abnormality or disease of the AV node producing acceleration of the AV conduction;

- AV dissociation: in single beats the position of the P wave may be coincidental; when present continuously the possibility of isorhythmic dissociation should be considered.

2. Normal P waves are present with a constant P-R interval; however, not all P waves are followed by QRS complexes: this indicates second degree AV block: it may take the form of a fixed relationship (2 to 1, 3 to 1) or intermittent and irregular falling out of QRS complexes (type II — Mobitz).

3. P-R interval varies with periodic lengthening of the interval and dropped beats — this is the classical Wenckebach phenomenon (type I of second degree AV block).

4. P waves and QRS complexes are unrelated to each other: if both are equidistant at different rates, complete AV dissociation can be diagnosed; if atrial complexes are equidistant but ventricular complexes show irregularity, the possibility of AV dissociation with capture should be considered. This can be proved if the ventricular complex "out of rhythm" with the others stands in a fixed relationship to the preceding P waves. Other forms of irregularity with dissociated P waves and QRS complexes indicate more complex types of arrhythmias.

5. Abnormal P waves are, as indicated, a reasonable evidence for ectopic origin of the rhythm. Their relationship to the QRS complexes

is variable and their diagnostic value regarding the location of the ectopic pacemaker is rather limited. Even the once widely accepted view that inverted P waves preceding QRS complexes signify "high" nodal rhythm and those following QRS complexes "low" nodal rhythm no longer holds true; its basic premise, that of identical antegrade and retrograde conduction velocity, is no longer valid.

In trying to carry the analysis of arrhythmias a step further, the following discussion contains additional information concerning various common arrhythmias.

1.   If the tracing shows a *regular* tachycardia, the following possibilities should be considered:

    a.   Supraventricular complexes are present:

- At rates up to 150 and with normal P waves, sinus tachycardia is most likely;

- If the rate is about 150 and P waves are not positively identified, atrial flutter should be suspected; the use of carotid sinus pressure or of a Valsalva maneuver to slow the ventricular response may unmask flutter waves;

- At rates above 160 in resting subjects ectopic tachycardia is almost certain; P waves may identify it as "atrial" or "nodal" (i.e., AV junctional)—upright P waves suggest the former, inverted the latter. Yet P waves are often indistinct and an overall diagnosis of "supraventricular tachycardia" may have to be made.

    b.   Ventricular complexes are present; here the differential diagnosis involves the following conditions:

- Sinus tachycardia with bundle branch block;

- Supraventricular tachycardia with bundle branch block;

- Supraventricular tachycardia with aberrant conduction;

- Ventricular tachycardia.

The importance of ruling out the first two conditions by means of control tracings is self-evident. The principal diagnostic difficulty lies in the differentiation between supraventricular tachycardia with aberrant conduction and ventricular tachycardia. None of the criteria is foolproof; the diagnosis has to be made on the basis of highest probability. Both ventricular tachycardia and junctional tachycardia can induce retrograde conduction, with inverted P waves showing a fixed relationship to the QRS complexes (not necessarily in a 1 to 1 ratio); or tachycardia can be associated with a retrograde block, in which case the dissociated atria obey sinus impulses. In the latter situation, fusion beats may appear, which strongly favor ventricular tachycardia. Other points in favor of ventricular tachycardia include the onset of tachycardia (if recorded) triggered by a ventricular ectopic beat, and the appearance of ventricular ectopic beats identical in configuration to those of the tachycardia before or after the paroxysm.

2.   If the tracing shows an irregular tachycardia, the following possibilities should be considered:

    a.   Supraventricular complexes are present:

- Atrial fibrillation;

- Multiple (unifocal) atrial premature contractions (usually some atrial activity other than f waves may be present);

- Chaotic atrial rhythm (multifocal supraventricular ectopic beats at a rapid rate);

- Supraventricular tachycardias (including atrial flutter) with variable conduction (less than 1 to 1 or 2 to 1 response).

    b.   Ventricular complexes are present:

- Atrial fibrillation with aberrant conduction or with bundle branch block is the most reasonable diagnosis.

3.   Arrhythmias occurring within the range of normal heart action (60 to 100):

    a.   The rhythm is regular; ectopic rhythm, shown by abnormal and misplaced P waves at moderate rates, includes:

- Junctional rhythm (with supraventricular complexes);

- Accelerated ventricular rhythm (with ventricular complexes).

Both types of rhythm could be escape rhythms, as will be discussed in the following chapters.

    b.   The rhythm is irregular; here a great many arrhythmias, from the simplest to the most complex, overlap. The following questions need to be considered:

- Are broad ventricular complexes aberrant supraventricular beats or ventricular ectopics?

- Is there some regularity of the appearance of abnormal beats: bigeminy, trigeminy, parasystole, or more subtle patterns?

- What is the dominant rhythm? (Occasionally sinus rhythm is interrupted by ectopic activity to such an extent that physiological beats are difficult to find.)

4. Bradyarrhythmias; here the following conditions should be considered:

- Sinus bradycardia (usually accompanied by sinus arrhythmia);

- Slow escape rhythms (junctional or idioventricular — see under 3, above);

- Sinus rhythm with bigeminy (the most deceiving is bigeminy with blocked atrial premature beats);

- Various forms of complete or incomplete AV block;

- Atrial fibrillation with high degree of AV block.

While in principle, the diagnosis of bradyarrhythmias is simpler than that of tachyarrhythmias, the practical importance of the precise diagnosis exceeds that in other arrhythmias. The error of inserting a permanent pacemaker in patients with digitalis toxicity or with atrial bigeminy may be more serious than that resulting from a confusion between atrial flutter and atrial tachycardia.

Arrhythmias, as indicated, appear in the form of single beats, groups, intermittently appearing beats or groups, or sustained abnormal rhythms. Inasmuch as the various causes of arrhythmias can affect more than one mechanism (e.g., impaired conduction *and* enhanced ectopy), complex disturbances of rhythm develop not infrequently. The diagnosis of arrhythmias may be difficult; especially since the conventional electrocardiogram provides a limited insight into electrophysiological events. Even the valuable addition of His bundle recording helps clarify only some arrhythmias. It should be emphasized, therefore, that the diagnosis of many arrhythmias is only inferential, based on deductions and accepting certain assumptions. Many complex arrhythmias are subject to more than one interpretation, and experts may disagree as to which one is correct.

Bibliography

Cranefield PF, Wit AL, Hoffmann BF: Genesis of cardiac arrhythmias. Circulation 47:190, 1973.

Damato AN, Lau SH: Clinical value of the electrogram of the conduction system, Prog. Cardiovasc. Dis. *13*:119, 1970.

Fisch C, Knoebel SB: Junctional rhythms. Prog. Cardiovasc. Dis. *13*:141, 1970.

Fisch C, Greenspan M, Anderson GJ, Exit block. Amer. J. Card. *28*:402, 1971.

Fisch C. Relationship of electrolyte disturbance to cardiac arrhythmias. Circulation *47*:408, 1973.

Han J: The concept of reentrant activity responsible for ectopic rhythms. Amer. J. Card. *28*:253, 1971.

Hecht HH, Kossman CE et al.: Atrioventricular and intraventricular conduction. Revised nomenclature and criteria. Amer. J. Card. *31*:232, 1973.

Kistin AD: Problem of differentiation of ventricular arrhythmias from supraventricular arrhythmias with abnormal QRS. Prog. Cardiovasc. Dis. *9*:1, 1966.

Marriott HJL, Menendez MM: A-V dissociation revisited. Prog. Cardiovasc. Dis. *8*:522, 1966.

Marriott HJL, Sandler IA: Criteria, old and new, of differentiating between ectopic ventricular beats and aberrant conduction in the presence of atrial fibrillation. Prog. Cardiovasc. Dis. *9*:18, 1966.

Pick A, Langedorff R: Recent advances in the differential diagnosis of A-V junctional arrhythmias. Amer. Heart J. *76*:553, 1968.

Pick A: Mechanism of cardiac arrhythmias: From hypothesis to physiological fact. Amer. Heart J. *86*:249, 1973.

Scherf D: Remarks on the nomenclature of cardiac arrhythmias. Prog. Cardiovasc. Dis. *13*:1, 1970.

18

Supraventricular Arrhythmias

ABNORMALITIES OF SINUS RHYTHM

Sinus tachycardia is, as stated in Chapter 17, primarily a manifestation of stimulation of the SA node by factors outside the heart. It is never a primary manifestation of cardiac disease or of a cardiac functional disorder. It may, however, represent a compensatory effort on the part of the circulatory system to maintain a better cardiac output in some forms of cardiac failure and in shock. Thus its importance in diagnosis involves the following approaches:

- Identification of its noncardiac causes: excitability, fever, hyperthyroidism, anemia, drugs, and others;

- Its recognition as a manifestation of occult cardiac failure or early shock (i.e., in acute myocardial infarction).

When no plausible explanation for persistent sinus tachycardia is found, the possibility of an increase in sympathetic drive should be considered. It is often advisable, in addition, to re-examine the tracing critically from the standpoint of possible misinterpretation of an ectopic tachycardia with P wave morphology similar to that of sinus tachycardia.

Sinus tachycardia very seldom requires direct therapy designed to reduce the heart rate. First, elimination of the underlying factor is the proper approach, if it is possible. Second, as a secondary manifestation of cardiac failure or shock it is compensatory, therefore desirable in such cases. Third, the only effective agent capable of slowing the SA node rhythmicity is propranolol; its use for this purpose is indicated only in rare cases of autonomic imbalance, in which the tachycardia becomes intolerable to the patient.

272

Sinus bradycardia, in contrast to sinus tachycardia, may under certain circumstances present itself as a manifestation of cardiac disease. In general, physiological slow automaticity in healthy individuals occurs more frequently than rapid rates. Young subjects may have rates as low as 40 beats per minute, often associated with sinus arrhythmias (both being manifestations of increased vagal activity). Its development in athletes has already been commented upon. In contrast to these physiological varieties and certain temporary conditions, mentioned in Chapter 17, sinus bradycardia may be a primary manifestation of pathological involvement of the SA node. Pathological sinus bradycardia has been referred to in recent years as evidence of the "sick sinus syndrome." Inasmuch as this entity almost always involves manifestations of disease of other portions of the conducting system, the discussion of this syndrome will be included in Chapter 20, dealing with conduction disturbances.

Sinus arrhythmias appear physiologically in conjunction with bradycardias, for the SA node automaticity at its lower range assumes a periodic variation of rhythm, usually related to respiratory phases. This phenomenon is exaggerated in children, in whom sinus bradycardia may be pronounced to the degree of producing activation of escape mechanisms. Sinus arrhythmias may also occur in conjunction with normal or faster than average rates. It is considered a normal variant of no significance. Its importance lies in recognizing it as such and not confusing it with more ominous forms of arrhythmias. Its diagnosis is contingent on demonstrating periodicity of rhythmic variation and gradual, rather than abrupt, changes of the rate.

Wandering pacemaker represents a variant of sinus arrhythmia and is also considered an innocent variation of the normal rhythmicity of the heart. It differs from sinus arrhythmia, in which the phasic irregularity is associated with normal P waves and a constant P-R interval, whereas wandering pacemaker shows different types of P waves and variable P-R intervals. In this arrhythmia, as in sinus arrhythmia, phasic periodicity and gradual change differentiate it from intermittently appearing ectopic rhythms. "Shifting pacemaker" is a term applied occasionally to abrupt rather than phasic change from a sinus to an atrial or AV junctional rhythm.

ECTOPIC BEATS

Supraventricular ectopic beats include the wide range of beats originating outside the SA node but maintaining the same mode of activation of the ventricles as physiological (i.e., sinus) beats. Such beats include those originating in the atria, in the region of the AV node, and in the bundle of His. As explained, the appearance of P waves and their relationship to the QRS complexes provide a guideline, but not a proof, of the site of origin of ectopic impulses.

The following variety of supraventricular ectopic beats can be differentiated:

1. *Atrial ectopic beats.* Such beats are almost always premature. They are characterized by abnormal P waves that have, however, the same axis as those of sinus beats. P waves in atrial ectopic beats may be indistinguishable from those in physiological sinus beats. Atrial ectopic beats also having the same P-R interval as normal beats have occasionally been termed "sinus premature beats." This name should be avoided, for it is exceedingly unlikely that the automaticity of the SA node would show nonperiodic abrupt changes: so-called "sinus premature beats" more likely represent ectopic beats originating in areas near the SA node. The P-R interval of atrial ectopic beats is variable. More often than not it is shorter than that of normal beats, but it may be the same length or longer. Atrial premature contractions occur as follows:

- As single premature beats;

- As repetitive beats occurring at random;

- As repetitive beats, regularly occurring (bigeminy, ectopics occurring every third or fourth beat, etc.);

- As multifocal ectopic beats showing multiform P waves and variable P-R intervals;

- As blocked atrial ectopic beats (appearing early in the cycle, finding the lower conducting system refractory).

Ectopic atrial beats represent, as a rule, an innocent type of arrhythmia. Frequently found in healthy individuals, they may or may not have an identifiable provoking factor (e,g., excitement, tobacco, coffee, etc.) Only rarely are they associated with organic cardiac disease in a manner that a causal relationship is implied. Such conditions include:

- Conditions with high proneness to atrial fibrillation (e.g., mitral stenosis), in which ectopic atrial beats may be the precursor of atrial fibrillation;

- Persistence of atrial ectopic beats in acute myocardial infarction may imply atrial involvement in the ischemic damage.

2. *AV junctional ectopic beats.* This variety of supraventricular ectopic beat is diagnosed when P waves show an abnormal axis (commonly superior, i.e., inverted in leads II, III, and AVF). The term of AV "junctional" (old terminology: nodal) is applied here within the broad context, recognizing that such beats could originate anywhere

from the lower portion of the atria (coronary sinus region of the right atrium, lower part of the left atrium) to the bundle of His. AV junctional beats may be encountered in the form of all varieties listed under atrial ectopic beats, but, in addition, such beats occur also as escaped beats, that is, not prematurely. AV junctional premature beats are much rarer than atrial ones: the pacemaking mechanism around the AV junction tends to generate ectopic rhythms much more often than ectopic single impulses. The reverse is true of atrial ectopic pacemakers. Such ectopic beats also bear no relationship to complex atrial arrhythmias (e.g., atrial fibrillation).

3. *Unidentified supraventricular ectopic beats.* Single beats or sequences of beats of supraventricular configuration in which atrial activity cannot be positively identified or morphologically separated from other electrocardiographic complexes are usually referred to by the above term. Obviously, they originate either in the atrium or within the upper conducting system; however, they have no distinctive features.

Treatment of supraventricular ectopic beats is seldom indicated. In this innocent arrhythmia, often merely a physiological variant, antiarrhythmic therapy is indicated only if a specific objective can be identified. However, should such arrhythmias be suspected of being related to the patient's mode of living or his use of various stimuli, recommendation for the appropriate change in habits is indicated as a preventive measure.

Antiarrhythmic therapy might be considered under the following circumstances:

- Some neurotic individuals are made uncomfortable by the heart's "skipping"; if reassurance is totally ineffective, suppression of arrhythmias may be tried.

- Arrhythmia may contribute to or perpetuate cardiac failure in patients with advanced myocardial disease. Its elimination may prove useful in the control of such patients' failure.

- Extreme bradycardia may be present as a result of atrial bigeminy with blocked premature contractions. Suppression of bigeminy may have a beneficial effect.

- Patients in whom atrial fibrillation is expected (i.e., after some cardiac operations or in patients under treatment to maintain sinus rhythm after electroshock conversion of atrial fibrillation), administration of antiarrhythmic agents or increase in the dose of such drugs already being given may be justifiable for repetitive atrial ectopic beats as precursors of atrial fibrillation.

- Whenever drug therapy is suspected of contributing to the

origin of supraventricular ectopy (or escape), reduction of the dose or discontinuation of such drug (digitalis, propranolol) is indicated.

SUPRAVENTRICULAR TACHYCARDIAS

Between ectopic beats and ectopic rhythms there is only a difference in degree. Tachycardias constitute the sequential appearance of ectopic beats originating in the atrium or in the broad region defined earlier within the context of AV junctional rhythm; as in ectopic beats, tachycardia can be electrocardiographically identified as "atrial," "AV junctional," or passed over without exact localization as "supraventricular." Inasmuch as rapid sustained rhythms may leave less opportunity to find telltale P waves, the overlap between atrial and AV junctional tachycardias is wider than that between single beats; hence more tachycardias are dismissed by the general term "supraventricular."

The great majority of tachycardias are paroxysmal in nature. They are characterized by an abrupt onset and termination. Their duration varies from a few seconds (a few successive ectopic beats) to weeks. As in ectopic beats, tachycardias more often than not are innocent, occurring in subjects without known cardiac disease. If they develop in patients who have organic cardiac disease, they may or may not have connotations relating them with the underlying condition. Among such relationships are the following:

- Conditions associated with atrial enlargement, in which paroxysmal tachycardias may appear, although atrial flutter and fibrillation occur more commonly: atrial septal defect, mitral stenosis, certain types of cardiomyopathy (e.g., "alcoholic");

- Acute conditions associated with possible atrial injury: acute myocardial infarction, the postoperative period following thoracic and cardiovascular operations;

- Drug effect and intoxication, particularly from digitalis.

In the majority of patients, when no evidence of cardiac disease can be found, paroxysmal tachycardias tend to recur. Proneness to paroxysmal tachycardia often develops in childhood or in youth and may persist for life. Sometimes such tendencies are familial. Paroxysmal tachycardias that occur in patients with Wolff-Parkinson-White syndrome and the related, rarer Lown-Ganong-Levine syndrome are of a special variety, but some patients with paroxysmal tachycardias and a normal interim electrocardiogram are occasionally found to have intermittent W-P-W complexes, thus suggesting that some forms of it, perhaps the familial ones, may represent variants, or a forme fruste, of one of these syndromes. Recent demonstration that many paroxysmal supraventricular tachycardias are caused by the re-entry mechanism rather than by enhanced automaticity of an ectopic focus adds weight to such speculation.

Effects of the Tachycardia. Paroxysmal tachycardia shows a wide range in rates: from less than 150 to over 300. Very rapid tachycardias often find the conducting tissues unable to function at the rapid rate, and a 2 to 1 ventricular response may take place, similar to that occurring in atrial flutter. The effect of the tachycardia depends upon three factors:

- Rapidity of the ventricular rate,

- Its duration,

- Whether or not underlying heart disease is present.

In healthy individuals paroxysmal tachycardia is most often a mere nuisance. Brief attacks at rates that are not excessive are occasionally not even noted by the subject; more prolonged attacks produce the discomfort of palpitation, which the patient upon reassurance by his physician learns to ignore. Effort tolerance during attacks vary: some can go about their normal activities; others may have to limit them. Occasionally copious diuresis occurs during such a paroxysm. Even prolonged attacks are unlikely to produce true cardiac symptoms, such as dyspnea, or evidence of cardiac failure. Such symptoms occur rarely, and only when the rate is very fast.

In the presence of *organic cardiac disease* paroxysms of rapid heart action may have serious, even disastrous, effects. The consequences of paroxysms depend upon the rapidity of the ventricular rate and the duration of the attack, and on the type and severity of the cardiac disease. Such paroxysms may produce the following:

- Aggravation of cardiac failure,

- Acute pulmonary edema,

- Shock-like state,

- Anginal attacks, prolonged ischemia.

Special Forms of Ectopic Tachycardias. There are a few special varieties of ectopic tachycardia that differ in some respects from the ordinary paroxysmal form. Among these are the following:

1. Paroxysmal tachycardia in infants: such arrhythmias are electrocardiographically identical with paroxysmal supraventricular varieties, but are more rapid, of longer duration (occasionally chronic), and

more resistant to therapy. The effect of such arrhythmia is more serious than in adults, so that they may even without known cardiac disease represent medical emergencies.

2.   Nonparoxysmal tachycardia: this chronic form of tachycardia occurs in infants, children, and adults (usually young ones). It may be associated with congenital heart disease but in the majority appears as an isolated clinical finding. Though not always alarming, circulatory effects of such tachycardia may be serious. After sinus rhythm is established, such patients require maintenance drug therapy. Sometimes tachycardia recurs regardless of therapy. Occasionally sinus rhythm cannot be established at all, suggesting the possibility that sinus automaticity may be defective.

3.   Repetitive supraventricular tachycardia represents a form of recurrent attacks of tachycardia, alternating with sinus rhythm. The rhythm changes continuously: a few sinus beats alternate with brief paroxysms of tachycardia. Such periods of atrial instability may occur episodically, with stable sinus rhythm in between, or be present continuously; they are often resistant to therapy.

4.   Paroxysmal tachycardia related to the pre-excitation syndromes. This will be discussed in Chapter 20.

Management of Tachycardias.   As explained, ectopic tachycardias, in terms of their clinical significance, present a broad spectrum, ranging from a minor nuisance to a life-threatening emergency. Consequently, the therapeutic approach to this problem has to be carefully thought out for each individual situation if the usual therapeutic equation (risk balanced by benefit) is to be observed. Therapy involves three approaches:

1.   Elimination or correction of identifiable exciting factors;

2.   Termination of the attack;

3.   Prevention of its recurrence.

The first of these may be the most rewarding, although precipitating factors are only occasionally identifiable. A survey of drugs and stimulants taken by the patient in the period preceding the paroxysms may be informative. Some patients have ceased to be susceptible to paroxysmal tachycardia after a chronic noncardiac disease has been eliminated (e.g., gallbladder disease, chronic urinary obstruction, and others).

The second and third of the above approaches to therapy are usually considered together as related therapeutic steps. Because of the wide range of available forms of treatment, specific therapeutic analysis needs to be done in each case. The following questions should be considered:

- How seriously does a paroxysm affect the patient (subjectively and objectively)?
- What are the frequency and duration of attacks?
- Is there information available regarding the patient's response to therapy in the past?

Methods of terminating attacks of paroxysmal supraventricular tachycardia include the following:

- Vagal stimulation. This is the most effective approach, though not uniformly successful. It involves several steps:

  a. Direct vagal stimulation by carotid sinus pressure;

  b. Pharmacological vagal stimulation (occasionally reinforced by additional carotid sinus pressure after the drug administration), including Prostigmin or edrophonium chloride;

  c. Indirect vagal stimulation via a pressor reflex, using pressor amines: phenylephrine, methoxamine;

  d. Methods now obsolete included, in the past, eyeball pressure or use of apomorphine.

- Intravenous administration of a rapid-acting digitalis preparation;

- Oral administration of quinidine, procainamide, or propranolol;

- Electroshock therapy;

- Mechanical induction of ventricular ectopic beats (this approach is practical only for paroxysms induced by catheter stimulation during cardiac catheterization);

- Pacing overdrive: this is obviously a drastic method suitable only for serious or life-threatening situations that are refractory to other forms of therapy.

Methods used for the prevention of attacks of tachycardia include the following maintenance drug therapy:

- digitalis
- quinidine
- procainamide

• propranolol

• combination of these drugs

The success of treatment of paroxysmal tachycardia depends often upon good collaboration between the clinician and the patient. Whenever possible, treatment should be made available to the patient at home. Only unusually serious attacks in normal individuals or attacks with known deleterious consequences in patients who have cardiac disease should be handled in the hospital. Mild attacks occurring frequently may often be managed without specific therapy, by instructing the patient to take a sedative and rest until the attack is terminated. Some patients take oral quinidine in doses of 0.2 to 0.4 every two hours for two or three doses to terminate attacks.

Electroshock therapy is obviously the most effective mode of therapy. Its use, however, in such benign arrhythmias as paroxysmal supraventricular tachycardia in healthy individuals should be restricted to extreme cases only (in terms of duration of the attacks, rapidity of ventricular rate, and its effect upon the patient). It is, of course, contraindicated if any suspicion exists that the attack may have been induced by digitalis.

In general, paroxysmal supraventricular tachycardia is much more often overtreated than undertreated; emphasis should be placed on its benign nature and the least therapeutic intervention possible.

ATRIAL FLUTTER

Atrial flutter occupies an intermediate place between atrial tachycardia and atrial fibrillation. Atrial tachycardia involves rapidly occurring, coordinated contraction of the atria; atrial fibrillation involves chaotic atrial activity without effective atrial systole. In atrial flutter, regular, very rapid atrial contractions take place, which are probably only borderline effective in terms of atrial transport function. The old controversy as to whether atrial flutter involves a continuous traveling wave-front "circus movement" or a rapidly discharging ectopic focus appears to have been resolved, at least in part, in favor of the former. The new impetus toward this view has been the demonstration that atrial tachycardias frequently involve a re-entry mechanism (a related form of "circus movement").

As in atrial tachycardia, atrial flutter may occur in individuals without known cardiac disease and in patients with organic disease. It occurs in a paroxysmal form with spontaneous termination, or may be a continuous, chronic process, when not treated. In general, flutter is less stable than fibrillation of the atria: even untreated atrial flutter may change into sinus rhythm or atrial fibrillation, leaving only a small proportion of patients in chronic flutter.

Electrocardiographic features of flutter were reviewed in Chapter 17. The atrial rate (F waves) ranges within a narrow zone of 220 to 340 beats per minute. The great majority of patients show ventricular responses to alternate F waves, producing a ventricular rate of 110 to 170 (2 to 1 response). Higher degrees of AV block with slower ventricular rates occur usually in response to therapy, only rarely spontaneously. Such higher degrees of block may be regular, producing a ventricular rate as a fraction of the flutter rate, or irregular, with varying degrees of block and an irregular ventricular rhythm. The great majority of cases of atrial flutter show a regular ventricular rhythm, the minority an irregular rhythm. The commonest is a flutter rate of 300 and a ventricular rate of 150.

Atrial flutter may develop at any age: its occurrence in childhood is rare but still more common than atrial fibrillation. Atrial flutter, as well as atrial fibrillation, occurs preferentially in some forms of disease. Among such relationships are the following:

- Conditions associated with proneness to atrial arrhythmias in general, but most commonly with atrial fibrillation (mitral stenosis, thyrotoxicosis, etc.);

- Congenital heart disease in adults, especially atrial septal defect;

- Diseases of the pericardium, especially invasion by tumors;

- Following cardiac or pulmonary operations.

Atrial flutter associated with organic cardiac disease may occur interchangeably with atrial fibrillation. Occasionally, especially in its paroxysmal form, flutter develops in some paroxysms, fibrillation in others. In general, some preferential appearance of atrial flutter in conditions involving the *right* atrium has been observed, with atrial fibrillation developing more often in conditions affecting the *left* atrium. Thus, mitral stenosis is much more commonly associated with atrial fibrillation; atrial septal defect, with atrial flutter. Tumor invasion or metastasis of the right atrium is more likely to produce atrial flutter; that of the left atrium, fibrillation.

Atrial flutter thus involves in the great majority of untreated patients a regular tachycardia with ventricular rate around 150/min. Carotid sinus stimulation produces in most patients an increase in the block, thereby reducing, for a period of a few beats, the ventricular rate to one half or less of the original response. The consequences of atrial flutter in healthy subjects are frequently even less bothersome to the patient than in supraventricular tachycardias, because the ventricular rate is usually slower than in that condition. In the presence of cardiac disease the effects of flutter are related to the tolerance of rapid rate and to some loss of atrial transport function. Systemic embolization constitutes a very rare risk associated with atrial flutter.

Management of atrial flutter consists—in common with the other atrial arrhythmias—of two steps: termination of the attack and prevention of its recurrences. In contrast to supraventricular tachycardias, which almost always are paroxysmal, the presence of atrial flutter in a patient does not always permit the differentiation between paroxysmal and established forms of this arrhythmia. An attack of atrial flutter in a patient who gives a history of having had previous brief attacks usually suggests the paroxysmal form, yet the paroxysmal form of this arrhythmia in some cases precedes the persistent form. Atrial flutter developing in a middle-aged individual for the first time and lasting more than 24 hours is likely to represent the persistent form.

The most effective means of terminating atrial flutter is electroshock therapy. This arrhythmia represents the most consistently responsive target of DC shock therapy, one sensitive to the small strength of the shock (25 to 50 joules, or watt-seconds). Nevertheless, the use of this major therapeutic procedure in paroxysmal atrial flutter—which because of its short duration is often of uncertain classification—should be discouraged in favor of drug therapy.

The principal drugs used for treatment of atrial flutter include digitalis, quinidine, propranolol, and procainamide. Digitalis decreases the ventricular rate by producing a higher degree of block but seldom terminates this atrial arrhythmia. Its action is less predictable in atrial flutter and requires much higher dosages than the similar effect exerted upon atrial fibrillation. Quinidine may restore sinus rhythm. Before atrial flutter is terminated by action of this drug the rate of the flutter waves decreases markedly. A well-advertised risk of quinidine therapy is the development of 1 to 1 ventricular response coincidental with the slowing of flutter waves to the 200 to 220 range, with a paradoxical increase in ventricular rate. This does occur, but is rare. The use of digitalis prior to quinidine administration is traditionally advocated to prevent such occurrence. At present propranolol is probably a much more effective agent to combine with quinidine. Procainamide has a weak action against atrial arrhythmias and its use is mainly for patients who cannot tolerate quinidine.

Maintenance drug therapy involves two situations: for patients who suffer from repetitive attacks of paroxysmal atrial flutter and in order to prevent relapses in patients who had been converted to sinus rhythm from established atrial flutter. In the first situation, quinidine, alone or combined with either digitalis or propranolol, may be used. The use depends upon the frequency of attacks: rare attacks probably justify no maintenance therapy at all. The second situation has to be treated individually and depends upon the circumstances. Healthy individuals developing atrial flutter without a provoking factor may be left without therapy after electroshock restoration of sinus rhythm; many such patients will not develop a recurrence at all; those who do are given maintenance therapy after repeat restoration of sinus rhythm. Patients with a precipitating factor that is temporary may be treated for an arbitrary time period, e.g., one or two months (in postoperative atrial flutter). Those with permanent cardiac lesions need continuous therapy. The dosages and drugs used need individual adjustment—usually by trial and error. In many cases atrial flutter relapses or changes into atrial fibrillation in spite of maintenance therapy.

ATRIAL FIBRILLATION

Atrial fibrillation represents the most common as well as the most serious disorder of the atria. Atrial activity in this condition is chaotic and uncoordinated, being tantamount to a complete loss of atrial function. Electrocardiographic features of atrial fibrillation have been mentioned in Chapter 17: irregular or occasionally regular atrial depolarization is recorded in the form of f waves at rates between 350 and 450.

Atrial fibrillation may develop in healthy individuals; in the majority of cases, however, organic disease of the heart is present. As in the other forms of arrhythmia, it may occur in the paroxysmal form or may become permanent. Occasionally, paroxysmal atrial fibrillation is present as a lifelong series of short episodes in otherwise healthy subjects. In the great majority of cases, however, paroxysmal atrial fibrillation is a precursor of permanent atrial fibrillation, antedating the persistent stage by years, months, or days.

The pathogenesis of atrial fibrillation involves more than a single factor. Trauma to the atrium has been established as an important cause of atrial fibrillation. As already mentioned in connection with atrial flutter, mechanical trauma during operations or cardiac catheterization may initiate atrial fibrillation. Trauma to the atrium, either acute or chronic, may well be the common denominator of all conditions associated with proneness to atrial fibrillation. The condition most often associated with chronic atrial fibrillation is mitral valve disease. In it chronic trauma initiates atrial fibrillation, which becomes a self-perpetuating process, producing atrial dilatation and eventual disintegration of the atrial musculature. The trauma to the left atrium is more pronounced in chronic mitral regurgitation than in mitral stenosis, hence a higher incidence of atrial fibrillation occurs in the former.

Other causes of atrial fibrillation include the following:

• Toxic conditions—hyperthyroidism, alcohol, hypoxia;

• Acute left atrial disease—acute myocardial infarction;

• Chronic left atrial disease—chronic congestive cardiac failure, constrictive pericarditis, tumor invasion.

The most important predisposing factor affecting the development and chronicity of atrial fibrillation, given a causative agent, is age. Atrial fibrillation is very rare in children; its incidence in response to comparable stimuli (e.g., open heart surgery) increases after the age of 20 in a linear fashion.

The *clinical features* of atrial fibrillation are related to three factors:

1. Rapid ventricular rate,

2. Loss of atrial transport function,

3. Complications—primarily systemic embolization.

Untreated atrial fibrillation produces irregular ventricular response to the fibrillating atria at an average of 3 to 1, that is, producing a ventricular rate between 150 and 200. If the ventricular rate is much slower than 150 beats/min., a suspicion regarding normal function of the AV node may arise. As in other tachyarrhythmias, the effect of the rapid ventricular rate varies depending upon the normal state of the heart or the extent of its abnormality. Atrial fibrillation is less well tolerated than other tachyarrhythmias of comparable ventricular rates: irregularity makes some beats ineffective (producing the well-known, clinically overemphasized "pulse deficit"). The loss of atrial transport function has a variable effect upon the circulation: in healthy individuals and in many diseased but compensated hearts such loss of function may be of minor significance. In critically balanced cardiac failure or in conditions in which low ventricular compliance requires a good "atrial kick," onset of fibrillation may bring about clinical deterioration by this mechanism alone (irrespective of ventricular rate).

The incidence of systemic embolization in atrial fibrillation is relatively high; its preferential occurrence in mitral valve disease in contrast to other conditions is well established, but non-mitral patients are not immune from such a complication. Cerebral embolism is by far the commonest (or most frequently recognized) site of embolization.

Management of atrial fibrillation involves three steps:

1. Control of ventricular rate during atrial fibrillation,

2. Termination of the attack,

3. Prevention of recurrences.

In addition, a fourth step may be considered in some cases: prevention of systemic embolization by anticoagulant therapy.

In contrast to other atrial tachyarrhythmias, the first two points often represent alternative options rather than sequential steps of treatment. Patients with atrial fibrillation can be arbitrarily divided into the following therapeutic groups:

1. Those with normal hearts and occasional paroxysms of atrial fibrillation. Here the choice lies between maintenance drug therapy for the prevention of paroxysms (quinidine and/or propranolol) and no interim treatment.

2. Those with established atrial fibrillation who show no other evidence of cardiac disease—the idiopathic form of this arrhythmia. "Lone" atrial fibrillation probably includes more than a single condition: there may be those with a real "electrical" accident as well as those with the disturbance of the rhythm as the first or only manifestation of cardiac disease (ischemic disease, degenerative disease of the conducting tissue, cardiomyopathy, etc.). Older individuals with idiopathic atrial fibrillation have a disappointingly high rate of recurrences after conversion to sinus rhythm. Consequently, the individual decision on therapy should be made along the guidelines submitted below.

3. Patients with established or paroxysmal atrial fibrillation who suffer from a cardiac disease *without* special propensity for this arrhythmia. Here restoration of sinus rhythm may be indicated in many cases.

4. Patients with established or paroxysmal atrial fibrillation who suffer from a cardiac disease *with* a special propensity for this arrhythmia. In these cases restoration of sinus rhythm is indicated only under special circumstances.

The decision-making process as to whether atrial fibrillation should be permitted to remain and therapy directed at optimal control of ventricular rate or whether sinus rhythm should be restored should be guided by the following clinical factors:

1. The older the patient, the lower the likelihood of permanently remaining in sinus rhythm after conversion from atrial fibrillation;

2. The larger the left atrium, the lower the likelihood of restoration and maintenance of sinus rhythm;

3. The greater the length of time the patient had atrial fibrillation, the lower the probability of restoration and maintenance of sinus rhythm.

4. In conditions associated with high proneness to atrial fibrillation a reasonable chance for successful maintenance of postconversion sinus rhythm is largely contingent upon improvement of the underlying condition (e.g., relief of mitral stenosis).

Thus, unqualified efforts to restore sinus rhythm should be made in younger patients with recent onset of atrial fibrillation and a small left atrium. Atrial fibrillation should not be converted to sinus rhythm in older patients with a very large left atrium and long-standing atrial fibrillation, even if a mitral valve operation has been successfully performed. Between these two extremes individual decisions are necessary. In patients who relapsed after successful restoration of sinus rhythm and optimal maintenance therapy has been administered, repeat attempts at conversion can be questioned.

The tools available for the various forms of treatment of atrial fibrillation are as follows:

- Control of ventricular rate: digitalis and propranolol are the two available agents. Propranolol is probably more uniformly effective, yet digitalis (in theory, at least) improves cardiac function, while propranolol worsens it.

- Restoration of sinus rhythm: electroshock therapy is the treatment of choice, unless small doses of quinidine can promptly restore sinus rhythm.

- Maintenance preventive therapy: quinidine is the most effective drug, with propranolol and procainamide less effective alternatives. Drug combinations have been tried with some claims of success.

- Termination of paroxysmal atrial fibrillation: quinidine in hourly or bihourly doses, possibly with propranolol as an alternative, is considered treatment of choice. An exception to this rule is in acute forms of atrial fibrillation occurring during cardiac catheterization; intravenous digoxin or deslanoside often terminates such attacks.

- Anticoagulation for the prevention of systemic embolization has not been standardized regarding its indications. The potential risk of such therapy probably precludes its routine use in all patients, even in all those with mitral valve disease. The indication for anticoagulant therapy is reasonably well founded in the prevention of recurrences in patients who have had a definite systemic embolic episode. If anticoagulation is not instituted in such patients, it should be considered, at least on a short-term basis, in those in whom restoration of sinus rhythm is contemplated. (Routine use of anticoagulants prior to restoration of sinus rhythm appears impractical and uneconomical in view of the uncertain benefits of such therapy.)

ECTOPIC RHYTHMS AT SLOW OR MODERATE RATES

The great majority of supraventricular arrhythmias are tachyarrhythmias, which have been discussed in the preceding sections. There are, however, some ectopic rhythms which fall into the range of cardiac rates between 50 and 100. Most of such "arrhythmias" illustrate the inadequacy of this term, for they show regular rhythm and normal or near-normal heart rate. Such disturbances of impulse formation involve three mechanisms:

- Escape rhythms at usual or accelerated rates,

- Slightly increased automaticity of an ectopic focus,

- Ectopic tachycardias with a high degree of AV block and lower ventricular rates.

Almost always ectopic rhythm in these categories originates in the AV junctional region (in its broad sense, as described above). The commoner forms of such ectopic rhythm at the range of its automaticity (50-60/min.) include the following:

- Congenital AV junctional rhythm; some patients never have sinus rhythm, a fact which suggests the possibility of congenital abnormality of the SA node or the internodal tracts. This can be an isolated finding or may occur in combination with certain congenital abnormalities (e.g., sinus venous type of atrial septal defect).

- Postoperative AV junctional rhythm: Patients who have had extensive manipulations in the right atrium may be left with permanent junctional rhythm, presumably caused by surgical trauma. Surgeons have now learned to avoid damage to atrial conducting tracts in the repair of transposition of the great vessels.

- "Idiopathic" acquired AV junctional rhythm develops in certain individuals.

- Toxic AV junctional escape rhythm (e.g., digitalis-induced).

- Postconversion AV junctional rhythm; following electroshock therapy escape rhythm may develop temporarily, or even permanently.

Patients with such arrhythmias should be approached with great caution. Since the escape rhythm is one developing "by default," every form of antiarrhythmic therapy may be contraindicated.

Another form of ectopic rhythm without tachycardia is a mildly increased automaticity of an AV junctional focus. Two possible consequences of such an activity of the ectopic pacemaker may develop: the ectopic rhythm may capture both the atria and the ventricles, producing the conventional form of a junctional rhythm; or the atria may remain under control of the SA node with the ectopic focus activating only the ventricle. The latter situation produces AV dissociation, which may be complete or incomplete, if an occasional atrial impulse, properly timed within the cardiac cycle, captures the ventricle and resets the automaticity of the ectopic focus.

Inasmuch as the accelerated AV junctional rhythm differs from the supraventricular tachycardia only in the rate of the impulse formation, circumstances of its occurrence resemble those of the tachycardias. The exception to this is the ectopic junctional rhythm associated with AV dissociation, which is one of the recognized forms of digitalis toxicity. The treatment of the accelerated AV junctional rhythm should be less aggressive than that of tachycardias, because such arrhythmias usually play a minor role as a factor in the clinical course of cardiac disease. In the case of digitalis intoxication, however, immediate termination of digitalis therapy is indicated, and sometimes active therapy may be needed.

Ectopic tachycardias with AV block and a moderate ventricular rate are encountered most frequently under two sets of circumstances:

- In association with disease of the conducting system,

- As a manifestation of digitalis toxicity.

This form of arrhythmia requires a careful analysis, in view of the fact that it is considered a particularly hazardous form of digitalis toxicity.

COMPLEX SUPRAVENTRICULAR ARRHYTHMIAS

In addition to the supraventricular arrhythmias discussed in the preceding section, there are rare forms of more complex arrhythmias. The complexity of such arrhythmias has no particular significance as to their etiology, association with heart disease, or gravity. Among the various rare forms four deserve mention here:

1. *Supraventricular parasystole.* Parasystolic rhythms originating in the atrium or the AV junction are much rarer than those developing in the lower part of the conducting system ("ventricular"). They compete with physiological beats for the capture of cardiac action. They are usually benign and have no special significance.

2. *Double tachycardias.* Here two ectopic foci with high automaticity

rate are present; the upper one—usually atrial—activates the atria, the lower—AV junctional—the ventricles. Retrograde block produces AV dissociation and prevents the two rhythms from interfering with each other. Such tachycardias are too rare to find relationship with any exciting factor. Digitalis intoxication may be the basis of some of these tachycardias.

3.   *Chaotic atrial rhythm* has been the term used for a combination of multiple multifocal ectopic beats and short runs of tachycardia. Such arrhythmias, rarely, may have a random distribution, or they may show repetitive patterns. There is no known specific cause of this arrhythmia.

4.   *Alternating bidirectional tachycardia.* This arrhythmia involves a regular AV junctional tachycardia with impulses alternately activating the ventricles via one and the other bundle branches, hence producing an alternation of right and left bundle branch complexes. This rare tachycardia is best known as a manifestation of digitalis intoxication, even though digitalis is not the only agent responsible for its occurrence.

Bibliography

Bailey GWH, Braniff BS, Hancock EW, Cohn KE: Relation of left atrial pathology to atrial fibrillation in mitral valvular disease. Ann. Int. Med. *69*:13, 1968.

Bellet S: Diagnostic features and management of supraventricular arrhythmias. Prog. Cardiovasc. Dis. *8*:483, 1966.

Evans W, Swann P: Lone auricular fibrillation. Brit. Heart J. *16*:189, 1954.

Neufeld HN, Wagenvoort CA, Burchell HB, Edwards JE: Idiopathic atrial fibrillation. Amer. J. Cardiol. *8*:193, 1961.

Probst P, Goldschlager NF, Selzer A: Factors influencing the development of atrial fibrillation in mitral stenosis. Circulation *48*:128, 1973.

Rosen KM: Junctional tachycardia: mechanism, diagnosis and management. Circulation *47*:654, 1973.

Selzer A, Kelly JJ Jr, Gerbode F, Kerth WJ, Blackley JE, Morgan JJ, Keyani K: Treatment of atrial fibrillation after surgical repair of the mitral valve. Ann. Int. Med. *62*:1213, 1965.

19
Ventricular Arrhythmias

Definition. In Chapter 17 the "ventricular" type of QRS complexes has been described: such abnormal complexes are characterized by an asynchronous activation of the two ventricles, producing significant delays within the lower portion of the conduction system. The term "ventricular" is one of convenience and tradition. The implication that ectopic rhythms originate in the ventricular myocardium is not definitely demonstrated. While electrophysiological studies indicate that in disease states any ordinary myocardial cell may assume the characteristics of a pacemaker cell and thus acquire the property of automaticity, it is much more likely that ventricular ectopy originates in the pacemaker cells of the lower part of the conduction system, i.e., the bundle branches, their secondary divisions, and the Purkinje network.

The difficulty of distinguishing between ventricular ectopy and that originating in the upper part of the conducting system associated with aberration has been discussed. There appears to be no foolproof criterion differentiating the two types of beats or rhythms — merely criteria indicating higher probability for one or the other mechanism. Such differentiation extends beyond academic purism: there are at least two implications of major importance in which ventricular rhythms differ from supraventricular rhythm with aberration:

- Different responses to drug therapy are observed (granted that there can be considerable overlap);

- The prognostic significance of ventricular rhythms can be much more grave, in view of the fact that they may be precursors of ventricular fibrillation.

ECTOPIC BEATS

Ventricular ectopic beats are almost always premature, signifying active pacemaking rather than an escape mechanism. A ventricular escape mechanism is rare in the absence of serious disturbance of the conducting system. Ventricular ectopy covers as wide a range as that of supraventricular ectopy: such beats occur in healthy subjects and in patients with a variety of cardiac diseases in response to many intrinsic or extrinsic stimuli. Although causes of ventricular ectopic beats cannot always be found, their common precipitating factors include the following:

- mechanical stimulation of the ventricular endocardium (during cardiac catheterization, pacemaker insertion),

- hypoxia,

- localized ischemia,

- acidosis,

- electrolyte imbalance (both hyperkalemia and hypokalemia may produce ectopy),

- drugs,

- other toxic agents,

- myocardial disease (acute or chronic).

Ventricular ectopic beats are encountered in a variety of forms, many of which have a higher risk in terms of overall prognosis or as manifestations of cardiac disease:

1. Occasional single premature ventricular contractions: These are the least significant, and occur with considerable frequency in healthy individuals. Criteria have been proposed regarding the minimum frequency of ventricular ectopic beats that would warrant initiating antiarrhythmic therapy. There is no solid data to make such standards valid on the basis of scientific evidence: the widely accepted criterion for coronary care units of 5 or 6 premature beats per minute as representing "significant" ectopy and a valid indication for therapeutic intervention is based on impression and opinion.

2. Recurrent ventricular ectopic beats may appear at irregular intervals of every second, third, or fourth beat, etc.: As stated above, there is speculative suggestion of a relationship between the frequency of ventricular ectopic activity and the prognosis, but not solid data.

3. Ventricular parasystole: Here a single ectopic pacemaker discharges regularly, competing with the physiological impulse formation. Exit block usually makes the ectopic pacemaker capture only occasionally ventricular activation. Parasystolic ectopy is basically a benign phenomenon that carries little serious connotation when compared with nonparasystolic ectopic beats occurring with comparable frequency.

4. Ventricular bigeminy (coupled premature beats with a fixed coupling period) represent one of the commonest forms of ventricular ectopy, occurring both in health and in cardiac disease. These ectopic beats are considered to be produced by re-entry phenomena. They represent a form of digitalis intoxication: this mechanism should always be suspected whenever the patient is taking this drug.

5. Early diastolic ventricular ectopic beats showing the R-on-T phenomenon are the most serious form of ventricular ectopy, since they may stimulate the heart during its vulnerable period and could trigger ventricular fibrillation.

6. Multiform ventricular ectopic beats, assumed to represent multifocal ectopy, are also a more ominous form of ventricular ectopy, although frequent multiform ventricular ectopic beats have occasionally been observed in healthy young individuals, apparently without serious prognostic implications.

7. Ectopic ventricular beats occurring during or after exercise present a suggestive evidence of ischemia. A wide overlap exists between healthy individuals and those with ischemic heart disease, so that the diagnostic and prognostic significance of such a finding is largely statistical, therefore only implied in individual cases. The appearance of more complex ventricular arrhythmias (multiform ventricular ectopic beats or short runs of ventricular tachycardia) steeply increases the probability of ischemic disease. Conversely, ventricular ectopic beats present at rest and disappearing during exercise imply, but do not prove, their benign nature.

The *significance* of ventricular ectopic beats varies with the circumstances of their occurrence, "the company they are in." Some guidelines for interpreting their significance are as follows:

- When found in young healthy individuals (often in teenagers), ventricular ectopic beats, particularly appearing in their more ominous forms, should alert one to a thorough search for the presence of cardiac disease. Such conditions as acute rheumatic fever and acute myocarditis may manifest themselves by this evidence of electrical instability of the myocardium. Search for drugs and toxic agents should also be undertaken. If a cause is not found, such an arrhythmia can be ignored, particularly if evidence is present that it represents a chronic feature in a given case. There is insufficient evidence linking isolated ventricular ectopy with ischemic disease to undertake coronary arteriography in young otherwise asymptomatic individuals.

- In patients with chronic cardiac disease, the appearance of ventricular ectopy should alert the clinician to the possibility that a specific factor capable of inducing this arrhythmia may be present; digitalis is always the prime potential culprit.

- In acute cardiac disease, e.g., myocardial infarction, ventricular ectopy is a manifestation of electrical instability of the myocardium; monitoring is then mandatory and therapy recommended.

The clinical effects of ventricular ectopy are analogous to those of supraventricular ectopy. Only in patients who are in such a critical state that any suboptimal factor may have a deleterious effect does the irregularity or the effective bradycardia produced by bigeminy aggravate heart failure or shock.

Management of ventricular ectopy involves two approaches:

- Elimination of provoking factors, if present;
- Antiarrhythmic therapy.

The first approach includes elimination of digitalis and other drugs or toxic agents, correction of electrolyte disturbance and hypoxia, and imposition of limits on amount of exercise, and similar steps.

The second approach offers the following agents:

- lidocaine (effective parenterally only, hence primarily suitable for in-hospital use),
- quinidine,
- procainamide,
- propranolol,
- diphenylhydantoin,
- bretylium tosylate (experimental).

The goal of antiarrhythmic therapy for ectopic ventricular beats is the prevention of more serious arrhythmias that may develop in the future. As mentioned, only under most unusual circumstances do ectopic beats affect the condition of the patient. The guidelines for therapy thus should be as follows:

- The first step is an appraisal of the potential seriousness of the arrhythmia. High priority is given the elimination of the more ominous forms of ectopy, e.g., frequent appearance of R-on-T beats, multiform ectopic beats. Low priority for therapy is in patients with simple, repeated ectopic beats.

- The therapy should have a measurable endpoint; some form

of monitoring can provide a qualitative (type of ectopy) and quantitative (number of ectopic beats) index of the effectiveness of therapy. Drug adjustment should be made until the desired effect is accomplished. If no effective therapy is found, the principle of treatment should be reappraised.

• More aggressive therapy is used for acute hospital care; caution should be applied to outpatient therapy. Some tentative views suggesting routine use of antiarrhythmic agents in all patients with ischemic heart disease are not acceptable at present in view of the definite risk of continuous antiarrhythmic therapy. However such therapy is justifiable in patients who demonstrate serious arrhythmias during treadmill exercise tests. Therapy here must be shown to be effective; i.e., there must be measurable evidence of diminished electrical instability on subsequent stress tests.

VENTRICULAR TACHYCARDIA

The relationship between ventricular ectopic beats and ventricular tachycardia is a quantitative one: whenever an ectopic focus discharges three or more sequential beats at a rapid rate, the term tachycardia can be applied. Some difference of opinion exists whether such runs of ventricular ectopic beats at rates under 100/min. should be termed "tachycardia" in view of the inherent low rate of automaticity within the pacemaker cells on the periphery of the conducting system. The preponderant opinion is that the term "tachycardia" should remain a designate of rates above 100. "Accelerated ventricular rhythm" is the term usually applied to slower ventricular ectopic rhythms.

Because of the kinship between single ventricular ectopy and ventricular tachycardia, it is clear that all factors producing ventricular ectopic beats are also capable of causing this form of tachycardia. A special variety of it has to be added, however: tachycardia enhanced by excessively slow rates in serious conduction disturbances. This form of "alternating tachycardia and bradycardia" will be discussed in the following chapter. It should also be mentioned that artifactual ventricular tachycardia may develop as a result of malfunction of an artificial pacemaker.

Ventricular tachycardia varies widely in terms of the rate and its duration. The rate of discharge of the ectopic focus may be as fast as 250, although most ventricular tachycardias are within the range of 130 to 170. Ventricular impulses may be conducted retrograde and activate the atria with 1 to 1 response, 2 to 1 response, or variable responses in a manner analogous to type I second degree AV block (Wenckebach). Retrograde block may also be present, in which case the atria remain under the control of the SA node, resulting in complete AV dissociation. The presence of AV dissociation often provides clinical signs enabling a bedside diagnosis of such tachycardia by means of observing the independent venous pulse at a slower rate than the arterial pulse and by the variability of the first heart sound. It has already been mentioned that AV dissociation does not prove ventricular origin of tachycardia, since infrajunctional tachycardias with aberration have many identical features.

Ventricular tachycardia can occur in the following forms:

1.   Sustained form: continuous tachycardia lasting until the end of a paroxysm or until termination by therapy;

2.   Repetitive form: runs of ventricular tachycardia of variable duration (usually short bursts), interrupted by sinus activity in terms of one or two beats up to periods of regular sinus rhythm;

3.   Short bursts of tachycardia associated with other evidences of electrical instability: uniform or multiform ventricular ectopic beats;

4.   Chronic ventricular tachycardia. Observations regarding chronicity of some forms of tachycardia date back to the time when few effective modes of termination of attacks were available. Such variety of tachycardia is now rare in a therapy-resistant form.

Clinical effects of ventricular tachycardia vary with its rate and duration. Even though many reports are available of ventricular tachycardia developing in normal individuals, it may be assumed that this form of arrhythmia is as a rule associated with cardiac disease. If the presence of disease is not evident, a concerted effort should be made to find a plausible cause of the tachycardia. One suspects that cases of ventricular tachycardia in healthy individuals in older writings may have been unrecognized cases of re-entry tachycardia due to a pre-excitation syndrome. During the tachycardia its circulatory effects will depend upon its rate and the extent of underlying heart disease. Such effects range from no detectable change to cardiogenic shock and may include various degrees of congestive failure and acute pulmonary edema. Considerable emphasis has been placed in the past upon the fact that ventricular tachycardia tends to be irregular, or at least is less consistently regular than the supraventricular variety. It is now generally agreed that ventricular tachycardia basically is regular except for very minor variations. The origin of the older view is traced to the misinterpretation of atrial fibrillation with very rapid ventricular response and broad complexes in patients with Wolff-Parkinson-White syndrome.

Management of ventricular tachycardia requires a great deal of thought and judgment. Inasmuch as ventricular tachycardia is only a small step away from ventricular fibrillation, aggressiveness in the therapeutic approach is justifiable. It is important to realize, however, that the patient with ventricular tachycardia more often than not has serious underlying cardiac disease, which may be unfavorably affected by misguided therapy of the arrhythmia.

Three steps constitute the therapeutic approach to ventricular tachycardia:

1. Prevention of the attack,

2. Termination of the attack,

3. Prevention of recurrences.

The first step has been discussed in detail in connection with ventricular ectopic beats, which constitute the precursor and early warning signs for ventricular tachycardia. This step includes the analysis and elimination of every possible factor influencing ventricular instability and active antiarrhythmic therapy.

Termination of the attack involves a variety of approaches:

• Drug treatment,

• Electroshock therapy,

• In extreme cases, when resistant to all forms of therapy, pacemaker overdrive or cardiac surgery.

Patients with ventricular tachycardia have to be continuously monitored. The drug of choice in sustained ventricular tachycardia is lidocaine in the form of continuous drip or intravenous bolus, or both. If this approach is unsuccessful, electroshock therapy is indicated. Such therapy may be the initial form of treatment, if the patient is in shock or in pulmonary edema. Electroshock therapy is contraindicated in the repetitive or intermittent form of ventricular tachycardia. Electroshock therapy is almost always effective in restoring sinus rhythm; however, its effectiveness may be nullified if either recurrence of the tachycardia or other forms of electrical instability develop after the successful termination of the attack. Repeated use of electroshock therapy is indicated only if each subsequent attack produces a life-threatening emergency.

Drug therapy of recurrent, intermittent, and repetitive ventricular tachycardia includes the agents listed in the section on ventricular ectopic beats. Lidocaine is the most widely used agent for intravenous therapy, probably the most effective, and the safest. Procainamide, related to lidocaine, is now less often used, for it offers few advantages over lidocaine and has a more pronounced hypotensive action. Propranolol may be very effective, though it requires caution in patients with cardiac failure. Diphenylhydantoin has been enthusiastically recommended by some investigators; its advantages over the other drugs have not, however, been demonstrated. It is frequently used as an alternate drug in patients who fail to respond to drugs previously used. Bretylium tosylate — the newest of these agents, not yet available for general use — may be in the same category, although its potential use has yet to be determined.

The use of drastic measures in treatment-resistant arrhythmias includes transvenous pacing. The artificial pacemaker inserted transvenously on a nonpermanent basis may capture the rhythm of the heart and terminate ventricular tachycardia and other evidences of electrical instability. Another rare method available in special situations is surgical excision of ventricular aneurysm. This drastic method is applicable to patients who, following acute myocardial infarction, develop persistent ventricular arrhythmias of the ominous variety (beyond the time of infarct healing), who are refractory to other forms of therapy, and in whom a resectable ventricular aneurysm can be demonstrated.

Oral antiarrhythmic therapy is used in patients who have recurrent or repetitive ventricular tachycardia over periods of time when continuous monitoring and intravenous therapy becomes impractical and whose general condition otherwise does not warrant acute care. Here quinidine is the drug of choice, with propranolol and procainamide as alternative drugs.

VENTRICULAR FIBRILLATION

Ventricular fibrillation represents the ultimate form of electrical instability affecting the ventricles. The separation of its more coordinated form, ventricular flutter, from the totally chaotic form, ventricular fibrillation, is of little practical importance, since both forms are incapable of maintaining a minimum cardiac output and thus are tantamount to circulatory arrest.

Ventricular fibrillation occurs in two forms, the difference between them being merely one of degree:

- Paroxysmal ventricular fibrillation, terminating spontaneously within a short enough time to permit the resumption of normal circulatory functions;

- Continuous ventricular fibrillation, fatal unless resuscitation is performed within a specific time limit.

Ventricular fibrillation produces an instant cessation of the circulation. Loss of consciousness occurs before there is time to develop evidence of cardiac failure or of hypoperfusion of other vital organs. As a rule, the patient drops to the ground without warning, and may or may not develop convulsive seizures.

It should be pointed out that ventricular fibrillation (and flutter) represents a progression of the electrical instability that produces, among other effects, ventricular tachycardia. Between ventricular tachycardia and fibrillation there is a difference of degree, with a blurred transition. From the practical standpoint the discussion here applies as well to extremely rapid forms of ventricular tachycardia, those producing instant cardiocirculatory arrest, as to true ventricular fibrillation.

The inevitability of a fatal outcome in ventricular fibrillation, unless instant help is available, has been dispelled by modern methods of monitoring cardiac rhythm; these methods have demonstrated the relative frequency of unrecognized paroxysms of ventricular fibrillation. Among conditions associated with such arrhythmia are the following:

1. Stokes-Adams syncope in patients with permanent or intermittent complete heart block has been shown to be caused with equal frequency by ventricular fibrillation as by cardiac standstill.

2. In ischemic heart disease paroxysmal ventricular fibrillation may develop during anginal attacks or during exercise, with or without chest pain.

3. Quinidine intoxication or intolerance may manifest itself as "quinidine syncope," which consists of repeated brief attacks of ventricular fibrillation.

The recognition and proper interpretation of paroxysmal ventricular fibrillation is obviously of paramount importance and is often lifesaving. While ventricular fibrillation is not the only cause of cardiac syncope, a high index of suspicion should be exercised that any unexplained abrupt loss of consciousness, or even repeated dizzy attacks, could represent paroxysms of ventricular fibrillation.

Causes of ventricular fibrillation include:

1. A true electrical "accident" consisting of premature contraction occurring during the critical vulnerable phase;

2. Mechanical stimulation, such as during cardiac catheterization and pacemaker insertion;

3. Ischemic electrical instability;

4. Severe myocardial disease;

5. A terminal event presumably due to severe hypoxia of the entire heart in massive myocardial infarction, and other catastrophic cardiac conditions and complications;

6. Drug effect, including that from digitalis, quinidine and others;

7. Electrolyte imbalance;

8. Severe disturbances of acid-base balance;

9. Hypothermia.

Treatment of ventricular fibrillation includes two steps: prevention and resuscitation. Preventive therapy includes all the steps discussed in connection with therapy of ventricular ectopic beats and ventricular tachycardia. Ventricular fibrillation is obviously the potentially fatal consequence against which such prophylactic therapy is directed.

Cardiac resuscitation involves defibrillation of the ventricles by means of electroshock therapy. Such a procedure may be performed in one of two ways: immediate application of the external shock, or delayed application following a period of external massage and oxygenation. Inasmuch as myocardial hypoxia perpetuates ventricular fibrillation to a point of nonresponsiveness to electroshock, immediate application of the shock is indicated only if it can be done within the first minute. This is possible if ventricular fibrillation occurs during cardiac catheterization, during induction of anesthesia, or in a coronary care unit if the appropriate equipment is close to the patient and the arrhythmia instantly discovered.

It should be pointed out that in some patients sinus rhythm may be restored by a mechanical stimulation—a sharp jolt to the precordial region. Resuscitative measures should always be initiated by such a maneuver. If ineffective, proper oxygenation with mouth-to-mouth breathing, followed by intubation and oxygen administration, should be started along with external cardiac massage. It is probable that correct application of the respiratory resuscitation is more important than the cardiac massage. Correction of acidosis is also of major importance in cases in which initial resuscitation is ineffective.

The success of resuscitative measures in patients with ventricular fibrillation is related to the skill with which resuscitation is applied and to the underlying condition. In myocardial infarction, which is by far the commonest condition in which resuscitation is performed, some authors suggest that this complication be divided into a "primary" and "secondary" form: electrical accident with a viable myocardium represents the former; ventricular fibrillation in cardiogenic shock and that caused by extension of the infarct, cardiac perforation, and other catastrophic events represent the latter. Obviously the ultimate success of resuscitation is possible only when the primary form is present.

Ventricular fibrillation represents the most common mechanism of instantaneous death and is assumed to be operative in all individuals who die suddenly and show no obvious cause of death. At present ventricular fibrillation is being successfully managed in acute conditions in patients under continuous monitoring. High-risk candidates for ventricular fibrillation are also being identified with increasing frequency; however, in cases in which the risk is a continuous one rather than confined to the course of an acute finite illness, the effectiveness of prophylactic therapy has not yet been conclusively demonstrated. Recent efforts to design automatic defibrillators that can sense ventricular fibrillation and administer the proper electroshock are being watched with interest. It remains to be seen whether current technology in the foreseeable future will permit a design that is safe, effective, and failproof.

IDIOVENTRICULAR RHYTHMS

The peripheral portions of the conducting system have an escape rate of their pacemaker cells of about 30 beats per minute. Pacemakers located higher, but below the His bundle, thus producing "ventricular" type complexes, have faster inherent automaticity, but as a rule it is below 50/min. Thus the escape rhythm that develops when impulses from above fail to reach the lower portion of the conducting system ranges from 30 to 50 beats per minute. Rates faster or slower than those indicate abnormality of such auxiliary pacemakers.

Slow escape rhythms at the appropriate rate qualifying for the term of "idioventricular" rhythm develop almost always in association with serious disturbances within the conducting system and therefore will be included in the discussion of the latter. The principal point of the discussion here is to distinguish the abnormal activity of the lower centers producing accelerated idioventricular rhythm. It has already been indicated that such forms of arrhythmia constitute a spectrum that extends into ventricular tachycardia. Thus many of the remarks regarding the causes and mechanism of ventricular tachycardia can be applied to this condition.

There is, however, one major difference between faster and slower ectopic ventricular rhythms. The slower ones often represent an *abnormal* escape mechanism, but nevertheless may constitute substitute rhythms that have developed by default. This is particularly true for such accelerated idioventricular rhythms occurring in the course of acute myocardial infarction. The moderate rate of such rhythms almost never taxes the circulatory state of the patient. Attempts to terminate such rhythms may or may not be successful, but if they succeed a more dangerous form of arrhythmia may develop. Thus it is generally conceded that in acute myocardial infarction such rhythms should *not* be treated either by drug therapy or by electroshock. They almost always spontaneously revert to a more normal mechanism.

Rarely, such accelerated idioventricular rhythms are present in patients as chronic states. If so it is more appropriate to assume that this represents an atypical form of a conduction disturbance rather than evidence of electrical instability of the ventricles. Treatment has to be individually considered and conservatively applied.

Bibliography

Cohn LJ, Donoso E, Friedberg CK: Ventricular tachycardia. Prog. Cardiovasc. Dis. *9*:29, 1966.

Koch-Weser J: Antiarrhythmic prophylaxis in ambulatory patients with coronary heart disease. Arch. Int. Med. *129*:763, 1972.

Lown B, Wolf M: Approaches to sudden death from coronary heart disease. Circulation *44*:130, 1971.

Selzer A, Wray HW: Quinidine syncope: paroxysmal ventricular fibrillation occurring during treatment of chronic atrial arrhythmias. Circulation *30*:17, 1964.

Surawicz B: Ventricular fibrillation. Amer. J. Cardiol. *28*:268, 1971.

20

Disturbances of Cardiac Conduction

Clinical conditions and syndromes in which disturbances of conduction play the principal role include those delaying the transmission of impulses from one part of the heart to another and those activating certain parts of the heart prematurely or out of sequence.

NONORGANIC CONDUCTION DELAYS

A number of toxic, environmental, and pathophysiological factors are capable of producing abnormal delays within the cardiac conducting system. These include:

- Drug effects (digitalis on total conducting system, quinidine on intraventricular conduction, etc.);

- Electrolyte disturbances (both hypokalemia and hyperkalemia may interfere with the normal spread of the excitation);

- Hypothermia;

- Myocardial ischemia;

- Vagal overactivity.

Such functional conduction disturbances are, as a rule, reversible when the exciting cause is eliminated. They account for many short-lasting conduction defects, including the "benign" form of heart block in inferior myocardial infarction.

CONGENITAL HEART BLOCK

Congenital heart block may involve various portions of the conducting system. It may be found as an isolated abnormality or in conjunction with various other forms of congenital cardiac disease.

The site of the involvement of the conducting system in congenital heart disease is almost always the upper portion of the conducting system, most commonly in the region of the AV node or the proximal portion of His' bundle. Conditions that show special predilection for association with heart block include:

- Corrected transposition of the great arteries;

- Malformation of the AV canal (endocardial cushion defects).

Congenital heart block has been reported in combination with most forms of congenital heart disease. The common forms of congenital conduction disturbances in general are:

- Simple AV conduction delay (first degree heart block);

- Complete AV block;

- Abnormal anatomy of bundle branches producing ventricular complexes that are wide and show marked superior orientation.

The two forms of *incomplete* heart block have no relationship to cardiac rhythm and therefore play no role in the patient's condition. *Complete* heart block is an important abnormality per se. It differs from most cases of acquired heart block in the following features:

- The ventricular rate is relatively fast: 45 to 60/min.;

- The rate accelerates during exercise;

- Ventricular complexes are of the supraventricular type.

These features, present in the great majority of patients with congenital heart block, indicate a high position of the escape pacemaker. There is some suggestion that congenital heart block may be due to an abnormality that does not permit the penetration of the SA impulses into the AV node. As a consequence of these features, the clinical effect of such block is less serious than that of other forms of complete heart block; Stokes-Adams attacks are very rare: Children usually show normal effort tolerance and in cases in which heart block is the sole lesion the prognosis may be excellent, involving a normal life expectancy, though not enough long-term studies are available to rule out the possibility that in older age some progression or adverse effect may occasionally develop. Therapy of congenital heart block is unnecessary, nor is there a reason to introduce restriction of activities. The rare instances in which development of syncope necessitates pacemaker insertion may actually represent a mechanism different from the common variety of congenital heart block.

TRAUMATIC HEART BLOCK

Interruption of the continuity of the conducting system occurs not infrequently as a result of trauma, particularly during cardiac surgery. Other traumatic factors include penetrating wounds of the heart and nonpenetrating trauma producing cardiac contusion and subendocardial hemorrhage and necrosis.

Surgical heart block was once a common complication associated with repair of intracardiac congenital defects. More recently surgical techniques have been improved to the extent that sutures are placed in areas away from the conducting system. Nevertheless, there is an unavoidable minimum of such accidents in congenital and acquired lesions in spite of all reasonable precautions. Operations susceptible to the production of damage to the conducting system include:

- Correction of lesions associated with AV canal malformation (septum primum type atrial septal defect, common AV canal);

- Repair of defects associated with corrected transposition of great vessels;

- "Total" correction of complete transposition of great vessels.

Rarely, heart block may be induced in the following operations:

- Aortic valve replacement;

- Operations for the relief of hypertrophic subaortic stenosis;

- Mitral valve replacement.

In congenital lesions damage to the conducting system often involves the uppermost portion of the system, i.e., the region of the AV node and the proximal part of the bundle of His. In such cases a stable escape rhythm at a reasonably fast rate (about 50/min.) and supraventricular complexes make this form relatively benign, not unlike that of the congenital variety.

Treatment of traumatic heart block involves usually, but not routinely, an artificial pacemaker. If a patient is found to be in complete heart block after an open heart operation, it is necessary first to determine whether organic and permanent damage to the conducting system has occurred, since, as indicated in Chapter 13, temporary and reversible heart block is much more common than a permanent block. If the heart block persists permanently, then pacemaker insertion should be considered in all patients except those showing the benign form, as defined in the preceding paragraph.

SPONTANEOUSLY ACQUIRED HEART BLOCK

Heart block acquired from causes other than trauma constitutes a common cardiac disorder. Recognizing the overlap and a certain arbitrariness in classifying spontaneously acquired heart block, one can distinguish the following general subdivisions:

1. Diseases of the conducting system secondary to anatomic lesions of the myocardium. In this category one includes heart block caused by myocardial infarction affecting the intraventricular septum and various infiltrating diseases: sarcoidosis, lues, rheumatoid arthritis, other granulomatous lesions, and cardiac tumors.

2. Primary disease of the conducting system or of adjacent fibrous structures ("fibrosis of the cardiac skeleton") affecting predominantly the lower division of it (in modern terminology, infra-His lesions). This is the commonest form of chronic complete heart block.

3. Primary disease of the conducting system involving its upper division (SA node and the region of the AV node). This form is responsible for the clinical picture of excessive bradycardias, slow escape rhythms, alternation of brady- and tachyarrhythmias. The term of "sick sinus syndrome" has been applied to some such cases.

With the exception of acute myocardial infarction, acquired heart block is basically a chronic, very slowly progressive disease. Once thought to be caused largely by chronic ischemic disease (as opposed to acute myocardial infarction), it is now believed that occlusive coronary artery disease plays an insignificant role in its origin, but rather that degenerative changes of the nonmuscular structure of the heart are the commonest cause of it. Such changes include also calcification of valve annuli.

The common variety — that involving the lower division of the conducting system — develops in one of two ways:

- Progression from lesser degrees of heart block into complete AV block;

- Progression from involvement of one fascicle of the lower division to two fascicles and then to complete AV block.

Heart block caused by involvement of the conducting system is seldom accompanied by signs or symptoms related to altered myocardial performance. Clinical symptomatology is basically dependent upon the effect of low cardiac rate; therefore patients in stages prior to the development of complete AV block often remain asymptomatic. Stokes-Adams syncope—the sudden loss of consciousness associated with failure of escape pacemakers (with or without subsequent ventricular fibrillation)—is the principal clinical manifestation of this disease. Such attacks may precede the stage of complete heart block developing in patients who after recovery show merely incomplete heart block or fascicular block, or they may occur periodically in patients who are in complete heart block. The appearance of permanent complete AV block often, but not always, brings about awareness of the slow rate and may reduce materially effort tolerance. There are patients, however, who are unaware of the change from sinus rhythm into complete heart block which may be incidentally discovered.

The natural history of acquired "idiopathic" heart block can be summarized by dividing the disease into stages:

1. Asymptomatic stage showing precursors of complete AV block, usually affecting individuals above the age of 60;

2. Appearance of complete AV block with its varied symptomatology (or without symptoms) but without syncopal attacks;

3. Stage of Stokes-Adams syncope.

As indicated, such a course is not invariable inasmuch as Stokes-Adams attacks may precede the development of complete AV block or appear with its onset.

Patients who have complete AV block in addition to another form of cardiac disease—e.g., valvular disease or ischemic heart disease—may tolerate the slow rate poorly. Aggravation of cardiac failure or its development may coincide with the onset of complete AV block irrespective of whether or not patients have Stokes-Adams attacks. In complete AV block secondary to a variety of diseases, as indicated above, the course, symptomatology, and prognosis vary in relation to the involvement of the heart by the primary condition.

Certain guidelines regarding the prognosis of complete AV block can be ascertained from the clinical and electrocardiographic picture. Thus:

1. The presence of supraventricular complexes, suggesting a bundle of His escape pacemaker, offers the best prognosis, especially if the inherent automaticity discharges at a rate above 45/min. Such patients may have no syncopal attacks at all.

2. Slower idioventricular rates and the bundle branch block type

of ventricular complexes usually indicate the "last line of defense" escape rhythm with a guarded prognosis.

3. The most ominous finding in complete AV block is the appearance of electrical instability in the form of ventricular ectopic beats, especially multiform. Here, pacemaker placement may be an emergency procedure.

Disease of the *upper division* of the conducting system is rarer, less well known, and more variable in its clinical manifestations than the complete heart block discussed above. Its recognition is relatively new and all its ramifications may not yet be known. Though termed by some "sick sinus syndrome," it is obviously a disease involving areas other than the SA node, for the excessive bradycardias are contingent upon malfunction or suppression of AV junctional escape rhythms and lower escape pacemakers.

Clinical manifestation of this syndrome includes the presence of excessive bradycardia, which more often is intermittent than continuous, or the alternation of bradycardia with tachycardia. Syncope may or may not occur in such attacks — some are characterized by subsyncopal states, such as sudden attacks of dizziness. Electrocardiographically, the presence of AV block is rare: sinus bradycardia or AV junctional bradycardia or both are usually found. The paroxysms of tachyarrhythmia usually are found to be atrial tachycardias, atrial flutter, or atrial fibrillation.

The episodic nature of such attacks, with normal clinical and electrocardiographic findings in between, may produce diagnostic difficulties. Monitoring by means of continuous recording electrocardiographic tape or by conventional coronary care type monitors may clarify the nature of obscure symptoms produced by this disease. If facilities are available, the overdrive-suppression test may be performed: artificial atrial pacing is performed at rapid rates and the rate of the resumption of the SA node automaticity is observed after cessation of pacing. It should be emphasized, however, that a normal SA node recovery time does not rule out the presence of periodic malfunction of the SA node and upper conducting system.

Management of bradyarrhythmias due to conduction disturbances involves drug therapy and the use of artificial pacemakers. The use of drugs has the serious disadvantage of their uncertain dependability for life-threatening attacks. Such agents as atropine and corticoids have been recommended in the past in acute states in hospitalized patients. Their value is unproven even as temporary measures. The use of isoproterenol provides us with an effective agent enhancing the automaticity of all centers and preventing their temporary failure. Yet, the inability to assure uninterrupted action of the drug makes this agent, too, unsuitable for chronic use by the patient at home.

Insertion of artificial pacemakers is thus the only foolproof therapy for symptomatic bradycardia. The wide popularity of standby type pacemakers is well deserved, for they prevent the occurrence of competing rhythm. In patients with chronic complete heart block and slow idioventricular rate—in which case the artificial pacemaker permanently remains the dominant one—fixed rate pacemakers are still occasionally used though their use is becoming obsolete.

Pacemaker insertion is a surgical procedure with its inherent cost, morbidity, and mortality. The indication for its use in bradyarrhythmias, both for temporary and permanent use, should be carefully spelled out:

1. Temporary pacing may become necessary in acute myocardial infarction and following open heart surgery for nonpermanent conduction disturbances. Its prophylactic use in anticipation of such disturbances is seldom indicated.

2. Permanent pacemaker insertion is mandatory in patients who have suffered documented Stokes-Adams type syncopal attacks.

3. Attacks of loss of consciousness or of dizziness that are not recorded or witnessed constitute an indication for permanent pacing, provided complete heart block or its precursor is present and a reasonable relationship between it and the attack is assumed. (Patients with conduction disturbances could have unrelated transient cerebral ischemic episodes!)

4. In patients with complete heart block who have no syncopal attacks but who are in poorly controllable cardiac failure, pacemaker insertion may improve the cardiac function, although such improvement is not uniform.

5. In asymptomatic patients with complete heart block, permanent pacing is optional. Prognosis guidelines listed above may help in case selection of suitable candidates. It should be remembered that in such patients the risk of dying during the first syncopal attack is relatively small and may not be balanced by the risk and nuisance value of pacing—which is then purely prophylactic.

6. Pacemaker insertion in asymptomatic patients with precursors of complete AV block (e.g., bifascicular block, particularly left anterior fascicular block combined with complete right bundle branch block) should be considered questionable. No longitudinal studies are available to demonstrate how high the probability of the development of complete heart block is; experience has shown that some such conduction disturbances may remain nonprogressive for many years.

PRE-EXCITATION SYNDROMES

Pre-excitation syndromes is a term applied to conditions in which the wave front of cardiac activation bypasses certain portions of the conducting system via abnormal communications, as already discussed. This term is preferable to "accelerated conduction," which has a narrower connotation, applicable only to some situations. Two distinct syndromes are now recognized; it is not yet entirely clear whether each syndrome represents a distinct pathophysiological and clinical entity, or whether each may include some as yet ill-defined entities. These two are:

1. Wolff-Parkinson-White syndrome — described originally to include apparently healthy individuals with "false" bundle branch block patterns and short P-R interval in the electrocardiogram who show proneness to paroxysmal tachyarrhythmias. The electrocardiographic factors are discussed in Chapter 6.

2. Lown-Ganong-Levine syndrome — described as one affecting apparently healthy individuals with normal ventricular complexes and abnormally short P-R intervals in the electrocardiogram, who have frequent attacks of tachyarrhythmias.

It has been postulated that the electrocardiographic abnormality of Wolff-Parkinson-White (W-P-W) syndrome is related to a functioning abnormal atrioventricular connection that can short-circuit the impulse from the proximal portion of the AV node to the ventricle, prematurely activating some portions of the ventricle but then meeting the wave front reaching the ventricle through the physiological channels. Thus the ventricular complex represents the fusion phenomenon, with the prematurely activated portion shown as delta-wave, but most of the ventricle activated in a normal fashion. The postulated abnormal communications include the bundles of Kent — a peripheral atrioventricular connection described in some animals and tentatively identified in some patients with W-P-W complexes. Other short-circuiting communications, identified by Mahaim and by James, are presumed to play a role in variants of the W-P-W syndrome and the Lown-Ganong-Levine syndrome.

Attacks of tachyarrhythmias occur when impulses pass from the AV node to the ventricle through the physiological pathway and then return to the AV node via the bypass — or vice versa. They represent the perfect example of re-entry tachycardias. This mechanism has been adequately documented by modern electrophysiological techniques. It involves regular tachycardias with supraventricular complexes, regular tachycardias with ventricular complexes, or atrial fibrillation with either type of complexes. Such attacks are often characterized by extremely rapid rates, often between 250 and 300/min. Atrial fibrillation not only is usually associated with the very rapid rate but, deprived of the protection of the bypassed AV node, may initiate fatal ventricular fibrillation; hence its appearance is of unfavorable prognostic significance.

It is assumed that the W-P-W syndrome is always congenital in origin. Theoretically the possibility, suggested by some, that acquired disease of the AV node may also produce pre-excitation cannot be ruled out, although this is supported largely by speculation. The fact that ventricular complexes with delta waves identical to those of the W-P-W syndrome may be provoked during cardiac catheterization has no bearing upon this discussion, as such complexes are fusion beats and need not in any way be related to the W-P-W syndrome.

Clinical Features. The incidence of W-P-W syndrome in the general population is not known, for it is most often an accidental finding. The propensity for the development of paroxysmal tachyarrhythmias is said to be present in about half of such patients, but it is likely to occur in a much smaller fraction than that, considering that many subclinical forms are presumably missed. The abnormal complexes in the electrocardiogram may be a permanent feature of such patients or may appear periodically or intermittently. The W-P-W syndrome is in a small number of cases — probably about 10 per cent — associated with organic heart disease, usually congenital in nature. As an isolated finding it may be familial. While associated lesions cover the spectrum of congenital heart disease, two conditions appear to have a preferential coexistence with W-P-W syndrome:

- Ebstein's anomaly,

- Hypertrophic subaortic stenosis (particularly its familial form).

The symptomatology is related to the presence or frequency of tachyarrhythmias or to a possible underlying cardiac lesion. The prognosis of W-P-W syndrome is good in principle, although sudden death due to arrhythmias is possible. (Its incidence is probably low, considering the common occurrence of the W-P-W syndrome.)

The recognition of the W-P-W syndrome from the electrocardiogram presents no difficulty in its typical forms; atypical features may present confusing differential diagnoses. Short P-R interval is usually helpful, but this feature may be absent in some cases. The most important diagnostic maneuver is the capability of normalizing the abnormal electrocardiogram. Though not always possible, temporary restoration of normal intraventricular conduction can often be accomplished by various methods: vagal stimulation, Valsalva maneuver, atrial pacing, or use of drugs such as atropine, autonomic stimulants or depressors, and digitalis. Such attempts have to be made on the basis of trial and error, for no predictable method of normalizing complexes is known. The introduction of His bundle recording has provided a reliable method of diagnosis of the W-P-W syndrome.

Management. The W-P-W syndrome requires no therapy per se, nor any form of restrictions of the patient's mode of living. Tachyarrhythmias present the major therapeutic problem, and often are a therapeutic challenge.

It has already been stated that tachyarrhythmias occur at a wider spectrum than in subjects without the W-P-W syndrome. In this disease, the cardiac rate is often faster and the response to therapy poorer. Though some attacks represent merely a nuisance, those with extremely rapid rates may produce serious symptoms, even without underlying heart disease (e.g., shock).

The treatment of tachyarrhythmias associated with W-P-W syndrome is analogous to that discussed in connection with other supraventricular tachyarrhythmias. Termination of the attack by means of antiarrhythmic agents or by electroshock therapy can be performed in persistent attacks and in those associated with serious consequences. The whole gamut of maintenance drugs of the antiarrhythmic series may be tried in the hope of finding the most suitable drug or drug combination. Unfortunately, there is a small group of patients with disabling arrhythmias who are resistant to all forms of therapy. Caution should be applied regarding the use of digitalis: it is contraindicated in patients with paroxysmal atrial fibrillation (Durrer, 1974).

With better understanding of the electrophysiological basis for the W-P-W syndrome, attempts have been made to treat resistant attacks surgically. These have included incisions in the region of the Kent bundle (located by means of electrophysiological "mapping" of the spread of excitation), sectioning of the bundle of His, and other similar procedures. In the small number of early trials there were successes as well as failures of these procedures. Recent results demonstrated frequent spectacular therapeutic successes occurring more predictably in institutions where sophisticated electrophysiological studies were performed prior to the operation. This technique appears promising for patients totally refractory to medical therapy.

Lown-Ganong-Levine syndrome is a rarer condition, not as well known as the W-P-W syndrome. It should be identified as such only if a definite tendency to tachyarrhythmias is demonstrated, for the mere presence of a short P-R interval may be due to a variety of other mechanisms. It is assumed that tachycardias in this syndrome are also of reentrant nature. Therapeutic approaches — and difficulties — in handling this syndrome are similar to those in the W-P-W syndrome.

Bibliography

Campbell M, Emanuel R: Six cases of complete heart block followed for 34 to 40 years. Brit. Heart J. 29:577, 1967.

Caracta AR, Damato AN, Gallagher JJ, Josephson ME, Vorghese PJ, Lau SH, Westura EE: Electrophysiological studies in the syndrome of short P-R interval, normal QRS complex. Amer. J. Cardiol. 31:245, 1973.

Durrer D., Schuilenberg RM, Wellens HJJ: Pre-excitation revisited. Amer. J. Cardiol. 25:290, 1970.

Durrer D, Wellens HJ: The Wolff-Parkinson-White syndrome. Europ. J. Cardiol. 1:347, 1974.

Gammon PG, Sellers RD, Kanjuh VI, Edwards JE, Lillehei CW: Complete heart block following replacement of the aortic valve. Circulation 33-34:Suppl. I-152, 1966.

Kaplan BM, Langendorff R, Lev M, Pick A: Tachycardia-bradycardia syndrome (so called "sick sinus syndrome"). Amer. J. Cardiol. 31:497, 1973.

Lenegre J: Etiology and pathology of bilateral bundle-branch block in relation to complete heart block. Prog. Cardiovasc. Dis. 6:409, 1964.

Lev M: Anatomic basis for A-V block. Amer. J. Med. 37:742, 1964.

Lev M: The pathology of complete A-V block. Prog. Cardiovasc. Dis. 6:317, 1964.

Lev M: Pathogenesis of complete A-V block. Prog. Cardiovasc. Dis. 15:145, 1972.

Newman BJ, Donoso E, Friedberg CK: Arrhythmias in the Wolff-Parkinson-White syndrome. Prog. Cardiovasc. Dis. 9:147, 1967.

Paul MH, Rudolph AM, Nadas AS: Congenital complete A-V block: Problems of clinical assessment. Circulation 18:183, 1959.

Rubenstein JJ, Schulman CL, Yurchak PM, DeSanctis RW: Clinical spectrum of the sick sinus syndrome. Circulation 46:5, 1972.

Scanlon PJ, Pryor R, Blount SG Jr: Right bundle-branch block associated with left superior and inferior intraventricular block. Clinical setting, prognosis, relation to complete heart block. Circulation 42:1123, 1970.

Part two

Diseases of the Heart and Circulation

21

Nosology, Etiology, and Special Features of Cardiac Disease

PROBLEMS RELATED TO CLASSIFICATION

Diagnostic approaches to a given subject, or even to individual cases, are greatly enhanced if a good classification is available. Cardiology was among the earliest of the fields of medicine in which a comprehensive classification was introduced. More than half a century ago it was recognized that pathological anatomy alone cannot serve as a basis for categorizing patients with cardiac disease. The then new classification represented a milestone in terms of simplification and modernization of thinking. It required that each case be recognized in terms of the etiology, pathological anatomy, physiology, and cardiac function. This classification has remained the basis for the currently used diagnostic terminology, although during the past two decades some deficiencies have become apparent. It had become evident that cardiology, when approached from a multidisciplinary standpoint, necessitates frequent crossovers between the various categories; many entities or even individual cases can no longer fit into neat "boxes." It is thus evident that some entities – or cases – can be best grouped along the line of etiology, others by their anatomic aspects, still others by means of pathophysiological disorders. For example, two patients with mitral regurgitation may be similar in terms of etiology, pathology, physiology, and impairment of cardiac function, and yet their prognosis and treatment would be entirely different if one represented the chronic form and the other the acute form.

Some of the standard etiological headings have now been eroded

315

by doubts: Should a patient with a congenital bicuspid aortic valve who develops aortic stenosis later in life be considered to have "congenital heart disease"? What etiological term should be used for chronic isolated aortic valvular disease—previously automatically placed in the "rheumatic" group?

Similarly, the anatomic classification presents difficulties in connection with many cases. How does hypertrophic subaortic stenosis or functional incompetence of valves fit into an anatomic classification?

Physiological classification represents the weakest link in the diagnostic chain. When the classification was first designed, physiological classification pertained to only two points: whether or not disturbance of cardiac rhythm and cardiac failure were present. Today, pathophysiology represents the most important aspect of recognizing clinical syndromes, stages of disease, and its complications and sequels, with such a wide variety of possible disturbances of cardiac function as to defy any simple cataloguing of them into a formal "classification."

The functional classification was discussed in Chapter 9. As a method of presenting patients' limitation of activities produced by symptoms, this classification revealed many inconsistencies and weaknesses which necessitated its recent revision. In its current form, referring to the overall status of the patient and to an estimated prognosis (rather than physician-imposed therapeutic limitations), it should be useful when widely adopted.

Classification of entities within specific disease categories presents difficulties similar to those mentioned in connection with the overall classification of cardiac diseases. As an example, in the classification of congenital heart disease, early classification initiated by Maude Abbott recognized "cyanotic," "late cyanotic," and "non-cyanotic" forms of malformations. Yet, as soon as more advanced physiological studies became possible, it became abundantly clear that the same anatomic entity presented itself sometimes in the cyanotic category, sometimes in the non-cyanotic, so that this consideration proved to be impractical. Later classifications of congenital heart disease proceeded along the line of high pulmonary arterial pressure vs. low pulmonary arterial pressure, or increased pulmonary blood flow vs. decreased pulmonary blood flow; other lines of division utilized various other features. However, exceptions were always found in sufficient numbers to suggest that a perfect classification of congenital heart disease may be unattainable.

The foregoing considerations are presented as a means of introducing some explanatory remarks regarding the structure and arrangement of cardiac diseases in the following chapters. Since a totally satisfactory classification of cardiac disease is unavailable, chapters in the second part of the book are arranged in a purely arbitrary manner — by grouping certain entities together in terms of convenience and logic. This presentation is not intended as a new classification. The four sections of Part Two of this book are as follows: acute diseases of the heart (Section IV), chronic diseases in which the principal disturbance is an increase in cardiac workload (Section V), chronic diseases affecting myocardial function and structure (Section VI), and a miscellaneous group of entities that do not fit into the other categories (Section VII). A break with tradition is represented by intermingling the various congenital lesions with other diseases in three sections rather than discussing them in a block.

The remainder of this introductory chapter deals with some etiological, epidemiological, and other aspects of cardiac disease which may be applicable to several of the forthcoming chapters.

CONGENITAL HEART DISEASE

The problems regarding the classification of congenital heart disease have already been discussed in the preceding section of this chapter. Nevertheless congenital malformations of the heart provide certain unique features of heart disease which will be briefly discussed here.

Etiology. Basically there are two principal factors responsible for the birth of a child with a malformed heart:

- Genetic abnormalities, including chromosomal aberrations and single gene mutations;

- Environmental factors.

Genetic abnormalities account for complex congenital malformations involving organs other than the heart. These may or may not fall into the category of well-defined congenital syndromes (e.g., Down's syndrome). In addition, some isolated congenital cardiac lesions show familial incidence, indicating a genetic factor.

Environmental factors involve the noxious effects of certain stimuli on the mother during early stages of gestation. The best known factors in human pathology are infections (German measles) and toxic agents (thalidomide), both of which have shown a high incidence of teratogenic effects upon the fetus. Experimental data indicate a broader number of teratogens, including thermal, bacterial, and toxic influences as well as dietary deficiencies.

At the present time a multifactorial theory of the etiology of congenital defects is gaining wide acceptance. According to this view, pure genetic and pure environmental factors account for only small fractions of the cases on the two extremes of the spectrum. In most cases the additive effects of these as well as those of other possible factors coexist.

From the practical standpoint it is important to recognize that the incidence of congenital cardiac lesions in siblings is, on the average, 2 per cent. The risk of recurrence shows some variation for the various lesions, although not a great deal. Even though the average parents of a child with congenital heart disease have one chance in 50 of having another malformed child, there are families with a much higher incidence of congenital heart disease.

Incidence. The incidence of congenital heart disease at birth is about 3 per 1,000; at school age it drops to about 1 per 1,000. At the present time, in the Western countries congenital heart disease accounts for the majority of patients with cardiac disease in the childhood age.

The distribution of the various congenital lesions at the time of birth shows a preponderance of lesions either totally incompatible with life or seriously impairing the chance of survival beyond infancy. Thus, the common complex malformations include the syndromes with transposition of great arteries, hypoplasia of either ventricle, and atresia of one of the cardiac orifices. The commonest among the simpler lesions is the ventricular septal defect. Lesions found in older children and adults include the following, according to Wood's figures:

(per cent)

- Atrial septal defect 23.5

- Ventricular septal defect 12

- Isolated pulmonary stenosis 11

- Coarctation of the aorta 10

- Tetralogy of Fallot 9.5

- Patent ductus arteriosus 9

- Aortic stenosis 6

Special Features. In spite of the already mentioned overlap between many congenital and acquired cardiac diseases, some features are found preferentially in congenital lesions to the extent that their presence may alert the clinician to the possibility of this group of diseases. They include the following:

1. Cyanosis. Cyanosis of congenital heart disease is usually of the central type, i.e., involving the entry of unoxygenated blood directly from the right to the left side of the heart, bypassing the lungs. Given an intracardiac or an aortopulmonary communication, the shunt ordinarily is directed from left to right by the pressure gradient or by differences in chamber compliances. Right-to-left shunt producing cyanosis can occur only under special circumstances such as:

- Transposition of the arterial trunks with venous blood ejected directly into the aorta;

- Obstruction to right ventricular outflow, reversing interventricular or interatrial pressure gradients;

- Development of pulmonary vascular disease, producing the same effect (usually late development);

- Isolated reversal of interatrial pressure gradients due to tricuspid disease (tricuspid atresia, stenosis, Ebstein's anomaly);

- Free mixing of oxygenated and deoxygenated bloods, such as occurs in single ventricle, total anomalous venous return, etc.

The degree of cyanosis varies from subliminal cyanosis, detected only during exercise or unusual circumstances, to severe cyanosis seen at a glance. The hypoxia which is the physiological basis for central cyanosis also stimulates the bone marrow and leads to polycythemia, which, in turn, accentuates the purplish blue color of the skin and the mucous membranes.

In the differential diagnosis of central cyanosis the following conditions other than cardiac malformations have to be considered:

- Pulmonary arteriovenous fistula (often congenital hemangioma of the lung);

- Right-to-left shunting through a patent foramen ovale (not congenitally abnormal) in end stages of various acquired diseases with severe right ventricular failure (without concomitant left ventricular failure);

- Severe hypoxia due to pulmonary disease.

2. Right-sided Cardiac Lesions. In view of the preferential involvement of the left ventricle in the great majority of acquired cardiac diseases the presence of an isolated right-sided lesion in a young patient should suggest the possibility of a congenital malformation of the heart. The diagnosis of congenital heart disease is supported by the following:

- Severe degree of right ventricular hypertrophy in the electrocardiogram (pattern resembling a postnatal electrocardiogram);

- Unusual cardiac shape in the roentgenogram;

- Increased pulmonary vascularity in the roentgenogram.

3. *Unusual Cardiac Murmurs.* Certain specific murmurs may arouse the suspicion of congenital cardiac disease. Among these are:

- Continuous murmurs,

- Ejection murmurs located in the pulmonary area,

- Pansystolic murmurs located along the left sternal borders.

4. *Associated Lesions.* Congenital malformations are often multiple, producing combined cardiac lesions and involving more than one organ. The presence of cardiac disease in an individual with a known congenital noncardiac malformation, e.g., cleft palate, should direct diagnostic consideration toward the possibility that heart disease is also of congenital origin.

Some complex congenital syndromes have a high incidence of congenital cardiac involvement and often show preferential appearance of a specific cardiac lesion. Among these are:

- Mongolism (Down's syndrome): 50 per cent incidence of cardiac disease; endocardial cushion defect is the commonest lesion;

- Turner's syndrome: coarctation of the aorta, ventricular septal defect;

- Ellis-van Creveld syndrome: single atrium, ventricular septal defect.

DISEASES DUE TO PATHOGENIC ORGANISMS

Pathogenic organisms can produce or contribute to the development of cardiac disease in two ways:

1. By directly affecting the heart;

2. By initiating an autoimmune tissue reaction which results in cardiac damage.

Direct etiological involvement of infectious pathogens accounts for only a small proportion of cardiac diseases. The most important is infective endocarditis, which will be discussed in a later chapter. Various pathogens may also produce diseases of the myocardium or the pericardium or may cause special situations in which the heart is involved. The more important examples are as follows:

- Involvement of the myocardium in various infectious diseases: diphtheria, salmonellosis, scarlet fever, tuberculosis;

- Viral myocarditis and/or pericarditis;

- Spirochetal and rickettsial myocarditis;

- Trypanosomiasis (Chagas' disease) — an infestation common in South America that produces a specific form of myocarditis;

- Helminthic involvement: trichinosis, echinococcosis, and schistosomiasis; the former two may produce myocardial involvement; schistosomiasis affects the heart secondarily by invading the pulmonary circulation and causing cor pulmonale.

Rheumatic fever represents the most important etiological entity related indirectly to a pathogenic organism. Though still subject to some controversy owing to many "missing links" in the chain of reactions, the most widely accepted view considers the rheumatic process an abnormal tissue reaction, presumably due to autoimmune mechanisms in a patient exposed to infection with a beta-hemolytic streptococcus.

Knowledge of the etiological factors affecting rheumatic fever is still incomplete. Certain facts appear reasonably well established:

- As a hypersensitivity phenomenon, rheumatic fever requires repeated exposure to the streptococcus; hence it is seldom found before the age of 3.

- There is almost always a "latent" period of two to three weeks between the streptococcal infection that triggers the attack and the clinical appearance of acute rheumatic fever.

- Once the patient recovers from an attack of rheumatic fever, he shows a high susceptibility to recurrence; each episode is triggered by streptococcal reinfection, but the attacks diminish with the passage of time and with the age of the patient.

- There is strong familial predisposition to the rheumatic reaction to streptococcal infection.

- Crowded living conditions, poor hygiene, faulty nutrition, and substandard medical care play an important role in the epidemiology of rheumatic fever, all these conditions increasing the susceptibility to and frequency and severity of rheumatic attacks.

- Recurrent attacks of rheumatic fever resemble earlier attacks: if a patient escaped carditis in the first attack he is unlikely to develop cardiac involvement in subsequent ones. As a corollary to this, the risk of permanent valve damage is highest in patients who showed definite cardiac involvement in the first attack.

There are many aspects of rheumatic fever that are as yet unknown or poorly understood. Some of these have to do with the marked change in the epidemiological picture of this disease:

- Once thought to be a disease of moderate climates, seldom occurring in the tropics, the reverse seems to be true at present: the incidence of rheumatic fever has markedly diminished in the Western nations but is a major health factor in the developing countries, most of which are in the tropics.

- Chronic manifestations of rheumatic heart disease appear frequently without any history of acute rheumatic fever. This is observed both in this country, where attacks of acute rheumatic fever now tend to be milder and less typical, as well as in the tropical countries, in which acute attacks occur with great severity and chronic valvular disease takes an accelerated form. As a possible explanation a subclinical form of rheumatic fever is suggested, namely isolated low-grade carditis without other acute manifestations of rheumatic fever. An altogether different etiology—viral disease—has also been suggested.

Reliable information regarding the incidence and variation in the clinical picture of rheumatic fever is very difficult to obtain. Neither its clinical features nor laboratory tests have sufficient specificity to establish the diagnosis beyond a reasonable doubt in all but truly "classical" cases. Furthermore, the diagnosis of the cardiac involvement in rheumatic fever (i.e., carditis) is based on signs, symptoms, and laboratory findings indicative of severe cardiac affliction, and hence is most likely to represent merely the visible top of an iceberg.

DISEASES DUE TO METABOLIC ABNORMALITIES

All human diseases related to metabolic disturbances are overshadowed by atherosclerosis, which is probably the number one health problem of today.

Atherosclerosis is a disease of the blood vessels. The significant locations of atherosclerosis as a cause of disease of organs other than the affected blood vessels include, in order of their clinical importance and frequency:

- coronary artery involvement,
- cerebral vascular involvement,

- peripheral vascular disease,

- renal arterial involvement,

- involvement of the aorta.

Coronary artery disease is the commonest and most serious manifestation of atherosclerosis and usually serves as a yardstick for the investigation of the etiological factors related to it. Most studies dealing with atherosclerosis use as its endpoint myocardial infarction, anginal syndrome, or sudden cardiac death.

Atherosclerotic lesions are initiated by an abnormal reaction between serum lipids and arterial intima, causing, in turn, a series of changes that eventually lead to the formation of intimal plaques and other abnormalities responsible for occlusive arterial disease.

Global epidemiology of atherosclerosis in general and of coronary arterial disease in particular shows a very high variation in the incidence and severity of this disease between geographical areas, races, and cultures. Many changes can be attributed to known risk factors; however, it is not entirely clear whether all risk factors have as yet been identified.

Risk factors include environmental influences and host factors. Environmental risk factors include the following:

1. Diet. The contribution of diets high in fats composed of saturated fatty acids and in cholesterol, possibly also with abundance of sugars, has been convincingly demonstrated in epidemiological studies.

2. Tobacco. Heavy smokers show a significantly higher incidence of coronary disease.

3. Absence of exercise. There is some suggestion, though not definitive evidence, that physical activity may delay the atherosclerotic process.

Host factors include:

4. Serum lipids. The level of cholesterol, of triglycerides, and of the various fractions of serum lipoproteins relates with the incidence and severity of coronary atherosclerosis. Hyperlipidemias fall into five categories described by Fredrickson and Levy, all of which are associated with increased risk of coronary disease. These are in part familial and hereditary and in part acquired alimentary factors.

5. Lipid metabolism. Individual patterns of lipid metabolism play an important role as a risk factor of atherosclerosis. They fall into three categories:

- Severe hereditary hyperlipidemias;

- Alimentary hyperlipidemia: given an average Western diet, some individuals increase postnatal serum cholesterol (usually under 200 mg./100 ml.) to the accepted "upper limit of normal" (in reality hyperlipidemic level) of about 250 mg./100 ml., while others remain in the low lipid range;

- Abnormal metabolism at normal lipidemic levels: some patients with familial premature coronary disease show serum lipids at the low normal level.

6. Height of arterial pressure. Hypertension has been identified as an important risk factor increasing the likelihood of coronary disease.

7. Diabetes. Premature atherosclerosis occurs frequently in diabetics. The exact nature of the relationship is not definitely known; it probably involves a combination of altered metabolism and changes in the arterial wall.

8. Obesity. Long suspected as a risk factor in the development of atherosclerosis, obesity is now considered a factor of minor importance, with some doubt of any increased risk at all.

9. Hormonal influences. Premenopausal women show a lower incidence of coronary artery disease, suggesting that estrogens exert some protective influence against atherosclerosis. Similarly, hyperthyroidism is associated with decreased and myxedema with increased tendency to atherosclerosis.

10. Stress. Stress has been implicated as an important risk factor. Yet, determination of the relationship between stress and coronary disease is hampered by the difficulty of measuring stress; hence this relationship can be considered only tentative.

11. Ethnic and racial factors have been suspected of contributing to the low incidence of atherosclerotic disease in some parts of the world. It is probable that factors other than diet and those listed above contribute to the fact that this disease is amazingly rare in some races, cultures, and geographical areas.

Other metabolic disorders may affect the heart but play a small role as an etiological factor in cardiac disease. They include:

- Amyloidosis as a cause of myocardial disease,

- Uremia as a cause of pericarditis,

- Hemochromatosis causing cardiomyopathy,

- Myocardial disease due to glycogen storage,

- Other metabolic diseases affecting the heart.

OTHER ETIOLOGICAL FACTORS CAUSING CARDIAC DISEASE

Atherosclerosis, rheumatic fever, congenital malformations, and hypertension account for the great majority of cardiac diseases. Other etiological factors will be discussed in connection with the various forms of heart disease in the subsequent chapters. A listing of the more important etiological factors other than the "big four" follows:

- Chronic pulmonary disease,

- Anemia,

- Trauma,

- Neoplasms,

- Drugs and toxic agents,

- Some endocrine malfunctions,

- Thiamine deficiency.

Bibliography

Blieden LC, Moller JH: Cardiac involvement in inherited disorders of metabolism. Prog. Cardiovasc. Dis. *16*:615, 1974.

Fontana RS, Edwards JE: Congenital cardiac disease. W. B. Saunders Co., Philadelphia, 1962, pp. 13–65.

Fredrickson DS, Levy RI, Lees RS: Fat transport in lipoproteins: An integrated approach to mechanisms and disorders. New Engl. J. Med. *276*:34, 94, 148, 215, 243, 1967.

Friedberg CK: Pathogenesis of atherosclerosis. *In* DISEASES OF THE HEART, 3rd Edition. W. B. Saunders Co., Philadelphia, 1966, pp. 651–675.

Kaplan MH, Frengley JD: Autoimmunity to the heart and cardiac disease. Current concepts of the relation of autoimmunity to rheumatic fever, postcardiotomy and postinfarction syndrome and cardiomyopathies. Amer. J. Cardiol. *24*:459, 1969.

Markowitz M, Gordis L: RHEUMATIC FEVER, 2nd Edition. W. B. Saunders Co., Philadelphia, 1972.

Nadas AS, Fyler DC: Congenital heart disease: general principles. *In* PEDIATRIC CARDIOLOGY, 3rd Edition. W. B. Saunders Co., Philadelphia, 1972, pp. 293–316.

NOMENCLATURE AND CRITERIA FOR DIAGNOSIS OF DISEASES OF THE HEART AND GREAT VESSELS, 7th Edition. Little Brown and Co., Boston, 1974.

Sellers TF Jr: An epidemiologic view of rheumatic fever. Prog. Cardiovasc. Dis. *16*:303, 1973.

Selzer A: Chronic cyanosis. Amer. J. Med. *10*:334, 1951.

Wood P: Congenital heart disease. *In* DISEASES OF THE HEART AND CIRCULATION, 3rd Edition. Eyre & Spottiswoode, London, 1968, pp. 354–360.

22

Myocardial Infarction

Definition. Acute myocardial infarction represents a mere episode in the natural history of ischemic heart disease. It is, nevertheless, a distinct clinical entity which manifests itself as an acute illness, terminating in recovery, in chronic illness, or in death—each outcome being independent of the occlusive disease of the coronary arteries which had initiated the infarction. Thus, myocardial infarction has its own natural history, course, and prognosis, justifying its independent coverage in the section *Acute Diseases of the Heart* separately from other aspects of ischemic heart disease to be presented in later chapters.

"Myocardial infarction" is a pathological term which has replaced the older terms "coronary thrombosis" and "coronary occlusion." This term is used in the clinical sense despite purely anatomic connotations. Yet, clinical and pathological aspects of myocardial infarction are not synonymous, but merely overlap to a great extent. For example, the pathological age of the infarct occasionally does not coincide with that estimated on the basis of the initial attack of pain, the anatomic change being either older or younger than the clinical counterpart.

From the clinical standpoint, myocardial infarction represents an arbitrary part of the spectrum of attacks of chest pain. Between the typical anginal attack and a classical myocardial infarction there are many intermediate forms that make ischemic heart disease a clinical continuum. It is undoubtedly an oversimplification to consider short attacks of ischemic chest pain as representing reversible ischemia, and long ones irreversible ischemia, i.e., myocardial infarction. Small infarcts may be clinically undetectable, masquerading as simple anginal attacks. Arbitrary division is necessary for the purpose of discussing myocardial infarction and angina pectoris. Thus, in this section the problems related to the unquestionable myocardial infarction will be discussed, leaving the various intermediate clinical syndromes referred

326

to as "unstable angina" and "pre-infarction angina" for the chapter on chronic ischemic heart disease.

CAUSES AND MECHANISMS

Infarction in general is by definition an ischemic necrosis of a portion of an organ caused by the cessation of flow in the perfusing endartery. Once considered an invariable consequence of a thrombotic complete occlusion of a coronary artery, myocardial infarction is now known to be caused by a variety of mechanisms.

In the great majority of cases occlusive coronary artery disease caused by *atherosclerosis* is the underlying basis for myocardial infarction. The following mechanisms may cause infarction of the myocardium:

- Thrombosis superimposed upon a stenotic area as a result of an atherosclerotic plaque in a coronary arterial branch. Recent studies indicate that thrombosis is relatively rare in patients dying early in myocardial infarction. A suggestion has been made that thrombosis may be the *effect* rather than the cause of the infarction — this is thus far merely an unproven hypothesis.

- Subintimal hemorrhage may abruptly narrow the lumen of a stenotic coronary artery, producing effective cessation of flow even though the vessel may not be totally occluded.

- The rupture of the lining of an atheromatous plaque may also produce further narrowing of an artery, causing critical reduction of blood flow.

- High degree of stenosis in a coronary artery may lead to myocardial infarction, either when it reaches a critical point of obstruction interfering with blood flow or when a factor reducing overall organ perfusion develops (e.g., fall in blood pressure).

In a small minority of cases nonatherosclerotic factors may lead to the development of myocardial infarction. They include the following:

- Embolism may occlude a coronary artery. Embolic myocardial infarction may develop under the following conditions:
  - in infective endocarditis;
  - from mural cardiac thrombi (atrial fibrillation, prosthetic cardiac valves);

- from iatrogenic causes (catheterization of the left side of the heart or the coronary arteries, cannulation during open heart surgery).

- Aortitis may occlude one of the coronary ostia. In the past, when luetic aortitis was common, this mechanism was occasionally encountered.

- Aortic dissection may extend into the coronary artery or may occlude an ostium.

- In the various forms of obliterative arteritis, involvement of the coronary arteries may lead to a myocardial infarction, but this is very rare.

The essential *pathological feature* of myocardial infarction is the necrotic change of the myocardium produced by one of the mechanisms discussed above. Myocardial necrosis is gradually replaced by fibrosis so that a firm myocardial scar is the permanent result of myocardial infarction. Replacement of necrotic tissue with fibrosis starts at once—the process is completed within six weeks from the onset.

The degree with which myocardial fibers are replaced with necrosis and then fibrosis varies a great deal, presumably relating to the extent and duration of the myocardial ischemia. Complete portions of ventricular wall may be affected by the infarction ("transmural") in some cases, some layers of it in others (the subendocardial layer of the myocardium is frequently involved—its blood supply makes it more vulnerable than the subepicardial portion); necrosis intermingled with healthy fibers may be present in still other cases. Transmural infarcts often involve the other layers of the heart: involvement of the endocardium frequently leads to the formation of mural thrombi; that of the pericardium, to localized pericarditis. Larger transmural infarcts may develop into aneurysms by the production of a discrete outward bulge of the infarcted area.

The size and location of the infarction vary. The majority of infarcts produced by occlusive changes in a major coronary arterial branch are 2 to 5 cm. in diameter. The left ventricle is primarily affected; involvement of the right ventricle or of the atria is uncommon—if present, it almost always represents an extension of a left ventricular infarction. The more typical locations are related to occlusion of one of the three branches of the coronary artery in patients with a balanced coronary circulation. They are:

- Anterior wall infarction—often extending into the septum (anterior descending branch);

- Inferior wall infarction (right coronary artery);

- Posterobasal myocardial infarction (right or circumflex branch);

- Lateral myocardial infarction (circumflex branch).

Larger infarcts may involve wider areas. This is commonly encountered in patients with slowly progressive coronary artery disease in which collateralization causes some branches to supply areas other than in their physiological distribution.

According to a widely accepted view, which is supported by experimental evidence but not conclusively demonstrated in human infarction, the size of the infarction may not be determined at the moment of the cessation of coronary blood flow. It is considered likely that the area that becomes immediately necrotic is surrounded by a zone of reversible ischemia, which may either recover or proceed into necrosis, depending on such factors as collateral coronary flow and maintenance of perfusion pressure, among others. It has been postulated that in cardiogenic shock following myocardial infarction unfavorable secondary influences extend the size of the infarction beyond its original size, producing a vicious circle.

Thus the critical pathological factors determining the course and prognosis of acute myocardial infarction relate to the following:

- Infarct size and location;

- Extent of involvement of the myocardium (transmural, subendocardial, partial wall necrosis);

- Anatomic sequels of the infarction:

  - mural thrombosis,

  - rupture of ventricular wall,

  - rupture of ventricular septum,

  - involvement of the atria,

  - involvement of the right ventricle,

  - involvement of the conducting system.

From the *pathophysiological* standpoint the necrotic area becomes noncontractile; the borderline ischemic zone may show paradoxical bulge during systole. The two principal immediate sequelae of myocardial infarction are:

1. Impairment of left ventricular function related to the size and location of the infarction;

2. Electrical instability initiating arrhythmias.

Myocardial dysfunction involves the entire range, from subclinical disturbance detectable only by special function tests to irreversible cardiac failure or cardiogenic shock. Cardiac malfunction may be aggravated and perpetuated by some of the secondary effects of the initial attack: nausea, vomiting, arterial hypotension due to severe pain, and effects of the drugs administered for the initial attack (e.g., morphine).

Cardiac function may be further affected by the sequels and complications of myocardial infarction, as mentioned above:

- ventricular aneurysms,

- septal perforation,

- mitral valve malfunction,

- serious arrhythmias.

Hemodynamic sequels to myocardial infarction include the entire spectrum of cardiac failure, as presented in Chapter 14. Complications related to mitral valve malfunction will be discussed in Chapter 34.

CLINICAL FEATURES, COURSE, COMPLICATIONS

The *initial attack* has as its characteristic feature chest pain. The pain may be typical of ischemic pain—in patients who had previously suffered from anginal attack the pain usually is similar to that of earlier attacks but more severe. Various patterns of onset may be observed:

1.   An attack unheralded by any previous symptoms may strike a patient "out of the blue."

2.   A patient may suffer an attack of severe pain after experiencing one or more minor attacks (often ignored) within 24 to 48 hours before.

3.   A patient may go through a stage of a series of attacks of "preinfarction angina" a few days or a week or two prior to the major attack.

4.   A patient with a stable effort angina may be seized suddenly by the severe attack.

5.   Patients with stable angina of effort may go through a stage of acceleration of the angina, leading crescendo into the severe attack.

The characteristic features of pain are described in Chapter 2. The intensity of the pain varies greatly. Some patients may experience relatively mild, though prolonged, chest pain; others suffer from excruciating, unbearable pain requiring drug intervention. Attacks of initial chest pain of acute myocardial infarction are frequently associated with pallor, perspiration, nausea, vomiting, dyspnea, faintness, and dizziness. The duration of the attacks varies as well; some last until relieved by medication (sometimes requiring more than one drug administration); others subside spontaneously and are gone by the time the patient reaches the hospital. Nitroglycerin is usually ineffective but occasionally may temporarily relieve the pain.

Atypical attacks of myocardial infarction occur frequently — no data, however, are available to determine the proportion of typical to atypical attacks. Atypical attacks of myocardial infarction fall into the following categories:

1. Chest pain is overshadowed by other symptoms: dyspnea, dizziness, nausea, faintness, and syncope. A careful interviewer may often obtain a history of an underlying typical or atypical chest pain.

2. Painless myocardial infarction may occur, with abovementioned symptoms heralding the attack but without any pain whatsoever.

3. Pain of atypical nature or location may mislead the patient and the physician alike (stabbing, pleural-like pain, pain limited to arms or neck, pain in the back of the thorax or the epigastrium, etc.).

4. Myocardial infarction may take place during surgical operations, with anesthesia preventing recognition of pain or other symptoms.

5. Truly subclinical myocardial infarction occurs but is probably rather rare. The patient may be discovered to have electrocardiographic evidence of healing or old myocardial infarctions without a clinical counterpart to account for it. Occasionally, a patient will recall "indigestion," ignored by him. Sometimes a complication of myocardial infarction (e.g., hemiplegia) brings the patient to the attention of a physician, who then recognizes a subclinical myocardial infarction as having preceded the onset of the complication.

The course of acute myocardial infarction is related to the direct consequences of the infarction and to secondary complications. The overall prognosis is also related to the extent of the coronary arterial involvement. Basically myocardial infarction is a self-limited disease with a reasonable prospect of recovery for a majority of patients.

The direct effects of acute myocardial infarction depend upon the extent and location of the myocardial involvement:

- Very severe myocardial damage usually results in early death.
- Severe myocardial damage may lead to cardiogenic shock.

• Moderate damage may cause clinically evident cardiac failure (appearing either at once or with some delay).

• Mild myocardial damage produces subclinical cardiac failure (detectable only by special tests) or normal cardiac function may be maintained throughout the acute stage.

Noncardiac consequences of myocardial infarction play a lesser role in the course and prognosis of the patient. They include:

• The initial effects of the infarction: nausea, vomiting, hypotension, perspiration;

• Fever and other constitutional reactions to the infarct;

• Disturbances of respiratory and renal functions.

The average-sized, uncomplicated myocardial infarction is associated with a benign course. Most patients are comfortable and feel well, once the initial pain subsides. Minor attacks of chest pain may occur repeatedly during the first few days. If more persistent or more severe pain follows myocardial infarction, the possibility of impending complication should be considered. Most patients experience no difficulties in resuming minor activities within two to three weeks after the attack and can become fully active six weeks following the onset.

From the standpoint of the course and prognosis, myocardial infarction can be conveniently divided into the following stages:

1. Prehospital stage, involving the onset of pain, circumstances immediately preceding its development, and the earliest sequels to the attack. The time from the onset of pain to the moment the patient is safely placed in a coronary care unit and has all therapeutic interventions available to him ranges from a half hour to several hours.

2. Early stage of myocardial infarction involves the response to initial therapy (usually pain medication). During the prehospital and early stage of myocardial infarction, the risk of electrical instability triggering off dangerous arrhythmias is highest. In this stage hypotension may develop, in which case it is important to discriminate between the causes of the fall in blood pressure, which may be due to infarction, reaction to drugs (or nausea), vagal effect, or incipient cardiogenic shock. Development of cardiac failure (e.g., pulmonary edema) in this stage is a serious sign, but does not necessarily presage irreversible cardiac failure.

3. Intermediate stage of myocardial infarction involves the first few days to a week—from the time the initial attack subsides (end of the early stage) to the time the patient is well enough to be transferred to intermediate or routine care. In most patients with uncomplicated

myocardial infarction this time period may involve freedom from symptoms. Even then, the first week after the attack represents the time of the highest incidence of complications.

4. Late stage includes the second and third week after the attack. In uncomplicated myocardial infarction the patient begins to ambulate during this period. The development of complications in this stage is uncommon.

Complications of acute myocardial infarction make this entity one of the most unpredictable cardiac diseases because of their number, variety, and unexpected appearance. The major complications of myocardial infarction are as follows:

1. Disturbances of rate and rhythm. This is the commonest sequel and complication of acute myocardial infarction and has the broadest potential implications regarding the outcome:

- Disturbances of the normal sinus mechanism: both sinus tachycardia and bradycardia may develop in myocardial infarction. Tachycardia is a distinctly unfavorable sign. Except in the presence of unusually severe febrile reaction, tachycardia almost always indicates a compensatory mechanism in the presence of major disturbance of cardiac function. Bradycardia occurs frequently in inferior myocardial infarction, mostly represents increased vagal activity, and is usually transient.

- Ventricular arrhythmias are common and are ominous. They are directly related to electrical instability originating in the ischemic and infarcted myocardium. They include:

  - single or occasional unifocal premature contractions,

  - multiform premature contractions,

  - repetitive premature contractions, those appearing in salvos,

  - ventricular tachycardia,

  - ventricular fibrillation.

Ventricular arrhythmias are the principal reason for monitoring patients in coronary care units — survival may depend on instant recognition and treatment of ventricular fibrillation.

- Atrial arrhythmias are less commonly encountered in myocardial infarction. Minor atrial arrhythmias, such as premature contractions, are of little consequence. Major arrhythmias — supraventricular tachycardias, atrial flutter, or atrial fibrillation — are potentially serious and require therapy. These arrhythmias often indicate extension of the infarction into the atrial musculature.

• Conduction disturbances appear less frequently than other disturbances of rhythm. They involve two principal types:

    a. Temporary conduction disturbance related to ischemia or temporary dysfunction of the AV node–His system; this variety almost always occurs in inferior myocardial infarction. It involves first and second degree heart block (the latter of the Wenckebach variety) and complete heart block. Degree of conduction disturbance may change from day to day or from hour to hour. The ventricular rate is usually normal or mildly reduced and the QRS complexes narrow.

    b. Permanent conduction disturbance occurs more often in anterior myocardial infarction and may be associated with septal involvement, with bizarre, wide QRS complexes, and with very slow ventricular rates. They may be preceded by bifascicular blocks. Their prognosis is very poor.

2. Consequences of extensive (and strategic) involvement of the left ventricular myocardium produce the following complications (some have been listed above):

• Ventricular aneurysm may develop early in the course of myocardial infarction (as early as 24 hours), and may produce gradual increase in cardiac size or a bulge. Clinically, aneurysms may be responsible for persistence of cardiac failure and may generate ventricular arrhythmias resistant to antiarrhythmic therapy.

• Mitral regurgitation can be produced by one of two mechanisms: abruptly, owing to rupture of a papillary muscle, or gradually, as a result of malfunction of the mitral valve from faulty contraction of the posterior papillary muscle and of the free wall of the left ventricle. The distinction between rupture of the base of the papillary muscle (rapidly fatal) and tear of one of the heads of the papillary muscle will be discussed in connection with mitral regurgitation.

• Rupture of the left ventricular wall may involve either the free wall, perforating into the pericardium, or the septum, perforating into the right ventricle. The former is rapidly fatal, except for rare instances when immediate surgical intervention is possible. Consequences of septal perforation depend on the size of the opening and the extent of the underlying myocardial infarction. A catastrophic deterioration of the patient's condition may ensue, though some such cases can be treated successfully by early operations. Smaller interventricular communications may be well tolerated and permit deferment of the operation till after the myocardial infarction is healed. Some patients may even retain reasonably good cardiac function without surgical closure of the defect.

3. Systemic and pulmonary emboli. Systemic emboli have their source in intracardiac mural thrombi. They occur mostly during the first two weeks of the infarction and involve most commonly cerebral and peripheral vessels. Pulmonary emboli are probably more frequent than they are clinically recognized. Their origin lies in deep venous thrombosis, which is now believed to be very common in acute myocardial infarction. Early ambulation and passive exercise appear to have effectively reduced the risk of this complication.

4. Respiratory complications are most likely to develop in patients who are seriously ill. They include hypoxia, bronchopneumonia, and atelectasis.

5. Cardiogenic shock occupies an intermediate place between a direct sequel of myocardial infarction and a complication. It is by far the most dramatic and ominous sequel to take place in patients with acute myocardial infarction. The exact definition of what represents cardiogenic shock is difficult to give because of a wide overlap between signs and symptoms related to shock and those directly due to the infarct itself. The mortality from shock and the successes of anti-shock therapy vary widely, the successes perhaps depending more upon the definition of shock than upon their merits.

The general features of cardiogenic shock have been presented in Chapter 14. Most of the clinical features of shock overlap with those of simple vasomotor collapse that may accompany the onset of acute myocardial infarction and may include severe pain and apprehension, sometimes aided by drugs given to combat the pain. Furthermore, "shock" is only too often equated with systemic arterial hypotension, which may develop in patients following acute myocardial infarction without any other evidence of true shock. For these reasons it is best to reserve the term "cardiogenic shock" for patients in whom hemodynamic measurements have been performed and a serious disturbance of cardiac function was demonstrated (low cardiac output with elevation of ventricular filling pressures and markedly reduced ventricular ejection fraction), and whose clinical features include evidence of organ hypoperfusion, such as mental obtundation and anuria. The mortality of patients in true cardiogenic shock has always been estimated at about 80 per cent. There is no evidence that any of the presently available conservative methods have reduced this high risk. Whether circulatory assist devices alone, or followed by revascularization procedures, will be able to salvage a higher proportion of patients in cardiogenic shock remains to be seen.

6. Mental disturbances. In many seriously ill patients, especially in the older age group, mental disturbances become apparent, particularly if hypoxia accompanies the illness. In myocardial infarction such manifestations are occasionally seen, although they do not approach the frequency of those encountered after open heart surgery. The manifestations of this disturbance include somnolence, agitation, confusion, and hallucinations. These disturbances are almost always reversible and seldom require therapy.

7. Extension of myocardial infarction. Early in the course of myocardial infarction further damage to the myocardium may develop by various mechanisms. First, the infarction for which the patient is hospitalized may represent a minor myocardial insult, and the major infarction may develop a few days later. Second, ischemic damage to the myocardium may develop in stages, over a period of several days. Third, two independent major infarcts could occur within the span of a few days with circulatory changes resulting from the first infarction aggravating ischemia produced by another coronary branch. Fourth, coronary embolism is a very rare, but possible, complication of acute myocardial infarction. Alertness regarding unusual persistence of chest pain while in the hospital and the development of unexplained symptoms (dyspnea, arrhythmias) may direct attention to this possibility.

8. Pericarditis. Localized pericardial involvement producing pericardial friction rub occurs commonly a few days after the onset. Generalized pericarditis is uncommon. In patients who are on anticoagulants hemorrhagic pericarditis may develop. Pericardial tamponade, if present, suggests the possibility of rupture of the free wall of the heart; its prompt recognition may be life-saving.

DIAGNOSIS

The diagnostic goals in acute myocardial infarction are threefold:

1. To establish or confirm the diagnosis of myocardial infarction;

2. To assess the extent of the damage of the heart;

3. To anticipate and recognize early the major complications.

Establishing the Diagnosis. The diagnosis of acute myocardial infarction involves the following problems:

- Mere confirmation of a typical attack;

- Differentiation of myocardial infarction from lesser ischemic attacks in patients with known ischemic heart disease;

- Differentiation of the nature of an attack of chest pain, distinguishing myocardial infarction from other cardiac or noncardiac pain, i.e., pericarditis, pulmonary infarct, dissecting aneurysm, pneumothorax, mediastinal emphysema, gastrointestinal pain, and thoracic wall pain;

- Recognition of atypical forms of myocardial infarction (principally painless).

The diagnostic contributions of the various signs and symptoms associated with the initial attack of myocardial infarction vary in their specificity and sensitivity:

Pain has the highest specificity if:

- It is typical in all respects;

- It is of long duration;

- It can be identified by a patient as similar to anginal pain but longer and more severe, or if it is similar to that of a previous myocardial infarction;

- It is associated with nausea, vomiting, pallor, perspiration.

Arrhythmia developing during attack of pain is not specific for myocardial infarction but helpful in separating ischemic pain from noncardiac pain.

Dyspnea and pulmonary edema when associated with chest pain are of moderately high specificity in indicating disturbance of left ventricular function.

Physical examination offers the following diagnostic points:

- Atrial (S4) gallop sound is a common finding in ischemia, hence may be of value in separating cardiac from noncardiac pain; its role is diminished by the occasional finding of S4 gallop sounds in normal individuals over the age of 50.

- Ventricular (S3) gallop sound is a more valuable sign indicative of cardiac failure. Its presence in patients suspected of having myocardial infarction adds probability to the diagnosis.

- Cardiac murmurs appear rarely during early stages of myocardial infarction, hence are of little value in the differential diagnosis.

• Pulmonary rales are of relatively low specificity and sensitivity: if present they support the diagnosis of the cardiac rather than the noncardiac origin of pain.

• Fall in arterial pressure has low specificity, though it occurs commonly in myocardial infarction.

Laboratory procedures often play the decisive role in the differentiation of acute myocardial infarction. The more important tests include;

• Radiography—chest film showing evidence of pulmonary vascular congestion is an important diagnostic aid in support of myocardial infarction especially if earlier films are shown not to have the pulmonary vascular changes.

• Electrocardiography is, of course, the most specific test for the detection of the myocardial damage caused by the infarction. A complete sequence of tracings showing the evolution of electrocardiographic changes characteristic of myocardial infarction is highly specific. Yet these evolutionary changes are not always present, even in proven transmural myocardial infarction. The important differential points involving the electrocardiogram include the following problems:

1. Differentiation of S-T deviations due to myocardial infarction from those occurring in variants of angina at rest, in ventricular aneurysm, after digitalis administration, in left ventricular hypertrophy, or in pericarditis.

2. The obliteration of the characteristic QRS changes by pre-existing electrocardiographic abnormalities: left bundle branch block, occasionally right-sided conduction defects, old myocardial infarction.

3. The diagnosis of nontransmural myocardial infarction may present difficulties because ST-T changes are of lower specificity than QRS abnormalities. Thus, problems may develop in differentiating myocardial infarction from pericarditis; S-T segmental depressions found in subendocardial infarction overlap with those produced by left ventricular hypertrophy or by digitalis.

4. Many atypical sequences of electrocardiographic changes may develop in acute myocardial infarction: they include accelerated evolution (the cycle of changes may be completed in 24 hours); delayed appearance of

changes (the electrocardiogram may remain normal during the first few days after the attack); the electrocardiogram may merely show nonspecific T-wave inversion with "minor" changes from day to day.

5. The presence of characteristic Q waves provides the most specific electrocardiographic change due to myocardial infarction. However, unless Q waves appear under observation in serial leads, they cannot time the infarct. False-positive Q waves are found rarely in severe right ventricular hypertrophy (in precordial leads) or in the pre-excitation syndrome.

6. The development of conduction disturbances may lower the specificity of the electrocardiogram.

- The contribution of vectorcardiography to the diagnosis of myocardial infarction is disappointing; occasionally, vectorcardiographic abnormalities may help in the differentiation between myocardial infarction and normal variants and those produced by other cardiac abnormalities. Vectorcardiographic abnormalities usually do not permit the separation between recent and old myocardial infarction.

- Erythrocyte sedimentation rate once played an important part in the diagnosis of acute myocardial infarction. It is a nonspecific test which can be considered of value only if myocardial infarction is the sole factor present that can produce its elevation. To be considered of any aid in the diagnosis, a significant rise in the sedimentation rate has to be recorded within the first 2 or 3 days after the suspected myocardial infarction.

- Serum enzymes. The determination of serum enzyme activity was introduced some two decades ago as one of the most important advances in the diagnosis of acute myocardial infarction. The importance of this series of tests cannot be overemphasized; yet, they have also been subject to occasional misuse owing to a too literal interpretation of the results. Several points need to be made to clarify the role of enzyme determination:

1. Enzymes released from the necrotic myocardium circulate in the serum in excess; hence their level becomes elevated above the normal range for each enzyme. Yet, serum elevation represents conditions similar to a clearance test: the level of the enzyme is related to the speed with which the enzymes are released and the rate of

their destruction. Thus slow release and rapid destruction in the course of myocardial infarction may cause the enzyme level to remain normal.

2. Technical considerations should always be taken into account when enzyme tests are being performed and results do not fit clinical factors. Since the test measures enzyme activity, the possibility of some inhibitors producing false-positive tests needs to be considered.

3. The specificity of enzymes is only fair: false-positive rises occur from the release of enzymes by the liver, skeletal muscles, and other organs, and may also be produced by hemolysis or as a result of intramuscular injection.

4. To be considered significant (rather than borderline), enzyme elevation has to be pronounced. Most enzymes rise after acute myocardial infarction to a range 2 to 10 times basal levels.

Among the serum enzymes, three have been widely accepted as suitable for routine clinical use in the diagnosis of acute myocardial infarction:

1. Serum glutamic oxaloacetic transaminase (SGOT) shows a rise a few hours after the infarction, reaches its peak $1\frac{1}{2}$ to 3 days after the onset, and then declines to the original level within 4 or 5 days.

2. Lactic dehydrogenase (LDH) increases above its original level within 48 hours, reaching a peak in 4 to 7 days, then falling off to return to normal within 2 weeks.

3. Creatine phosphokinase (CPK) increases within a few hours to reach a peak in 24 hours, then returns to normal within 3 to 4 days.

Each of the three enzyme tests has false-positive and false-negative results. The CPK test has the highest sensitivity but only medium specificity. The fact that each enzyme has a different speed of clearance is of considerable diagnostic help. First, the test most likely to provide the answer can be selected at the appropriate time. Second, the use of two or of all three tests may offer very strong diagnostic support if sequential rises occur at appropriate times after the initial attack.

• Isoenzymes have been introduced in an attempt to increase the specificity of the tests. At present the fractionation of the

LDH permits the separation of the "myocardial fraction," thereby eliminating false-positive results stemming from hepatic congestion. Isoenzyme determination does increase the specificity of the test, but its interpretation has to be made with the same caution as that of enzymes in general. More recently fractionation of CPK has also been used to provide isoenzymes more specific for myocardial tissue.

Diagnostic points derived from the *clinical course* may be of supplemental value in confirming the presence of acute myocardial infarction. They include:

- Fever and leukocytosis. These are nonspecific constitutional reactions which usually appear one to two days after the onset and last for several days afterward. They may help differentiate myocardial infarction from lesser ischemic episodes and from noncardiac thoracic wall pain.

- Delayed appearance of signs of cardiac failure: gallop sounds, pulmonary rales, radiographic evidence of pulmonary vascular congestion, and other signs may provide confirmation of cardiac involvement and confirm the diagnosis of myocardial infarction in many situations.

- Pericardial friction rub has moderate specificity in confirming myocardial infarction in an appropriate setting.

Invasive diagnostic procedures are as a rule not indicated for the confirmation of acute myocardial infarction. Occasionally, the measurement of intracardiac pressures by means of a flow-directed balloon catheter may help confirm the presence of subclinical cardiac failure and, in some situations, throw the weight of diagnosis in favor of myocardial infarction. The role of invasive procedures such as cardiac catheterization and angiocardiography lies in the clarification of some of the complications of myocardial infarction, to be discussed later.

Assessment of Extent of Myocardial Damage. It is important from the prognostic standpoint, both in terms of the immediate survival and recovery and in terms of the probability of postinfarctional rehabilitation and resumption of an active life, to determine the extent of damage. Attempts at an accurate delineation of the size of the infarction are now being made in research laboratories, using complex "mapping" of electrocardiographic precordial changes and quantification of some specific isoenzymes. These procedures are at present not suited for routine clinical use; furthermore, their accuracy has yet to be definitely established.

The available means of evaluation of the extent of myocardial damage from the infarct are crude and often misleading. They include:

- The magnitude of electrocardiographic changes in the routine leads; extensive appearance of Q waves or disappearance of R waves in several leads suggests larger myocardial infarction than in cases with less pronounced changes. This relationship, however, is very crude since the electrocardiogram exaggerates changes in some locations and minimizes those in other locations. Vectorcardiographic changes do not increase the accuracy in estimating the size of the infarcts.

- The magnitude of enzyme rises. In a crude sense, enzyme elevation to levels 10 times normal imply larger infarcts than those producing enzyme levels twice normal. This relationship is also rather crude: it can be demonstrated for groups of cases, but in an individual patient it has to be accepted cautiously.

- The magnitude of the constitutional reaction. High fever, severe leukocytosis, pronounced elevation of the erythrocyte sedimentation rate—all suggest extensive damage. Yet, individual reactions vary so that this relationship is even more inaccurate than the others.

- Evidence of cardiac failure. Appearance of signs of cardiac failure is probably the strongest diagnostic point in favor of significant cardiac damage. It does not matter whether such changes occur at once, or with some delay, except that a gradual deterioration of the circulatory status provides a serious prognostic clue. The signs in question are persistent sinus tachycardia, persistent hypotension, prominent gallop sounds, persistent pulmonary rales, and pressure rise in the caval system.

Recognition of Complications. The major complications of acute myocardial infarction have been listed above. Inasmuch as the complications play a critical role in the prognosis of acute myocardial infarction, altertness for their early recognition is of paramount importance, especially since some complications can be successfully treated. The diagnostic approaches to complications include the following:

Arrhythmias. Early recognition of arrhythmias is easy in the coronary care unit. The various arrhythmias are displayed on the monitor and recorded in strips. The following points need special attention:

- Overall trends—the increase or decrease of ectopy; the response to therapy;

- Correct diagnosis of the arrhythmia — especially differentiation between supraventricular and ventricular ectopy; in many situations it is advisable to use all possible means of differentiation — even the application of esophageal or atrial leads. Similarly, the precise mechanism of conduction disturbances may have to be clarified.

Cardiac Failure. It is important to differentiate between cardiac failure secondary to the infarction and that initiated by a complication. Serial physical examinations and daily chest roentgenograms provide good means of monitoring the state of the circulation. Direct monitoring via a central venous catheter or flow-directed balloon catheter has considerable merit, although its routine use should be discouraged and it should be reserved only for patients whose clinical course is less than optimal. Two points need to be considered: First, central venous pressure is a poor index of the left ventricular competence — which is of paramount importance in myocardial infarction. Second, intracardiac pressure monitoring is reliable in institutions with an adequate caseload and staff experienced in hemodynamics. Its use in small coronary care units is not justified, for the findings can be too easily misinterpreted and false conclusions drawn. Whenever cardiac failure develops abruptly, a high index of suspicion that a complication is present should prevail.

Shock. This dreaded complication was discussed above and some diagnostic difficulties were already pointed out. The following questions should be considered in patients who are hypotensive and show some signs of shock:

- Is the patient really in shock or merely hypotensive?

- Is there any possible cause for a simple vasomotor collapse rather than cardiogenic shock (e.g., severe pain, nausea, drug administration)?

- If shock is present, can a specific cause be identified? (This is particularly important in delayed development of shock.)

- Could shock be due to pericardial tamponade?

Patients with early signs of shock should be monitored by means of intracardiac catheters. The patient's life may depend upon immediate intervention, if and when a specific cause of shock is identified. Therefore, it is advisable to transfer patients who are in early shock, or even those who merely show progressive fall in arterial pressure beyond that expected in myocardial infarction, to cardiac centers with all facilities available (large-volume laboratory, experienced surgical team).

Systemic Embolization. A high index of suspicion serves to alert the physician to the possibility of systemic embolization. Unexplained pain in the abdomen or in the extremities or changes in the patient's mental status call for the differentiation between unimportant incidents and sequels to the infarction, on the one hand, and the presence of systemic emboli, on the other.

Deep Venous Thrombosis and Pulmonary Emboli. Frequent examination of the extremities, palpation of the veins, and tests for the Homans sign are indicated during the initial stages after myocardial infarction. Chest pain of pleural character and sudden change in respiratory rate should make one suspicious of pulmonary emboli.

Anuria. Three conditions should be considered in patients who are severely oliguric or anuric:

- inability to empty the bladder,

- fluid retention from latent cardiac failure,

- renal tubular damage from low perfusion pressure.

Differentiation may be aided by the use of an indwelling catheter, and by monitoring the level of arterial blood pressure.

Pulmonary Complications. Arterial hypoxia is occasionally present after myocardial infarction even in the absence of obvious respiratory problems. Seriously ill patients may have respiratory distress, which requires treatment. Atelectasis and pneumonia may develop in patients after myocardial infarction — these need to be differentiated from pulmonary infarcts.

Appearance of Cardiac Murmurs. The two major complications, presented above, include rupture of the ventricular septum and rupture of the head of the papillary muscle. Lesser degrees of mitral regurgitation related to temporary or permanent malfunction of the mitral valve seldom produce loud murmurs and are unlikely to produce a change in the patient's condition (careful auscultation revealed in some series that more than half of random patients with acute myocardial infarction develop apical systolic murmurs). The appearance of a loud systolic murmur is usually associated with an abrupt deterioration in the condition of the patient, ranging from a fall in arterial pressure to appearance of signs of cardiac failure to outright shock. If such change takes place the diagnosis of the underlying condition should be made at once, even if the condition is not serious enough to consider immediate surgical intervention. The simplest diagnostic approach is to use a flow-directed balloon catheter, which can:

- Identify septal perforation by showing an oxygen step-up in the right ventricle,

- Suggest mitral regurgitation by showing tall V waves in pulmonary "wedge" pressure.

Recurrent Ischemic Type of Chest Pain. As stated, in the great majority of patients, little or no chest pain is present during the course of acute myocardial infarction, once the initial attack has subsided, even if the patient had suffered severe recurrent pain prior to the infarct. Recurrence of chest pain may be present occasionally without apparent reason and without affecting the outcome. However, more often recurrent chest pain may presage a continuing ischemic process, extension of the infarction, or the threat of a new, second infarction. Patients who have continuing pain should be more carefully supervised, left longer in the coronary care unit, and have frequent 12-lead electrocardiograms recorded, if possible, during attacks of pain.

Diagnostic Approaches

In a serious, life-threatening disease such as myocardial infarction the importance of an orderly approach to the diagnostic evaluation is self-evident. The various possible steps have been discussed and the respective importance of each explained. It remains now to summarize diagnostic options as they present themselves in different situations:

1. Given a patient with a "classical" myocardial infarction, the diagnostic workup can be relatively simple. With high probability of the diagnosis of myocardial infarction on clinical grounds, laboratory diagnosis can merely include two or three serial electrocardiograms to record the evolutionary changes and two or three enzyme determinations. Further steps consist merely of careful monitoring, provided the patient's clinical course is uncomplicated. Assessment of the severity of damage and alertness for the development of complications should be routine for all patients with known myocardial infarction.

2. Many patients suffer their first attack of anterior thoracic pain which is consistent with, but not characteristic of, acute myocardial infarction, and no other findings implicating the heart are present. A brief diagnostic hospital workup is justified in those in whom the diagnosis of myocardial infarction is not confirmed. This may include:

- Daily electrocardiograms for three days;
- Daily enzyme determination for three days (with the first sample drawn immediately after admission);
- Clinical observation, with special attention to cardiac abnormalities.

3. Patients with previous effort angina who are admitted with severe chest pain at rest should be investigated, concentrating upon serial electrocardiographic changes (particularly the development of Q waves), enzyme rises, and signs of cardiac failure.

4. Patients admitted with unusually severe chest pain and signs of either shock or vasomotor collapse should be investigated not only from the standpoint of acute myocardial infarction but also regarding other possible conditions. The diagnosis of myocardial infarction may appear the most obvious one, and yet some such patients turn out to be suffering from dissecting aneurysm, massive pulmonary embolism, or even perforation of a viscus. Active search for many possibilities should be instituted rather than passively waiting to rule out myocardial infarction.

5. Patients who have typical myocardial infarction and who, after a satisfactory initial course, begin to deteriorate present a real challenge to the clinician. The various clinical signs of deterioration include:

- persistent or increasing arrhythmias,
- development of sinus tachycardia,
- appearance of dyspnea, signs of pulmonary edema,
- acute or gradual development of cardiac failure,
- fall in arterial pressure,
- shock,
- increasing chest pain.

The various diagnostic procedures discussed in the preceding sections should be utilized. Monitoring of all possible indices is recommended. Complete diagnostic study, including cardiac catheterization, left ventriculography, and coronary arteriography may be indicated if the possibility of surgical treatment is being considered. Possible operations include:

- aneurysmectomy for cardiac failure,
- aneurysmectomy for intractable arrhythmias,
- septal repair,
- mitral valve replacement,
- repair of external cardiac rupture,
- coronary revascularization for continuing ischemia.

PROGNOSIS

The prognosis of acute myocardial infarction involves three issues:

1. The probability of survival from the attack;

2.   The degree of impairment of cardiac function after the attack;

3.   The possible progression of coronary occlusive disease.

In general the risk of patients hospitalized with acute myocardial infarction is reasonable. It is widely recognized that the highest risk of dying occurs within the first hour after the onset of an attack. Various statistics place the percentage of fatalities taking place within the first hour at from 35 to 80 per cent of all deaths from acute myocardial infarction. Thus the hospital population encompasses a select group with an average of about 15 per cent mortality. It is further acknowledged that the majority of hospital deaths — at least 60 per cent — take place within the first 24 hours after admission. The introduction of coronary care units led to a reduction — though not complete elimination — of "electrical deaths," i.e., those due to ventricular fibrillation. Their contribution will be discussed below.

Causes of death vary: some patients die as a result of damage to the myocardium so extensive that it is unable to carry the circulatory load. Many patients succumb, however, to one of the complications of myocardial infarction.

Inasmuch as survival and recovery from the attack are contingent upon many factors other than the initial myocardial insult, the prognosis can be discussed only in broadest terms, indicative of trends rather than reasonable estimates of the outcome in individual cases. Some clinical findings bear definitive relationships to the outcome; others are of little prognostic value:

- Signs of cardiac failure are perhaps the most important indications of the seriousness of the condition, yet complete restoration of cardiac function and good recovery may occur in spite of the presence of cardiac failure during the acute stage.

- Development of cardiac enlargement as determined by radiography is also considered an unfavorable sign.

- Persistent arterial hypotension calls for a guarded prognosis.

- Indices estimating the size of myocardial infarction bear some relationship to the outcome, though they are of lesser importance than disturbances of cardiac function; the difficulty in their interpretation has been commented upon.

- Arrhythmias occurring during the first few days after the attack are the result of electrical instability; they bear relationship to the immediate course but have little influence upon the late outcome.

- Persistent arrhythmias throughout the entire course of myocardial infarction (including persistent conduction disturbances) may be ominous and presage problems after recovery from the acute stage.

• The persistence of ischemic type chest pain is significant in terms of a possible extension of the infarction; it does not necessarily indicate continued anginal attacks after recovery.

• The severity of the initial attack of pain and of the accompanying signs and symptoms has only a minor relationship to the outcome.

• The extent of electrocardiographic changes is of minor predictive value regarding the outcome of the attack; however, the development of serious conduction defects is considered an unfavorable sign.

• Complications influence the prognosis in accordance with their nature, magnitude, and permanency.

The restoration and maintenance of adequate cardiac function after recovery from an attack of acute myocardial infarction are primarily related to the severity of myocardial damage. It has been pointed out that the presence of cardiac failure during the acute stage and the development of cardiomegaly diminish the prospect for the resumption of good effort tolerance. However, it should be emphasized that the *absence* of cardiac failure or enlargement does not constitute a definite sign that the patient had escaped permanent myocardial damage; many patients show no evidence of circulatory embarrassment until they stress themselves when resuming normal activities after the attack. In addition to delayed development of cardiac failure, postinfarctional mitral regurgitation may not be apparent until after the patient is fully active.

Thus, the survivors from acute myocardial infarction fall into the following categories:

1. Patients who make a complete recovery and regain full health and an asymptomatic state;

2. Patients who make a good recovery in terms of cardiac function but whose activities are limited by recurrence of effort angina;

3. Patients who end up with a compromised cardiac function, ranging from mild limitation of activities to total disability, or "cardiac invalidism";

4. Patients whose clinical disability is related both to ischemic pain and to cardiac malfunction.

A good deal of effort has been put into categorizing patients with acute myocardial infarction into prognostic groups. More or less favorable groups have been identified without difficulty—using criteria presented above—although these groups should be accepted merely as overall trends. Prognostication in individual cases is unreliable except on the two extreme ends of the spectrum.

Remarks pertaining to the course and prognosis of acute myocardial infarction presented in this chapter apply not only to patients who come down with their first myocardial infarction but to those with repeated infarcts as well. Unless the myocardium is already seriously compromised from previous myocardial infarcts, subsequent attacks are subject to the same diagnostic and prognostic guidelines as the first infarcts. The few minor differences (e.g., electrocardiographic diagnostic difficulties) have been pointed out.

THERAPY

Acute myocardial infarction is a self-limited disease. It is not unusual to discover accidentally past myocardial infarcts in patients who either had no clinical indications of the infarction or who misinterpreted warning signs and went about their usual lives during the acute stage of myocardial infarction without any ill effects whatsoever. Even in typical cases of acute myocardial infarction, patients often feel very well after the initial chest pain has subsided and are frequently skeptical regarding all the "fuss" about their illness. Thus, active therapy of acute myocardial infarction requires specific *goals* that can be summarized as follows:

1. To control the initial attack;

2. To insure best possible healing of the infarct;

3. To maintain patient morale;

4. To prevent complications;

5. To treat evident ill effects, consequences, and complications;

6. To facilitate complete rehabilitation after the attack.

Several of these objectives are thought to be partially fulfilled by the widely accepted concept of treatment in the *coronary care unit* (CCU). As in all forms of therapy, it is necessary to review the contribution of the coronary care unit in terms of the risk-vs.-benefit therapeutic equation. The principal contribution of the coronary care unit is its monitoring facility. The introduction of closed-chest massage and external defibrillation of the heart made it possible to salvage many patients who develop ventricular fibrillation. Experience has shown that ventricular fibrillation in acute myocardial infarction is more often than not an electrical "accident" which bears no relationship to the severity of the disease and its prognosis. The monitoring of cardiac rhythm permits instant recognition of ventricular fibrillation and thereby an almost perfect salvage rate from a given attack of ventricular fibrillation. While the actual figures are difficult to obtain because of inability to provide perfect randomization, it is certain that a significant reduction of mortality from acute myocardial infarction has taken place (though probably not as great as some of the statistics indicate). While no one can argue against this advantage of coronary care units, voices are occasionally heard recommending home treatment of those patients with myocardial infarction who are in the best prognostic categories in order to avoid the psychological trauma. One should not minimize the possible adverse effects of the anxieties of patients exposed to the frightening equipment, aware of their own heart beats (particularly if mild and innocent arrhythmias are present), witnessing the care of seriously ill neighbors, seeing some patients die. Many of the newer CCU's are designed to minimize these adverse features. It is probable, however, that the safety of the coronary care unit outweighs these disadvantages. Furthermore, the appropriate psychotherapy can offset the negative aspects of the unit in all but the most neurotic patients. The second major disadvantage of the CCU is its underutilization. The pressure from patients and physicians—the prestige factor—has produced conditions in which even the smallest hospital is obligated to have a CCU. The potential safety of the unit is contingent upon the availability of well-trained personnel whose decisions in emergencies are based upon judgment that comes not only from training but also from constant practice. This is not always fulfilled in the "part-time" CCU which may offer false security to patients.

A coronary care unit in an active cardiological center offers facility beyond that of rhythm monitoring aimed at the prevention and treatment of ventricular fibrillation. A good coronary care unit should also offer excellent facilities for the monitoring and treatment of other features of myocardial infarction and have the capability for the early detection of anticipated complications, as outlined above. These facilities are as a rule not available in smaller CCU's. It should be clearly understood that emphasis is often placed on cardiac rhythm and other aspects of myocardial infarction are too often disregarded. The importance of early recognition of problems other than the arrhythmia and of transferring patients who are suspected of having them to more complete facilities cannot be overemphasized.

The success of the coronary care unit concept led to the consideration of the possibility that treatment could be provided before the patient reaches the coronary care unit. As already indicated, the majority of deaths from acute myocardial infarction occur within minutes or hours after the onset—most of them before the patient can reach a hospital facility. Some deaths undoubtedly represent myocardial damage too extensive for survival, but others are presumed to be due to "electrical accidents" and early intervention might prevent some of these fatalities. "Prehospital care" has been approached from the standpoint of special ambulances, mobile coronary care units, and even self-administration of drugs by patients. Technical difficulties in the execution of the various plans are great, perhaps insurmountable. They include:

- The time lost by the patient until he recognizes the nature of his pain;

- The time necessary to reach the patient (under various traffic conditions);

- The expense and availability of maintaining trained teams within reach of anyone reporting suspected cardiac pain;

- The overselling of the alertness and anticipation of attack to patients with known coronary disease.

The success of the various prehospital plans for patients with acute myocardial infarction remains to be demonstrated. Pilot studies are encouraging but their wide application has not been evaluated. Some simplified partial plans appear more realistic (i.e., telemetry during ambulance transport) and may at least dent the high attrition rate of patients in early stages of myocardial infarction.

The Initial Attack.   Wherever the patient is first seen — his home, the emergency room, a medical office, or the coronary care unit — the first step in therapy is control of the pain in the initial attack. Some patients who have suffered from attacks of ischemic pain in the past tend to use nitroglycerin — often several tablets. Nitroglycerin is considered by some contraindicated in acute myocardial infarction as an agent that may precipitate fall in arterial pressure. Definitive studies to prove this point are not available, and whether nitroglycerin actually can harm a patient is subject to doubt; it is almost always ineffective. Strong analgesic drugs such as morphine or similar synthetic drugs are usually needed; the intravenous route is preferable. It should be noted, however, that control of pain offers a mixed blessing. Narcotics and other similar drugs may enhance or even initiate gastrointestinal upset (nausea and vomiting) with its concomitant vagal stimulation, as well as hypotensive episodes, overlapping with or aggravating similar symptoms produced by the pain itself. Individual judgment and careful clinical observation should guide the clinician as to the use, the choice, and the dosage of pain-killing drugs.

If the patient is seen outside the coronary care unit, the decision should be made as to whether other forms of therapy are needed. Some investigators advocate prophylactic use of an antiarrhythmic agent (lidocaine bolus) to cover the period until the time the patient is connected with a monitor. This therapy is by no means universally accepted. Many authorities object to the use of antiarrhythmic agents without specific indications. Occasionally patients show mild to moderate bradycardia (rates of 50 to 70) attributed to vagal overactivity. The administration of atropine has been recommended and may be effective. Yet, recently objections have been raised to the use of atropine because of its potential harm.

Once the patient is in a coronary care unit, monitoring is initiated and an intravenous drip is started. Oxygen administration is a time-honored therapy in the early stages of myocardial infarction. In patients who show no respiratory distress and who are comfortable and free of pain, the use of oxygen may be questioned. If in doubt, a determination of oxygen tension in arterial blood may be used as a guide to the need for oxygen therapy.

Rest. The question of rest has been subject to change over a period of decades. Once it was considered standard therapy to remain for six weeks on absolute bed rest and another six weeks on partial rest, but periods of bed rest have been gradually shortened to the point at which one wonders whether early activity is not being now overemphasized. The disadvantages of prolonged bed rest are well recognized; "good-risk" patients with acute myocardial infarction seem to show no ill effects from early ambulation. Nevertheless it is prudent to recommend at least one week of rest in bed, during which there may be short periods of rest in bedside chairs; the use of a commode may begin within 48 hours after the onset. Gradual ambulation may begin during the second week. In uncomplicated myocardial infarction patients are often discharged from the hospital during the early part of the third week after the attack.

Psychotherapy. Psychotherapy represents an extremely important, yet often neglected, aspect of treatment of myocardial infarction. It is preferable that the patient's physician rather than a psychiatrist undertake this aspect of therapy. The purpose of psychotherapy is as follows:

- To explain the need for treatment in a special setting for a patient who basically feels fit;

- To prepare the patient for loss of time from his usual activities;

- To discuss the various options regarding his fate after the acute attack — presenting the situation in as optimistic terms as seem prudent.

Well-managed psychotherapy often permits immunization of the patient against some of the negative aspects of the coronary care unit, while at the same time setting the stage for good rehabilitation.

Treatment of Untoward Sequels and Complications. The whole spectrum of complications listed in earlier parts of this chapter must be considered. Therapy of myocardial infarction can be approached from an aggressive standpoint or from a conservative standpoint. In the author's opinion a conservative approach has more merit, within the guidelines of the therapeutic principle (risk vs. benefit), unless either the aggressive approach is justified by irrefutable evidence in its favor or the situation is desperate enough to justify the risks.

Antiarrhythmic Therapy. This may be approached as prophylaxis in patients who show only mild and innocent arrhythmias (e.g., few ventricular ectopic beats per minute) or as remedial therapy against serious arrhythmias. Lidocaine has established itself as the first-choice antiarrhythmic drug, having the advantage of immediate action when administered by intravenous drip, a reasonable opportunity to titrate the dose on the basis of its effects, and the immediate termination of its action when the drip is turned off. Its prime target is ventricular arrhythmias. If lidocaine is ineffective, other antiarrhythmic agents that can be used parenterally include propranolol, procainamide and diphenylhydantoin. Quinidine should only be used orally but may be useful when drug combinations are necessary for the control of more serious arrhythmias.

Life-threatening or persistent arrhythmias may require drastic steps if simpler measures fail. Sustained tachycardias (supraventricular or ventricular), atrial flutter, or atrial fibrillation may be terminated by electroshock therapy; its prime indications are for those cases in which rapid rates appear to produce hypotension, dyspnea, or other untoward effects. In life-threatening ventricular arrhythmias that are totally refractory to drug therapy and unsuitable for electroshock because of their recurrent nature, the extreme measure of atrial or ventricular overdrive pacing has to be considered. If even this treatment fails, emergency operations might be taken under consideration: aneurysmectomy or revascularization of the coronary arteries or both procedures. These operative procedures require cardiac catheterization and angiographic studies prior to their performance.

Atrial arrhythmias may require no therapy if only occasional atrial premature contractions occur. Attacks of atrial flutter or atrial fibrillation may be treated with digitalis (particularly atrial fibrillation) unless poor tolerance of rapid ventricular rate compels one to perform electroshock treatment to attain immediate conversion. Rapid supraventricular tachycardias may be handled in the same fashion.

Conduction disturbances complicating acute myocardial infarction fall into two categories. The "benign" type occurs in inferior myocardial infarction; first, second, or third degree heart block may develop. Occasionally all three degrees of block appear sequentially. A relatively normal ventricular rate (faster than 50) and narrow QRS complexes identical with those present prior to the conduction disturbance are characteristic for this form of heart block. Heart block of this variety is almost always transient; treatment may not be necessary unless even the mildly reduced ventricular rate is poorly tolerated, in which case a temporary demand pacemaker may be inserted. Routine insertion of a standby pacemaker in the early stages of this type of conduction disturbance should be discouraged, especially in institutions where pacemakers are only occasionally inserted, because the risk of the procedure probably outweighs the risk of syncopal attacks. In contrast, heart block occurring in anterior myocardial infarction is usually permanent; it is often characterized by bizarre, wide QRS complexes and excessively slow ventricular rates (30 to 40). It may be preceded by bifascicular and trifascicular block. This type of heart block carries a poor prognosis; pacemaker insertion is indicated, but even with it the mortality is very high.

Treatment of Cardiac Failure. The aggressiveness of therapy directed against cardiac failure is a subject of controversy. Digitalis is considered by some the drug of choice; even prophylactic routine administration of digitalis has been suggested, though fortunately not widely accepted. Considering the negative aspects of digitalis therapy in seriously ill patients, as explained in Chapter 11, it is believed that other forms of therapy should take precedence over digitalis in the treatment of cardiac failure. Furthermore, when cardiac failure manifests itself merely by the presence of gallop sounds and pulmonary rales, treatment may be altogether omitted, provided the patient is carefully watched clinically and his intracardiac pressures are monitored in the coronary care unit. If more than minimal signs of cardiac failure appear, diuretics may control them adequately and should be first tried alone; only if failure persists is digitalis indicated, with the appropriate precautions.

As mentioned above, severe progressive cardiac failure strongly suggests the presence of a serious complication; the possibility of surgical intervention should be considered, first clinically (see above), then by means of a complete hemodynamic-angiocardiographic study. Progressive cardiac failure, irreversible by medical treatment, represents a situation desperate enough to require open heart surgery, even if myocardial infarction is but a few days along.

Treatment of Shock. Drug therapy for cardiogenic shock is often ineffective. A rational approach to shock therapy requires a reasonable knowledge of the underlying physiological mechanism. Hypovolemic shock may be at least temporarily alleviated by volume expanders. Shock associated with severe arteriolar constriction may respond to the administration of alpha-adrenergic blocking agents or other vasodilators (phentolamine, nitroglycerin, nitroprusside); shock associated with low peripheral arteriolar resistance, to pressor amines. It is believed that inotropic agents, such as isoproterenol or digitalis, may be more harmful than useful because they increase myocardial oxygen consumption, an effect which could outweigh their inotropic benefits. Recently released dopamine has shown promise in the treatment of cardiogenic shock, but its role has not yet been completely defined.

Present experience has not yet clarified the role of circulatory assist devices in cardiogenic shock. Although it is clear that artificial devices can maintain the circulation in spite of the "pump failure," no evidence has been presented that during the short period the artificial circulation is maintained the heart can acquire improved function that will enable it to assume a more adequate performance when the assist is terminated. The possibility that early use of assist devices may cut the vicious circle of progressive cardiac damage and prevent irreversible changes in the myocardium is at this time purely hypothetical, without direct support derived from studies in man. One wonders how many of the "successes" of circulatory assists merely involve patients with simple vasomotor collapse who would have recovered without any therapy. A promising lead is being investigated at present: the use of assist devices to carry patients until surgical revascularization can be performed to improve coronary perfusion.

Respiratory Problems. Treatment of respiratory problems ranges from management of mild hypoxia, easily corrected by the administration of oxygen, to the use of respirators for the management of serious respiratory distress. The two guiding principles in instituting respiratory therapy are:

- Reduction of the work of breathing,

- Correction of impaired gas exchange.

Respiratory problems may be a part of overwhelming cardiorespiratory failure, such as occurs in shock, or may be the result of complications such as pneumonia, atelectasis, or pulmonary infarction. The treatment of the underlying condition should be carried on concurrently with respiratory supportive therapy.

Anticoagulant Therapy. Prevention of thromboembolism in acute myocardial infarction has been a subject of debate for more than a quarter of a century. Originally recommended for the protection of the patient from the threat of systemic emboli due to mural thrombosis and from secondary coronary thrombosis, it is now considered likely that anticoagulation is mostly effective against deep venous thrombosis and pulmonary emboli. Whether the risk of anticoagulant therapy is justifiable on a routine basis, in the light of reduced risk of phlebothrombosis with almost immediate seating of patients in bedside chairs and early ambulation, has not been settled. A compromise solution widely used is to limit anticoagulant therapy to patients falling into the "poor risk" category and to omit therapy in good risk cases of myocardial infarction. The strongest indication for anticoagulant therapy is the suggested presence of phlebothrombosis or pulmonary infarcts.

Surgical Therapy.   The principal surgical procedures applicable to acute myocardial infarction have already been listed above. In spite of considerable enthusiasm by some surgeons, open heart surgery during acute myocardial infarction should be performed only after most thorough considerations of the pros and cons. Such glib suggestions as routine infarctectomy or early revascularization of all patients immediately after the initial attack deserve no serious consideration. The therapeutic equation regarding surgery in acute myocardial infarction involves the patient whose life is endangered to such an extent that the relatively high risk of open heart surgery is the lesser evil.

The most urgent indication for surgery is intractable cardiac failure or shock related to a definite complication of myocardial infarction. Four such complications come under consideration:

- External rupture of the heart,

- Perforation of the ventricular septum,

- Rupture of a head of a papillary muscle,

- Aneurysm.

The first of these represents a dire emergency with little time to spare. Large perforations are immediately fatal. Smaller ones produce hemopericardium with tamponade, which may temporarily act as a hemostatic factor. Here the diagnostic acumen of the clinician is at a premium. In the presence of pericardial tamponade with hemopericardium, surgical exploration may be life-saving.

Septal perforation produces a wide range of consequences. Deferment of septal repair until the infarction is healed improves the chances of survival and success. Thus, immediate operations are indicated only if patients fail to respond to medical therapy.

Similar considerations apply to acute mitral regurgitation. Aneurysm is a less well defined reversible cause of cardiac failure in the acute stage of myocardial infarction. However, aneurysmectomy may be considered as a means of containing life-threatening arrhythmias unresponsive to drug therapy.

The risk of these operations is high, much greater than comparable operations performed electively. Their performance should always be considered a desperate, life-saving effort.

The operation about which least information is available regarding its risk, indications, and success rate is the revascularization procedure performed on patients with acute myocardial infarction who continue having ischemic pain. Here the possibility is suggested that another infarction may be prevented by the operation. Perhaps the only criterion that one can use is the presence of a very severe stenotic lesion in a major coronary artery supplying areas other than the infarcted one.

Rehabilitation. The rehabilitative management of patients recovering from myocardial infarction is an often neglected part of the therapy. Along with early psychotherapy, rehabilitation often determines whether or not the patient who recovers physically will be capable of resuming an active life. Excess caution may be responsible for crippling neuroses in middle-aged individuals, neuroses which often cause permanent disability. Neurotic disability is seen not only in patients who have recovered from an attack of acute myocardial infarction but also in individuals who have been hospitalized for a suspected myocardial infarction in which the diagnosis was never established.

The essence of a good rehabilitation program should include the following points:

- Reduction of the time of rest after the initial attack;

- Early ambulation;

- Graded resumption of activity;

- Careful observation of the patient during the critical period that he resumes an active life; one should be especially alert for the presence of arrhythmias with exercise, the development of cardiac failure after resumption of activities, and the appearance of mitral regurgitation;

- Return to work as early as possible, considering the individual patient's occupation.

The question as to whether a formal standard exercise program performed under medical supervision is superior to one individually recommended by the physician has not been definitely settled.

Bibliography

Edwards JE: What is myocardial infarction? Circulation *40*, Suppl IV:5, 1969.

Chandler AB, Chapman I, Erhardt LR, Roberts WC, Schwartz CJ, Sinapus D, Spain DM, Cherry S, Ness PM, Simon TL: Coronary thrombosis in myocardial infarction. Amer. J. Cardiol. *34*:823, 1974.

DeSanctis RW, Block P, Hutter AM Jr: Tachyarrhythmias in myocardial infarction. Circulation *45*:681, 1972.

Fulton M, Julian DG, Oliver MF: Sudden death and myocardial infarction. Circulation *40*, Suppl IV:182, 1969.

James TN: Sudden death related to myocardial infarction. Circulation *45*:205, 1972.

Kuller L, Lilienfeld A, Fisher R: An epidemiological study of sudden and unexpected deaths in adults. Medicine *48*:341, 1967.

Levine HD, Young E, Williams RA: Electrocardiogram and vectorcardiogram in myocardial infarction. Circulation *45*:457, 1972.

Lown B, Selzer A: The coronary care unit. Amer. J. Cardiol. *22*:297, 1968.

Mundth ED, Buckley MJ, Daggett WM, Saunders CA, Austen WG: Surgery for complications of acute myocardial infarction. Circulation *45*:1279, 1972.

Rotman M, Wagner GS, Wallace AG: Bradyarrhythmias in acute myocardial infarction. Circulation *45*:703, 1972.

Scheidt S, Ascheim R, Killip T: Shock after acute myocardial infarction. A clinical and hemodynamic profile. Amer. J. Cardiol. *26*:556, 1970.

Sobel BE, Shell WE: Serum enzyme determinations in the diagnosis and assessment of myocardial infarction. Circulation *45*:471, 1972.

Stokes J III, Dawber TR: The "silent coronary." The frequency and clinical characteristics of unrecognized myocardial infarction in the Framingham study. Ann. Int. Med. *50*:1359, 1959.

Wolk MJ, Scheidt S, Killip T: Heart failure complicating acute myocardial infarction. Circulation *45*:1125, 1972.

Whalen RE, Ramo BW, Wallace AG: The value and limitations of coronary care monitoring. Prog. Cardiovasc. Dis. *13*:442, 1971.

23
Rheumatic Fever

Definition. Rheumatic fever represents a clinical entity caused by abnormal tissue reaction related to autoimmune mechanisms produced by exposure to hemolytic streptococci. It involves several organs and tissues, the heart being one of them. The heart, however, plays a unique role, in that damage initiated by the acute process often persists and progresses into a lifetime affliction. The acute cardiac involvement in rheumatic fever manifests itself by changes in the endocardium, the myocardium, and the pericardium. Myocardial and pericardial changes are, as a rule, ephemeral; endocardial involvement initiates the chronic rheumatic process that culminates in valvular heart disease.

ETIOLOGY AND PATHOLOGY

Etiological consideration of the rheumatic state has been presented in Chapter 21. The hypersensitivity reaction represented by acute rheumatic fever shows certain similarities to other conditions believed to be related to hyperimmune mechanisms: serum sickness, rheumatoid arthritis, systemic lupus erythematosus, polyarteritis, and other forms of collagen-vascular diseases.

Rheumatic fever is a disease of the young, affecting primarily populations between the ages of 3 and 20. The familial predisposition and influence of crowding, poor hygiene, inadequate diet, and other factors have been commented upon previously.

The principal target organs of rheumatic fever are the following:

- large joints,
- heart,
- central nervous system (chorea),
- lungs (rheumatic pneumonia),

- skin (erythema marginatum),

- serous membrane (pleurisy, pericarditis),

- subcutaneous tissues (rheumatic nodules).

Pathological changes produced by rheumatic activity include, as the most characteristic feature, Aschoff bodies, consisting of collections of reticuloendothelial cells, lymphocytes and fibroblasts, with a necrotic center filled with amorphous eosinophilic material. These are most commonly encountered in the myocardium, but may be found in other organs as well. The lesions upon the cardiac valves are characteristic and include fine translucent vegetations composed of fibrin and platelets located upon the edges of the valve leaflets, along the line of valve closure. Acute rheumatic valvulitis is basically not a destructive process. While acute incompetence of valves may develop, the permanent valve damage represents the later scarring process, which is not directly related to rheumatic activity but merely initiated by it. Pericardial involvement is largely nonspecific, consisting of fibrinous exudation, usually, but not always, associated with pericardial effusion.

NATURAL HISTORY

The diagnostic problems in recognizing atypical cases of rheumatic fever make it very difficult to develop a good perspective of the entire spectrum of this disease. Only more typical cases are recognized with reasonable probability. This difficulty is compounded by the changing picture of acute rheumatic fever. Some 30 years ago there were geographical areas in this country with a high incidence of rheumatic fever; these areas included the Northeastern seaboard, the Great Lakes area and the Rocky Mountain area. In these areas acute rheumatic fever not only was endemic but occurred usually in its classical form, often with great virulence. In other parts of the country rheumatic fever was less frequently encountered and tended to appear in atypical, milder forms. Today the incidence of rheumatic fever has diminished dramatically, the endemic areas have been obliterated, and rheumatic fever appears mostly in milder forms in all areas. In contrast, high incidence and great severity of rheumatic fever can be observed in developing countries; in some of them rheumatic fever and its sequelae rank high among serious public health problems.

Typical cases of rheumatic fever involve three stages:

- Streptococcal infection—sore throat or upper respiratory infection;

- Latent period of two to three weeks;

- Development of clinical manifestations of rheumatic fever.

The clinical course of the initial attack of rheumatic fever (stage 3, above) may proceed along the following courses:

- A single attack of four to eight weeks' duration, with recovery;

- Acute onset with a prolonged months-long subacute, lingering course;

- A recurrent, cyclic course with several short-term (weeks) exacerbations, separated by weeks or months of apparent recovery;

- Subclinical or ill-defined subacute illness;

- Widely separated acute attacks, often seasonal, with recoveries, the repeat attacks frequently precipitated by streptococcal re-exposure.

The three principal clinical manifestations of rheumatic fever are:

- arthritis,

- chorea,

- carditis.

1. Arthritis, in rheumatic fever, usually takes the form of acute migrating polyarthritis. Large joints are, as a rule, involved, usually one or two at a time. Their involvement varies from severe immobilizing arthritis with effusion and periarthritic inflammatory changes to mere arthralgias without objective changes in the joints. Characteristically, arthritis is nonsuppurative. The "migration" of arthritis occurs in short succession — usually a few days, with prompt healing of the previously involved joints. The knees, ankles, shoulders, and elbows are most commonly involved in the process. In older individuals there is some tendency toward involvement of small joints. As a rule the acute process heals without residua.

2. Chorea may occur in combination with other clinical manifestations of acute rheumatic fever but more often develops alone. It may take a protracted course, lasting for months. It is seldom accompanied by clinically recognizable acute arthritis or carditis, yet chronic rheumatic heart disease develops in a significant proportion of patients whose only manifestation of the rheumatic state was an attack of chorea.

3. Carditis is the most important clinical feature of rheumatic fever in that it determines the long-term outcome of this disease. As indicated, cardiac involvement affects all three layers of the heart pathologically. Clinically, pericarditis is most easily perceived; involvement of

the myocardium and endocardium may or may not be readily detected. Yet, in severe cases myocardial disease or endocardial disease leads to more serious clinical manifestations. Overt attacks of rheumatic carditis often determine the duration of the acute stage of the disease. Evidence of cardiac involvement often persists after the febrile episode or arthritic manifestations have long cleared. Two most serious consequences of acute rheumatic carditis are:

- Cardiac failure—caused by myocardial involvement;

- Acute valvular incompetence—caused by endocardial changes, often aggravated by left ventricular dilatation due to myocarditis.

In the past irreversible cardiac failure leading to death occurred not infrequently; now it is very rare. Occasionally valve incompetence is sufficiently life-threatening that surgical treatment has to be considered.

The great majority of cases of rheumatic fever at the present time are mild, often atypical. The diagnosis of carditis may be difficult to establish and even the basic diagnosis of rheumatic fever may be in doubt. Patients with known rheumatic heart disease frequently have no recollection of attacks of rheumatic fever. Sometimes retrospectively "growing pains" are considered attacks of rheumatic fever, although such history has to be accepted with skepticism (see also Chapter 3). Thus, undoubtedly, subclinical rheumatic carditis occurs commonly. There is little doubt that the clinical diagnosis of rheumatic carditis is made mostly because of the high index of suspicion developed in patients in whom arthritis and an acute febrile illness draw attention to the possibility of rheumatic fever. If involvement of joints is missing, the diagnosis of carditis may be impossible to arrive at.

Once the diagnosis of carditis is established, observations regarding the duration of the acute state is made on the basis of cardiac signs. Among the various indices of carditis, to be presented later in this chapter, tachycardia is probably the most persistent index of activity.

As stated, cardiac involvement in the first attack of rheumatic fever makes it likely that carditis will also develop in subsequent attacks, if they occur. Patients who have residual valvular heart disease from an attack of rheumatic fever may develop cardiac failure during subsequent attacks because of the additive effect of myocardial involvement from carditis.

The long-range sequels of rheumatic fever will be discussed in connection with valvular heart disease. It should be pointed out, however, that there is often a long latent period between the acute attack or attacks and the fully developed valvular heart disease; during this period no evidence of cardiac involvement may be apparent, or a trivial apical systolic murmur may be found.

DIAGNOSIS

The diagnosis of acute rheumatic fever involves two important questions:

1. Can the illness be identified as rheumatic fever?

2. If so, is rheumatic carditis present?

Except for chorea, which is characteristic in itself, the diagnosis of acute rheumatic fever may be difficult, even when it appears in a fairly typical form. The traditional Jones' diagnostic criteria help in a general way, though they cannot be considered absolutely accurate (i.e., the presence of two major criteria or one major plus two minor criteria *prove* the diagnosis of rheumatic fever): These criteria merely indicate a high probability of the presence of rheumatic fever. Jones recognized five major manifestations of rheumatic fever:

- polyarthritis,

- carditis,

- chorea,

- subcutaneous nodules,

- erythema marginatum.

The minor manifestations of rheumatic fever are as follows:

- history of previous definite rheumatic fever,

- evidence of preceding streptococcal infection,

- fever,

- elevated sedimentation rate, leukocytosis, positive C-reactive protein,

- arthralgia (as contrasted with true arthritis),

- prolonged P-R interval in the electrocardiogram.

Each of the major manifestations of rheumatic fever has a moderate to fair specificity. Minor manifestations have a low specificity, but serve well as supportive points in the differential diagnosis.

A differentiation of each major manifestation of rheumatic fever involves a variety of other diseases:

- Arthritis has to be distinguished from more acute forms of rheumatoid disease, from arthritis due to pyogenic organisms, particularly Neisseria, from various allergic forms of arthritis, and from traumatic arthritis.

- Carditis will be discussed in more detail later; it manifests itself by a variety of nonspecific signs of cardiac involvement.

- Chorea should be differentiated from hysterical manifestations in children and from Huntington's chorea.

- Rheumatic nodules develop also in rheumatoid arthritis and other related conditions.

- Erythema marginatum, though characteristic in itself, may resemble various other erythematous skin lesions when in less typical form.

In general, rheumatic fever is often confused with a variety of febrile illnesses in which manifestations such as joint pains and the presence of cardiac murmurs are too readily accepted as implicating the heart and suggesting rheumatic fever. Allergic reactions such as serum sickness and certain drug sensitivity phenomena may be confused with acute rheumatic fever.

Laboratory confirmation of the diagnosis is not available in a direct manner. The most specific test is the elevation of the titer of anti-streptolysin O. This specific antibody for the beta-hemolytic streptococcus demonstrates, if present in excess, that the host has been exposed to a recent streptococcal infection. The test, however, bears no relationship to rheumatic fever, that is, cannot distinguish individuals who respond normally to streptococcal invasion from those who are hypersensitive to it and develop a rheumatic reaction. Thus the value of antistreptolysin O test lies in the following:

- In children, since large segments of the childhood population are exposed to streptococcal infection, an elevated anti-streptolysin O titer is of little diagnostic value; a low anti-streptolysin O titer may be used against the probability that the disease in question is rheumatic fever.

- In adults an opposite approach may be taken; the rarity of high ASO titers in the adult population makes its presence a point supporting (but not proving) a diagnosis of acute rheumatic fever.

- A significant rise in ASO titer during the early stage of an illness suspected of being rheumatic fever increases the probability of this diagnosis, even in children.

The use of laboratory tests such as the erythrocyte sedimentation rate and the C-reactive protein test is limited by the low specificity of these tests. They are occasionally used for longitudinal follow-up of patients who show a prolonged course of rheumatic fever with transition into a subacute state. Even in these cases a high erythrocyte sedimentation rate and a positive C-reactive protein test are very sensitive; they often remain abnormal at a time when all other evidences of activity have subsided. There is no valid evidence to consider these tests alone as decisive enough in determining the presence or absence of rheumatic activity.

CARDITIS

The diagnosis of carditis is contingent upon finding an abnormality caused by rheumatic involvement of the pericardium, the myocardium, the endocardium, or a combination of these. Clinical manifestations of involvement of the various parts of the heart include the following:

1. Pericardium:
   - pericardial friction rub,
   - clinical evidence of pericardial effusion,
   - radiographic evidence of pericardial effusion,
   - echocardiographic evidence of pericardial effusion,
   - electrocardiographic signs suggestive of pericarditis.

2. Myocardium:
   - evidence of cardiac failure,
   - persistent tachycardia, out of proportion to the fever,
   - evidence of cardiac enlargement (clinical or radiographic),
   - non-organic murmurs (mid-diastolic mitral rumbling murmur, possibly transient mitral regurgitation),
   - electrocardiographic abnormalities (ST-T changes, QRS abnormalities, first degree heart block),
   - arrhythmias.

3. Endocardium:
   - development of mitral or aortic regurgitation.

The nonspecificity of these various clinical manifestations of carditis is obvious and their importance lies with their development during a new acute illness otherwise suggestive of rheumatic fever. One sees only too often patients with obvious congenital heart disease who give a history of "rheumatic fever" which was based on an acute febrile illness in the course of which a heart murmur was found for the first time. A few special differential points are worthy of mentioning:

- Pericarditis is not rare in children and adolescents, either alone or in combination with other generalized illnesses: its specificity is relatively low.

- All manifestations of myocardial involvement may occur in nonrheumatic myocarditis.

- Changing murmurs, e.g., those signifying the development of aortic or mitral regurgitation, are less specific as evidence of an acute cardiac problem than generally believed. Murmurs may vary from day to day without obvious reason; early diastolic murmurs of aortic regurgitation are occasionally heard on some days but not on others.

- Some patients develop signs and symptoms suggestive of rheumatic fever with the implication that it is their first attack. Examination reveals definite evidence of mitral stenosis or aortic stenosis. While it is true that a stenotic lesion cannot appear during a first attack of rheumatic fever, one cannot justifiably conclude that heart disease here is unrelated to rheumatic fever. Some such patients may have acquired valve disease as a result of previous unrecognized attacks — the attack in question may be a recurrence.

THERAPY

The goals of therapy in acute rheumatic fever are:

- control of streptococcal infection,
- treatment of manifestations of rheumatic fever,
- treatment of carditis,
- prevention of recurrences of rheumatic fever,
- prevention of chronic valve damage.

The control of streptococcal infection consists of *penicillin therapy*. The question as to whether patients whose streptococcal infection is promptly brought under control are less likely to develop the rheumatic reaction than those who receive late therapy or none at all has not yet been answered. There is convincing evidence, however, that the *prevention* of streptococcal infection protects the host from rheumatic fever. The suggested possibility that the mildness of rheumatic fever and the reduction of its overall prevalence in the Western world are the result of wide use of penicillin for any infection cannot be considered a proven fact, inasmuch as other epidemiological factors may also be playing a part in this change. The wide use — perhaps overuse — of antibiotics may have affected either individual exposures to streptococcal infection or may have altogether reduced the streptococcus as a widely prevalent pathogen.

Penicillin therapy still plays an important role in the management of rheumatic fever:

- Early treatment of streptococcal infection is important even if it is not known whether it will or will not affect the later rheumatic reaction.

- Penicillin treatment is recommended for the attack of acute rheumatic fever, immediately after the diagnosis is established. The rationale for the therapy is the suggestion by some that the rheumatic reaction is perpetuated by the presence of viable streptococci in the body, even if the original streptococcal infection that triggered the attack of rheumatic fever is long gone.

- Continuous penicillin therapy is recommended for all who have recovered from the attack of rheumatic fever as a means of preventing subsequent recurrences.

An alternate antistreptococcal agent which may be used in patients who show evidence of penicillin sensitivity is one of the sulfonamide drugs, particularly sulfadiazine.

The therapy of acute rheumatic fever by means other than antibiotics depends upon the severity of the disease. The guiding principles of therapy include the following measures:

- rest,

- salicylates,

- steroids,

- treatment of cardiac failure,

- cardiac surgery.

The question of rest is as empirical and unsupported by solid evidence of benefit as in many other diseases in which rest is recommended. The theory that the presence of carditis can never be ruled out since only the most obvious instances of cardiac involvement can be detected is undoubtedly correct. Nevertheless, whether there is a beneficial effect in prescribing rest for all patients with rheumatic activity because of the possibility of carditis is uncertain, even doubtful. One can occasionally encounter patients with chronic heart disease whose disability (often more properly referred to as poor conditioning) is related not to the valve disease but to having spent a year in bed during formative years and then been forbidden to participate in all but minor activities. It is also interesting to note that a large proportion of patients with rheumatic mitral stenosis give no history of acute rheumatic fever and have no recollection of any prolonged illness. It is logical to assume that these patients "walked through" subclinical attacks of rheumatic carditis that affected their mitral valves in a similar manner as in some patients with acute myocardial infarction who remained active during the period of their infarcts. There is no evidence that patients who do not rest during carditis end up with more severe valvular damage, die earlier, or show any ill effects of their neglect.

Recommendations regarding the timing and the extent of rest in the treatment of acute rheumatic fever can be made only on the basis of common sense, for no valid data to support its value or test its importance are available:

• It would appear logical that in severe attacks of rheumatic fever a reasonable period of rest is indicated, whether or not clinical evidence of carditis is present. Part of the rest will be automatic, necessitated by the arthritis; if arthritis is not disabling, rest should be enforced during significant elevation of the temperature.

• If evidence of carditis is present a reasonable period of rest is probably indicated. The enforcement of rest gets higher in priority as the signs of carditis become more ominous: persistent tachycardia and signs of cardiac failure have the highest priority; evidence for cardiac enlargement and pericarditis the next priority; purely laboratory evidence of carditis (e.g., the electrocardiogram) the lowest priority.

• There appears to be no valid reason to be guided in the length of rest by such laboratory findings as elevation of erythrocyte sedimentation rate or positive C-reaction protein.

• It is important to take into consideration the effect of long periods of rest on the psyche of a youngster with acute rheumatic fever. Psychological support and occupational therapy are important.

• No arbitrary guidelines are available regarding the return to normal activities (usually return to school). Individual judgments have to be made, but it may be wise to consider whether keeping a child from participation in at least the ordinary school activities may not be in the long run more harmful than the possible effect of the rheumatic fever.

Salicylates and corticosteroids represent anti-inflammatory drugs used in acute rheumatic fever. The former have few side effects and are used preferentially in milder cases. The latter are more effective and may have to be used in rheumatic fever with severe clinical manifestations. Either of the two groups of drugs can promptly control acute rheumatic fever. In very severe affliction corticoids may be life-saving. The questions as to whether corticoids can actually abort an attack, prevent or arrest carditis, and protect the heart from long-range valve damage have not been definitely answered. The Anglo-American ten-year cooperative study produced results suggesting only symptomatic improvement by both drugs. Thus, at present there is insufficient evidence to recommend routine use of steroids in acute rheumatic fever—their role is to control the clinical manifestations of disease and in most cases mild symptomatology requires no such therapy. The duration of therapy varies: inasmuch as most attacks do not exceed six weeks, drugs can be tapered off after four to six weeks of therapy. One can, however, expect a recrudescence of the disease in some patients after withdrawal of the therapy.

Therapy of cardiac failure developing during acute rheumatic carditis should combine steroid treatment with the conventional measures of sodium restriction, digitalis, and diuretics.

Cardiac surgery should be considered only in extreme situations in the course of rheumatic carditis. There are few recorded cases in which a severe mechanical overload of rheumatic valvular disease (e.g., mitral regurgitation) superimposed upon rheumatic myocarditis produced desperate situations with cardiac failure unresponsive to any form of medical therapy. Mitral valve replacement has produced dramatic improvement in cardiac function with eventual elimination of rheumatic activities. Mitral valve replacements should never be considered lightly in children and young adults, especially if there is—as in rheumatic fever—an element of a self-limited reversible process. Thus, consideration of such drastic steps can be made only when the situation is really desperate and the probability of death high in response to a medical regimen.

Bibliography

Besterman E: The changing face of acute rheumatic fever. Brit. Heart J. *32*:579, 1970.

Bland EF: Declining severity of rheumatic fever. A comparative study of the past four decades. New Engl. J. Med. *262*:597, 1960.

Feinstein AR, Spanuolo M: The clinical patterns of acute rheumatic fever: A reappraisal. Medicine *41*:279, 1962.

Joint Report by the Rheumatic Fever Working Party (U.K. and U.S.A.): The natural history of rheumatic fever and rheumatic heart disease. Ten year report of a cooperative clinical trial of ACTH, cortisone, and aspirin. Circulation *31*:457, 1965.

Jones criteria (revised) for guidance in the diagnosis of rheumatic fever. Circulation *32*:664, 1965.

Markowitz M, Gordis L: RHEUMATIC FEVER, 2nd Edition. W. B. Saunders Co., Philadelphia, 1972.

Nadas AS, Fyler DC: Acute rheumatic fever. *In* PEDIATRIC CARDIOLOGY, 3rd Edition. W. B. Saunders Co., Philadelphia, 1972, pp. 141–158.

Sievers J, Hall P: Incidence of acute rheumatic fever. Brit. Heart J. *33*:833, 1971.

Wood P: Rheumatic fever and acute rheumatic carditis. *In* DISEASES OF THE HEART AND CIRCULATION, 3rd Edition. Eyre and Spottiswoode, London, 1968, pp. 573–599.

24
Myocarditis

Definition. Acute myocarditis represents a nonspecific inflammatory disease of the myocardium. A special form of myocarditis is rheumatic myocarditis, which was discussed in the preceding chapter, and which plays a unique role in the pathogenesis of chronic cardiac disease. Myocarditis may appear as an involvement of the myocardium in general infections or in diseases affecting other organs, or it may be a primary disease of the heart. The cause of myocarditis may or may not be evident.

ETIOLOGY AND PATHOLOGY

The various etiological agents that can cause myocarditis have been listed in Chapter 21. The majority of known pathogenic organisms causing human disease have been implicated in producing myocardial changes that may or may not be of clinical significance. Myocarditis can develop at any age, from the neonatal period to old age. Among the various etiological forms of myocarditis there are a few that occur often enough to be considered of some importance, outside the range of single-case reports. These include:

- Diphtheritic myocarditis, once an important cause of cardiac disease, is rare today since diphtheria has been partly eradicated in many parts of the world;

- Viral myocarditis—this is probably the principal cause of primary myocarditis and "idiopathic" myocarditis. Coxsackie virus is one of the commoner pathogens;

- Protozoal myocarditis due to Trypanosoma causing Chagas' disease is a relatively common form of heart disease in South America.

Pathological changes of myocarditis are largely nonspecific and differ from the characteristic picture seen in rheumatic myocarditis. The commonest finding is the disintegration of some myocardial fibers, usually scattered diffusely throughout the myocardium, with cellular infiltration by lymphocytes. As a rule, extension into the pericardium and endocardium is not present.

NATURAL HISTORY

Both the relative rarity of acute myocarditis and the variability of its clinical picture preclude any characteristic clinical features. In general terms, one can divide myocarditis into three varieties:

- Subclinical myocarditis accompanying infectious diseases,

- Clinically significant myocarditis occurring in association with other infectious diseases,

- Myocarditis appearing as an isolated disease.

The great majority of patients with clinically significant myocarditis recover without known sequelae. In some, persistent electrocardiographic abnormalities or continuing reduction of effort tolerance has been suggested as representing residua from the acute attack of myocarditis; this relationship is, at best, conjectural. Occasionally chronic cardiomyopathy has its origin in acute myocarditis. How often this occurs is not definitely known, nor is it recognized whether or not some idiopathic cases of chronic cardiomyopathy may be initiated by subclinical acute myocarditis. Fatal cardiac failure occurs occasionally. Rarely, myocarditis may be the cause of sudden death.

DIAGNOSIS

The diagnosis of myocarditis depends upon alertness and a high index of suspicion. A search for occult myocardial involvement in patients with general infections often yields postive results. The principal diagnostic critera are similar to those discussed in connection with rheumatic carditis:

- Electrocardiographic abnormalities;

- Changes in heart sounds; development of murmurs;

- Arrhythmias;

- Signs of cardiac enlargement;

- Signs of cardiac failure;

- Persistent sinus tachycardia.

The *electrocardiogram* has been the most consistently valuable tool for the discovery of subclinical myocarditis. In various viral infections, such as poliomyelitis, mumps, influenza, infectious hepatitis, infectious mononucleosis, and others, serial electrocardiograms may show changing ST-T abnormalities. Occasionally, more extensive electrocardiographic changes may be found, such as Q waves resembling those of myocardial infarction, or intraventricular conduction defect (particularly left bundle branch block). These changes, however, are more likely to be associated with clinical signs of myocarditis.

Auscultatory findings include a decrease in the intensity of the first sound, the appearance of gallop sounds, and the development of nonorganic cardiac murmurs.

Cardiac enlargement may be detected by clinical means or by radiography. If enlargement is evident in serial chest roentgenograms, the differentiation between cardiac dilatation and pericardial effusion has to be made. Helpful in this situation are the abovementioned auscultatory findings, which then make the diagnosis of myocarditis highly probable.

Arrhythmias may represent the first indication of myocardial involvement; the whole range of ventricular arrhythmias occurs in acute myocarditis.

Cardiac failure may develop at any stage of acute myocarditis. The manifestations of failure range from subtle signs that have to be searched for, e.g., transient pulmonary rales, gallop sounds, and pulsus alternans, to overt clinical evidence of combined left and right ventricular failure. As indicated in connection with myocardial infarction, serial chest roentgenograms provide an excellent means of detecting early left ventricular failure.

Sinus tachycardia along with ectopic rhythms may be the finding that alerts the clinician to the possibility of cardiac involvement.

The recognition and differentiation of acute myocarditis may be a diagnostic challenge which requires a high index of suspicion. Myocarditis may develop under a variety of circumstances, hence the diagnostic approaches may vary widely:

- Myocarditis as the primary disease may develop as an acute illness with clear-cut cardiac symptoms: dyspnea on effort, paroxysmal dyspnea, fatigability; clinical evidence of cardiac failure may be apparent and a febrile course may be an indication of the infectious nature of the disease. The differential diagnosis includes the consideration of other acute illnesses involving the heart: rheumatic fever, acute pericarditis, infective endocarditis, and—more remotely—myocardial infarction. If myocarditis is the most likely diagnosis, a survey of potential etiological factors should be made.

- Myocarditis unassociated with other manifestations of disease may be subclinical, with vague symptoms, such as lassitude and palpitations. Arrhythmias may represent the tip-off for the cardiac disease; occasionally, an equally subclinical underlying cause may be detected, e.g., infectious mononucleosis.

- In the course of the various acute infectious diseases, including the communicable childhood infections, alertness to the possibility of cardiac involvement has invariably demonstrated that myocarditis is more common than recognized. As stated, serial electrocardiograms and frequent physical examinations have led several investigators to detect some evidence of myocarditis in an appreciable proportion of random cases. In the great majority of patients myocarditis detectable only by instrumental means is of no clinical importance; however, patients who have either arrhythmias or more pronounced indications of cardiac involvement should be observed more carefully than those in routine cases of infectious disease.

PROGNOSIS

The prognosis of acute myocarditis is uncertain: the pathological change in the myocardium cannot be clinically assessed, and its reversibility vs. nonreversibility is impossible to judge. Furthermore, too few controlled observations have been made in acute myocarditis to provide even a rough idea regarding the routes that myocarditis can take. It has already been indicated that most patients make a complete recovery. Unlike rheumatic fever, myocarditis does not affect the endocardium and, as far as is known, has no capability of initiating chronic valvular disease. Nevertheless, during the active stage of myocarditis its potential seriousness and uncertainty regarding the outcome should not be underestimated.

THERAPY

There are no specific therapeutic approaches to acute myocarditis except in the very rare cases of infections with organisms amenable to direct attack (e.g., tuberculosis). The treatment thus consists of rest, monitoring, antiarrhythmic therapy, and control of cardiac failure.

Arrhythmias are probably the most potentially significant sequels of myocarditis that require special attention. Sudden death may occur in myocarditis and may take place in patients with overt signs of myocarditis as well as in patients with unrecognized myocarditis. Sudden death most likely represents "electrical" death, hence is, at least in theory, sometimes preventable. Thus, patients, who show any evidence of disturbance of cardiac rate and rhythm probably require as careful monitoring as those with myocardial infarction, and usually for longer periods of time. Antiarrhythmic therapy administered to such patients is indicated along the guidelines of therapy for myocardial infarction.

Treatment of cardiac failure is analogous to that of acute rheumatic carditis. It is questionable whether failure evident only by subtle signs needs attention other than rest and mild dietary restriction. Overt cardiac failure requires the usual therapy with digitalis and diuretics.

Bibliography

Abelmann WE: Myocarditis. New Engl. J. Med. 275:832, 944, 1966.
Pruitt RD: Acute myocarditis in adults. Prog. Cardiovasc. Dis. 7:73, 1964.
Sanders V: Viral myocarditis, Amer. Heart J. 66:707, 1963.

25

Pericarditis and Cardiac Tamponade

Definition. This chapter deals with those acute diseases of the pericardium which are of major clinical import. It includes discussion of primary and secondary forms of pericarditis and of acute cardiac tamponade, but does not consider simple pericardial effusions without cardiac consequences.

ETIOLOGY

A great variety of disease processes involve to a significant extent the pericardium. The more important etiological factors include the following:

1. Pericarditis due to infectious pathogens:

   • viral pericarditis,

   • tuberculous pericarditis,

   • septic and purulent pericarditis,

   • fungal pericarditis.

2. Pericarditis due to immune reactions:

   • some forms of "idiopathic" pericarditis,

   • post-cardiotomy pericarditis,

   • pericarditis of rheumatic fever,

   • post-myocardial infarction syndrome,

   • pericarditis following trauma (as a late sequel).

3. Pericarditis due to systemic diseases:
   - rheumatoid arthritis,
   - systemic lupus erythematosus,
   - polyarteritis,
   - scleroderma.

4. Pericarditis by contiguity:
   - acute myocardial infarction (during the infarction),
   - neoplastic invasion,
   - lymphoma,
   - some forms of tuberculous pericarditis,
   - mediastinitis.

5. Traumatic pericarditis:
   - penetrating trauma,
   - iatrogenic (various forms of puncture, catheterization, pacemaker placement),
   - radiation pericarditis.

6. Cardiac tamponade due to hemopericardium:
   - external penetrating trauma,
   - internal trauma (catheter or needle perforation),
   - rupture of a ventricle (myocardial infarction),
   - rupture of the intrapericardial portion of the aorta (dissecting or plain aneurysm),
   - a complication of anticoagulant therapy.

7. Toxic pericarditis:
   - uremic pericarditis,
   - pericarditis due to drugs and other toxic agents.

PATHOLOGY AND PATHOPHYSIOLOGY

Anatomic abnormalities of the pericardium in the various acute diseases of the pericardium consist mostly of nonspecific inflammatory and fibrinous reactions of the pericardium. Both the epicardial and parietal layers are usually involved. Extension of the inflammatory reaction to the subepicardial portion of the myocardium occurs frequently: it is believed that the electrocardiographic abnormalities found in pericarditis are produced by subepicardial myocarditis. Specific pathological abnormalities are found in tuberculous pericarditis as well in those related to other granulomatous processes and neoplasms.

The pericardial fluid is most commonly a clear exudate in viral and reactive types of pericarditis. Sanguineous fluid is occasionally present in "nonspecific" types or in tuberculous pericarditis; it is common in neoplastic and traumatic forms.

Pericarditis—regardless whether dry or exudative—produces no significant alterations of cardiac function except when tamponade is present. The clinical manifestations of pericarditis include:

- pain,
- pericardial friction rub.

Cardiac tamponade is related to the following factors:

- the speed of accumulation of pericardial fluid (or blood),
- the compliance of parietal pericardium.

The consequence of pericardial tamponade is interference with diastolic filling of the heart owing to an increase in intrapericardial pressure. The principal consequences of this are:

- increase in systemic venous pressure,
- reduction in cardiac output, often associated with a fall in systemic arterial pressure,
- "paradoxical pulse," a respiratory variation of the systemic arterial pressure with a fall in pressure occurring during inspiration.

The magnitude of these changes determines the urgency of the situation, which ranges from a life-threatening emergency to the occurrence of mild symptoms.

CLINICAL PICTURE

The overall symptomatology and laboratory findings in acute pericardial disease include the following:

1. *Pain* is a very common though not an invariable symptom of acute pericarditis. It ranges from a mere discomfort to excruciating

pain. In spite of some overlap with ischemic pain, it has distinctive features which may suggest the pericardial origin of the pain. These are:

- a sharp component in the pain,
- aggravation of the pain in respiration,
- lessening or relief of pain with change in body position (particularly when leaning forward).

2. Respiratory distress is rare and occurs only when very large pericardial effusions are present.

3. Nonspecific symptoms of an infectious process include fever, malaise, and lassitude. Viral pericarditis may be preceded or accompanied by an upper respiratory infection.

4. Physical examination of the heart often reveals the presence of pericardial friction rub. This valuable sign may be ephemeral; its detection is often related to the frequency with which physical examination is performed. Pericardial friction rub often disappears when large effusions develop, hence it may be present in early and late stages of pericarditis but not in between. Determination of cardiac size by percussion has too low specificity to be of value: The position of the apical impulse may help determine whether cardiac enlargement or pericardial effusion is responsible for cardiac enlargement (detected by radiography). Diminished intensity of cardiac sounds is of value only if a change develops under observation. Inasmuch as only a small proportion of patients with acute pericardial disease develop any degree of cardiac tamponade, elevation of systemic venous pressure, reduction of pulse pressure, and a paradoxical pulse are not common findings in pericarditis. It is essential, however, that these signs be frequently looked for in all patients suspected of having pericarditis, since early detection of cardiac tamponade is of utmost importance.

5. Examination of other organs and systems may provide important information regarding the etiology and nature of pericarditis, or of pericardial effusion.

6. Electrocardiographic changes of pericarditis include serial S-T segment changes that differ from those of myocardial infarction by their concordant nature, i.e., *no* reciprocal S-T elevation-depression is found in anterior vs. inferior or posterior vs. lateral leads, respectively. At a later stage T-wave inversion is present and may involve most leads. The extent and duration of electrocardiographic changes show wide variation: at times they can be detected only by taking one or two tracings every day. When present in their typical form, these changes have good specificity and add great weight to the diagnosis of pericarditis.

7. Radiography is helpful in revealing enlargement of the car-

diac shadow. Sudden, pronounced changes in cardiac size are more likely to represent pericardial effusion than cardiac dilatation. The alleged characteristic changes in the shape of the heart associated with pericardial effusion are of low specificity and therefore of little diagnostic help.

8. Contrast radiography is a highly specific test differentiating cardiac dilatation from enlargement of the cardiac shadow due to other causes (pericardial effusion or solid tissue, such as tumor). As contrast media, radiopaque substance or gas (carbon dioxide) can be used, injected into the blood stream directly or via a catheter.

9. Radioisotope scanning provides an alternate method of visualization of cardiac chambers within the overall cardiac shadow, thus determining the presence of fluid or solid medium outside the heart.

10. Echocardiography constitutes the most important and specific as well as the simplest noninvasive method of detection of pericardial fluid. It is capable of distinguishing fluid from solid medium in the pericardial space and can also be used to estimate roughly the amount of the effusion. The importance of this technique cannot be overemphasized: it should be used as a screening method and a means of longitudinal follow-up, whenever any clinical point suggests the possibility of pericardial effusion. It is important, however, to remember that cardiac failure from any cause may be associated with a pericardial effusion; thus the interpretation of echocardiographic findings has to be done in the context of other clinical information helpful to the decision, whether pericardial disease is the primary problem or a secondary complication of cardiac failure.

11. Cardiac catheterization is of little diagnostic value in acute pericardial disease. Catheterization of the right side of the heart has been used to estimate the distance between the cavity of the right atrium (with the catheter placed against its lateral wall) and the border of the cardiac shadow. Yet contrast radiography or isotope scanning displays this point more reliably than the cardiac catheter.

12. Other laboratory tests (hematological, bacteriological, immunological, etc.) are of importance in the differential diagnosis of pericarditis against other similar conditions, and as a means of detecting possible etiological factors.

13. Diagnostic paracentesis of the pericardium (i.e., *not* performed to relieve high intrapericardial pressure) should be undertaken with specific goals in mind, inasmuch as this procedure carries a certain risk. Its value is in the diagnostic evaluation of the following:

- the diagnosis of purulent pericarditis or the possibility of culturing pathogenic organisms in patients who either run high fever or are very ill;

- to establish or confirm the diagnosis of tuberculous pericarditis;

- to establish the diagnosis of hemopericardium;

- when tumor is suspected;

- to examine the pericardial fluid in long-standing pericarditis.

NATURAL HISTORY OF ACUTE PERICARDIAL DISEASE

Idiopathic "Benign" Pericarditis. This is a clinically defined entity of undetermined etiology, which often—though not always—takes a benign course. In some cases viral origin is demonstrated; in many more it is suspected but not proved. It is probable that viral pericarditis accounts for many of these cases. Coxsackie virus is a common pathogen. Some cases may fall into the category of immunoreactive pericarditis without a detectable initiating factor.

Pericarditis affects individuals of any age, from childhood on. The attack may have an abrupt onset or may affect the patient gradually over a period of a few days; it may or may not be preceded by or associated with an upper respiratory infection; if it is, it may take the form of pleuropericarditis. Chest pain in association with generalized symptoms (fever, malaise, etc.) is the principal manifestation of the illness in the great majority of patients. Signs of pericardial tamponade do occur occasionally but are rare. Examination reveals in most patients the presence of a pericardial friction rub: pericardial effusion is usually, but not always, present. The duration of this illness ranges from a few days to three to four weeks.

The severity of the illness manifests itself in one of two ways:

- sudden fluid accumulation producing cardiac tamponade,

- severe general signs of infection.

The course of acute idiopathic pericarditis varies:

- The majority of patients recover completely;

- A minority—about one quarter—develop one or more recurrent attacks;

- Some patients may enter a subacute stage, lingering for months, with eventual recovery;

- In a few constrictive pericarditis may develop.

Immunoreactive Pericarditis. Autoimmune reactions, usually initiated by some form of injury to the heart in general and the pericardium in particular, cause a form of pericarditis which resembles idiopathic "benign" pericarditis and, in all probability, overlaps with it in some instances. Pericarditis most frequently appears as the only site of the reaction, but occasionally, pleurisy, arthritis, and other signs manifest themselves in addition. The injury initiating the reaction may include the following conditions:

- Acute myocardial infarction;

- Surgical trauma associated with all forms of thoracic operations involving the pericardium;

- Penetrating thoracic trauma;

- The possibility that recurrences of idiopathic pericarditis may involve a tissue reaction to the original trauma of a viral pericarditis must also be considered.

No reliable figures are available as to the number of patients with each of these conditions susceptible to pericarditis; it seems to represent a small fraction. The time interval between the injury and the reaction varies from a few weeks to several months.

The clinical course of immunoreactive pericarditis is similar to that of idiopathic benign pericarditis during its acute stage. It differs in its late outcome in that subacute or chronic stages are unlikely to be present, but recurrences are the rule. This form of pericarditis is basically a cyclic disease with remissions after each attack and exacerbations developing weeks or months later. As a rule the first attack is the most severe one; subsequent ones tend to be progressively milder. The number of recurrences may vary from one to several, but usually three or four attacks complete the "reaction."

Tuberculous Pericarditis. Tuberculous infection by contiguity from mediastinal nodes is more often responsible for tuberculous pericarditis than blood stream infection as a part of miliary tuberculosis. Tuberculous pericarditis tends to be less acute than the idiopathic form, although temperature elevation may be considerable, and "swinging" fever may be present. Tuberculous pericarditis is associated with a protracted course, entering a subacute and a chronic stage as a continuum.

Purulent Pericarditis. Pyogenic infection of the pericardium develops either as a part of septicemia, by contiguity from purulent mediastinitis, or as a complication of surgical and invasive procedures involving the pericardium. Its course is related to that of the overall infection and the aggressiveness of therapy, which almost always requires pericardial drainage in addition to antibiotic treatment.

Acute Pericardial Tamponade. The potentially disastrous consequences of rapid rise of intrapericardial pressure interfering with cardiac filling requires prompt recognition and action. Cardiac tamponade is a short-term condition: it represents by definition a state in which pericardial fluid accumulates faster than the pericardial sac can stretch to accommodate it. Thus, unless this disproportion is checked, death is likely to ensue. Tamponade is as a rule progressive unless checked by intervention. Only occasionally a state of equilibrium is reached at a point of tolerable interference of cardiac function; for example, when the high intrapericardial pressure can inhibit further fluid accumulation or seal off a leak. Causes of tamponade have been listed above; hemopericardium outweighs in frequency tamponade due to rapid accumulation of exudate.

Other Forms of Pericarditis. The course of uremic pericarditis, of pericardial effusion in the course of systemic diseases, of neoplasms, and of various infections other than those discussed above depends on the underlying disease. Pericardial tamponade is rare in such cases and pericardial involvement plays a relatively small part in the prognosis.

DIAGNOSIS

Diagnostic problems in acute diseases of the pericardium include the following:

1. Differentiation of isolated pericarditis from other acute illnesses associated with chest pain;

2. Identification of the type of pericarditis, with special attention to those requiring specific therapy;

3. Immediate recognition of cardiac tamponade.

The most important and difficult differential diagnosis is between acute pericarditis and myocardial infarction:

Points of similarity:

- Anterior chest pain is the characteristic initial symptom in both;

- Pericardial friction rub occurs in both;

- Electrocardiographic changes have definite similarity;

- Serum enzyme elevation may occur in both.

Differential points:

- Pain of pericarditis and that in myocardial infarction overlap only in atypical cases; in the majority, a reasonable differentiation can be made from the history;

- Pericardial friction rub is likely to occur early in pericarditis, and with delay in myocardial infarction;

- Pronounced elevation of serum enzymes does not occur in pericarditis;

- Electrocardiographic difficulties arise only in atypical cases;

- In the presence of significant pericardial effusion myocardial infarction can be easily ruled out;

- Any evidence of cardiac failure is in favor of myocardial infarction.

Other conditions involved in the differential diagnosis of anterior thoracic pain include:

- dissecting aneurysm,

- pulmonary embolism,

- mediastinal emphysema,

- thoracic wall pain,

- pleurisy,

- pain originating in the gastrointestinal tract.

Once the diagnosis of acute pericardial disease appears reasonably well established, differentiation of the etiological factor is important only as guidance to therapy. The highest priority in the initiation of specific therapy should be given to two types:

- tuberculous pericarditis,

- purulent pericarditis.

In both of these, background information may aid in the diagnosis. Evidence of pulmonary tuberculosis or miliary tuberculosis offers important diagnostic help; positive tuberculin skin test is somewhat helpful but not as important as a negative skin test is in making tuberculous etiology unlikely. Purulent pericarditis almost always is associated with an obvious point of entry of the infection or with generalized septicemia. The most important diagnostic test lies in the examination of the fluid obtained by diagnostic pericardiocentesis. Purulent pericarditis can be recognized at once. Tuberculous pericarditis depends upon demonstration of tubercle bacilli in the fluid, positive culture, or positive animal inoculation test. Inasmuch as cultures and animal tests require weeks of waiting, pericardial biopsy may be performed to provide an earlier answer.

The diagnosis of cardiac tamponade may be easy in typical cases, but considerable difficulties have been encountered in atypical cases. The principal diagnostic signs consist of elevated systemic venous pressure, low pulse pressure of the arterial blood pressure, and the paradoxical pulse. However, the effects of tamponade upon the arterial side of the circulation may be so mild as to make findings inconclusive. Differentiation presents difficulty in some specific situations:

- Very abrupt development of the tamponade, with the patient going into shock and the arterial pressure becoming unobtainable;

- Tamponade developing as a complication of cardiac catheterization, particularly in patients with aortic stenosis, may be associated with very little blood in the pericardial space and yet lead to a critical effect. Even a pericardial tap may then be inconclusive because of the small amount of blood in the pericardium;

- Rarely, dehydration—particularly following excessive diuretic therapy—may lead to a condition of tamponade accompanied by minimal elevation of venous pressure;

- Tamponade developing in patients who have serious cardiac disease may be indistinguishable from the effects of cardiac failure. The detection of pericardial fluid in such cases does not constitute evidence that tamponade exists. The deciding factor may be cardiac catheterization during which pressure in the cardiac atria are monitored while the needle is in the pericardial sac, observing the relationship of atrial to intrapericardial pressures and recording the effect of removal of pericardial fluid.

THERAPY

The goals of therapy include the following:

- General supportive therapy of idiopathic "benign" pericarditis;

- Specific therapy against known and responsive pathogens;

- Immediate relief of cardiac tamponade;

- Prevention of recurrences and of chronic constrictive pericarditis.

In milder cases of pericarditis a reasonable period of rest with an optional use of salicylates suffices. For pericarditis associated with severe constitutional reactions, especially in cases with the immunoreactive etiology, corticosteroids often have a dramatically suppressive effect. Steroid therapy should never be instituted lightly: it is reserved for cases unresponsive to other forms of therapy. Pericardial tap is not indicated for therapeutic purposes regardless of the size of the effusion except when evidence of tamponade is present, or in the rare cases when the amount of fluid is large enough to produce mechanical pressure effects within the thorax.

Antituberculous therapy is indicated in patients in whom the diagnosis of tuberculous pericarditis is established. It is occasionally used on presumptive evidence of tuberculosis, especially following the use of corticosteroids: there are cases of tuberculous pericarditis in which the clinical diagnosis cannot be made with certainty.

Antibacterial therapy for purulent pericarditis is usually indicated in combination with surgical drainage of the pericardium.

Cardiac tamponade requires immediate relief of intrapericardial pressure by drainage. Needle tap may suffice in "medical" cases with rapid accumulation of exudate, but this often needs to be periodically repeated. In surgical forms of tamponade pericardial tap has to be performed even if the diagnosis of the origin of hemopericardium is not yet clearly established. In cases of minor trauma the initial bleeding may have stopped and the situation may be brought under control by a single pericardiocentesis. Immediate surgical exploration may be indicated if continuous bleeding into the pericardium is suggested or demonstrated.

Therapy directed at the prevention of recurrent attacks or of the development of chronic constriction is limited; no effective medical means are available. Though corticosteroids may control and abort attacks of pericarditis, the overall consequences and the side effects of continuous steroid therapy for recurrent pericarditis preclude the chronic use of such therapy in all but extreme cases.

Surgical removal of the parietal pericardium has been used occasionally for treatment of subacute or persistently recurring cases. The justification for surgical therapy is well demonstrated in the subacute stage of tuberculous pericarditis. A high probability of eventual pericardial constriction exists here, which might be prevented by pericardiectomy. The role of pericardiectomy for recurrent pericarditis has not been definitely established.

Bibliography

Dressler W: Post-myocardial infarction syndrome. Arch. Int. Med. *103*:28, 1959.

Feigenbaum H: Echocardiographic diagnosis of pericardial effusion. Amer. J. Cardiol. *26*:475, 1970.

Ito T, Engle MA, Goldberg HD: Post-pericardiotomy syndrome following surgery for non-rheumatic heart disease. Circulation *17*:549, 1958.

Robinson J, Brigden W: Immunological studies in the postcardiotomy syndrome. Brit. Med. J. 2:706, 1963.

Robinson J, Brigden W: Recurrent pericarditis. Brit. Med. J. 2:272, 1968.

Shearn MA: The heart in systemic lupus erythematosus. Amer. Heart J. 58:452, 1963.

Shabetai R, Fowler NO, Guntheroth WG: The hemodynamics of cardiac tamponade. Amer. J. Cardiol. 26:480, 1970.

Spodick DH: Acute cardiac tamponade—pathophysiology, diagnosis and management. Prog. Cardiovasc. Dis. 10:64, 1967.

Spodick DH: Differential diagnosis of acute pericarditis. Prog. Cardiovasc. Dis. 14:192, 1971.

Surawicz B, Lesseter KC: Electrocardiogram in pericarditis. Amer. J. Cardiol. 26:471, 1970.

26
Infective Endocarditis

Definition. Infective endocarditis represents an acute or subacute disease of the endocardium caused by invasion and growth of pathogenic organisms, almost always bacteria or fungi.

ETIOLOGY AND PATHOLOGY

Organisms causing infective endocarditis can be isolated and identified in at least 80 per cent of clinically diagnosed cases. Virtually every known organism has been at one time or another described as the cause of infective endocarditis. However, pathogens most frequently involved in cases of endocarditis include the following:

- *Streptococcus viridans* (alpha-hemolytic streptococcus),
- Other strains of streptococci,
- *Staphylococcus aureus* or *albus.*

Certain special relationships regarding the etiology of infective endocarditis have been observed:

- Staphylococcal endocarditis occurs often in hospital-acquired infections (frequently penicillin-resistant organisms cause the disease);
- Pneumococcal endocarditis may develop in debilitated individuals as a complication of pneumonia;
- Gram-negative organisms may cause endocarditis in older patients following urological operations or manipulations;
- Fungal infections (Candida) may develop after cardiac operations.

During the pre-antibiotic era *Streptococcus viridans* was the offending organism in the overwhelming majority of cases, as many as 80 to 90 per cent. Early in the penicillin era *S. viridans* endocarditis continued as the predominant pathogen, but its sensitivity to antibiotic therapy made the cure rate very high. In recent years the order of the involved pathogens has changed and *S. viridans* now accounts for less than 50 per cent of the cases. Furthermore, a high proportion of antibiotic-resistant organisms is involved in the production of endocarditis, reducing the cure rate and making treatment more difficult.

The pathological picture of endocarditis involves inflammatory vegetations that consist of fibrinous structures mixed with platelet and blood cell aggregations and with the pathogenic organisms. In contrast to rheumatic endocarditis or other noninfectious processes, vegetations of infective endocarditis are friable and tend to embolize, either as bacterial microembolisms or as macroembolisms with portions of the vegetations. The localization of the vegetations is most common on cardiac valves, on orifices, on abnormal communications, and on previously damaged areas of the endocardium.

The consequences of the endocarditis process consist of the following:

- Its effect upon the valve structure and function;

- Its effect upon structures other than the valves;

- The secondary effects of embolism.

The direct effects of endocarditis vary in the extent of damage to the affected structure. As a rule, subacute involvement with organisms of not too high virulence produces only mild damage; virulent microorganisms may produce changes that were referred to in the older writings as acute ulcerative endocarditis; here valve perforation is common. Among the lesions produced by endocarditis are the following:

- aortic regurgitation due to perforation of leaflet,

- aortic regurgitation due to lesser destructive lesions,

- mitral regurgitation due to destruction or perforation of the mitral leaflet,

- mitral regurgitation due to rupture of chordae tendineae,

- regurgitant lesions of the pulmonary and tricuspid valves,

- perforation of nonvalvular structures (e.g., rupture of aneurysm of sinus of Valsalva).

Secondary lesions related predominantly to microembolization are:

- embolic myocarditis, myocardial abscesses,

- mycotic aneurysms of the aorta and other large arteries,
- focal embolic glomerulonephritis.

Larger embolisms of fragments of vegetations produce the following:

- cerebral infarction,
- coronary embolism with myocardial infarction,
- emboli to various organs within the systemic circulation,
- peripheral arterial emboli,
- pulmonary emboli and infarcts in right-sided endocarditis.

PATHOGENESIS

In the great majority of cases pre-existing cardiac disease represents the predisposing factor in the host. The exact incidence of endocarditis developing upon *normal* cardiac valves is unknown: pathological series reporting a high proportion of cases in which this was thought to be the case may be biased: Endocarditis on undamaged valves is likely to be caused by virulent organisms and thus more often fatal than that affecting patients with pre-existing disease. Almost every form of endocardial, valvular, or arterial disease affecting the intima may be susceptible to infection. However, lesions can be divided into higher and lower risk categories in terms of probability of endocarditis.

The risk of endocarditis is high in lesions associated with turbulent flow and those producing high velocity jets. Such lesions as mitral regurgitation, aortic regurgitation, and ventricular septal defect show a relatively high incidence of infection. Patent ductus arteriosus and coarctation of the aorta also may develop endarteritis upon these lesions. Stenotic lesions of the aortic and pulmonary valves or orifices have a somewhat lower probability of infection; mitral stenosis rarely develops endocarditis; atrial septal defect is virtually immune from endocarditis. Subclinical lesions, such as bicuspid aortic valves, may develop infection. The location of the vegetation is related to the direction of the blood flow: in aortic regurgitation vegetations develop on the ventricular side of the cusps; in ventricular septal defect vegetations may be found on the right ventricular border of the defect, or occasionally on the "jet lesions," on the right ventricular endocardium opposite the right ventricular opening of the defect. Endocarditis may even develop in postmyocardial infarctional mural thrombi.

The precipitating factor of endocarditis is presumed to be bacteremia due to the infecting organism. Inasmuch as bacteremias occur very commonly under many circumstances, only a very small proportion of bacteremias lead to the initiation of infective endocarditis, even in high-risk individuals. The following events have been frequently observed prior to the onset of endocarditis:

- dental extraction or extensive manipulation of the teeth,

- urinary tract manipulations and operations,

- parenteral drug self-administration in addicts,

- pregnancy and puerperium,

- cardiac operations.

In an appreciable number of patients the source of infection is not apparent.

CLINICAL PICTURE

The symptoms of infective endocarditis vary greatly; they are most typically related to the infection, and include:

- feverishness,

- malaise,

- headaches,

- chills,

- night sweats or excessive perspiration in general.

Cardiac symptoms are uncommon; chest pain, dyspnea, and palpitations are apt to signify secondary involvement of the myocardium rather than the effect of endocarditis.

Other symptoms may result from embolic phenomena involving the central nervous system, the splanchnic organs, or the extremities.

Signs of infective endocarditis include evidence of a valvular or congenital lesion in the majority of cases. The critical issue in terms of cardiac examination is a comparison of the findings before the onset of the infection and at the time when it is brought under control. Development of new lesions, aggravation of existing lesions, or change in the mode of how the lesion is tolerated can have an important bearing upon the natural history and the outcome.

Signs of the infection are evident by the following findings:

- pallor,

- splenomegaly,

- petechiae,

- Osler's nodules,

- clubbing of digits.

Signs pointing to major embolic complications include the following:

- development of neurological signs,

- gross hematuria,

- signs of embolism in peripheral arteries.

Laboratory tests produce important diagnostic support for endocarditis:

- Blood culture growth of a pathogen represents the most important diagnostic finding;

- Anemia occurs frequently;

- Other laboratory findings—elevated erythrocyte sedimentation rate, leukocytosis, abnormal serum protein—may be present in infective endocarditis, but their specificity is too low to play an important role in differential diagnosis;

- Radiography, electrocardiography, and other cardiac diagnostic procedures are of importance only for the detection or the monitoring of progressive cardiac damage; in the majority of cases in which no new damage to the heart is produced these tests play a minor role.

NATURAL HISTORY

The natural history of infective endocarditis depends upon:

1. The virulence of the pathogen,

2. The duration of the infection up to the time it is brought under control,

3. The extent of new damage to the heart,

4. The embolic complications,

5. The response to therapy.

In the older writing a distinction was made between "acute endocarditis" and "subacute endocarditis" (also termed "endocarditis lenta"). Acute forms were most often produced by virulent organisms and have certain common features:

- Acute endocarditis often affected previously intact valves;

- Septicemia with involvement of other organs by the infection was common;

- Early and severe damage to cardiac valves was frequently found;

- High fever with "swinging" septic temperature elevations was the rule.

In subacute endocarditis a low grade infection was often inconspicuous, the diagnosis difficult to make; the following features contrasted with the acute form:

- *Streptococcus viridans* was almost always the offending organism;

- Pre-existing valvular or congenital heart disease was the rule;

- Anemia was a constant feature;

- Low-grade temperature elevations were usually present; even an afebrile course could take place;

- The onset of the disease was often very insidious: weeks or months may have elapsed before its recognition.

The changing pathogenesis of infective endocarditis and the role of the antibiotics in its treatment (these drugs were occasionally used without any awareness of the presence of endocarditis) obliterated the differences between acute and subacute forms, leaving them merely as the extreme ends of a spectrum. Today, cases fulfilling the abovementioned criteria are in a small minority—most cases fall in between.

From the standpoint of the infection, the disease can be divided into three stages:

1. The period prior to the time the diagnosis is established,

2. The stage of active antibiotic therapy,

3. The post-therapy stage of surveying the success of the cure of the infection.

The initial stage may be of crucial importance: the difference between an early diagnosis and a delay may determine curability, preservation of cardiac function, and survival. It is the subacute, insidious variety of infective endocarditis which offers the most difficulties to the clinician.

In general, the feasibility of total eradication of the infection determines survival. In rare instances, if drug therapy is incapable of accomplishing a cure, surgical excision of an infected valve may save the patient's life.

Cardiac consequences often present serious problems which may have bearing upon the immediate future of the patient or may have delayed effects. The following problems may arise:

- The original cardiac lesion remains unchanged (at least no clinical evidences of its progression are found);
- Progression of the lesion results from endocarditis, but the patient does not show functional deterioration;
- Progression or extension of the original lesions produces cardiac failure, which is manageable by medical means;
- Intractable cardiac failure requires surgical correction of the cardiac lesion, either as an emergency or electively.

Long-range consequences of the complications of infective endocarditis include permanent neurological damage from cerebral embolisms and chronic renal disease.

DIAGNOSIS

The diagnostic goals in infective endocarditis are as follows:

- To establish the diagnosis of infective endocarditis,
- To identify the pathogenic organism,
- To recognize complications and relapses,
- To monitor and evaluate cardiac lesions.

The diagnosis of infective endocarditis requires the recognition of an endocardial lesion, the demonstration of an active infection, and the establishment of a reasonable relationship between the two.

The great majority of cases of infective endocarditis develop, as stated, upon existing prior cardiac lesions. The knowledge of the presence of a lesion with a high risk of endocarditis constitutes a background upon which the diagnosis can rest. In the absence of clear-cut signs of high-risk cardiac lesions, a search for discrete cardiac murmurs, not necessarily characteristic for any cardiac lesion, is important in order to recognize subclinical lesions. Only rarely is infective endocarditis associated with normal cardiac findings and then its diagnosis can be considered only tentative.

The diagnosis of the infection depends upon its severity. Given an acute febrile illness, the main task is to find a connecting link between this illness and the cardiac abnormality. In patients with a low-grade fever the diagnosis of the infection needs to be made. Findings providing strong support for the diagnosis of endocarditis include the following:

- petechiae,
- splenomegaly,
- Osler's nodes,
- clubbing of digits.

Laboratory test findings aiding in the diagnosis include the following:

- positive blood cultures,
- anemia,
- hematuria,
- elevated sedimentation rate.

Additional diagnostic points may be obtained from the history:

- if the infection develops after dental operations,
- if preceded by various intravascular manipulations,
- if following open heart operations,
- if initiated by urological procedures.

Common differential problems include the following situations:

1. Patients with valvular or congenital lesions susceptible to endocarditis develop an acute febrile illness. Here the diagnostic possibilities are:

- infective endocarditis,
- intercurrent infection,
- acute rheumatic fever (in valvular diseases).

2. Patients run a febrile course or a recrudescence of fever after open heart operations (particularly after valve replacement). The differentiation (see also Chapter 13) includes the following:

- infective endocarditis,
- postoperative pyogenic infection (e.g., wound),
- intrathoracic complications,
- postcardiotomy syndrome.

3. Low-grade febrile disease lingers in a patient who has minimal and nondiagnostic cardiac findings (e.g., a minor systolic murmur).

The differential diagnosis requires consideration of the following:

- infective endocarditis,

- systemic diseases, such as systemic lupus erythematosus, or scleroderma,

- lymphoma or other forms of occult neoplasm,

- cardiac myxoma,

- low-grade infectious processes: tuberculosis, infectious mononucleosis, etc.

The high priority findings supporting the diagnosis of infective endocarditis include the following:

- positive blood culture,

- development of new cardiac lesions (e.g., aortic regurgitation), under observation,

- the appearance of the various embolic complications.

As stated, some patients fail to show positive blood cultures or present inconclusive bacteriological findings. If this occurs and none of the more specific findings appear in support of endocarditis, the diagnosis may be considered presumptive but with sufficient probability to justify the institution of a full therapeutic regimen.

The *isolation of the pathogenic organism* depends upon the bacteriological examination. It is the most important diagnostic proof of infective endocarditis and an essential step for optimal therapy. The reliability of the bacteriological examination involves the following factors:

- bacteriological laboratory facilities and experience,

- adequate number of blood cultures drawn,

- properties of the pathogenic organism.

False-positive blood cultures may involve contaminants. Growths containing saprophytic organisms or normal inhabitants of human flora (e.g., coagulase-negative *Staphylococcus albus*) should be accepted as pathogens only if repeated cultures taken at different times grow this same organism. It is furthermore important to remember that truly positive blood cultures do not prove infective endocarditis but merely demonstrate bacteremia. It is generally recognized that transient bacteremia occurs under many circumstances without producing ill effects in normal individuals; transient bacteremias occurring in patients with cardiac lesions thus can be accepted as evidence of cardiac infection only if supported by other strong clinical evidence.

Negative blood cultures occur in endocarditis, as stated, in from 10 to 20 per cent of cases. Undoubtedly the yield of positive blood cultures may be increased by impeccable bacteriological technique (including the use of special media) and by increasing the opportunity of drawing samples at the point of maximum shower of pathogens. Various rules have been suggested as means of increasing the yield of positive cultures. Yet, it has not been definitely demonstrated that drawing more than four or five blood cultures, that obtaining culture during the height of temperature elevation, or that culturing arterial blood increases the yield of correct bacteriological diagnoses.

The diagnostic acumen of the clinician is important in following the course of infective endocarditis. After this disease is definitely diagnosed, the following events need recognition and analysis:

- complications of endocarditis, particularly emboli,

- the diagnosis of untoward effects of therapy,

- the diagnosis of cardiac sequels of the infection.

Major embolic complications, such as cerebral, splanchnic, or peripheral arterial emboli, are usually self-evident; lesser emboli may manifest themselves as recrudescences of fever, ill-defined symptoms, and so on. Such events need to be differentiated from relapses of the infection or escapes and failure of antibiotic therapy, or drug reactions.

Therapy of infective endocarditis often necessitates the use of toxic drugs; evidence of toxicity or untoward drug reactions may produce renal failure, toxic effects upon the blood, drug fever, and other possible therapy-related complications that need to be differentiated from natural complications of the disease. The similarity of the two types of complications may necessitate an interruption of the therapy or a change of drugs.

Early detection of deteriorating cardiac lesions or developing new lesions is of importance from the standpoint of prognosis and therapy. The diagnostic evaluation has to consider not only the type of the lesion but its quantification and hemodynamic effects. Sudden acute aortic regurgitation initiated by the perforation of an aortic leaflet caused by endocarditis may produce intolerable cardiac overload and lead to cardiac failure severe enough to require an emergency operation.

THERAPY

Therapeutic objectives concerning infective endocarditis are as follows:

1. The prevention of endocarditis in patients at risk;

2. A complete cure of the infection;

3. Prevention of cardiac damage and of complications;

4. Treatment of the cardiac consequences of the infection;

5. Surgical treatment, where indicated.

Prevention of infective endocarditis requires the use of antibiotics during procedures known to be the cause of transient bacteremias in all patients who are considered susceptible to this disease. This includes:

- all patients with valvular heart disease and with congenital lesions with the possible exception of atrial septal defect;

- patients with undiagnosed cardiac murmurs.

The most important potential triggering point for infection is traumatic dental work; urological infections constitute the second priority. The prophylactic use of antibiotics in open heart surgery has been debated for a long time; the evidence seems to point against the rationality of the routine use of antibiotics. Prophylactic therapy prior to catheterization and angiocardiographic procedures has been tried and generally shown to be ineffective (or unrewarding); its use is being discouraged.

The cure of an existing infection involves the following steps:

- the bacteriological diagnosis,

- the test of sensitivities of the pathogen to various antibiotics,

- the therapy,

- the monitoring of the bactericidal capability of the patient's serum against the pathogen followed by an appropriate dosage adjustment,

- post-therapy observation to insure the completeness of the cure.

Once a pathogenic microorganism has been cultured from the blood of the patient, the dosage schedule of the appropriate drug with a reasonable sensitivity to the pathogen should be designed in a way that is likely to accomplish bactericidal blood levels. Its effectiveness is gauged by:

- regression of the signs of the infection (temperature fall, relief of symptoms, patient's well-being, etc.)

- in vitro demonstration of bactericidal drug concentration of the patient's serum against the pathogen,

- absence of relapses after the treatment is terminated.

The duration of therapy has to be set arbitrarily, since the minimum time necessary to cure infective endocarditis is not known. It is usually considered advisable to start with parenteral therapy for at least a two-week period, to be followed by another two weeks of oral drug administration. In general, the length depends upon the type of the organism, its sensitivity to antibiotics demonstrated in vitro, the level of bactericidal action of the patient's serum attained during the therapy, and the type of the lesion. Longer than average periods of antibiotic therapy, usually arbitrarily set at six weeks, are considered necessary in the following circumstances:

- infection with organisms with low pathogenicity (e.g., coagulase-negative staphylococci),

- infection with organisms other than bacteria (e.g., fungi),

- infection in patients with foreign material in the heart (artificial valves, other prostheses, patches).

As stated, in about 20 per cent of patients with bacterial endocarditis blood cultures remain negative in spite of repeated tests done in the best bacteriological laboratories. Treatment of endocarditis in these patients is just as important as in those with proven etiological factors; antibiotic therapy has to be initiated in an arbitrary manner and continued under the guidance of its effect upon the fever, and on the symptoms. Therapy for unknown pathogens has to be performed under two possible circumstances:

1. In patients in whom the diagnosis is definitely established (e.g., overt signs of infection with several confirmatory clinical findings of bacterial endocarditis, as discussed above);

2. In patients with a merely presumptive diagnosis (low-grade signs of infection in patients with lesions susceptible to endocarditis, but without any confirmatory signs of endocarditis).

In the first category a full course of therapy is considered necessary and is often extended to a six-week period, even if signs of endocarditis are brought under control immediately after the initiation of therapy. In patients with a presumptive diagnosis of endocarditis therapy is often handled individually; no rational guidelines are available or can ever be expected because the diagnosis can only be arbitrarily guessed. Some experts recommend that any unexplained febrile episode of more than seven days in a patient with a cardiac lesion known to be susceptible to endocarditis should be diagnosed presumptively as infective endocarditis and treated with the standard therapy. There are no data to enable one to argue either for or against this recommendation.

The "standard" therapy of endocarditis in patients with an unknown pathogen consists in most centers of:

- Parenteral therapy with large doses of penicillin (or penicillin-like synthetic drugs) for at least four weeks. The usually recommended dose is 20 million units per 24 hours.

- The addition of 1 to 2 grams of streptomycin during the first 10 days of the treatment; gentamicin is occasionally substituted for streptomycin.

The protection of a patient with infective endocarditis from extension of cardiac damage and from the various complications of the infection (mostly related to embolic phenomena) rests entirely on early diagnosis and immediate institution of effective therapy. No secondary form of treatment is available other than the rare use of cardiac surgery. Anticoagulant therapy has been shown to be not only ineffective but potentially harmful.

Treatment of cardiac consequences of endocarditis relates to two problems:

1. Cardiac failure produced by the development of a more severe valvular lesion or by the production of a new lesion;

2. Cardiac failure due to myocardial involvement — either major embolism (myocardial infarction) or myocarditis caused by the organism.

If the lesion leading to cardiac failure is primarily *endocardial,* conventional therapy of failure should be initiated with the knowledge that the damage is permanent; then if medical therapy is entirely ineffective, a surgical approach — valve replacement — must be considered. *Myocardial* lesions are, as a rule, not amenable to surgical therapy; however, they may be considered potentially reversible upon eradication of the infection, and therefore a conservative approach is indicated.

Surgical therapy of infective endocarditis or its consequences involves the following problems:

1. Removal of the nidus of infection in patients in whom the best antipathogenic therapy is shown to be ineffective. Not all lesions can be surgically attacked; this approach has the following priorities:

- Infection presumed to be located upon foreign material in the heart or great vessels has the highest priority;

- Infection involving the mitral or aortic valve that has produced new lesions upon either valve has the next highest priority;

• Other presumably accessible foci of infection are the third priority.

The number of cures accomplished by surgical removal of the infected areas in patients thought to be intractable provides good evidence that this radical approach is rational. It is important to consider, however, that there is a large number of failures as well, including patients in whom the entire infected area cannot be resected as well as those who undergo complete removal of infected parts but who later suffer relapses. Thus, surgery predicated primarily upon the potential care of intractable infection is to be considered only a last resort.

2. Valve replacement for intractable cardiac failure almost always involves the aortic or the mitral valves. Indications for valve replacement include emergency situations and elective operations.

> • Emergency valve replacement performed during the active stage of the infection should be considered only in life-threatening situations, unless the infection is unresponsive to therapy and both hemodynamic and bacteriological indications for the operation coexist.

> • Every effort should be made to defer operations until the infection is cured: first, the risk of the operation is higher during the active infectious stage; second, the placement of a prosthesis in an infected area provides a potentially serious problem; third, the possibility of a temporary myocardial factor in the production of cardiac failure needs to be considered.

> • Elective valve replacement after a bacteriological cure should be reserved for patients in whom there is convincing evidence that the overload of the new lesion cannot be tolerated. Even severe acute mitral or aortic regurgitation produced by infective endocarditis may permit compensatory cardiac hypertrophy to overcome the initial failure and restore reasonable compensation.

Bibliography

Braniff BA, Shumway NF, Harrison DC: Valve replacement in active bacterial endocarditis. New Engl. J. Med. *276*:1464, 1967.
Buchbinder NA, Roberts WC: Left-sided valvular active infective endocarditis. A study of 45 necropsy patients. Amer. J. Med. *53*:20, 1972.
Cohn LH, Roberts WC, Rockoff SD, Morrow AG: Bacterial endocarditis following aortic valve replacement. Circulation *33*:209, 1966.
Finland M, Barnes MW: Changing etiology of bacterial endocarditis in the antibiotic era. Experiences at Boston City Hospital 1933–1965. Ann. Int. Med. *72*:341, 1970.

Roberts WC, Buchbinder NA: Right-sided valvular infective endocarditis. A clinicopathological study of 12 necropsy patients. Amer. J. Med. *53*:7, 1972.
Weinstein L, Rubin RH: Infective endocarditis — 1973. Prog. Cardiovasc. Dis. *16*:239, 1973.
Weinstein L, Rubin RH: Treatment of infective endocarditis — 1973. Prog. Cardiovasc. Dis. *16*:275, 1973.
Weinstein L, Schlesinger JJ: Pathoanatomic, pathophysiologic and clinical correlations in endocarditis. New Engl. J. Med. *291*:832, 1122, 1974.

*V. Diseases Primarily Increasing Cardiac Workload*_____

27

Atrial Septal Defect

Definition. This chapter deals with interatrial communications large enough to produce significant circulatory derangement as a result of increased pulmonary blood flow. They include (Fig. 27–1):

- septum secundum type atrial septal defect;

- its variant, sinus venosus type atrial septal defect;

- septum primum type atrial septal defect with intact ventricular septum but including valve clefts.

Excluded are the following:

- patent foramen ovale, clinically silent or insignificant;

- right-to-left shunts through a patent foramen ovale secondary to right-sided cardiac lesions;

- endocardial cushion defects involving the ventricular septum.

Associated cardiac lesions other than the atrial septal defect are included in the presentation only if atrial septal defect is the clinically preponderant lesion; among these are partial anomalous venous return, mild pulmonary stenosis, and mitral valve disease.

As indicated in Chapter 21, atrial septal defect is the commonest congenital cardiac lesion in adults and in older children. The great majority of patients exhibit the secundum type atrial septal defect. Septum primum type defects account for from 10 to 20 per cent of the total number. There is a preponderance of female over male patients.

PATHOLOGY AND PATHOPHYSIOLOGY

The atrial septal defect of the secundum type is located generally in the posterior portion of the septum, in the overall region of the fossa ovalis. The defects vary widely in size and exact location. The majority of defects are located in the fossa ovalis and encompass the foramen. Some defects represent merely a widely patent foramen ovale without the valve-like flap. The spectrum of sizes of atrial septal defects ranges from wide patency of the foramen ovale (usually about 1.5 cm. in diameter) to a total absence of the atrial septum (single atrium). Multiple defects are occasionally found. Atrial septal defect located at the uppermost portion of the atrial septum, near the orifice of the superior vena cava, is termed "sinus venosus type." It plays a special role because of its common association with partial anomalous venous return and accounts for some 8 per cent of atrial septal defects.

Associated lesions (within the restrictions of this discussion) with secundum type atrial septal defect include the following:

- Anomalous drainage of pulmonary veins from the right lung (either to the right atrium or to the superior vena cava, the latter variety being especially characteristic for the sinus venosus type of atrial septal defect);

- Persistent left superior vena cava is occasionally present;
- Mitral valve cleft — characteristic for septum primum type defect — is very occasionally associated with a secundum type atrial septal defect;

- Mucoid degeneration of mitral cusps;

- Mild valvular pulmonary stenosis;

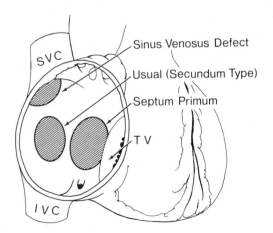

Figure 27–1. Diagrammatic presentation of three commonest types of atrial septal defect, as viewed from the right atrium. (TV — tricuspid valve; SVC — superior vena cava; IVC — inferior vena cava.)

- Mitral stenosis and/or regurgitation due to deformity of leaflets.

Septum primum atrial septal defect is of different embryological origin than secundum type defect, being an endocardial cushion type of malformation. It is located in the anterior portion of the septum, adjacent to the tricuspid leaflet. Its unique features are:

- An association with an abnormal location and course of the AV node and the bundle of His;

- A common association with clefts in the mitral valve;

- Frequent clefts or other deformities of the tricuspid valve.

The physiological consequence of communications between the atria is a left-to-right intracardiac shunt through the defect. The normal pressure differential between the two atria is but 3 or 4 mm. Hg. In large atrial septal defect even this small gradient may be obliterated and the pressure in the two chambers equilibrated. Left-to-right shunt is not caused by higher pressure in the left atrium but rather by the lower resistance to diastolic filling of the more compliant right ventricle, with the two atria serving as a common reservoir. These dynamic conditions have the following consequences:

- Low velocity flow does not produce cardiac murmurs; it makes the development of infective endocarditis extremely rare;

- There is usually no direct relationship between the anatomic size of the defect and the magnitude of the shunt;

- Significant left-to-right shunt may not develop immediately after birth but rather may increase gradually over a period of months, in line with the normal postnatal relationship of the respective compliances of the two ventricles.

The hemodynamic consequences of the left-to-right shunt include an increase in right ventricular output without the concomitant rise in left ventricular output (Fig. 27–2). The pulmonary blood flow becomes two, three, or four times larger than the systemic blood flow, increasing the workload of the right ventricle (volume overload) and producing right ventricular hypertrophy and dilatation. The large reserve capacity of the pulmonary capillary bed can easily accommodate the increased flow without increasing resistance to flow, hence pulmonary arterial pressure as a rule remains normal even if the flow increases four times.

Pulmonary hypertension may develop in atrial septal defect as a secondary complication. In secundum type atrial septal defect it develops almost always in the adult age; it may then progress rapidly. Early pul-

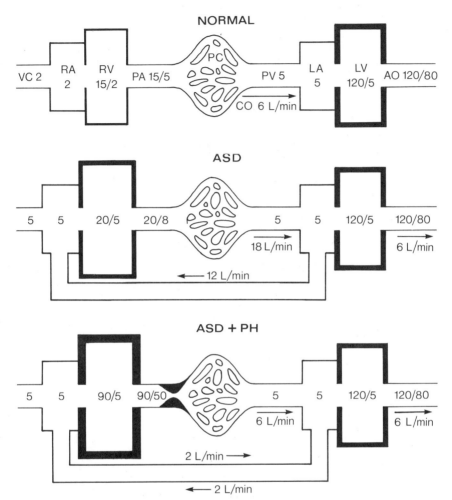

Figure 27-2. Hemodynamic diagram showing sequentially circulatory segments between the caval system and the aorta with the respective pressures and the cardiac output. *Upper diagram*, normal circulation. *Middle diagram*, atrial septal defect: in this example a three-to-one left-to-right shunt is present; pressures are normal. *Lower diagram*, an example of atrial septal defect complicated by severe pulmonary hypertension producing a balanced bidirectional shunt. (VC — vena cava; RA — right atrium; RV — right ventricle; PA — pulmonary artery; PV — pulmonary veins; LA — left atrium; LV — left ventricle; AO — aorta; ASD — atrial septal defect; PH — pulmonary hypertension.)

monary hypertension develops occasionally in primum type atrial septal defects. Pulmonary hypertension is caused primarily by irreversible intimal changes in the pulmonary arterioles which may be the result of the long-standing increase in pulmonary flow that produces this reaction in susceptible individuals.

Shunt reversal producing significant arterial hypoxemia is most commonly encountered as a late complication of atrial septal defect in patients who develop severe pulmonary hypertension, thereby reversing resistances to flow and ventricular compliances. Occasionally, uncomplicated atrial septal defect may be associated with hypoxemia due to bidirectional shunting related to two other possible mechanisms:

- Streamlining of inferior caval blood directed into the fossa ovalis similarly to that of the fetus; the blood is thus ejected into the left atrium;

- Free mixing of oxygenated and caval blood in large defects, e.g., in a single atrium.

Cardiac failure rarely develops in secundum type atrial septal defect prior to the fifth or sixth decade of life. The mechanics of the two ventricles being filled from a functionally single atrial reservoir, with blood automatically directed toward a chamber that can handle it best, provides a very efficient circulatory pump. There is still a controversy as to whether cardiac failure in atrial septal defect represents malfunction of the left or the right ventricle — a difference that may be more semantic than real. In primum type atrial septal defect cardiac failure may develop early in life; the difference here is probably related to malfunction of atrioventricular valves, particularly the tricuspid.

NATURAL HISTORY

In general, the natural history of atrial septal defect is influenced by the following:

1. The consequences of prolonged volume overload of the right ventricle;

2. The effects of increased flow upon the pulmonary circulation;

3. Complications resulting from the above;

4. Associated lesions and their sequelae.

Secundum Type Atrial Septal Defect

Infancy and Early Childhood. As stated, postnatal adaptation of the heart and circulation produces circumstances that make the presence of an interatrial communication of little consequence as a cause of left-to-right shunt during the postnatal period and early infancy. However, the respective resistances and compliances on the two sides of the heart may facilitate right-to-left shunt as a continuation of the fetal circulation after birth. Thus patients with atrial septal defects may demonstrate transient cyanosis in the early postnatal period more frequently than those with other left-to-right shunting lesions.

Atrial septal defect is seldom recognized during infancy. During early childhood the great majority of children are asymptomatic; only rarely some evidence of decreased effort tolerance presents itself. However, there is increased susceptibility to upper respiratory infections, including pneumonias; whether such infections bring about cardiac failure is uncertain. Most children with atrial septal defect are diagnosed on the basis of abnormal auscultatory findings or abnormal chest roentgenograms rather than on the basis of symptoms.

Late Childhood and Adolescence. Patients in this age group, who have not been previously diagnosed and operated upon, continue a benign course. The tendency to respiratory infections usually subsides. If limitation of activities exists, it is often minor, manifested as "tiredness"; it may be difficult to distinguish limitations of activities due to symptoms related to the atrial septal defect from those produced by deconditioning caused by excessive limitation of activities.

Early Adult Life. During the third decade of life the majority of patients remain asymptomatic. However, in patients susceptible to the development of increased pulmonary vascular resistance, this complication may progress rapidly, producing altered signs, increasing symptomatology, and eventually cyanosis.

Middle and Late Adult Life. During the fifth and sixth decades of life many patients develop disability, even though some remain asymptomatic and may live a normal span of life. The basis of disability is the development of cardiac failure, which is usually associated with, and possibly triggered by, atrial arrhythmias. Chronic atrial flutter or fibrillation, as a rule, accompanies the signs of cardiac failure.

Associated Lesions and Complications. The effects of the various associated lesions and complications of the secundum type atrial septal defect vary widely in their influence upon the course of the natural history:

1. *Pulmonary hypertension* represents the most serious complication of the atrial septal defect. It develops in some 15 per cent of patients in the third or fourth decade of life. Often rapidly progressive, it may render the patient inoperable and eventually reverse the interatrial shunt, producing hypoxemia, cyanosis, polycythemia, and their sequels. Patients who develop this complication may still remain asymptomatic for some years. They may survive a decade or two with progressive limitation of activities, eventually developing right ventricular failure. Some die as a result of the thrombotic complications that may develop from the polycythemia. Occasionally, rupture of the pulmonary artery represents the terminal event.

2. *Mitral stenosis* develops in patients with atrial septal defect more frequently than in patients with a random combination of two cardiac lesions. Once thought to be the result of coexisting rheumatic heart disease, it is now considered to be a direct effect of the atrial septal defect: stresses upon the atrioventricular rings resulting from large interatrial shunting produce altered flow patterns through the mitral valve which may traumatize this valve, eventually leading to fibrotic changes. The combination of atrial septal defect and mitral stenosis, known also as *Lutembacher's syndrome,* may follow the course of an uncomplicated atrial septal defect (leading to atrial fibrillation and cardiac failure in late middle life) or may proceed along the pattern of natural history of pure mitral stenosis.

3. *Mitral regurgitation* may be produced by valve clefts. They will be discussed in connection with the primum type atrial septal defect. Mild regurgitation may also be caused by mucoid degeneration of the mitral valve, manifested by a midsystolic click and late systolic murmur.

4. *Pulmonary stenosis* of mild degree has little influence upon the natural history of the atrial septal defect.

5. *Partial anomalous venous drainage and persistent left superior vena cava* represent anatomic malformations of no clinical significance. They may, however, present problems to the cardiovascular surgeons at the time of atrial septal repair; hence the knowledge of their presence is of importance.

6. *Ectopic rhythms* occasionally associated with atrial septal defect, particularly with the sinus venosus type, play a very small role in the natural history of this condition. The cardiac rate may be somewhat slower than the average; however, responses to exercise and other sympathetic stimuli are normal. The importance of this complication lies in its recognition as an associated congenital lesion rather than an acquired complication, so that the clinician will not be tempted to treat it.

7. *Paradoxical embolism* represents a potential danger in any patient with intracardiac communications. Fortunately its incidence is very low.

Primum Type Atrial Septal Defect

This variety of atrial septal defect is a more serious congenital lesion than the commoner secundum type defect. Hemodynamically, the magnitude of the interatrial shunt shows a similar range and the consequences are identical. The difference in the course stems from the associated lesions and special characteristics.

- Congenital abnormalities of the conducting system produce electrocardiographic patterns of bifascicular block; occasionally first degree AV block may also be present. As a rule this associated anomaly plays no significant role in the course; yet, occasionally patients may develop complete heart block — in childhood or later in life.

- Clefts in the atrioventricular valves vary in their contribution to clinical problems; some are completely silent (found only at operation); others may produce unimportant apical systolic murmurs; still others cause significant valvular regurgitation, which may be evident since infancy, or may develop at any time in life. The additive effect of valvular incompetence may lead to cardiac failure early in life: the tricuspid valve probably contributes more to this effect than the mitral valve.

- Pulmonary hypertension tends to develop more often and earlier in life than in the secundum type atrial septal defect.

- Cyanosis may appear early in life, with or without concomitant pulmonary hypertension. It is estimated to be present in 10 per cent of cases.

- The risk in surgical correction of this type of defect is higher than in the secundum type because of the possibility of damage to the conducting system and to atrioventricular structures.

Postsurgical Course

The natural history of patients who undergo surgical treatment of atrial septal defect depends upon the age at the operation. In principle, the operation comes close to being a curative one, inasmuch as the anatomic lesion is totally corrected. In practice, a number of problems may arise in the life of operated patients.

Patients *operated on in childhood* for the correction of secundum type atrial septal defect, as a rule, have no significant problems. Clinical evidence suggests that hypertrophy and dilatation of the right ventricle from the shunt regress after the shunt is eliminated. Occasionally children are left with an ectopic site of impulse formation (usually a junctional rhythm), stemming presumably from damage to the internodal tracts or the S-A node. As far as one can judge, a permanent junctional rhythm does not have serious consequences. Patients who show *congenital* ectopic rhythms in association with atrial septal defect will, of course, continue to have them after repair of the defect.

Patients *operated on in adulthood* for uncomplicated atrial septal defect of the secundum type usually do well and also come close to a "cure." However, their postoperative course may be more stormy: they show a high incidence of postoperative atrial arrhythmias that can extend into months after the operation; furthermore, at least 10 per cent of them develop postcardiotomy syndromes (see Chapter 13). In most, the susceptibility for postoperative arrhythmias gradually diminishes and eventually disappears. In some, a lifelong tendency to atrial arrhythmias may develop—some may eventually get chronic atrial fibrillation. Thus, the operation not only may not protect patients from this complication of atrial septal defect but may occasionally increase the risk of its appearance.

Patients operated on in the presence of *pulmonary hypertension* demonstrate a wide range of consequences. Those with purely hyperkinetic pulmonary hypertension (i.e., normal pulmonary vascular resistance) are expected to show a fall of pulmonary arterial pressure to normal after elimination of the shunt. Most of them do. Yet, occasionally mild residual pulmonary hypertension persists. How many of these will eventually develop more severe pulmonary hypertension later in life is not known; this possibility should, however, be considered and the patient followed appropriately. Patients who already have elevated pulmonary vascular resistance prior to the operation but still have operable shunts (a ratio of two to one or greater) will usually be left with pulmonary hypertension of lesser degree. In them the operation accomplishes the prevention of rapid progression of pulmonary vascular disease and shunt reversal, but may merely be a form of palliation. The probability of further progression of pulmonary hypertension, at a slower pace, exists in these cases. There are some cases on record in which pulmonary vascular resistance falls after closure of defects, but they represent a small minority.

Patients operated on *later in life*, at the time of disability and cardiac failure, often show significant improvement; yet, the operation carries a higher risk and offers merely palliation. In such cases pros and cons of surgical therapy have to be carefully weighed.

In *septum primum* type atrial septal defect, not only does operation carry higher risk but various additional problems may arise:

- Surgical damage to the conducting system may require the placement of a pacemaker.

- Clefts associated with evident valve incompetence may require valve replacement.

- Surgical suturing of "silent" valve clefts may eventually produce serious disease of that valve.

- "Silent" valve clefts left alone at the time of the surgery may initiate severe valve incompetence after the operation, possibly from altered anatomic relationship of the annuli secondary to closure of the defect.

• Unoperated patients stand a small risk of acquiring complete AV block, and this tendency would not be influenced by surgical repair of the septal defect.

In spite of these additional problems patients operated upon for the primum type atrial septal defect may do as well as those with the secundum defect. Other problems that may arise in their postsurgical course are identical with those discussed above in connection with the secundum defect.

DIAGNOSIS

Case Finding. Atrial septal defect is less often recognized early in life than most other congenital cardiac lesions. The reasons for this have been mentioned in the preceding sections and need only be recapitulated here:

• It may be virtually silent in infancy;

• It takes a benign course in most cases;

• It does not produce a pathognomonic cardiac murmur.

Since the majority of patients with this lesion are asymptomatic, case finding depends usually upon detection of abnormalities during routine examination or medical care for unrelated conditions. The wide variability of the various features makes case finding related to auscultatory abnormalities in some cases, to radiographic features in others, or to electrocardiographic changes in still others. Adults with unrecognized atrial septal defect are often passed over as having "rheumatic heart disease" because of a superficial resemblance to mitral valve disease. Diagnostic features in some adolescents may be so close to the normal range that only sophisticated diagnosticians may direct some patients for study and find large left-to-right shunts.

Objectives of Diagnostic Evaluation. It is worth reiterating that blood flow through the atrial septal defect does not produce a murmur; all clinical findings — physical, electrocardiographic, roentgenographic — are related to large pulmonary flow. It is thus evident that small atrial septal defect is not diagnosable and that whenever the diagnosis is made, a significant derangement of the circulation exists. Thus the clinical spectrum of atrial septal defect involves a range from moderate to very large left-to-right shunt. The objectives of diagnostic evaluation should be therefore reviewed from the standpoint that each patient is a potential surgical candidate. They include:

- The definitive diagnosis of atrial septal defect with differentiation from similar lesions;

- Recognition of its type (primum, secundum, sinus venosus);

- Recognition of its sequels and complications;

- Search for associated significant lesions.

Physical Findings. The following signs are associated with atrial septal defect (in order of their specificity):

1. A "fixed" widely split second sound occurs in most, though not all, patients with this lesion. Its frequency is higher in childhood (probably above 90 per cent) than in adult life. The pathognomonic quality of this sign is lessened by the following differential difficulties:

- "Fixed" splitting involves some respiratory variation; therefore there is an inevitable overlap with other forms of wide splitting of the second sound;

- Rarely, unexplained wide, "fixed" splitting occurs without atrial septal defect;

- Mitral opening snap may be mistaken for wide, fixed splitting.

2. Delayed diastolic flow murmurs originate in the tricuspid valve owing to the large volume of flow through it. They are heard at the lower left sternal border, occasionally close to the apical region. These murmurs are of higher frequency and shorter than the mitral diastolic rumbles, sometimes presenting a scratchy quality. They have occasionally been mistaken for murmurs of mitral stenosis, although this differentiation is not difficult. They may overlap with extracardiac noises. These murmurs have a very good specificity but low sensitivity, for they are more often absent than present (an incidence of 30 per cent, according to Wood) (Barber et al., 1950).

3. Systolic ejection murmur at the upper left sternal border is the result of increased flow through the pulmonary orifice. It varies in intensity from trivial murmurs, even those heard only after exercise, to very loud and long murmurs suggesting significant pulmonary stenosis. The ejection murmur is the most sensitive — present in close to 100 per cent of cases — but not a very specific clinical sign. It overlaps with the innocent ejection murmur so often found in healthy children and adolescents, with organic pulmonary stenosis, and with atypical aortic stenosis (including hypertrophic subaortic stenosis). Its specificity is

very low if the murmur is of low intensity; it is moderate if the murmur is loud.

4.   Hyperactive precordial motion is frequently found in atrial septal defect due to exaggerated excursion of the overactive right ventricle. Present in patients with very large shunts, this sign is merely a supporting clinical feature, because of the frequent occurrence of increased precordial motion in normal young individuals due to the high output caused by excitement or due to a thin chest wall. There is also an overlap with various hypercirculatory states and with valve incompetence.

5.   Early diastolic murmur of semilunar valve incompetence is rare in atrial septal defect; it originates in the pulmonary valve, and the incompetence is almost always related to complicating pulmonary hypertension.

The clinical diagnosis of atrial septal defect may be easy and reliable if a combination of the above signs is present. Given a patient who shows the first four signs described above, the diagnosis is virtually certain; with three of these four signs it is highly probable. The presence of one of two of the findings makes the diagnosis contingent upon laboratory studies.

Radiological Features.   The large pulmonary flow causes an increase in the size of the right heart chambers without concomitant enlargement of the left side of the heart, and enlargement of the pulmonary artery with an increase in pulmonary vascularity extending into the periphery of the lung fields. The aortic knob is usually small. These first two radiographic features vary widely, ranging from discrete changes overlapping with the normal variation to a highly characteristic picture with cardiomegaly and a very large pulmonary artery and branches. As a rule more pronounced radiographic changes are found in adults, lesser changes in children, but in each age group there is wide variation. Among the crucial diagnostic points are the following:

- Absence of left atrial enlargement, a feature which separates atrial septal defect from mitral valve disease with pulmonary hypertension;

- Absence of left ventricular enlargement (not always easy to determine), which separates this lesion from shunts at ventricular and aortopulmonary levels;

- Differentiation of high pulmonary flow from the effects of pulmonary hypertension (the former characterized by vascularity in the periphery of the lungs).

Electrocardiographic Features. The characteristic electrocardiographic finding in secundum type atrial septal defect is the presence of incomplete right bundle branch block. This is a rather sensitive finding, present in at least 90 per cent of cases; its specificity is moderate—right bundle branch block is not an uncommon finding in other lesions and occurs in normal individuals. "Incomplete right bundle branch block" represents a broad range, from a minor right-sided conduction delay (evidenced by a terminal R' in leads V_1 and V_2) to a fully developed block in the right bundle with the duration of QRS complexes less than 0.12 second. It is the latter type that adds more weight to the diagnosis of atrial septal defect; minor delays occur too often in normal individuals.

The electrocardiogram represents the principal diagnostic tool in the differentiation of the septum primum atrial septal defect from its other forms. Characteristically, in all endocardial cushion defects there is a delay in the activation of the portions of the left ventricle supplied by the anterior division of the left bundle. Consequently a superior orientation of the QRS axis in the limb leads occurs, usually combined with right bundle branch block. The axis ranges from $-30°$ to $-90°$ and beyond. Prolonged AV conduction (first degree heart block) often accompanies these changes. The patterns of bifascicular block described above give high specificity to the presence of endocardial cushion defect (but does not discriminate whether ostium primum atrial septal defect is present alone or in combination with other abnormalities).

Given a patient with atrial septal defect who shows an abnormal P wave axis (superior) indicative of ectopic pacemaker, the probability is high that this is the sinus venosus type. Yet the sensitivity of this finding is low, for only some patients with this type of defect have abnormal impulse formation.

Vectorcardiographic studies have served to amplify the differentiation of the primum from the secundum type of atrial septal defects, based on the features described above. It has not been established that vectorcardiography provides a more reliable diagnostic tool in this respect than the conventional electrocardiogram.

Phonocardiography. This may be of diagnostic aid in atrial septal defect as a means of differentiating the late component of the second heart sound from other early diastolic sounds (e.g., mitral opening snap) and in observing the degree of respiratory relationship of the aortic and pulmonary closure sounds.

Echocardiography. This has established itself as an important noninvasive diagnostic aid in atrial septal defect. It may demonstrate:

- enlargement of the right ventricular chamber,

- paradoxical motion of the septum.

The reliability of echocardiographic studies is moderately good and this method serves as a confirmation of the clinical diagnosis. There is, however, the inevitable overlap in that both of these findings may occur in tricuspid regurgitation and also in patients showing left bundle branch block. Furthermore, occasional false-negative tests have been reported in which a normal echocardiogram was recorded in patients with sizable shunts from atrial septal defects.

Cardiac Catheterization. This procedure is a sine qua non as part of the diagnostic evaluation of all congenital defects. In atrial septal defect it can establish the diagnosis with reasonable accuracy, leaving only a very small fraction of cases doubtful. It also is an important, though not necessarily decisive, aid in the differentiation of the various types of atrial septal defect.

The basic diagnostic feature of atrial septal defect is a step-up in oxygen content of blood samples drawn from the caval system and those from the right atrium. Inasmuch as clinically recognizable atrial septal defect involves major shunts, the oxygen differential is usually clear-cut, leaving no doubt as to its validity. Caval samples can be drawn from both the superior and inferior vena cava, or, more often, just from the superior vena cava, the oxygen content of which correlates well in normal individuals with that in the pulmonary artery (i.e., mixed venous blood). In addition, direct entry into the left atrium is usually possible in atrial septal defect. Measurement of the pulmonary arterial pressure constitutes an important part of the evaluation. The following differential points are noteworthy:

- In atrial septal defect with smaller shunts (e.g., two-to-one) oxygen figures may be inconclusive because of streamlining of oxygenated and unoxygenated blood. Use of qualitative measures such as the hydrogen inhalation test may be necessary to make the presence of a shunt definitely demonstrated.

- The presence of a shunt may not differentiate atrial septal defect from isolated anomalous venous return. Even though right atrial drainage of pulmonary veins occurs usually in conjunction with atrial septal defect, occasionally it may be the sole lesion. The differentiation is aided by angiocardiography.

- The entry of the catheter into the left atrium does not constitute the proof of a significant defect but may be due to probe patency of the foramen ovale. Catheterization from the leg veins permits preferential crossing of the foramen ovale; hence traversing of the septum from the arm is more diagnostically significant.

- The course of the catheter entering the left atrium may help differentiate a secundum type defect (higher curve) from a primum type defect (low arching of the catheter, just in the region of the tricuspid valve).

- Streamlining of oxygenated blood entering the right atrium just above the tricuspid valve in the primum type defect may cause the oxygen step-up to be detected only in the right ventricle—a finding also supporting the lower defect but requiring differentiation from ventricular septal defect.

- The entry of a catheter into a pulmonary vein does not prove the existence of partial anomalous pulmonary drainage, because the catheter may enter the vein via the left atrium (a fact not always easy to detect on fluoroscopic observation). The exception is the anomalous right superior pulmonary vein draining into the superior vena cava in conjunction with the sinus venosus defect.

Angiocardiography. This procedure plays a more limited role in the diagnosis of atrial septal defect than in other congenital lesions. It serves primarily as a means of investigating the possibility of associated lesions. The commonest problem requiring angiocardiographic examination is the question of pulmonary venous drainage: injection of the contrast medium into either of the pulmonary branches usually establishes the point of entry of the pulmonary veins into the atria.

Differential Points in Diagnostic Evaluation. The differential diagnosis of atrial septal defect involves a wide spectrum of acquired and congenital lesions as well as the separation from normals. The following are the common conditions with which atrial septal defect may be confused:

1. In children and adolescents:

    - Innocent cardiac murmurs or other borderline findings in healthy individuals,

    - "Straight back syndrome,"

    - Mild pulmonary stenosis,

    - Idiopathic dilatation of the pulmonary artery,

    - Total anomalous venous return,

    - Other shunting lesions,

    - Rheumatic mitral regurgitation,

    - Aortic stenosis or hypertrophic subaortic stenosis.

2. In adults:

   • Mitral valve disease,

   • Other congenital lesions with shunts,

   • Cor pulmonale,

   • Pulmonary hypertension from any cause, including idiopathic variety.

Indications for Invasive Studies. The general guidelines for the selection of cases for cardiac catheterization are presented in Chapter 8. Atrial septal defect, being primarily a potentially surgical lesion, requires that the diagnosis be arrived at by all available means; hence cardiac catheterization is a presurgical requisite. Even if the clinical diagnosis is established with certainty — as is sometimes possible — recording of pulmonary arterial pressure and investigation of the pulmonary venous drainage and of possible associated lesions justify the study. The most serious dilemma is presented by young subjects in whom one or two findings vaguely suggest the possibility of atrial septal defect but in whom probabilities point against any organic cardiac disease. Here the decision as to who should and should not be catheterized is one of judgment and experience of the diagnostician. There should at least be a reasonable possibility of the presence of a congenital lesion to justify cardiac catheterization in healthy, asymptomatic subjects. It is axiomatic that all noninvasive laboratory studies, including echocardiography, should be performed before cardiac catheterization is recommended.

THERAPY

Problems involved in treatment of atrial septal defect include the following:

   • selection of patients for surgical treatment,

   • timing of the operation,

   • medical management of unoperated patients,

   • treatment of complications,

   • postsurgical therapy.

The general objectives of surgical treatment of atrial septal defect are as follows:

   • elimination of right ventricular volume overload imposed by the shunt,

- relief of symptoms, disability, and respiratory infections caused by the large pulmonary flow,

- prevention of pulmonary hypertension,

- prevention of arrhythmias (late in life),

- prevention of cardiac failure.

These objectives, which for the most part fall into the category of preventive rather than remedial treatment, nevertheless constitute a firm basis for operating on virtually all patients with atrial septal defect in view of the very low surgical risk (estimated at 1 per cent in experienced surgical units) and the almost curative nature of the operation. The crucial point is whether the effects of atrial septal defect are ever small enough to justify withholding the operation. The answer to this question is not definitive, because virtually all diagnosable atrial septal defects have shunts of sufficient magnitude to alter circulatory dynamics. Yet, occasionally atrial septal defects with smaller shunts are diagnosed (often as an accidental finding in patients investigated for another condition). In considering this question, it is generally estimated that shunts with less than a two-to-one ratio are unlikely to lead to significant consequences and may be left unoperated. This general rule applies to ventricular and aortopulmonary shunts, and should probably also be applied to atrial septal defect.

The timing of the operation depends upon many factors, some of an individual and personal nature. It is important to appreciate the fact that pulmonary hypertension is unlikely to develop before the end of the second decade, and that the peak frequency of this complication falls in the third decade of life. Thus, operation should not be postponed beyond the age of 18, unless important reasons for the delay are evident. In general the operation is recommended as soon as the diagnosis is established; small children recover more quickly from the effects of the operation than older ones and are less likely to have even the minor complications (e.g., arrhythmias) that may be present at older ages. In patients who are symptomatic early operation is, of course, indicated.

The question on the other end of the spectrum is: When are patients inoperable? One group of patients in the inoperable category are those with severe pulmonary hypertension who have either balanced or reversed interatrial shunts. Patients with pulmonary hypertension who have sizable left-to-right shunts are always considered surgical candidates. It is doubtful, however, whether operations should be performed in those with shunts of a ratio of $1\frac{1}{2}$ to 1 or less, for reasons explained above. In general, patients with severe pulmonary hypertension (and elevated pulmonary vascular resistance) are routinely operated upon if the shunt is 2 to 1 or greater. Those with shunts between 2 to 1 and 1½ to 1 are in the "gray zone" in which individual decisions have to be weighed carefully.

Elderly patients with large left-to-right shunts and normal pulmonary vascular resistance are operated upon routinely, regardless of whether or not arrhythmias and cardiac failure are present. The high incidence of these complications makes it justifiable to operate even if patients happen to be completely asymptomatic. It is well to remember, though, that the risk in such patients is higher than the overall 1 per cent figure, that the rate of postoperative complications and sequels is relatively high, and that the operation is no longer "curative" in this group. Nevertheless, the benefits appear to outweigh the risks.

In *septum primum* type atrial septal defect, surgical considerations differ from those indicated above. The more serious clinical conditions and accelerated rate of progression make these patients more urgent surgical candidates. Some patients have to be operated upon very early in life. The higher risk of the operation is usually balanced by the fact that the operation is more often remedial than prophylactic. Yet, in children with primum type defects who are asymptomatic and do not show very large interatrial shunts, some consideration should be given to conservative management, especially if the available surgical team does not have wide experience in handling this type of lesion.

Decisions regarding clefts in atrioventricular valves are difficult: they may be perplexing, both in situations in which valve incompetence is present and in those in which they are clinically "silent." Here surgical experience is at a premium.

Medical treatment of atrial septal defect can be summarized as follows:

1. Prevention of infective endocarditis is generally not indicated in patients with the secundum type atrial septal defect, since the incidence of this complication is virtually nil. In those with the primum type defect the usual measures should be applied.

2. Use of antibiotics as prophylaxis for children susceptible to repetitive respiratory infections has been recommended by some; the efficacy of this measure has not been demonstrated. Early surgical closure offers a more satisfactory solution.

3. No limitation of activities needs to be imposed beyond those produced by the patient's symptoms.

4. Inoperable patients with severe pulmonary hypertension are not amenable to any meaningful therapy. The use of anticoagulants has not been demonstrated to be of definite value, although it is widely applied for want of any other therapy.

5. Postoperative arrhythmias require symptomatic treatment sim-

ilar to therapy for comparable arrhythmias occurring in patients with other conditions. In those who develop persistent atrial fibrillation, control of rate is probably preferable to attempts to restore sinus rhythm, in view of anatomic changes and the size of cardiac atria.

Bibliography

Barber JM, Magidson O, Wood P: Atrial septal defect with special reference to the electrocardiogram, the pulmonary arterial pressure and the second heart sound. Brit. Heart J. *12*:277, 1950.

Campbell M: Natural history of atrial septal defect. Brit. Heart J. *32*:820, 1970.

Craig RJ, Selzer A: Natural history and prognosis of atrial septal defect. Circulation *37*:805, 1968.

Cohn LH, Morrow AG, Braunwald E: Operative treatment of atrial septal defect: Clinical and hemodynamic assessment in 175 patients. Brit. Heart J. *29*:725, 1967.

Dexter L: Atrial septal defect. Brit. Heart J. *18*:209, 1956.

Kamigaki M, Goldschlager N: Echocardiographic analysis of mitral valve motion in atrial septal defect. Amer. J. Cardiol. *30*:343, 1972.

Okada R, Glagov S, Lev M: Relation of shunt flow and right ventricular pressure to heart valve structure in atrial septal defect. Amer. Heart J. *78*:781, 1969.

Selzer A: Defects of the cardiac septums. J.A.M.A. *154*:129, 1954.

Selzer A, Lewis AE: The occurrence of chronic cyanosis in cases of atrial septal defect. Amer. J. Med. Sci. *218*:516, 1949.

Sommerville J: Ostium primum defect: factors causing deterioration in the natural history. Brit. Heart J. *27*:413, 1965.

Steinbrunn W, Cohn KE, Selzer A: Atrial septal defect associated with mitral stenosis. The Lutembacher syndrome revisited. Amer. J. Med. *48*:295, 1970.

Weyn AS, Bartle SH, Nolan TB, Dammann JF Jr.: Atrial septal defect—primum type. Circulation *32*(Suppl. III):13, 1965.

Zaver AG, Nadas AS: Atrial septal defect, secundum type. Circulation *32*(Suppl. III):24, 1965.

28

Ventricular Septal Defect

Definition. Ventricular septal defect is defined as a congenital malformation of the heart involving a communication between the two ventricles, namely a localized opening in the ventricular septum. Defects vary considerably in size, but even the largest involve only a small portion of the septum, thus excluding total absence of the septum (single ventricle). Ventricular septal defect is a lesion that occurs more often in combination with other cardiac malformations than alone. However, in this chapter only isolated defects of the ventricular septum will be discussed. The commonest associated lesion is stenosis of the outflow tract from the right ventricle (tetralogy of Fallot), which will be discussed in a later chapter. Excluded from this discussion also is acquired perforation of the ventricular septum secondary to myocardial infarction or to trauma. The ventricular septal defect is the commonest congenital lesion in infants (after the postnatal period) and in small children.

The clinical syndromes associated with interventricular communications involve a wide range, from a small left-to-right shunt and normal right-sided pressures to large communications with right-to-left shunts and severe pulmonary hypertension (Eisenmenger complex).

The most important single factor determining the natural history of ventricular septal defect is the response of the pulmonary vasculature. A critical dividing line separates smaller defects with a preserved pressure differential between the ventricles from large defects in which right ventricular pressures are equilibrated with left ventricular pressures. Consequently the two general categories will be discussed separately in regard to their clinical picture.

PATHOLOGY AND PATHOPHYSIOLOGY

Defects of the ventricular septum are the commonest congenital malformation of the heart at birth. They occur alone, or in combina-

421

tion with other malformations, as part of specific clinicopathologic syndromes. The usual site of the defect is the base of the heart—the region of the membranous septum. The commonest location of the defect on the left side of the ventricular septum is underneath the aortic valve; it opens in the right ventricle below the crista supraventricularis, behind the curtain of the tricuspid valve (Fig. 28–1). Less common are "supracristal" defects, located on the left side below the aortic valve as well, but opening above the crista supraventricularis on the right side, i.e., in the outflow tract, below the pulmonary valve. Defects in the muscular septum, located most frequently in the lowest part of the septum, near the apex, between muscular trabeculae, are the rarest (less than 10 per cent).

The defects vary in size from minute—almost pinpoint—openings to large defects involving the entire region of the membranous septum. However, it should be stressed that the largest defects still involve only a small portion of the ventricular septum, measuring not more than 2 to 3 cm. in diameter. Total absence of the ventricular septum does not represent the end of the spectrum of sizes (as it does in atrial septal defect), but is an entirely different type of malformation, almost always associated with malposition of the great vessels and a rudimentary ventricle.

While combined malformations are not included in this discussion, one lesion should be mentioned as a secondary abnormality to ventricular septal defect: aortic regurgitation due to a prolapse of the septal leaflet of the aortic valve. This lesion is usually acquired and progressive; it occurs most frequently when the defect is located high, just underneath the aortic valve leaflets.

The most important hemodynamic determinant of the ventricular septal defect is its size in relation to the size of the aortic opening. Inasmuch as there is a large systolic pressure gradient between the two ventricles, a sizable communication between them would provide a low resistance exit and thus would make ejection into the aorta impossible if normal pressure relationships were preserved.

The principle of "double outlet ventricle" can best be illustrated by a simple experiment involving a sphygmomanometer. With the cuff around the patient's arm, the pressure in the manometer cannot be raised by squeezing the rubber bulb unless the valve is at least partially closed. An open valve provides the low-resistance outlet from the system. There is a critical point in closing the valve, at which pressure can be raised in the system even though some air escapes through a partially open valve. The contracting left ventricle, given two large outlets—the aorta and the large defect—can only eject into the aorta if the pressure in the right ventricle equals that in the left; thus the two ventricles become a single pump with equilibrated pressure. This presupposes pulmonary hypertension or pulmonary stenosis. On the other hand, a small opening offers enough resistance to flow (similar to a

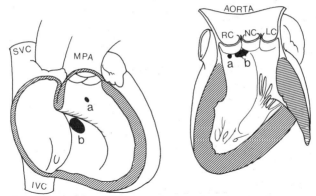

Figure 28-1. Diagrammatic presentation of two ventricular septal defects, as viewed from the right ventricle (left diagram) and from the left ventricle (right diagram). a—small supracristal defect; b—large infracristal defect. (SVC—superior vena cava; IVC—inferior vena cava; MPA—main pulmonary artery; RC—right coronary cusp; NC—noncoronary cusp; LC—left coronary cusp—of the aortic valve.)

partly closed sphygmomanometer valve) to permit a normal pressure differential. It has been shown that the critical dividing line between equilibrating and nonequilibrating ventricular septal defect is reached when the systolic size of the opening exceeds 1.5 cm. in diameter for the adult heart (1 cm.^{2} per M.^{2} of body size); this roughly represents 30 to 40 per cent of the area of the open aortic orifice.

In *nonequilibrating* ventricular septal defect the shunt is a direct function of the size of the defect. The driving force is the pressure gradient between the two ventricles in systole. The formula of Gorlin and Gorlin applicable to valve stenosis can also be applied to ventricular septal defects of the nonequilibrating variety, so that the size of the defect can be calculated from hemodynamic data. Nonequilibrating defects show a wide range of shunt sizes, which are directly related to the systolic size of the defect. Small communications may involve shunts too small to be detected by oxygen step-up in the right heart chambers; they can be diagnosed only by the qualitative hydrogen inhalation test. Large communications—those just below the critical point of equilibration—produce large shunts that may increase the pulmonary flow three- to four-fold.

Hemodynamic consequences of ventricular septal defect of the nonequilibrating variety vary with the size of the shunt (Fig. 28-2). Small defects exert no load upon the circulation, therefore are of no hemodynamic consequence. Large defects increase the pulmonary blood flow. However, in contradistinction to atrial septal defect, in which the load is carried entirely by the right ventricle, here both ventricles are involved; the left ventricle ejects its full load into the aorta

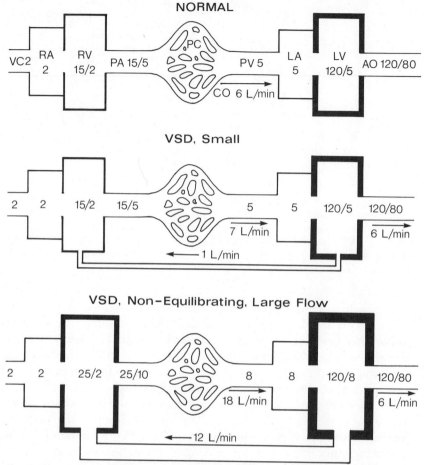

Figure 28–2. Hemodynamic diagram showing the normal circulation (*upper tracing*); an example of a small ventricular septal defect (VSD), with no hemodynamic consequences (*middle diagram*); a "small" (i.e., non-equilibrating) ventricular septal defect with a three-to-one left-to-right shunt with its hemodynamic consequences (*lower diagram*).

and the shunted blood into the right ventricle; the right ventricle ejects the increased amount into the pulmonary artery. Thus volume overload of both ventricles is present. The dividing line between the hemodynamically insignificant and significant ventricular septal defect is at a level of about a two-to-one shunt.

The nonequilibrating ventricular septal defect preserves a pressure differential between the two ventricles; however, in some cases pulmonary hypertension may secondarily and progressively increase in a manner analogous to that of late hypertension occurring in atrial septal defect. If this occurs, then ventricular septal defect may become indistinguishable from the equilibrating variety (Fig. 28–3), unless either the pulmonary hypertension is mild, or — as happens occasionally — the pressure in the right ventricle is higher than that in the left.

The *equilibrating* ventricular septal defect is invariably associated with pulmonary hypertension. (Those combined with pulmonary stenosis are not included in this discussion.) Pulmonary hypertension is present since birth: in infancy and early childhood the pulmonary arterial pressure is maintained at its systemic level by the high flow ("hyperkinetic pulmonary hypertension" — see Chapter 40); the magnitude of the shunt (thus of the pulmonary flow) is determined not by the size of the ventricular septal defect but by the respective resistances in the systemic and pulmonary circuits. The low pulmonary resistance in the postnatal period — permitting large left-to-right shunt — usually increases slowly and gradually, changing the hyperkinetic type of pulmonary hypertension into the high resistance variety. As a consequence, the left-to-right shunt gradually diminishes and eventually may lead to shunt reversal (Eisenmenger's complex). The timing of this change — i.e., from large left-to-right shunt into balanced shunt, then into right-to-left shunt — varies greatly. It may start as early as the second or third year of life. In the majority of cases, however, hyperkinetic pulmonary hypertension persists through early childhood, occasionally even through adolescence. The importance of this change in its effect upon the natural history and surgical management of the large ventricular septal defect will be discussed later.

The hemodynamic consequence of the pulmonary hypertension combined with the initial left-to-right shunt is the imposition of an overload upon the right ventricle in excess of that of the large left-to-right shunt alone Thus right ventricular hypertrophy may predominate early and become more severe as the resistance in the pulmonary circuit increases.

NONEQUILIBRATING VENTRICULAR SEPTAL DEFECT

Clinical Picture

Natural History. The *small ventricular septal defect* that exerts no hemodynamic effects upon the circulation is an eminently benign lesion. Recognized by its characteristic murmur, small communications are not associated with any other detectable abnormality. The only risk involved in this lesion lies in its susceptibility to infective endocarditis. A significant number of such communications close spontaneously; many, probably the majority, persist through life.

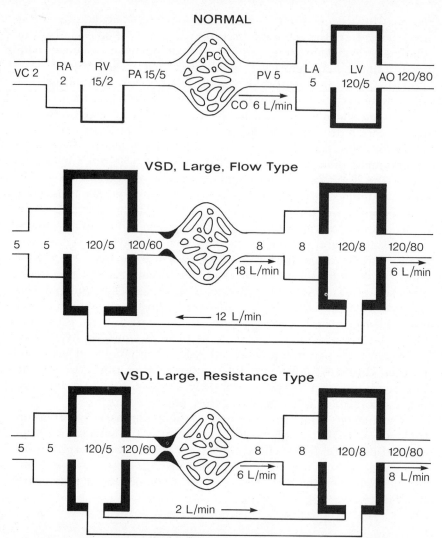

Figure 28–3. Hemodynamic diagram showing the normal circulation (*top*), and two examples of large (equilibrating) ventricular septal defects: High-flow type with a three-to-one flow (*middle diagram*) and high resistance type with a shunt reversal (a 2 liter right-to-left shunt) (*lower diagram*).

The *larger nonequilibrating ventricular septal defect* imposes an overload upon the circulatory system. The natural history of this type of communication is not well known; it may well merge in infancy with the "large" defect and then separate from it with growth (defects tend to become smaller with aging, seldom, if ever, larger). In childhood, the natural history parallels that of other left-to-right shunts of appreciable magnitude. Clinical disability may be present, but the majority of patients remain asymptomatic. Cardiac enlargement and electrocardiographic abnormalities attest to the significant nature of the abnormality and bring such patients within the group in which surgical correction is undertaken. While no exact figures are available, it is probable that patients in this category may develop pulmonary hypertension earlier, perhaps also more often, than those with atrial septal defect. Survival to old age — a relatively common occurrence in atrial septal defect — is unusual in this disease.

The postsurgical course of patients operated upon for nonequilibrating ventricular septal defect is also less well known than that of the much commoner atrial septal defect. Atrial arrhythmias are less often encountered in the immediate postoperative period, or in the later course. Many patients are left with a permanent complete right bundle branch block; occasionally complete heart block of surgical origin requires the insertion of a pacemaker. The long-range course of patients operated on in childhood or early adult life requires further follow-up. The unanswered questions involve the late effects of right ventriculotomy, if any, and the long-range effects of the damage to the right side of the conduction system.

Diagnosis

Case Finding. The essential and most characteristic feature of interventricular communications of the nonequilibrating type is a loud holosystolic murmur located along the left sternal border. Its intensity and location make it difficult to overlook, even at perfunctory examinations; hence the discovery of this lesion occurs as a rule early in life, often immediately after birth. The great majority of patients who are discovered as having this lesion are at the asymptomatic stage.

Objectives of Diagnostic Evaluation. With the clinical diagnosis often established beyond reasonable doubt by simple clinical examination, the evaluation has the following specific objectives:

- Definitive confirmation of the diagnosis of ventricular septal defect;
- Determination of the magnitude of the shunt;
- Evaluation of the effects of the lesion upon the pulmonary circulation;
- Search for significant associated lesions.

Physical Findings. The *small* ventricular septal defect (pulmonary to systemic flow ratio of 1½ to 1 or less) is characterized by a sole abnormal finding: the loud holosystolic murmur. The murmur is located along the left sternal border; the usual infracristal location of the defect makes the point of maximum intensity at the lower part of the border; supracristal ventricular septal defects may produce murmurs located in the second and third intercostal space, left sternal border. The murmur is of grade 4 to 6 intensity and is usually associated with a systolic thrill—an expression of the lower frequencies of this harsh murmur. It is most often localized to a relatively small area and shows no specific radiation. The apical impulse, the precordial motion, and the cardiac sounds are all normal and no other abnormalities are, as a rule, present.

Larger nonequilibrating ventricular septal defects show holosystolic murmurs identical with those described above, this feature being related to a high velocity flow between ventricles driven by a high pressure differential. However, clinical evidence of increased cardiac workload here becomes apparent, its extent determined by the size of the shunt. The findings then may include the following in addition to the characteristic murmur:

- Forceful apical impulse, suggesting left ventricular hypertrophy and hyperkinesia;

- Increase in overall precordial motion;

- S3 gallop sound;

- Mid-diastolic rumbling apical murmur resulting from increased flow through the mitral valve;

- Wide splitting of the second sound (less constantly encountered).

Radiological Features. Normal cardiovascular shadow is expected in the small ventricular septal defect. In larger communications of this category, varying degrees of cardiomegaly and increase in size of the pulmonary vessels are found. The diagnostic points include the following:

- Cardiac enlargement involves both sides of the heart, often all four chambers;

- Increased pulmonary vascularity is present, associated with prominence of the pulmonary artery and its principal branches.

Electrocardiographic Features. A normal electrocardiogram can be expected in patients with small ventricular septal defect; larger defects produce variable electrocardiographic changes that may include the following:

- pattern of left ventricular hypertrophy,

- pattern of biventricular hypertrophy,
- "balanced" pattern showing merely T-wave abnormalities,
- rarely, right ventricular hypertrophy.

Vectorcardiographic examination does not present any characteristic features beyond the above patterns.

Phonocardiography and Echocardiography. These play less important roles in the diagnosis of this lesion than in atrial septal defect.

Cardiac Catheterization. The detection of a left-to-right shunt is the principal objective of cardiac catheterization in small ventricular septal defect. Shunts with less than 20 per cent of the systemic flow cannot be reliably detected by the oxygen method. They are diagnosed by the hydrogen inhalation method. Larger shunts can be diagnosed by detection of a step-up in oxygen content in samples drawn from the right atrium compared with those obtained from the right ventricle. The accuracy of the test may be enhanced when several samples are drawn from each area and the results averaged, thereby minimizing the effects of streamlining of blood flow. It has been mentioned in connection with the ostium primum type atrial septal defect that the oxygen step-up in that lesion may first be found in the right ventricle. The differentiation of ventricular septal defect from low atrial septal defect may not be possible by means of cardiac catheterization alone; however, concomitant clinical features permit the establishment of the overall diagnosis of either lesion with considerable accuracy.

The essential feature of the larger nonequilibrating ventricular communications is a differential pressure gradient between the two ventricles. Cardiac catheterization may be the only means of separating the nonequilibrating ventricular septal defect with large shunt from the equilibrating variety. This differentiation will be discussed in connection with the latter variety. Readings of pulmonary arterial pressure that are normal or elevated to a modest degree (less than 75 per cent of the systemic pressure in systole) clearly place the lesion in the nonequilibrating variety.

Angiocardiography. Direct visualization of the ventricular defect can be accomplished by angiocardiography. The estimation of the size of the defect is at best approximate and can be done more reliably by means of oxygen determination. However, the location of the defect as shown by angiocardiography may be of importance, particularly in patients in whom surgical treatment is contemplated.

Differential Points in Diagnostic Evaluation. The differential diagnosis of the ventricular septal defect of the nonequilibrating variety includes the following problems:

1. Differentiation of the small ventricular septal defect from innocent murmurs should present no difficulties because innocent mur-

murs are of the ejection variety and the VSD murmur is a holosystolic one; however, inexperienced clinicians commonly confuse the two types of murmurs.

2. Mitral regurgitation may be difficult to differentiate from ventricular septal defect at all levels; trivial mitral regurgitation and small ventricular septal defect both show holosystolic murmur as the only abnormality; the location of the murmurs differs but there may be an area of overlap. Larger ventricular septal defect and moderately severe mitral regurgitation resemble each other in respect to the systolic murmur, the S3 gallop, and the diastolic rumbling murmur, and in many of the radiographic and electrocardiographic details. An echocardiographic study—or if necessary cardiac catheterization—can resolve the diagnostic dilemma.

3. Other shunting lesions—atrial septal defect, patent ductus arteriosus—show some clinical features in common with the small ventricular septal defect, but, in general, differentiation is not too difficult.

4. The presence or absence of pulmonary stenosis in addition to the ventricular septal defect may be difficult to determine on clinical grounds, because the ejection murmur of pulmonary stenosis may blend with the holosystolic murmur of the ventricular septal defect.

Indications for Invasive Studies. The need for complete evaluation of all patients with significant left-to-right shunt is evident; the "gray zone" group of patients includes those in whom a small, nonsurgical ventricular septal defect can be diagnosed with reasonable certainty on clinical grounds. Approaches to this problem vary in different institutions. It is felt that a simple right-sided cardiac catheterization that would establish the diagnosis of ventricular septal defect and confirm its trivial nature is always worthwhile; the negligible risk is well justified by the benefit of a definitive diagnosis.

Therapy

The objectives of therapy for nonequilibrating ventricular septal defect are as follows:

1. Selection of candidates for surgical treatment,

2. Selection of the optimal timing for the operation,

3. Prevention of infective endocarditis,

4. Optimal management of nonsurgical cases.

Goals of surgical treatment include the prevention of pulmonary hypertension and of hemodynamic sequels of cardiac overload. The additional potential benefit, that of preventing infective endocarditis, does not balance the risk of the operation in those patients who do not show any evidence of circulatory overload, and thus in whom this would represent the sole reason for operating. It is generally agreed that ventricular septal defect with shunts of less than 1½ to 1 do not require surgical closure. Shunt ratios of 2 to 1 or larger, on the other hand, affect hemodynamics significantly and such patients are, as a rule, considered surgical candidates. The in-between zone—those with ratios of 1½ to 2—need individual decisions based on the presence or absence of clinical evidence of increased circulatory load. It should be reiterated, as explained in Chapter 8, that calculation of shunts is subject to considerable error, hence the magnitude of the clinical consequences of the shunt may be a better guide for the selection of patients for surgery than the actual shunt figures.

Now that the frequency of spontaneous closure of the defects has been definitely demonstrated, the timing of the operation presents considerable difficulty. On the one hand, large left-to-right shunt may bring about early pulmonary hypertension and render the patient inoperable; on the other hand, it is now known that spontaneous closure may occur at any time, not merely during infancy. Perhaps the most logical approach is to follow patients carefully, subjecting them to periodic right-sided cardiac catheterizations. Medical management is justifiable if the pulmonary arterial pressure is normal, but its rise—even small—detected on serial studies, would constitute an indication to proceed with the operation. During the intervals between hemodynamic studies, management should be guided by careful clinical observation geared at finding changes by means of noninvasive techniques.

The prevention of infective endocarditis requires the standard approach of penicillin prophylaxis prior to and after dental procedures and any other conditions potentially associated with bacteremias.

Medical treatment other than the abovementioned penicillin therapy involves mainly prudent regulation of activities; in general, no restrictions need be imposed on patients with shunts too small to require operation; all desired physical activities, pregnancy, and incidental surgical operations should be permitted and the patient assumed to represent a normal risk, save for the possibility of the infection.

LARGE (EQUILIBRATING) VENTRICULAR SEPTAL DEFECT

Clinical Picture

Natural History. In the presence of a large ventricular septal defect the left ventricle becomes a "double outlet ventricle" from which the ejection can take two pathways. The proportion of blood ejected into the aorta and that ejected into the right ventricle and pulmonary artery, as already mentioned, relates to the respective resistances within the periphery of the systemic and pulmonary circuits. The presence of this situation at birth imposes conditions that may interfere with the normal postnatal adaptation. Thus, the large ventricular septal defect seriously affects the circulation during the neonatal period and later in infancy.

Physiological changes in the pulmonary circulation during the postnatal period involve a fall in pressure and result in regression of the thickness of the media of the pulmonary arterioles. This normal sequence occurring in the presence of a large ventricular septal defect would enhance the "flooding" of the lungs, since most of the blood would be ejected from the left ventricle into the low-resistance pulmonary circulation. Thus, the pressure in the right ventricle must be kept at systemic levels as a condition for survival; therefore, pulmonary hypertension exists in those with large ventricular septal defect since birth and is maintained partly by increased tone of the pulmonary vasculature and partly by increased pulmonary flow (i.e., left-to-right shunting). A certain number of infants, unable to adapt their pulmonary vasculature to the defect, die in the early postnatal period.

The relationship between the pulmonary arteriolar tone and the pulmonary blood flow in maintaining pulmonary pressure at systemic levels determines the natural history of the large ventricular septal defect during the first year of life. Infants with very large shunts develop cardiac failure with or without respiratory infections. They may respond to medical treatment, but some die unless either a palliative operation restricting pulmonary flow is performed (pulmonary arterial banding) or definite correction is feasible in infancy. Infants with more modest left-to-right shunts but higher pulmonary vascular resistances may sail through the first year of life without apparent ill effects.

Experience has shown that toward the end of the first year of life adaptive changes in the pulmonary circulation begin to appear which make ventricular septal defect more tolerable. Some defects close spontaneously. Some reduce the pulmonary shunt by elevating pulmonary resistance to the extent that their circulation is no longer overtaxed. Thus after the first year of life children who did not undergo surgical treatment improve, often becoming asymptomatic.

All children with large ventricular septal defects have severe pulmonary hypertension; the great majority still have large left-to-right shunts. The natural course of the disease in those who do not show spontaneous closure of the defect is a gradual increase in pulmonary vascular resistance with a corresponding fall in pulmonary flow. It is obvious that this process involves a slowly progressive change from an operable cardiac defect to an inoperable one. Thus, the critical issue is the timing of this change. Although not enough longitudinal studies have been performed to provide the final answer, evidence available suggests that only a small minority of young children develop severe vascular changes; in the majority this occurs in late childhood or early adult life.

Gradual progression of the process of pulmonary vascular disease leads to a change from a left-to-right shunt to a balanced shunt and then to a right-to-left shunt. Once a significant right-to-left shunt is established, the patient may develop overt cyanosis, polycythemia and clubbing of digits ("Eisenmenger complex"). It appears paradoxical, but patients with large ventricular septal defect and high pulmonary vascular resistance tolerate the lesion well. Many patients are asymptomatic or only mildly limited in their activities for a long period of time. Survival into middle age is common, and a few live into their fifties and beyond.

The principal complications of large ventricular septal defect include the following:

- Infective endocarditis (rarer than in the small ventricular septal defect);

- Consequences of pulmonary hypertension: right ventricular failure, pulmonary artery rupture;

- Consequences of polycythemia (in Eisenmenger complex): thrombotic phenomena.

Diagnosis

Case Finding. Patients with large ventricular septal defect are detected under a variety of conditions. Many are diagnosed after birth either because of the murmur or when they develop postnatal cardiac failure (which occasionally precedes the appearance of the murmur). Many escape detection and are recognized later in life, sometimes when shunt reversal is already present.

Objectives of Evaluation. In large ventricular septal defect the presence of pulmonary hypertension is often self-evident. Evaluation of the patient serves the purpose of establishing the definitive diagnosis, differentiating from other forms of pulmonary hypertension — with or without congenital lesions — and, most of all, of determining the ratio of systemic to pulmonary resistance as the index of operability.

Physical Findings. The holosystolic murmur is still the hallmark of the large ventricular septal defect, although its presence is not as constant as in smaller defects and its features may be less characteristic.

The location of the murmur is similar to that of smaller communications; however, its intensity is often lower. Some patients present themselves with soft murmurs. Occasionally the murmur may be altogether absent—most frequently in defects with balanced shunts or right-to-left shunts. Apical diastolic rumbling murmurs occur only in patients with large left-to-right shunts, thus are less often found in adults with large ventricular septal defect than in those with smaller defects. Severe pulmonary hypertension often makes the pulmonary valve incompetent, producing early diastolic blowing murmurs along the upper left sternal border. Pulmonary hypertension is evidenced by a loud second component of the second heart sound; the narrow splitting often produces the effect of a single booming second sound. Ejection sounds are also commonly present. Motion of the precordium may provide some information regarding the flow-resistance relationship; exaggerated precordial motion suggests large flow; discrete parasternal lift, high resistance.

Radiological Features. Evidence for pulmonary hypertension is provided by the enlargement of the pulmonary artery and its principal branches. The enlargement of the pulmonary vessels ranges from a modest degree to giant, aneurysmal enlargement of the various segments of the pulmonary arterial tree. Abrupt tapering off of smaller central branches is seen in high resistance pulmonary hypertension, and increased vascularity extending into the periphery of the lungs in high flow pulmonary hypertension. The cardiac size also varies from modest to severe cardiomegaly. All four cardiac chambers may participate in the enlargement.

Electrocardiographic Features. In the presence of systemic pressure in the pulmonary circulation the electrocardiogram shows right ventricular hypertrophy or biventricular hypertrophy. The former is likely to appear with high resistance pulmonary hypertension; the latter with high flow pulmonary hypertension. This may be corroborated by vectorcardiography.

Other Noninvasive Tests. Phonocardiography adds little to the diagnosis beyond documentation of the various auscultatory findings. Echocardiography is not consistently helpful in the differential diagnosis of ventricular septal defects, although certain subaortic defects may be shown directly by this technique.

Cardiac Catheterization. The critical point in establishing the diagnosis of the large ventricular septal defect is the demonstration of equilibrated pressure in the two ventricles. It should be emphasized that "equilibration," i.e., equality of systolic pressures in the two ventricles, may not be as easy to demonstrate as might be expected. Firstly, it requires simultaneous recording of pressure from both ventricles inasmuch as pressures vary from minute to minute. Secondly, the practice of recording systemic pressure from a systemic artery and right-sided systolic pressure from the pulmonary artery may introduce some apparent differences, since systolic pressures in the arteries are not always identical with those in the respective ventricles. Thus, it is assumed that if pressures are within 25 per cent of each other, the probability of equilibration is good. An additional point may be made in recording simultaneously pulmonary arterial and systemic arterial pressures during a Valsalva maneuver and showing that the pressure changes in the four stages occur simultaneously (in nonequilibrated circulations there is a slight delay between right- and left-sided pressures in the responses to the maneuver).

The second objective of the study is the evaluation of left-to-right shunt. The ratio of systemic to pulmonary flow indicates shunt magnitude, yet sampling of blood from the pulmonary artery may not give representative "mixed" venous blood because of streamlining, so that conventional calculations in ventricular septal defect may be subject to error. Some investigators doubt the accuracy of shunt calculation to such an extent that they consider the intensity of holosystolic murmur a better index of large pulmonary flow than calculated values of shunt and resistance (Hollman et al., 1963).

The third objective of the hemodynamic study is the detection and estimation of right-to-left shunt at the late stages of ventricular septal defect. The mere presence of arterial oxygen unsaturation does not prove shunt reversal, because pulmonary hypertension may cause interference with the intrapulmonary gas exchange. Shunt reversal can be demonstrated by dye dilution curves or by angiocardiography.

Angiocardiography. Angiocardiographic studies permit the determination of the location of the defect and of the direction of the shunting, therefore often are of crucial diagnostic importance.

Differential Points in Evaluation. The differentiation of conditions which can be confused with the large ventricular septal defect depends upon the stage of the disease. In patients with large left-to-right shunt the differentiation from other shunting lesions has to be made. In high resistance type ventricular septal defects, various forms of pulmonary hypertension and other cyanotic congenital lesions need to be considered in the differentiation.

Indications for Invasive Studies. The need for establishment of the diagnosis in patients with a serious congenital cardiac defect is axiomatic; hence cardiac catheterization studies are routinely indicated. In overtly cyanotic patients who obviously are not surgical candidates, a differentiation from other, correctable lesions is essential. However, the most important role of cardiac catheterization is the longitudinal following of infants and young children. The timing of the operation may determine permanent curability, and yet operating too early may not be advisable in view of the possibility of spontaneous closure of the defect.

Therapy

Therapeutic problems related to the large ventricular septal defect include the following:

- management of the patient during the first year of life,
- determination of operability and the timing of the operation,
- management of the inoperable patient.

During the postnatal period the diagnosis of a ventricular septal defect imposes the obligation of a very careful follow-up during the critical first months of life. Development of cardiac failure provides the clinician with the option of three choices:

- medical treatment,
- palliative surgical treatment (pulmonary arterial banding),
- total surgical correction.

Medical treatment offers advantages. Firstly, the critical time period of circulatory difficulty is finite: toward the end of the first year tendency to failure decreases or disappears; secondly, the rate of spontaneous closure is high; thirdly, many infants respond to digitalis and sodium restriction more dramatically than do adults.

If medical treatment is unsuccessful, surgical therapy has to be considered. Total correction of the defect offers obvious advantages over a palliative operation, which will require reoperation later in life. Yet, the risk of operating on an infant is unduly high in all but a few highly specialized infant surgical units.

In patients who survive the critical early period of life, surgical therapy is indicated because, unlike those with the atrial septal defect, all patients are likely to become inoperable. The timing depends upon two factors: the age at which the risk reaches the plateau of lowest level, and the probability of spontaneous closure. It has been mentioned already that these two considerations produce a dilemma which may be resolved only if large numbers of patients are followed longitudinally.

The determination of operability is based on the probability that a sufficiently large left-to-right shunt is present to permit significant fall of pulmonary arterial pressure after the defect is closed. Fall in pulmonary vascular resistance has been observed in isolated cases. However, whereas in patients with mitral valve disease high pulmonary vascular resistance is reversible, no consistent data are available that such reversibility exists in pulmonary vascular disease associated with cardiac shunts. The preponderance of evidence points in the other direction: namely, that pulmonary vascular disease in this situation is irreversible except for isolated cases. Thus, in large ventricular septal defect surgical goals have been more modest than those in some other congenital lesions (including the smaller interventricular communications), inasmuch as some degree of pulmonary hypertension usually remains after shunt elimination. It is generally assumed that shunts with flow ratios of 2 to 1 or larger are benefited by closure of the defect. The difficulty of shunt calculation has been commented upon; hence surgical decisions may be more difficult here than in other lesions.

Inoperable patients require as a rule little medical care. Many remain asymptomatic for many years. No known measures are available to prevent the progression of pulmonary vascular disease or of the resulting complications. Anticoagulant therapy has been tried and generally abandoned. Polycythemia, if severe, may require occasional phlebotomies, but the effects of these procedures are not always beneficial. Late stages of the disease may involve the development of cardiac failure, in which case conventional measures are applied. Patients may also die as the result of thrombotic complications or rupture of a pulmonary arterial vessel.

VENTRICULAR SEPTAL DEFECT AND AORTIC REGURGITATION

Aortic regurgitation is usually not an associated congenital malformation but an acquired sequel to certain types of interventricular communications. It is likely to occur in defects located high, just underneath an aortic leaflet. The leaflet, usually the noncoronary cusp, losing its support, enlarges, becomes redundant, and prolapses, making the valve incompetent. This complication may develop regardless of the size of the interventricular communication; hence it may be associated with large as well as with nonequilibrating ventricular septal defect.

Aortic regurgitation is as a rule progressive. The presence of ventricular septal defect is usually detected in the postnatal period; the diastolic murmur of aortic regurgitation appears later, most frequently after the age of two. At first, the murmur may be the only sign of aortic regurgitation; gradually the pulse and pressure may increase and the fully developed picture of severe aortic regurgitation may become apparent.

This combination of lesions is often poorly tolerated; cardiac failure may develop early in life. Some patients, however, manage to remain asymptomatic and reach adulthood without difficulty. Nevertheless, the aortic lesion tends to be progressive and the patient may eventually develop serious disability.

The physical findings combine the characteristic features of both lesions. If aortic regurgitation appears with nonequilibrating ventricular septal defect (the majority), evidence for left ventricular hypertrophy appears early and in more severe form than with the defect alone. The combination of the holosystolic murmur and the early diastolic murmur—both located in the same area of the thorax—produces a mumur very similar to, though not identical with, the continuous murmur. It resembles more closely the murmur of ruptured sinus of Valsalva than that of patent ductus arteriosus. Peripheral signs of aortic regurgitation—wide pulse pressure and collapsing pulses—characterize all three lesions: large ducts, sinus of Valsalva aneurysm with rupture, and this lesion.

Treatment of this combination of lesions presents a therapeutic dilemma. Closure of the ventricular septal defect alone in patients with mild aortic regurgitation may leave the patient with a more severe aortic lesion. Corrective surgical procedures upon the prolapsing leaflets have been largely unsuccessful. Valve replacement combined with the closure of the defect is the surgical treatment of choice. Yet, one hesitates to place an artificial valve in a child or an adolescent, in view of all the uncertainty regarding its long-range fate, especially in cases with milder degrees of aortic regurgitation. Difficult individual decisions have to be made, therefore: whether to recommend operation and when. Such decisions should be guided by the disability of the patient and the rapidity of the progression of the lesions.

Cardiac catheterization and angiocardiography are, as a rule, performed for the study of the ventricular septal defect. The additional presence of aortic regurgitation cannot be directly quantified by catheterization, although its effect upon left ventricular performance has an important bearing upon the evaluation. Angiocardiography permits estimation of the severity of aortic valve incompetence and is essential in the differentiation of ventricular septal defect with aortic regurgitation from patent ductus arteriosus with a large shunt, and from rupture of a sinus of Valsalva aneurysm.

POSTSURGICAL PROBLEMS IN VENTRICULAR SEPTAL DEFECT

Patients who undergo surgical treatment for ventricular septal defect represent a population in which the principal lesion has been eliminated but the cardiac condition not necessarily cured. A large range of problems affects the course of such patients:

1. The role of ventriculotomy is as yet unknown. Patients who had a smaller ventricular septal defect repaired and who have normal pulmonary arterial pressure usually have normal circulatory dynamics. Yet, in the few patients who had postoperative studies, the cardiac output was often abnormally low during exercise; it is implied, though by no means proved, that cardiac function in such patients may be slightly

depressed. Clinically this appears inconsequential; the crucial question is whether with advancing age it will remain so. The answer to this question is not yet available.

2. An analogous question pertains to the role of complete right bundle branch block that is produced surgically in the majority of patients who undergo ventricular septal repair. The possible role of this acquired conduction defect in the production of complete heart block late in life can only be surmised.

3. Inasmuch as many patients operated upon for ventricular septal defect also have pulmonary hypertension, the problem of pulmonary vascular disease can be looked upon in terms of two stages:

- Patients with large flow and normal or near normal resistance represent a population analogous to those with atrial septal defect. Here the fall of pulmonary arterial pressure can be anticipated and return to normal is probable. A small number, however, may gradually develop pulmonary hypertension in spite of the fact that its initiating cause has been eliminated.

- Patients with elevated pulmonary vascular resistance will show residual pulmonary hypertension (as stated, reduction of pulmonary resistance represents an exception rather than the rule). In many, stationary, moderate pulmonary hypertension persists without further progression. In some, progressive pulmonary hypertension persists after a temporary postoperative fall, in which case the closure of the defect merely protects the patient from shunt reversal and cyanosis. Yet, it appears, although definitive comparison is not available, that patients with the Eisenmenger complex may take a more benign course than those with isolated severe pulmonary hypertension; hence the operation may be counterproductive in such cases. Finally, there are patients in whom the calculation of the shunt ratios was faulty and in whom the pulmonary arterial pressure is never altered by the operation. These patients, more consistently than the preceding group, may be worse off than if they were never operated upon.

Bibliography

Cartmill TB, DuShane JW, McGoon DC, Kirklin JW: Results of repair of ventricular septal defect. J. Thorac. Cardiovasc. Surg. 52:586, 1966.

Edwards JE: Functional pathology of the pulmonary vascular tree in congenital cardiac disease. Circulation 15:164, 1957.

Halliday-Smith KA, Olsen EGJ, Oakley CM, Goodwin JF, Clelland WP: Ventricular septal defect and aortic regurgitation. Thorax 24:257, 1969.

Hoffman, JIE, Rudolph AM: The natural history of ventricular septal defect in infancy. Amer. J. Cardiol. 16:634, 1965.

Hollman A, Morgan JJ, Goodwin JF, Fields H: Auscultatory and phonocardiographic findings in ventricular septal defect. A study of 93 surgically treated patients. Circulation 28:94, 1963.

Nadas AS, Thilenius OG, LaFarge CG, Hauck AJ.: Ventricular septal defect and aortic regurgitation: Medical and pathologic aspects. Circulation 29:862, 1964.

Rudolph AM: The changes in the circulation after birth. Circulation 41:334, 1970.

Selzer A: Defect of the ventricular septum. Arch. Int. Med. 84:798, 1949.

Selzer A: Defects of the cardiac septums. J.A.M.A. 154:129, 1954.

Selzer A, Lacqueur GA: The Eisenmenger complex and its relation to the uncomplicated defect of the ventricular septum. Arch. Int. Med. 87:218, 1951.

Wood P.: The Eisenmenger syndrome or pulmonary hypertension with reversed central shunts. Brit. Med. J. 2:701, 1958.

Wood P, Magidson O, Wilson PAO: Ventricular septal defect with a note on acyanotic Fallot's Tetralogy. Brit. Heart J. 16:387, 1954.

29

Aorticopulmonary
Communications

Definition. Included in this discussion is the persistence of the fetal ductus arteriosus and its rare variant, the aorticopulmonary septal defect (aorticopulmonary window). It will not include combinations of congenital malformations in which patency of ductus arteriosus coexists with other lesions.

PATHOLOGY AND PATHOPHYSIOLOGY

The fetal duct normally connects the aortic arch just beyond the origin of the right subclavian artery with the main pulmonary artery at the point of origin of the left pulmonary artery. In most subjects the ligamentum arteriosum—a residuum of the closed duct—can be identified. Persistent patency of the duct constitutes one of the common congenital anomalies. The duct varies in length, width, and location: the average length is 2 to 4 cm., the average width 1 to 1.5 cm. The commonest type of patent ductus arteriosus is a small communication between the two great vessels; less often an abnormally large "widely patent ductus arteriosus" connects the trunks. Patent ductus is often a part of complex cardiac malformations and may play an important role as a condition of survival (e.g., in some forms of transposition of the great vessels, or in pulmonary atresia).

The aorticopulmonary septal defect represents an opening between the first portion of the ascending aorta and the main pulmonary artery. The size of the opening varies, usually being between 1 and 3 cm. in diameter. It is most commonly located just above the two sets of valves.

In a manner analogous to that of the ventricular septal defect, ducts can be classified as "small" and "large" according to the effect they exert upon the pulmonary circulation.

Small ducts are the site of left-to-right shunts between the aorta and the pulmonary artery. Inasmuch as a pressure gradient exists between the two arterial trunks throughout the cardiac cycle, continuous flow through the duct takes place.

As in the ventricular septal defect, the magnitude of flow is a direct function of the size of the communication (Fig. 29–1). Small communications have no hemodynamic consequences. Larger communications provide a low-pressure exit from the arterial system that may profoundly alter circulatory dynamics. In normal subjects the

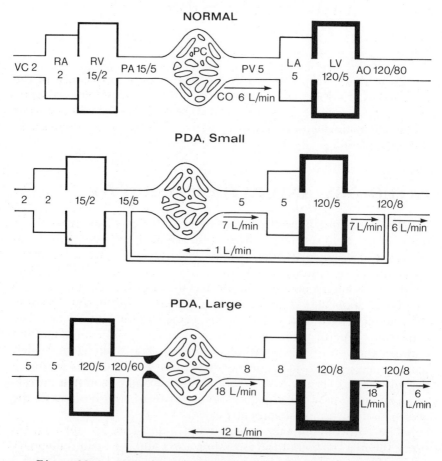

Figure 29–1. Hemodynamic diagram showing the normal circulation *(top)* and two examples of patent ductus arteriosus (PDA): small duct, without hemodynamic consequences *(middle diagram);* large duct with a large flow (three-to-one left-to-right shunt) and pressure equilibration *(lower diagram).*

closed arterial system (between the aortic valve and the arterioles in the periphery) acts as a hydraulic filter ("Windkessel") which changes intermittent pumping action into constant capillary flow. The presence of a leak in this system, such as occurs in patent ductus arteriosus (also in aortic regurgitation or in arteriovenous fistulae), causes the premature emptying of the arterial system, which is compensated by a more abrupt left ventricular contraction, by a higher systolic level of pressure, a lower diastolic pressure, and a rapid fall in arterial pressure. Increased workload upon the left ventricle is imposed by these changes as well as by the larger stroke volume (which includes the forward flow as well and the volume of blood re-entering the pulmonary circulation via the duct).

When the duct is still larger, elevated pressure in the pulmonary artery is required as a condition of survival — in a manner analogous to the equilibrating type of ventricular septal defect. As in the latter, the high pressure in the pulmonary circuit may be maintained by increased pulmonary flow derived from the ductal shunt, by high pulmonary arteriolar resistance, or by a combination of both. The flow through the duct in this variety may thus be left-to-right, balanced, or right-to-left. In cases with shunt reversal, the anatomic position of the duct causes unoxygenated blood from the pulmonary artery to enter directly into the descending aorta.

Hemodynamic consequences of the patency of ductus arteriosus justify three distinct clinical syndromes:

1. Small duct with negligible hemodynamic effects;

2. Intermediate-sized duct with evidence of left ventricular overload and peripheral effects upon the pulse pressure and pulse contour;

3. Large duct with pulmonary arterial pressures at systemic levels.

The aorticopulmonary septal defect usually fits into the third category; only in the minority of cases is there a pressure gradient between the two arterial trunks, placing them in the second category.

SMALL DUCTUS ARTERIOSUS

Natural History. Basically a benign lesion, small ducts have no measurable adverse effects upon cardiovascular function. Their only clinical significance lies in their being a potential nidus for infective endocarditis. There are no known effects of this type of patent ductus arteriosus upon life expectancy in patients except for the above infection.

Diagnosis. The diagnosis of small ducts is based entirely upon the presence of a continuous murmur at the upper portion of the left anterior hemothorax. By definition, other physical signs, radiographic signs, and the electrocardiogram are all normal.

In its characteristic form the continuous murmur provides at least a 95 per cent probability of correctly identifying patent ductus arteriosus. On this basis in some cardiac centers children are subjected to surgical closure of the duct without further studies. Whether the remote risk of performing an unnecessary thoracotomy in the small minority of cases with ductus-like murmurs originating elsewhere justifies routine invasive studies remains a matter of individual preference.

Conditions that may be confused with the small patent ductus arteriosus include the following (assuming that the murmur is the only abnormality):

- Venous hum; experienced diagnosticians are unlikely to confuse the two conditions, but such errors are common. Various maneuvers can obliterate the venous hum but not the ductus murmur;

- Coronary arteriovenous fistula: the murmur may be identical with that of a ductus; its location is usually different, the former being lower upon the thorax;

- Anomalous origin of the coronary artery from the pulmonary artery: continuous murmurs are not always present; if they are the resemblance to the duct may be great;

- Branch stenosis of the left pulmonary artery: continuous murmurs are occasionally present; location of the murmur tends to be more lateral than the duct.

Invasive studies include cardiac catheterization and angiocardiography. Oxygen step-up cannot be expected to provide a reliable answer in small ducts; rarely, the duct may be entered by the catheter. The diagnosis depends upon a positive hydrogen inhalation test; yet, this test will not discriminate between a small duct and the origin of the left coronary artery from the pulmonary artery. The final diagnosis can be made only by means of retrograde arterial catheterization and aortographic demonstration of the duct.

Treatment. Even though the hemodynamic effects of small ducts are totally inconsequential, it is generally believed that the risk of surgical closure of the duct in children and young adults is less than that of possible infective endarteritis of the duct. This is based upon the considerations that surgical mortality of closure of the duct during the childhood period in experienced hands is about 0.25 per cent, and that the thoracic operation outside the pericardium carries no known long-range consequences or harm to the patient. It should be made clear, however, that this is merely an opinion and not a proven fact, but the opinion seems reasonable, especially since appropriate data can no longer be collected to present the final evidence. In middle age and beyond, closure of small ducts may be questioned because the risk of the operation is higher.

If surgery is not performed, patients should be instructed in the usual preventive measures against endocarditis.

INTERMEDIATE-SIZED DUCTUS ARTERIOSUS

Natural History. Infants with persistent sizable ducts often develop serious cardiac difficulties in the postnatal period. Inasmuch as it is not possible to differentiate intermediate-sized ducts from large ducts during infancy — the distinctive differential features develop only after infancy — the postnatal problems of the duct will be discussed in connection with large ducts.

Larger ducts may not be apparent in early infancy; the continuous murmur often is first heard between the first and the fourth year of life. As in other left-to-right shunting lesions, the effects upon patients vary: some may exhibit repeated respiratory infections; some show mild to moderate effort intolerance, though seldom overt cardiac failure; most remain asymptomatic.

In adults, the hemodynamic effects of patent ductus arteriosus of intermediate size resemble those of aortic regurgitation. In both defects, the overload upon the left ventricle may be considerable, and yet it is well tolerated. Effort intolerance and then failure may appear toward early middle age. Patent ductus arteriosus has, however, in addition to its effect upon the left side of the heart, high pulmonary blood flow. It may be assumed that some patients will develop pulmonary hypertension as a result of pulmonary plethora. The evidence for this can only be surmised from the occasional patients found to have pulmonary hypertension, but not at systemic levels. Patients showing severe pulmonary hypertension may be assumed to belong in the category of "large" duct. The principal complication of this lesion is infective endocarditis. Rarely, aneurysms of the ducts may develop.

It is axiomatic that patients in this category should undergo surgical treatment as soon as the diagnosis is established, considering that a curative operation at a low risk is available.

The postsurgical course is usually uneventful. The potential sequelae of opening the pericardium and of a cardiac incision are absent; not even the remote risk resulting from the use of the cardiopulmonary bypass need be feared. The operation can be considered a curative one unless it is postponed long enough to permit irreversible left ventricular hypertrophy to take place, in which case residual impairment of cardiac function may be present.

Diagnosis. The characteristic continuous murmur makes the bedside diagnosis of this lesion easy; hence the majority of patients are recognized early in life. There is a significant number of patients, however, in whom the diagnosis is altogether missed; some do not undergo physical examinations, and in others the diagnosis is incorrectly made (often aortic regurgitation on a rheumatic basis). These patients may be discovered at any age, occasionally seeking medical care for cardiac symptoms.

Physical signs include the continuous "machinery" murmur, which often is louder than that of small ducts, even though there is no good correlation between the size of the duct and the intensity of the murmur. An S3 gallop sound and an apical mid-diastolic rumbling murmur due to increased flow through the mitral valve are commonly present. Reversed splitting of the second sound may be heard in many cases. Palpatory evidence of left ventricular hypertrophy and increase in overall precordial motion are also common clinical findings. Right ventricular lift is not encountered in this category of ducts.

Peripheral pulses may be bounding or collapsing of the waterhammer variety. The diastolic pressure is low.

Radiographic studies usually reveal cardiac enlargement of variable degree; the enlargement involves only the left heart chambers. In addition, prominence of the pulmonary arterial tree is present, including increased vascularity extending into the periphery of the lungs. The aortic arch tends to be more prominent than in intracardiac shunts.

The *electrocardiogram* may show left ventricular hypertrophy; occasionally normal ventricular complexes or nonspecific patterns are found. Right ventricular hypertrophy is a strong point against the diagnosis of intermediate-sized ducts. Vectorcardiography adds little to the differential diagnosis.

Invasive diagnostic studies are indicated routinely, for each patient in whom the clinical diagnosis is made becomes a surgical candidate. The purpose of the special studies is to confirm the clinical diagnosis and to differentiate patent ductus arteriosus from the few other conditions that provide similar clinical findings, primarily aorticopulmonary septal defect, ruptured aneurysm of the sinus of Valsalva, and the combination of ventricular septal defect with aortic regurgitation.

Cardiac catheterization should provide evidence for the duct in the form of considerable oxygen step-up in the pulmonary artery over that of right ventricular blood samples. The calculation of pulmonary flow is virtually impossible, since nowhere does blood from the right ventricle and that shunted from the aorta reach a homogeneous mixture from which a representative sample may be obtained. Pulmonary arterial pressure is normal or may be elevated, but not at systemic levels. The most important means of confirming the diagnosis on cardiac catheterization is to enter the duct and demonstrate its course (as contrasted with the location of the communication in aorticopulmonary septal defect, which may give identical catheterization findings). This is possible in about 25 per cent of cases in the intermediate-sized duct.

Angiocardiography establishes the definite diagnosis and provides information regarding the size and location of the duct.

Treatment. Surgical therapy is, as stated, the correct treatment of intermediate-sized ducts. It should be performed at any age, as soon as the diagnosis is established, unless specific contraindications are present.

LARGE PATENT DUCTUS ARTERIOSUS

Natural History. Large ducts tax the circulation during the postnatal adaptive period to the extent that infants may go into severe cardiac failure during the first few weeks of life. Early diagnosis and surgical ligation of the duct is then lifesaving. As in ventricular septal defect, the course of patients with large ducts later takes a more favorable turn. With the "obligatory" pulmonary hypertension, the pulmonary vasculature may display a wide spectrum of responses: some show high pulmonary flow, others high pulmonary resistance, with all transitions in between. Early reversal of the shunt may occur — some patients develop cyanosis of the lower part of the body in early childhood. In general, the course of the large duct parallels that of the large ventricular septal defect: a certain number of patients remain asymptomatic; some show impairment of effort tolerance, some go into overt cardiac failure; frequent respiratory infections, often initiating cardiac failure, are also common. In older children and adults the disability varies: it may range from total lack of symptoms to serious limitations of activities. The fact that the physical findings of large ducts are less characteristic than those of smaller ones makes it easy to miss the correct diagnosis. In a number of patients this correctable lesion is found at the time when pulmonary hypertension has changed from high-flow to high-resistance, thus making prospects of successive surgical correction more remote. Some are recognized only at the stage of balanced or reversed shunts, then being altogether beyond the point of surgical help. Cyanosis, when present as a result of shunt reversal, involves fewer problems than when produced by intracardiac shunt, because hypoxemia here affects only the lower part of the body. However, polycythemia and its secondary consequences may affect the natural history of such cases.

The course of large ducts ligated surgically differs from that of smaller communications. Pulmonary hypertension present since birth precludes a complete cure, inasmuch as some functional abnormality of the pulmonary circulation is likely to persist. Whether patients whose ducts were ligated in the neonatal period would remain entirely normal is not known, but logically this group appears to be the only one in which good prospects for complete cure exist. The degree of residual pulmonary hypertension depends upon the respective contributions of high flow and high resistance to the maintenance of pulmonary hypertension prior to the operation. Patients with purely hyperkinetic pulmonary hypertension (i.e., with normal pulmonary arteriolar resistance) are expected to show a fall of pulmonary artery pressure to near normal levels after ligation of the duct. Yet, some hyperreactivity may remain, and the possibility of progressive pulmonary vascular disease later in life should always be considered. Marginal surgical candidates, i.e., those with small net left-to-right shunts, respond to the operation in an unpredictable way, since shunt calculations are particularly inaccurate in this group. In a sense, the postoperative response—the eventual level of the pulmonary arterial pressure—tells the story on whether or not the operation was well advised.

The eventual outcome of patients who either were inoperable or in whom the operation was unsuccessful resembles that of severe pulmonary hypertension. Right ventricular failure and rupture of a pulmonary artery represent the commonest causes of death. The effects of cyanosis and polycythemia play, as stated, a lesser role in the course of this lesion.

Diagnosis. The large duct is more difficult to recognize because the characteristic continuous murmur is almost always absent. Most patients show loud systolic murmurs, but some may show insignificant murmurs or none at all. In symptomatic patients the diagnosis of a cardiac lesion is obvious, but its identification may present considerable difficulties. In asymptomatic patients abnormal radiographic or electrocardiographic findings often direct attention to cardiac disease.

Physical findings. In patients with shunt reversal the differential cyanosis—involving the lower part of the body but sparing the brachiocephalic circulation—may be a pathognomonic finding. All patients with clinical evidence for pulmonary hypertension should be carefully screened for this clinical sign. In general, the physical diagnosis varies with the magnitude and the direction of the shunt through the duct.

The auscultatory findings include the following:

- A typical continuous ductus murmur is only occasionally found in this type of duct.

- A holosystolic murmur similar to that of the ventricular septal defect but located higher upon the chest wall is usually present in patients with high-flow pulmonary hypertension.

- Those with balanced or reversed shunts may show noncharacteristic systolic murmurs, often of the ejection variety (originating in the dilated pulmonary artery); in reversed shunt the murmur is often absent.

- Early diastolic blowing murmurs of pulmonary valve incompetence are commonly found.

- Apical rumbling—mitral flow—murmurs are uncommon; if present, they suggest a large left-to-right shunt.

- The first sound is often followed by a loud ejection sound.

- The second sound shows narrow splitting and accentuation of its late component (appearing as a single loud second sound).

- Atrial (S4) right-sided gallop sound occurs frequently.

- Palpatory evidence of right ventricular lift is usually present.

- Hyperkinetic precordial motion may be present in patients with high-flow pulmonary hypertension.

- Those with left-to-right shunt may show rapid rising pulses and wide pulse pressure; truly collapsing pulses are uncommon.

- Pulses are normal or small in patients with reversed shunt.

Radiographic findings include evidence for pulmonary hypertension. Pulmonary arteries are very large. The radiologic picture of the peripheral pulmonary vasculature depends upon the predominance of high flow or of high resistance. Cardiac size varies: patients with high resistance—especially those who acquired it early in life—may show normal or near-normal cardiac shadows, displaying usually some evidence of right ventricular enlargement. Those with high flow may show considerable degree of cardiomegaly, involving the right heart chambers or all cardiac chambers.

Electrocardiography displays characteristically the pattern of right ventricular hypertrophy, which is also present in the vectorcardiogram. These findings obviously have little discriminatory and differential value except in pointing to the presence of pulmonary hypertension.

Invasive diagnostic procedures are required in all cases to establish or confirm the diagnosis and to determine the preponderance of flow or resistance in the maintenance of high pulmonary arterial pressure.

Cardiac catheterization permits the direct entry of the catheter into the duct in a much higher percentage of cases than in patients without pulmonary hypertension. In those with shunt reversal the duct can be entered in virtually 100 per cent of cases. After the presence of a duct is established, the demonstration of pulmonary hypertension and of equilibration of pressures (similar to that in the large ventricular septal defect) represents the next priority of the test. The demonstration of the shunt by oxygen step-up may give misleading results: the common occurrence of incompetent pulmonary valve makes oxygenated blood spill into the right ventricle; hence findings overlap with those of ventricular septal defect. This difficulty is compounded by the occasional occurrence of a combination of large ventricular septal defect and large duct (especially in infants). In the presence of shunt reversal the crucial test consists of drawing simultaneously samples from the right brachial artery and a femoral artery and demonstrating significantly lower oxygen content in the latter. Indicator dilution curves may also be used.

Angiocardiography plays the decisive role in demonstrating large ducts. In left-to-right shunts injection of the contrast medium in the arch of the aorta, and in right-to-left shunts into the pulmonary artery, will demonstrate the location and size of the duct. An estimation of the magnitude and the predominant direction of the shunt can also be made by this technique.

Differential points in the diagnosis have been discussed in connection with the various procedures. As in other lesions complicated by pulmonary hypertension, it is necessary to identify the type of the underlying lesion as well as to distinguish between congenital heart disease combined with pulmonary hypertension and "primary" pulmonary hypertension. Confusion of the large duct with rheumatic heart disease is less common than in smaller ducts; nevertheless, some overlapping features may make this differentiation difficult on clinical grounds alone.

Perhaps the most critical differential diagnosis needs to be considered in infants who develop cardiac failure in the postnatal period. A high index of suspicion that patent ductus arteriosus causes failure often pays off, this being the most important surgically correctable lesion in this age group. It is important, however, to recognize that the demonstration of a large duct by aortography is not enough; coexisting lesions inoperable in infancy (e.g., large ventricular septal defect) have to be ruled out before duct ligation is undertaken.

Treatment. The optimal therapy of a large duct is early surgical closure of the duct; the timing is of essence. The principles of surgical results have already been discussed and it was pointed out that the operation in pulmonary hypertensive ducts is not curative, as it may be in simple ducts, except, perhaps, when operated upon in infancy. The success of therapy is thus contingent upon the earliest possible elimination of this lesion; therefore diagnostic skill is at premium.

The most important problem of therapy is the decision making in patients of the marginal group: in view of the spectrum that ranges from purely hyperkinetic pulmonary hypertension (good surgical prospects) to high resistance pulmonary hypertension (inoperable patients), those in the intermediate group require difficult individual decisions. It has already been explained that shunt calculation in ducts has much lower reliability than in atrial septal defect or in ventricular septal defect. A combined assessment is necessary in large ducts, taking into consideration the presence and intensity of the systolic murmur, the presence of peripheral signs of hypercirculatory state, and findings in cardiac catheterization and angiocardiography. Even the best estimates may be wrong and there is a certain amount of "trial and error" in predicting success of the closure of large ducts with marginal surgical indications. Yet, a conservative approach to the selection of patients is advisable because:

- Operations performed in patients with resistance higher than that calculated on the basis of cardiac catheterization may not only be ineffective but may produce rapid deterioration and death.

- Unoperated patients with high resistance may have many years of productive life ahead of them.

Medical therapy of patients with large ducts is of limited value. In infants, the dilemma of carrying the patient on a medical regimen that was expounded in connection with the large ventricular septal defect is not present because surgical closure of the duct can be performed easily at any age. Thus, the diagnosis of an isolated large duct calls for an immediate operation. Only unusual circumstances may provide reasons for not performing surgical closure of a large duct in patients as soon as recognized. Patients considered inoperable are permitted to engage in activities that their limitations allow; yet, young patients should be advised against choosing an occupation or hobbies requiring especially strenuous physical effort. When the patient enters the stage of cardiac failure, the usual methods are used to control it, as well as one can.

AORTICOPULMONARY SEPTAL DEFECT

The physiological consequences of this lesion are identical with those of patent ductus arteriosus. Its commonest size corresponds to that of a large duct; occasionally smaller communications are present analogous to those in the intermediate-sized duct. The clinical picture is identical with ducts of the corresponding sizes. The importance of this rare lesion lies in its requiring a more involved, technically difficult open heart operation rather than simple extrapericardial closure of the duct; hence preoperative identification of this lesion and its diagnostic differentiation from the duct are essential. The majority of patients, showing equilibrated pressures in the arterial trunks, do not display a continuous murmur. The importance of angiographic differentiation of the anatomic lesion in patients with the physiological findings of the large duct who are to be operated upon is self-evident, even though the statistical odds against finding a defect rather than a patent duct are several hundred to one. In those with shunt reversal or balanced shunt the differentiation is merely of academic interest. In the few patients with smaller shunt through the defect, the quality of the continuous murmur can provide a clue: the murmurs have been described as located lower on the chest wall and sounding more superficial. In all other respects aortico-pulmonary septal defect overlaps with patent ductus arteriosus of equivalent size.

Bibliography

Campbell M: Natural history of persistent ductus arteriosus. Brit. Heart J. 30:4, 1968.

Fairley GH, Goodwin JF: Patent ductus arteriosus in adult life. Brit. J. Dis. Chest. 53:263, 1959.

Espino-Vela J, Cardenas N, Cruz R: Patent ductus arteriosus with special reference to patients with pulmonary hypertension. Circulation 37–37(Suppl. V):45, 1968.

Hultgren H, Selzer A, Purdy A, Holman E, Gerbode F: The syndrome of patent ductus arteriosus with pulmonary hypertension. Circulation 8:15, 1953.

30
Right-Sided Outflow Obstruction

Definition. Obstructive lesions in the outflow tract of the right ventricle or in the pulmonary arterial system constitute a large segment of congenital malformations of the heart. They are more often present in combination with other lesions than alone, and some of the combinations produce entities with specific clinical connotations. In this chapter various clinical entities will be discussed; as a rule, right-sided outflow obstruction constitutes the sole or the important factor influencing the natural history; in some, as a part of a spectrum, pulmonary stenosis is less important but nevertheless these entities will be included here to aid in a balanced presentation of this subject. Arbitrary division into clinical syndromes has been made; it should be recognized, however, that they are merely parts of a continuum.

The following clinical entities (perhaps better referred to as "sub-entities") will be discussed:

1. Mild valvular pulmonary stenosis (including idiopathic dilatation of the pulmonary artery);

2. Severe isolated valvular pulmonary stenosis;

3. Valvular pulmonary stenosis with patency of the foramen ovale and right-to-left shunt;

4. Isolated infundibular pulmonary stenosis;

5. Pulmonary outflow obstruction with ventricular septal defect (tetralogy of Fallot and related syndromes);

6. Supravalvular pulmonary arterial obstruction, including branch stenoses of the pulmonary artery;

7. Secondary right ventricular obstruction.

Not included in this presentation are more complex congenital malformations in which pulmonary stenosis or pulmonary atresia is present.

ETIOLOGY

In these entities congenital heart disease accounts for the great majority of cases, yet a variety of acquired rare lesions produces some of the clinical syndromes in question. Among these are the following:

- Acquired hypertrophy of the right ventricular outflow tract (usually crista supraventricularis), occurring in cardiomyopathy or secondary to valvular stenosis;

- Obstruction of the outflow tract from aneurysm of the ventricular septum;

- Right ventricular tumors (including myxoma);

- Valvular pulmonary stenosis in the carcinoid syndrome.

PATHOLOGY AND PATHOPHYSIOLOGY

Valvular pulmonary stenosis is almost always congenital. Milder degrees involve fusion of the commissures between the cusps of the pulmonary valve; severe pulmonary stenosis usually presents itself in a characteristic form as fibrous membrane composed of the completely fused three cusps (with commissures no longer identifiable), which bulges into the pulmonary artery; a round central opening constitutes the communication between the right ventricle and the pulmonary artery. Viewed from the pulmonary artery, the stenotic valve resembles cervix uteri. In older adults this structure may become thick; calcifications are rare but do occur. Associated with valvular pulmonary stenosis, but only partly related to the severity of the obstruction, is poststenotic dilatation of the pulmonary artery, involving primarily the main pulmonary artery but sometimes extending into the right and left branches. Long-standing severe pulmonary stenosis may cause secondary myocardial fibrosis in the right ventricle.

Infundibular pulmonary stenosis varies a great deal: it may involve a mere hypertrophy of the crista supraventricularis with functional rather than anatomic obstruction; fibrous narrowing may separate the infundibular chamber from the lower part of the outflow tract. While valvular pulmonary stenosis is more often the sole lesion, infundibular pulmonary stenosis is usually associated with other lesions, particularly the large ventricular septal defect. Infundibular stenosis seldom produces poststenotic dilatation of the pulmonary artery.

Tetralogy of Fallot represents the combination of the large ventricular septal defect with pulmonary outflow obstruction. Both components of this lesion are most frequently produced by the same developmental error: failure to close the ventricular septum associated with unequal division of the arterial trunks. Thus, pulmonary outflow obstruction may be manifested by the *hypoplasia* of the pulmonary orifice and the pulmonary artery, rather than by a discrete obstruction. If obstruction is present, it is more often infundibular, or it may be a combined infundibular and valvular stenosis; Severe pulmonary valvular stenosis as described above is unusual in association with large ventricular septal defect. In some patients the infundibular right ventricular stenosis is acquired and is clearly secondary to the effects of the large ventricular septal defect: many authenticated cases are reported in which infants are born showing ventricular septal defect as the sole lesion but then develop the infundibular obstruction characteristic of tetralogy of Fallot. Thus, this has to be recognized as an alternate mechanism for the development of this syndrome. Pathologically as well as clinically, tetralogy of Fallot represents a wide range of combinations, from a very severe pulmonary stenosis (or hypoplasia), producing a large right-to-left shunt, to mild obstruction, merely reducing somewhat the impact of the large ventricular septal defect.

In addition to tetralogy of Fallot, which is the commonest syndrome involving right ventricular outflow stenosis with intracardiac shunting, two other conditions are encountered:

- Patency of the foramen ovale (not necessarily a congenital atrial septal defect but merely a failure of postnatal closure caused by the right-sided obstruction present at birth) may produce the site of significant right-to-left shunt in severe valvular stenosis;

- Valvular pulmonary stenosis (of the "primary" variety) may coexist with a small ventricular septal defect;

- Mild valvular pulmonary stenosis may be present in combination with an atrial septal defect (see Chapter 27).

Supravalvular obstruction is rare within the main pulmonary artery. Gradients between the main pulmonary artery and the right and left branches are frequently found in children; this, however, is merely caused by flow patterns and does not represent a significant true obstruction.

Stenosis of pulmonary arterial branches is a common lesion; it appears in two forms: as a discrete narrowing at the junction between the main pulmonary artery at the branches, or as multiple obstructing lesions within the principal branches, often present also in the secondary branches.

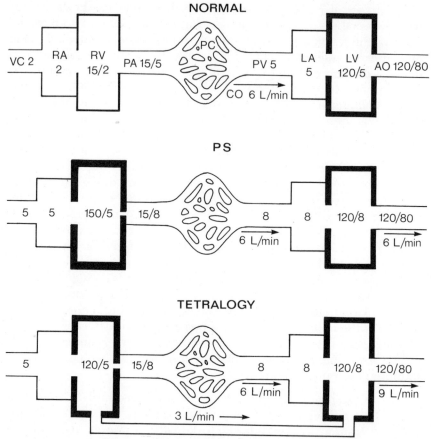

Figure 30-1. Hemodynamic diagram showing the normal circulation *(top)*; an example of severe valvular pulmonary stenosis (PS) with closed septa *(middle diagram)*, and an example of tetralogy of Fallot with a moderate right-to-left shunt through the ventricular septal defect *(lower diagram)*.

Acquired diseases producing right ventricular obstruction have already been mentioned. Hypertrophy of the ventricular septum, associated with cardiomyopathy or as an isolated lesion, may produce outflow obstruction within *both* ventricles. The familial form of this lesion is somewhat more apt to affect the right ventricle as well as the left.

Obstruction by tumor involves both pedunculated myxoma and solid tumors (teratoma, fibrosarcoma, etc.). Aneurysms of the ventricular septum may bulge into the right ventricle, imitating infundibular stenosis; some of those originate in the sinus of Valsalva and may eventually rupture into the right ventricle. Finally, endocardial sclerosis produced by carcinoid syndrome may produce pulmonary stenosis; this is caused by sclerotic changes in the leaflets; it is unlikely to be a severe obstructive lesion.

Right ventricular outflow stenosis introduces *resistance to the flow of blood,* which is expressed as a pressure gradient across the valve or at other points of obstruction (Fig. 30–1). For any given flow there is an inverse relationship between the area of the narrowest point and the square root of the pressure gradient. Thus, outflow obstruction causes right ventricular systolic hypertension proximally to the stenosis. Given a case in which no abnormal communications exist between the two sides of the heart, right ventricular hypertension is the only abnormality; hypertrophy of the right ventricular myocardium as a rule compensates for the increased workload. Elevation of diastolic right ventricular pressure indicative of cardiac failure is rare except in severe degrees of stenosis.

In the presence of intracardiac communications, pulmonary stenosis may exert secondary effects in a variety of ways:

1. During the postnatal period severe pulmonary stenosis may prevent the normal sealing of the foramen ovale. An anatomically open foramen ovale, often found in normal subjects, is of no consequence because higher pressure in the left atrium seals the competent valve made out of the flap covering the foramen; however, pulmonary stenosis reverses the pressure relationship in the atrium: right-to-left shunt takes place with ease. Severe pulmonary stenosis produces right ventricular hypertrophy and may enlarge the size of the right atrium, thereby facilitating still wider opening of the foramen and thus increasing the size of the shunt. This mechanism may produce large right-to-left shunt, resulting in severe hypoxemia.

2. In tetralogy of Fallot resistance of outflow from the right ventricle provides the means of maintaining systemic pressure in the right ventricle (essential because of the equilibration) without evoking increased pulmonary arterial pressure (see Chapter 28). Thus, the addition of pulmonary stenosis exerts a highly significant favorable prognostic influence in the large ventricular septal defect by protecting the patient from pulmonary vascular disease. (This principle is used as the basis for the palliative operation of "banding" the pulmonary artery, i.e., producing artificially pulmonary stenosis.) The resistance at the point of obstruction determines the magnitude and the direction of the shunt; hence tetralogy of Fallot involves a wide spectrum, from cases with mild pulmonary stenosis and large left-to-right shunt to those with severe pulmonary stenosis and large right-to-left shunt, including all intermediate degrees.

3. Valvular pulmonary stenosis combined with small ventricular septal defect coexist as two unrelated lesions. The magnitude of the shunt is influenced only to the extent that right ventricular hypertension may reduce the gradient, thereby diminishing the driving pressure. If pulmonary stenosis is severe, the flow across the defect may thus be considerably reduced, and may even cease altogether. Some cases are reported in which severe pulmonary stenosis increases right ventricular pressure to a level higher than the left (this could not occur in large ventricular septal defect because of the equilibration effect), in which case right-to-left shunt may occur owing to a true reversal of the pressure gradient.

Supravalvular obstruction introduces a pressure gradient above the pulmonary valve; such gradients are almost always small and not enough proximal pressure elevation is present to introduce a significant load upon the right ventricle. The exception is the presence of congenital multiple branch stenoses of the pulmonary artery. The sum total of the obstructions may elevate the resistance to flow into the lungs, producing moderately severe to severe pulmonary hypertension. These patients then behave like those with primary pulmonary hypertension; the large number of the obstructive lesions as well as their peripheral location often make this lesion inoperable.

An important hemodynamic issue, as yet unsolved, concerns the question as to whether or not right ventricular obstructive lesions progress with the growth and development of the child or later in life with aging. Not enough appropriate longitudinal studies are available to provide a definitive answer to this question. From those studies that have been made, the impression is that pulmonary stenosis is largely stationary, i.e., a patient with mild or moderate pulmonary stenosis is unlikely to develop severe pulmonary stenosis (and thus a larger gradient and severe load upon the right ventricle) later in life.

THE CLINICAL SYNDROMES

Mild Valvular Pulmonary Stenosis

Included in this category are patients with a pressure gradient of not more than 40 mm. Hg without coexisting additional lesions.

Natural history. The benign nature of this group of cases is supported by the already mentioned impression gained by a few longitudinal studies that valvular pulmonary stenosis is nonprogressive. The extent of the right ventricular overload ranges from none to mild; its clinical implications are negligible. Along with most congenital lesions, with the sole exception of the atrial septal defect, susceptibility to infective endocarditis represents a significant risk to the patient. It is probable, however, that the site of pulmonary stenosis is less often the site of infection than in ventricular septal defect and patent ductus arteriosus.

The *diagnosis* of milder forms of pulmonary stenosis involves the lower half of the spectrum of this obstructive lesion. Case finding is easy because of the prominence of the cardiac murmur. Inasmuch as patients virtually always are asymptomatic, discovery of the lesion is almost always accidental, contingent upon a "check-up" or examination in connection with problems other than cardiac disease.

The diagnosis can be made wih reasonable probability on clinical grounds, supported by noninvasive laboratory methods. Invasive evaluation may be indicated as a means to determine the severity of the obstruction and its differentiation from other lesions and from innocent murmurs.

Physical examination includes the following findings:

- Palpatory examination reveals no abnormality or only mild right ventricular lift;

- The first sound is followed by an ejection sound;

- The second sound shows wider than average splitting with the normal respiratory variation;

- An ejection systolic murmur is present at the upper left sternal border, usually in the second and third intercostal spaces.

Radiological diagnosis is based on the presence of poststenotic dilatation of the pulmonary artery; enlargement of right heart chambers is seldom present in milder forms of pulmonary stenosis. The degree of the pulmonary arterial dilatation varies from mild to gross, and may even include aneurysmal enlargement.

Electrocardiographic findings range from a normal record to moderate degree of right ventricular hypertrophy. A mere right axis shift, or the presence of modest R waves in right precordial leads is the most frequently encountered finding. Other noninvasive diagnostic methods add little to the diagnosis of mild pulmonary stenosis.

Cardiac catheterization establishes the diagnosis by demonstrating a systolic pressure gradient between the right ventricle and the main pulmonary artery. The study should include the various steps necessary to rule out intracardiac shunts. The role of *angiocardiography* is a minor one; it may serve as means of localization of the obstruction whenever suspicion is aroused that isolated infundibular stenosis may be present.

The *differential diagnosis* of mild pulmonary stenosis involves as the commonest similar conditions the following:

- Atrial septal defect; the similarity of the physical findings is considerable; the principal differential point is the respiratory variation of the pulmonary valve closure in pulmonary stenosis. Radiographic and electrocardiographic features also offer considerable overlap.

• Mild aortic stenosis may present some difficulties if the location of the murmur is atypical (which commonly occurs in small children) and if the obstruction of either outflow tract is mild enough not to give evidence for right vs. left ventricular hypertrophy.

• Milder degrees of hypertrophic subaortic stenosis show some superficial similarities to pulmonary stenosis.

• The innocent cardiac murmur is commonly confused with mild pulmonary stenosis; the difference often has to be settled by invasive studies, since the milder forms of pulmonary stenosis may have all normal findings except for the overlapping murmur.

• Idiopathic dilatation of the pulmonary artery. This clinical syndrome has findings virtually identical with those of mild pulmonary stenosis: pulmonary ejection murmur, ejection sound, and dilatation of the main pulmonary artery. The question has not been answered as to whether this represents a congenital weakness of the main pulmonary arterial wall or is merely a very mild pulmonary stenosis with no measurable gradient and in which there is an unusual degree of post-stenotic dilatation of the pulmonary artery.

The treatment of mild pulmonary stenosis requires merely the usual preventive measures to protect the patient from infective endocarditis. No restrictions are necessary; as soon as the diagnosis is proved, full reassurance can be given to the patient and his family. It is sometimes important to keep patients with moderate pulmonary stenosis from the hands of eager cardiac surgeons.

Severe Valvular Pulmonary Stenosis

Severe valvular pulmonary stenosis is a lesion that may profoundly affect the circulation. A primarily right-sided lesion, it leads to right ventricular hypertrophy and eventually right ventricular failure. However, even in cases of very severe pulmonary stenosis, the natural history is more benign than in equivalent degrees of other congenital lesions. The reason for this is the sparing of the pulmonary circulation, which is neither subjected to high pressure nor congested. The symptomatology of patients with severe valvular pulmonary stenosis who enter a symptomatic stage varies. Dyspnea may be present (its mechanism is not entirely clear); weakness and angina-like chest pain occur in some; syncope is rare but has been reported in some patients. Patients may be restricted in their activities by a very low cardiac output, which produces excessive fatigability. The clinical findings in the presence of restricted cardiac output may include severe peripheral cyanosis (i.e., associated with normal arterial oxygen saturation). Nevertheless, some recent observations (based on a small number of cases, to be sure) implied that the prognosis of severe valvular pulmonary stenosis may be better than hitherto assumed. An exception to the basically benign course is severe pulmonary stenosis with closed septums in infants. Here the lesion may be poorly tolerated and may produce emergencies.

Severe pulmonary stenosis is considered a surgical lesion; it is generally recommended that patients have pulmonary valvotomy performed even if they are asymptomatic. The proof of the benefit of this approach is not available — recently a plea has been made to consider for surgical treatment only symptomatic patients and not to set criteria on the basis of measurement (e.g., patients with systolic pressure in the right ventricle in excess of 100, or with transpulmonary gradients over 80 mm. Hg). The indications may have to be revised, although in the absence of good longitudinal studies one cannot expect a sound scientific basis for the selection of patients for surgical treatment.

Postsurgical problems may not be trivial in patients in this category, First, pulmonary valve incompetence commonly results from valvotomy. Second, valvotomy may only partially relieve the obstruction; in some patients there is a secondary point of obstruction related to the severe hypertrophy of the outflow tract producing hypertrophic subpulmonary stenosis that becomes evident only when the valvular obstruction is relieved. In the majority, but not in all patients, this secondary hypertrophy gradually recedes and the pressure gradient disappears. The monitoring of this process may be accomplished noninvasively by observation of the regression of the electrocardiographic changes of right ventricular hypertrophy, a reliable index of hemodynamic improvement. Nevertheless, the occasional finding of patients who are left with still severe pulmonary stenosis after undergoing pulmonary valvotomy has made some surgeons combine valvotomy with the resection of the infundibular muscle. This usually relieves the obstruction satisfactorily but at a price; it may require ventriculotomy (rather than the more benign transpulmonary approach) and often produces complete right bundle branch block, discussed in Chapter 28. Thus the operation for pulmonary stenosis does not nearly approach the curative status of that for atrial septal defect.

The *diagnosis* of severe valvular pulmonary stenosis may often be made by simple clinical examination and noninvasive tests. The prominence of the systolic murmur makes it likely that cases would be discovered early in life. In most, the diagnosis is made during an asymptomatic stage.

The objectives of the diagnostic evaluation involve the confirmation of the clinical diagnosis, the assessment of the severity of the obstruction, the detection or ruling out of associated lesions, and the differentiation from some rare conditions in which overlap of the clinical findings exists.

Physical examination reveals the following findings:

- Jugular venous pulse usually shows "giant" a waves.

- A pronounced and sustained left parasternal lift is present, produced by the hypertrophic right ventricle.

- The first sound is followed by an ejection sound (an important differential point separating valvular stenosis from infundibular stenosis, in which this sound is not heard).

- The pulmonary valve closure (late component of the second sound) is considerably delayed and diminished in intensity. The aortic valve closure may be encompassed by the murmur, hence may not be audible over some areas of the thorax.

- An S4 gallop sound is heard at the xiphoid area and the lower left sternal border.

- A loud (grade IV to VI) intensity ejection murmur is heard in the second and third intercostal space, left sternal border. The diamond-shaped murmur is of long duration, starting immediately with the ejection sound and overriding the aortic component of the second sound. A systolic thrill is almost always present at the corresponding area of the thorax.

Radiographic examination reveals as the most characteristic finding poststenotic dilatation of the pulmonary artery. Inasmuch as most patients with severe pulmonary stenosis show concentric hypertrophy of the right ventricle, cardiomegaly may be absent, though some landmarks may point to right ventricular hypertrophy. In some patients, moderate and even gross cardiomegaly may be present. Radiographic appearance of normal or reduced peripheral lung vascularity provides a means for the differentiation from shunting lesions, but the specificity of these findings is fairly low.

The electrocardiogram is of considerable value in supporting the diagnosis of severe valvular pulmonary stenosis:

- Prominent P waves are usually present — a distinguishing feature from tetralogy of Fallot and from other forms of right ventricular hypertrophy.

- Evidence of severe right ventricular hypertrophy is present, i.e., very tall R waves in V_1 and V_2 (often qR waves), deep S waves in V_5 and V_6, in addition to right-sided axis shift.

The vectorcardiogram shows the main portion of the QRS loop directed inferiorly, anteriorly, and rightward; an exaggerated P loop directed anteriorly may be present.

Cardiac catheterization provides the means of evaluating the severity of pulmonary stenosis; The formula by Gorlin and Gorlin permits a reasonable measurement of the pulmonary valve area. It requires that the cardiac output and the pressure gradient be measured almost simultaneously (withdrawal from the pulmonary artery to the right ventricle is made while the determination of cardiac output is being performed). The important point during the study is to investigate the possibility of shunts. Right-to-left shunts need to be considered if cyanosis is clinically present; arterial oxygen saturation and indicator dilution curves usually permit this point to be settled. Left-to-right shunts are investigated by serial oxygen sampling and by the hydrogen inhalation test. It should be mentioned that the evidence for shunt in either direction may be missing if perfect balance of resistance is present in connection with large ventricular septal defect. Here the Valsalva test, with simultaneously recorded pressures in the right ventricle and a systemic artery, may be given, indicating whether true equilibration through a ventricular septal defect exists, or whether coincidentally the pressure in the two ventricles are at similar levels. The diagnostic study should also include an exercise test. Inasmuch as cardiac output increases during exercise the gradient across the pulmonary valve is expected to rise with it. The height of the peak systolic pressure during exercise may provide an index of the load upon the right ventricle.

Angiocardiography supplements cardiac catheterization. The goals of the examination include:

- An injection of contrast material into the right ventricle to outline the point of obstruction (in obvious valvular stenosis the additional presence of hypertrophy of the infundibular region may have surgical implications);

- Angiocardiographic examination provides an additional method to evaluate the possibility of right-to-left shunts;

- In suspected, but not definitely proven, ventricular septal defect, left-sided injection helps to settle this point.

Differential diagnosis presents difficulty only if atypical features are present. The conditions to be considered are as follows:

- Tetralogy of Fallot;

- Small ventricular septal defect of the supracristal variety;
- Atrial septal defect combined with mild pulmonary stenosis;
- Isolated infundibular stenosis;
- Rare forms of secondary right ventricular obstruction.

In establishing the diagnosis by noninvasive examination, the following differential points are helpful:

- Evidence of right atrial overload (jugular pulse A waves, atrial gallop sound, tall "gothic" P waves in the electrocardiogram) discriminates against tetralogy of Fallot and all other conditions not associated with pulmonary hypertension, but not against primary pulmonary hypertension.

- The presence of an ejection sound is a strong point for the presence of valvular stenosis, and against infundibular stenosis.

- The length of the systolic ejection murmur and the delay in pulmonary valve closure are indices of the severity of pulmonary stenosis.

- Wide splitting of the second sound with good respiratory variation and diminished late component supports the diagnosis of pulmonary stenosis.

- Radiographic evidence for poststenotic dilatation of the pulmonary artery is a point in favor of valvular pulmonary stenosis.

Treatment of severe pulmonary stenosis usually involves surgical relief of the obstruction. The dilemma involved in the selection of patients has already been discussed in connection with the natural history of this lesion. The trend toward a less aggressive surgical approach is emphasized.

In selecting patients for surgical treatment symptoms provide the first priority. It is necessary to relate the symptoms to pulmonary stenosis by making other causes of disability unlikely and by demonstrating the severe degree of pulmonary stenosis. If surgery is contemplated in patients without overt disability, the following findings may suggest that an operation is indicated:

- low cardiac output with peripheral cyanosis,
- elevated right ventricular diastolic pressure.

As mentioned, a special situation develops in infants with severe stenosis. Infants who develop right ventricular failure from valvular pulmonary stenosis may deteriorate rapidly. It is generally considered that cardiac failure associated with pulmonary stenosis represents a surgical emergency. Infants even respond poorly to the invasive studies that establish the diagnosis—surgical treatment may have to be instituted immediately after the diagnostic test. The low cardiac output resulting from cardiac failure may reduce the intensity of the systolic ejection murmur so as to make the clinical diagnosis difficult. It is thus necessary to have a high index of suspicion that noncyanotic infants with severe electrocardiographic evidence of right ventricular hypertrophy may have this treatable lesion.

Medical treatment of pulmonary stenosis has little to offer. Asymptomatic patients need only minor restrictions and protection from infective endocarditis. Inasmuch as this lesion never reaches an inoperable stage, management of a disabled unoperated patient comes under consideration only if unusual circumstances contraindicate surgical treatment. Conventional therapy for cardiac failure is all there is to offer to such patients.

Valvular Pulmonary Stenosis with Patent Foramen Ovale

This syndrome, which has on occasion been termed "the trilogy of Fallot," presupposes right-to-left shunt, which only occurs in the presence of severe degree of right ventricular outflow obstruction. Thus clinical features, including symptomatology, physical findings, and radiographic and electrocardiographic findings, are identical with those of the severe valvular pulmonary stenosis and closed septums, except for the addition of hypoxemia, cyanosis, polycythemia, and clubbing of digits.

While it is probable that right-to-left shunting through the foramen ovale is present since infancy, overt cyanosis usually makes its appearance with some delay: in early childhood, late childhood, or adolescence. Cyanosis is progressive: it appears first only during effort or otherwise intermittently, then permanently with the color becoming more intensely cyanotic. Symptoms appear earlier than in patients with pulmonary stenosis of equivalent degree and closed septum; the disability may be severe. Life-threatening complications resulting from hypoxia and secondary polycythemia (see below—tetralogy of Fallot) make prognosis of this lesion poorer than in pure pulmonary stenosis of comparable degree.

The principal problem in differential diagnosis of this lesion is its separation from the tetralogy of Fallot. The main points of the differentiation include the following:

- The presence of atrial overload (see above) almost always indicates closed ventricular septum.

- Classical high-amplitude ejection murmurs in the pulmonary area are uncommon in tetralogy.

- Radiographic evidence of poststenotic dilatation of the pulmonary artery favors valvular pulmonary stenosis with patent foramen ovale.

- Electrocardiographic patterns of advanced right ventricular hypertrophy also favor valvular pulmonary stenosis.

Treatment of pulmonary stenosis with patent foramen ovale is surgical, namely pulmonary valvotomy and closure of the foramen ovale. Progression of the cyanosis and the possibility of sequels and complications related to severe hypoxemia call for a more aggressive attitude in this syndrome than in the noncyanotic valvular pulmonary stenosis. The establishment of the diagnosis of severe pulmonary stenosis and the detection of hypoxemia (even above the threshold of cyanosis) due to atrial shunting are recognized as indications for early operation.

Isolated Infundibular Pulmonary Stenosis

As indicated, infundibular pulmonary stenosis occurs in the overwhelming majority of cases in combination with other lesions, primarily with ventricular septal defect. Because of this, it is necessary to have a high index of suspicion for the presence of an additional lesion, should the diagnosis of isolated infundibular pulmonary stenosis suggest itself.

The natural history of pulmonary stenosis is related to the severity of the obstruction and the possibility of secondary shunting: the location of the obstruction is immaterial to the course. Thus, the importance of this lesion lies in its presenting atypical features that could divert the clinician's attention from the recognition of a significant pulmonary outflow tract obstruction.

The important differential point between valvular and infundibular pulmonary stenosis is based on the following characteristics of infundibular stenosis:

- The ejection systolic murmur may be located lower, at the left sternal border (third and fourth intercostal spaces).

- The ejection sound is absent.

- Poststenotic dilatation of the pulmonary artery is not present in the radiograph.

It should be pointed out, however, that the differentiation between isolated infundibular stenosis and the noncyanotic form of tetralogy of Fallot may be difficult as well. The following points are noteworthy:

- In milder forms of infundibular pulmonary stenosis the presence or absence of ventricular septal defect may be very difficult to determine noninvasively.

- In severe infundibular pulmonary stenosis the earmarks presented above in association with severe valvular obstruction are usually helpful (atrial overload, advanced electrocardiographic changes).

Given a patient in whom clinical findings suggest isolated infundibular pulmonary stenosis, the diagnostic approach should include the following considerations:

- Determination of whether or not intracardiac shunts are present;

- Investigation of the possibility of secondary obstruction produced by septal aneurysm, tumor, etc.;

- Investigation of the possibility of coexisting left-sided ventricular obstruction (hypertrophy, subaortic stenosis).

Some noninvasive tests may shed some light in this direction, e.g., echocardiography. However, cardiac catheterization and angiocardiography are virtually always needed to make the definitive diagnosis. Inasmuch as the problem at issue is one of anatomic change rather than pathophysiologic changes, angiocardiography plays the crucial role in the differentiation.

Pulmonary Outflow Obstruction with Ventricular Septal Defect

The term "tetralogy of Fallot" has established itself in the terminology of congenital heart disease with such firmness that it is probably futile to point out its lack of logic; first, one of the four components of tetralogy is incorrect (overriding of the aorta); one is secondary to the main problem (right ventricular hypertrophy); hence the term is misleading. Second, it was originally described in connection with severely cyanotic patients; hence its application to the whole spectrum of pulmonary stenosis with ventricular septal defect is not justified. However, bowing to the entrenched custom, the spectrum of this combination of defects will be referred to as the cyanotic and the noncyanotic forms of Fallot's tetralogy.

The spectrum of tetralogy involves the pathophysiological effect of pulmonary outflow obstruction. Severe obstruction produces shunt reversal; mild obstruction represents merely a minor variant of the pure "large" ventricular septal defect. The natural history and clinical features of the "blue" and "pink" varieties of Fallot's tetralogy differ to such an extent that they must be discussed separately.

The Cyanotic Form of Tetralogy of Fallot

Natural History. Tetralogy of Fallot is the commonest cyanotic cardiac lesion in children and adults. Its variability can best be illustrated by pointing out that it may become a common medical-surgical emergency in infancy and childhood on the one hand, but that many patients survive to middle age or even old age and may lead reasonably comfortable lives on the other hand. The course of the disease is related primarily to the magnitude of the right-to-left shunt, thus the severity of right-sided outflow obstruction.

Cyanosis is seldom evident immediately after birth. It is apt to appear in infancy or childhood and to progress henceforth. First evident during exercise or with crying, it eventually establishes itself as a permanent feature, varying from a mildly bluish hue to deep purple cyanosis. Hypoxia in children may be severe: arterial oxygen saturation in the 50 per cent range or even lower is not uncommon. Cyanotic children are usually dyspneic; characteristically they squat—squatting permits somewhat better arterial oxygenation. Many have periodic attacks of deep cyanosis which may be associated with loss of consciousness. Angina-like pain has also been occasionally observed. Infants and young children showing these symptoms and signs represent the group cases in whom surgical treatment (palliative or corrective) is a condition for survival. Further along the spectrum, children may show only mild and intermittent cyanosis, may retain good effort tolerance, and may remain in reasonably good condition, although some delaying effect of the serious cardiac lesion upon growth and development (but not necessarily upon mental status) is usually evident.

Unoperated adults vary in their course. Some limitation of effort tolerance is the rule, but many remain within a stable status, capable of functioning with some adjustment to their limitations. As stated, survival into the sixties is not rare.

Complications of Fallot's tetralogy include the following:

- Infective endocarditis—commonly located at the pulmonary valve;

- Paradoxical embolism: the entry of venous blood directly into the aorta provides the background for systemic embolization from peripheral venous thrombosis;

- Cerebral abscess occurs commonly—its incidence increases in a general way with the severity of cyanosis;

- Thrombotic phenomena represent the common complication of all cyanotic lesions associated with polycythemia; their frequency increases with the severity of the polycythemia.

Postsurgical course varies a great deal. Two types of operations are offered to children with tetralogy of Fallot: a palliative operation (Blalock-Taussig anastomosis or other shunting procedures) returns incompletely oxygenated blood into the lungs thereby reducing hypoxemia; "total correction" of the lesion provides relief of right-sided outflow obstruction and closure of the ventricular septal defect, but by no means represents a curative procedure.

The effect of the palliative operation upon the course ranges from mild improvement to dramatic change in color and symptoms. Most children can function better; their growth and development improve and they can now wait for the optimal age to have the definitive operation performed. The potential untoward effect of the operation relates to "flooding" of the lungs produced by too large an anastomosis. This possibility occurs almost exclusively with the use of a direct aorticopulmonary artery anastomosis, in which the surgeon selects the size of the connection between the aorta and the pulmonary artery. In the Blalock-Taussig procedure the size of the subclavian artery limits the amount of the shunt flow. Too large shunts created by the surgeon may produce left ventricular failure — not unlike the conditions existing in the large patent ductus arteriosus in infancy. Rare cases are reported in which the Blalock-Taussig anastomosis or the direct aorticopulmonary anastomosis is well tolerated and effective, but over the period of years induces pulmonary vascular disease and pulmonary hypertension. This is, of course, only possible in patients who fail to undergo the second, definitive operation, during which the anastomosis is closed.

Another rare untoward effect of shunting operations may develop in patients with very severe pulmonary stenosis, in whom the pulmonary orifice may become atretic and all the pulmonary flow courses through the anastomosis.

Results of the definitive operation are also variable. Several factors stand in the way of making this operation a curative one:

- The pulmonary outflow tract and the main pulmonary artery are frequently hypoplastic. Even if the obstruction is eliminated some impediment to right ventricular outflow persists.

- The pulmonary valve is often sacrificed. Pulmonary regurgitation is basically a benign lesion so that valve replacement is not ordinarily done; nevertheless, it may exert some effect toward depressing cardiac performance.

- Potential disadvantages of right ventriculotomy and the

frequently induced bundle branch block have already been discussed in connection with closure of simple ventricular septal defect.

• Rarely, complete AV block may be caused by the operation.

Patients, in general, perform well, especially in light of their previous disabilities; yet, their performance, clinically and hemodynamically, seldom approximates that of healthy subjects.

Diagnosis. The presence of cyanosis makes the detection of Fallot's tetralogy early in life the rule; only occasionally, delayed development of cyanosis leads to late recognition of this lesion.

Physical diagnosis permits the establishment of the diagnosis in a reasonable number of cases. The important diagnostic features are as follows:

• Venous pressure is normal—jugular venous *a* waves are rare.

• Palpatory findings may reveal a right ventricular lift, but with less regularity than in valvular pulmonary stenosis.

• The first sound is normal; an ejection sound may be present (if it is, it originates in the dilated aorta).

• An ejection systolic murmur is almost always present; it may be absent in severely cyanotic children with markedly diminished flow through the pulmonary outflow tract.

• The systolic murmur is located lower than in valvular pulmonary stenosis; it is of lesser intensity, ranging from grade II to IV, being very loud only in the minority of the cases; its peak occurs earlier than in pulmonary stenosis.

• The second sound is loud and single, representing only aortic valve closure; a faint, delayed pulmonary valve closure sound is only occasionally heard, though it may be recorded in the phonocardiogram.

• Cyanosis and clubbing of digits are usually obvious.

The diagnosis based on physical examination involves basically a cyanotic patient; in the presence of cyanosis the diagnostic possibilities are limited to such an extent that the presence of most of the findings listed above provides a high probability of a correct diagnosis; these same findings in a noncyanotic patient would be inconclusive.

Laboratory examination includes the presence of polycythemia, which is usually mild to moderate.

The electrocardiogram shows more often than not normal P waves; tall, abnormal P waves are uncommon. Ventricular complexes reveal mild degree of right ventricular hypertrophy or biventricular hypertrophy; moderate right axis shift, diphasic precordial QRS complexes and prominent S waves in left-sided leads are commonly present.

The roentgenogram shows most often a normal-sized or mildly enlarged cardiac shadow. The pulmonary artery shadow is small, providing a concavity of the left cardiac border; right ventricular hypertrophy may produce elevation of the apical arch, giving the appearance of the "coeur en sabot" that is traditionally associated with tetralogy. Typical sabot-type heart shape is seen, however, only in some patients and is not the rule (nor is it specific for this lesion).

Cardiac catheterization permits the demonstration of pressure equilibration between the two ventricles; pressure gradient across the pulmonary valve, along with the magnitude of pulmonary flow, determines the severity of pulmonary stenosis. In some patients it may be difficult to enter the pulmonary artery, the cardiac catheter being guided preferentially into the aorta. The respective contribution of the shunts can be made from the appropriate blood samples. The site of right-to-left shunting may be demonstrated with the aid of indicator dilution studies; the possible coexisting left-to-right shunt can be diagnosed by oxygen step-up. Cardiac catheterization plays an important role in patients who underwent palliation by means of an anastomotic operation prior to a contemplated total correction. The knowledge of pulmonary arterial pressure is often of crucial importance, especially in older children and adults, for the presence of pulmonary hypertension may require some revision of surgical plans.

Angiocardiography represents the basic diagnostic tool for the definitive evaluation of tetralogy of Fallot. In contrast to many other congenital cardiac lesions, Fallot's tetralogy shows a wide range of anatomic variations or sequels of the lesion and of associated malformations, the knowledge of which is important from the medical and surgical standpoints. Angiocardiographic examination includes the following necessary details:

- The site of the outflow obstruction and the size of the outflow tract and of the pulmonary artery;

- The location of the ventricular septal defect;

- The possible presence of an additional foramen ovale (this combination is sometimes referred to as "pentalogy of Fallot");

- The position of the aortic root and aortic arch (true dextroposition of the aorta is occasionally present);

- Associated lesions may be present (e.g., absence of one pulmonary branch).

Differential diagnosis of the cyanotic form of tetralogy of Fallot involves other cyanotic lesions. In infants and small children the whole gamut of rare congenital cyanotic lesions has to be considered; in older children and adults the problem is simpler, for only occasional survival of patients with the more complex cyanotic lesions occurs. The more important cyanotic lesions to be considered include the following:

- Pulmonary stenosis with patent foramen ovale; the differentiation has already been presented;

- Reversed shunts in intracardiac or aorticopulmonary communications: the presence of clinical features pointing out severe pulmonary hypertension in this group makes the clinical differentiation with tetralogy usually easy;

- Ebstein's anomaly: there is relatively little overlap between this lesion and tetralogy, except in atypical cases;

- Transposition syndromes: the wide range of abnormalities and combination of defects make the differentiation between it and tetralogy difficult in the infant age group;

- Pulmonary atresia: this is really the end of the spectrum of severe tetralogy; the differentiation is purely on the basis of angiographic studies;

- Tricuspid atresia: here the presence of left ventricular overload puts this lesion in a different category from most other cyanotic congenital lesions.

Treatment. The treatment of cyanotic tetralogy is primarily surgical. It is generally agreed that in children above 10 kg. of body weight the definitive corrective procedure is the treatment of choice. In smaller children the use of a single operation offers many advantages over the performance of the palliative procedure first, then to be followed by the corrective operation. However, consideration of the risk makes the decision contingent upon the experience of the given institution with infant surgery.

In considering definitive surgery, a knowledge of the anatomic conditions may serve to guide the decision and even the type of operation. Patients with severe hypoplasia of the right ventricular outflow tracts and of the main pulmonary artery may not present good prospects for total correction. In such patients palliative operation may be the preferable procedure; there is some thought (though no definitive evidence) that an increase of pulmonary flow by the shunting operation may help to increase the size of the pulmonary artery, thereby making the patient a better candidate for complete correction at an older age. It is probable that in some cases total correction should not be attempted at all.

Medical treatment involves first of all a careful follow-up. Children may deteriorate rapidly: alertness of the family to ominous symptoms may be lifesaving. Patients with Fallot's tetralogy seldom develop cardiac failure; problems in the course of the disease include complications related to hypoxia. Cyanotic attacks may be treated with oxygen; beta-adrenergic blocking agents (propranolol) have a sound theoretical base as preventive agents for these attacks. Regulation of the hemoglobin carrying capacity may be of importance: mild anemia may produce serious symptoms, even if anemia is only relative (absence of polycythemia); excessive polycythemia may require phlebotomy. Preventive measures against infective endocarditis have to be observed carefully; the susceptibility of tetralogy to infection is relatively high.

Noncyanotic Tetralogy of Fallot

Within the spectrum of the tetralogy of Fallot all grades of pulmonary outflow obstruction are included. Somewhere in the center is the dividing line between the cyanotic and noncyanotic forms, in which equal resistances to outflow from the two ventricles—functioning as a single pump—balance the flow so that approximately the same amount is ejected into either circuit. Beyond this dividing line, lower resistance in the right side of the circulation causes a predominant left-to-right direction of flow through the ventricular septal defect. This group of patients thus has the following features:

- Systemic pressure level in the right ventricle;

- Normal or mildly elevated pressures in the pulmonary artery (beyond the stenosis);

- Left-to-right shunt through the large ventricular septal defect;

- Increase in pulmonary blood flow determined by the degree of pulmonary outflow obstruction (i.e., resistance to flow at this point);

- Biventricular hypertrophy.

In essence, noncyanotic tetralogy resembles the large ventricular septal defect except for the fact that the pulmonary vasculature is protected from the ravages of high pressure by the outflow obstruction, thus preventing the most serious consequence of the large ventricular septal defect.

The overall course is more benign than either the ventricular septal defect or the cyanotic variety of tetralogy of Fallot. Children in whom the pulmonary flow is large may have respiratory infections or, even evidence of cardiac failure, but the course of the disease in them resembles more the benign course of the atrial septal defect than that of large ventricular septal defects.

There are no satisfactory longitudinal studies of the tetralogy of Fallot that investigate the causes of late onset of cyanosis. Undoubtedly, noncyanotic tetralogy of Fallot may change into the cyanotic form during late childhood or adolescence. This implies that the pulmonary outflow obstruction has become more severe. Yet it would appear unlikely that this progression would involve a major change, but rather that patients with marginal shunts progress into right-to-left shunts. In uncomplicated large ventricular septal defect, pulmonary arteriolar disease may progress to such an extent that a large left-to-right shunt gradually becomes totally reversed. Such progression of resistance at the outflow tract probably cannot occur and one can assume that patients with sizable left-to-right shunts will never become cyanotic.

The diagnostic features of noncyanotic tetralogy consist of a combination of the findings of large ventricular septal defect and of pulmonary stenosis, more closely resembling the former:

- Venous pressure is normal; no exaggerated *a* waves are encountered;

- Right ventricular lift is present, combined with hyperactive precordial motion (related to the magnitude of the shunt);

- The presence of an ejection sound is inconstant;

- The second sound may be widely split;

- The murmur of right ventricular outflow obstruction (ejection) and that of interventricular flow (holosystolic) blend into a harsh very loud (grades 4 to 6) murmur and thrill, located at the third and fourth intercostal space, left sternal border;

- In the presence of large shunts an apical S3 gallop or diastolic rumble may be present;

- Radiographic features include at least moderate cardiac enlargement with prominence of the pulmonary vessels and increased vascularity;

- Electrocardiography shows biventricular hypertrophy or right ventricular hypertrophy of modest degree.

Cardiac catheterization can establish the diagnosis by showing equilibration of pressure in the ventricles, combined with a left-to-right shunt and a right ventricular outflow pressure gradient. The magnitude of the shunt is of considerable importance in the decision regarding surgical treatment. With a smaller left-to-right shunt it may be important to test the effects of exercise, namely, to determine whether or not shunt reversal occurs during exercise.

Angiocardiographic examination permits the delineation of the outflow obstruction in the right ventricle. The demonstration of the ventricular septal defect is usually of lesser importance.

The differential diagnosis of the noncyanotic tetralogy involves other left-to-right shunting lesions, particularly if the pulmonary flow is increased. In cases with balanced shunts isolated infundibular pulmonary stenosis overlaps with the noncyanotic tetralogy; invasive studies are often necessary to distinguish between these two lesions.

Surgical correction of noncyanotic tetralogy is as a rule simpler than that of the cyanotic variety. Problems related to the reduced size of some vessels do not occur. Protection of the pulmonary vasculature by pulmonary stenosis makes the timing of the operation less important than in the large ventricular septal defect. Thus the operation approaches the status of closure of the intermediate-sized ventricular septal defect and, except for the consequences of ventriculotomy and the conduction system damage, comes close to being curative. On this basis routine correction of the noncyanotic variety of tetralogy is tempting, yet one cannot help wondering whether the benign course of most cases might not justify a more conservative approach—leaving them alone.

Medical therapy has little to offer; the usual protection from endocarditis should be instituted; no major restrictions are necessary.

Pulmonary Branch Stenosis

Branch stenosis of the pulmonary artery occurs more often in association with other congenital malformations (e.g., complex malformations, including those produced by the rubella syndrome) than as an isolated lesion. This lesion is of clinical importance on two counts:

- As a cause of systolic or continuous murmurs over the thorax which may present perplexing diagnostic problems;

- As a cause of severe pulmonary hypertension.

Isolated unilateral branch stenosis or milder bilateral stenosis, most often located at the point of origin of the two branches from the main pulmonary artery, may cause:

- systolic ejection murmur;

- systolic murmur with delayed onset, overriding the second sound;

- a continuous murmur resembling that of patent ductus arteriosus.

Murmurs are located higher than those of valvular pulmonary stenosis; they often radiate laterally, below the clavicles, and may be well audible in the suprascapular region of the back. Clinical examination may reveal no abnormalities other than the murmur; radiographic and electrocardiographic examination usually shows normal findings. Invasive studies are often unnecessary unless the possibility of more serious lesions is raised, in which case simple right-sided cardiac catheterization demonstrating a significant gradient at the bifurcation of the pulmonary artery may settle the matter. The conditions producing similar murmurs include:

- patent ductus arteriosus,

- coronary arteriovenous fistula,

- other intrathoracic arteriovenous fistula.

Angiocardiographic studies are usually unnecessary unless multiple areas of obstruction are suspected.

Pulmonary hypertension produced by branch stenosis of the pulmonary artery is almost always caused by the coexistence of several areas of obstruction extending into the periphery of the pulmonary arterial branches. Here the clinical findings are related to the severity of pulmonary arterial pressure elevation. This is a rare cause of pulmonary hypertension and not enough observations are reported to know the course and natural history of this entity.

Clinical examination may reveal the physical signs of pulmonary hypertension; when these are combined with continuous murmurs over the upper portions of the thorax, a clinical diagnosis of multiple branch stenoses of the pulmonary arteries may be suspected. Cardiac catheterization may reveal multiple areas of abrupt pressure changes, usually showing normal pressure in the periphery of the pulmonary arterial system, hence implying that the pulmonary vasculature is healthy. Angiocardiography shows areas of obstruction usually associated with poststenotic dilatation of the portions of the pulmonary branches just beyond the stenosis.

Surgical correction has been attempted in cases with more centrally located obstructive lesions. The nature of this disease makes pulmonary hypertension theoretically correctable; yet technical difficulties in relieving all major obstructions makes results uncertain, even doubtful.

Secondary Right Ventricular Outflow Obstruction

Conditions other than congenital malformation of the infundibular of the right ventricle may cause obstructive lesions that overlap with subpulmonary stenosis. To reiterate, the lesions in this category include:

- septal hypertrophy (often obstructing both chambers),

- tumors of the right ventricle,

- aneurysms of the septum.

Physiologically these obstructive lesions exert the same effects as congenital obstructive lesions. Their recognition can be made only by a study of the anatomic detail and implied by associated events. Diagnostic points suggesting conditions other than congenital heart disease include the following.

1. Reliable evidence that the murmur (or other evidence of cardiac disease) was not present at birth and during early childhood;

2. Rapid progression of the obstructive process;

3. Familial history of cardiomyopathy or of hypertrophic subaortic stenosis.

4. Presence of left ventricular muscular outflow obstruction in addition.

If suspicion exists that right ventricular outflow obstruction is not congenital in origin, the critical study is angiocardiography. Selective visualization of the right ventricular cavity should be made; simultaneous biventricular injection may be helpful: aortograms to visualize the sinuses of Valsalva are also indicated. It should be mentioned that the presence of an extraneous obstruction other than septal hypertrophy justifies a more aggressive surgical approach than in cases of congenital infundibular stenosis.

Bibliography

Abrahams DG, Wood P: Pulmonary stenosis with normal aortic root. Brit. Heart J. *13*:519, 1961.

Eldridge F, Selzer A, Hultgren H: Stenosis of a branch of the pulmonary artery. An additional cause of continuous murmurs over the chest. Circulation *15*:865, 1957.

Gasul BM, Dillon RF, Vila V, Hait G: Ventricular septal defects: their natural transformation into those with infundibular stenosis or into those with cyanotic or noncyanotic type of tetralogy of Fallot. J.A.M.A. *164*:847, 1957.

Gottsman MS, Beck W, Barnard CN, O'Donovan TG, Schrire V: Results of repair of tetralogy of Fallot. Circulation *40*:803, 1969.

Johnson LW, Grossman W, Dalen JE, Dexter L: Pulmonic stenosis in the adults: Long-term follow-up results. New Engl. J. Med. *287*:1159, 1972.

Kirklin JW, Wallace RB, McGoon DC, DuShane JW: Early and late results after intracardiac repair of tetralogy of Fallot: 5 year review of 337 patients. Ann. Surg. *162*:578, 1965.

Levine OR, Blumenthal S: Pulmonic stenosis. Circulation 32 (Suppl III): 33, 1965.

Moller I, Wennonvold A, Lyngborg KF: Natural history of pulmonary stenosis. Long term follow-up with serial heart catheterization. Cardiology *50*:193, 1973.

Selzer A, Carnes WH, Noble CA, Higgins WH Jr., Holmes RO: The syndrome of pulmonary stenosis with patent foramen ovale. Amer. J. Med. *6*:3, 1949.

Selzer A, Carnes WH: The role of pulmonary stenosis in the production of chronic cyanosis. Amer. Heart J. *45*:382, 1953.

Taussig HB, Crocetti E, Eshaghpour E, Keinonen R, Yap N, Bachman D, Momberger N, Kirk H: Fifteen-year follow-up on the first 6 years of the Blalock-Taussig operation. *In* Kidd BSL and Keith JD (Ed.): CONGENITAL HEART DEFECTS. Charles C Thomas, Publisher, Springfield, Ill, 1971, p. 83.

Tinker J, Howitt G, Markman P, Wade DG: The natural history of isolated pulmonary stenosis. Brit. Heart J. *27*:151, 1965.

Wood P: Attacks of deeper cyanosis and loss of consciousness (syncope) in Fallot's tetralogy. Brit. Heart J. *20*:282, 1958.

Watson H, Lowe KG: Functional adaptation of the right ventricular outflow tracts in congenital heart disease. Brit. Heart J. *27*:408, 1965.

31

Left-Sided Outflow Obstruction

Definition. Obstructive lesions within the left ventricle and the aorta include several well-defined entities of congenital or acquired origin. The largest group in this category, valvular aortic stenosis, has been arbitrarily divided into three subsections; this division is related to their respective natural histories, an important criterion being the age at which symptoms are most likely to appear. Thus the following groups are included:

- Congenital valvular aortic stenosis,

- Valvular aortic stenosis ("rheumatic") of middle age,

- Senile calcific aortic stenosis,

- Congenital fixed subaortic stenosis,

- Hypertrophic subaortic stenosis,

- Supravalvular aortic stenosis,

- Coarctation of the aorta

Among these entities is one included here with qualifications: hypertrophic subaortic stenosis. This lesion overrides two areas: obstructive left ventricular outflow disease and primary myocardial disease with septal hypertrophy; thus it could be included with justification in either section. However, the obstructive nature of this lesion affects its natural history more profoundly than does myocardial disease; hence it is incorporated into this chapter.

ETIOLOGY, PATHOLOGY AND PATHOPHYSIOLOGY

Valvular stenosis of the aortic cusps is often of uncertain etiology: even pathological examination cannot always determine the original process that produced the lesion. The most clear-cut etiological entity in this category is congenital aortic stenosis with an obvious malformation of the valve and with clinical evidence of the telltale systolic murmur present since birth.

Patients who develop signs of aortic stenosis in early middle life are often assumed to have rheumatic heart disease. Only a small number give a history of acute rheumatic fever, although, of course, lack of history does not preclude the rheumatic etiology. Yet, the present emphasis upon secondary changes in the leaflets superimposed on a congenital bicuspid aortic valve brings out the possibility that at least some such patients have aortic stenosis with a congenital background.

The calcific aortic stenosis of old age is now regarded as being predominantly due to a degenerative process developing in patients who were either born with bicuspid aortic valves or have acquired some deformity of it. Mild rheumatic valve damage is one of the mechanisms by which secondary changes are produced, with gradually developing fibrosis and calcium deposition leading to severe stenosis.

The widely accepted theory of development and progression of aortic stenosis suggests that the valve may be traumatized by abnormal flow patterns, initiated by any congenital or acquired deformity of valve cusps, as a result of which the leaflets are incapable of opening completely during systole (Edwards, 1962). Thus, bicuspid aortic valve — in which the systolic aortic orifice is oval rather than triangular — is one of the background conditions which alter flow patterns in a manner that eventually produces the obstruction. As a corollary of this theory it may be assumed that aortic stenosis is always a progressive, self-perpetuating lesion. Bicuspid aortic valve may be the mildest deformity that alters flow patterns — it takes 50 to 70 years before thickening of the valve reaches the critical point of clinically significant stenosis.

Congenital heart disease accounts for three other entities:

- Fixed subaortic stenosis, in which a fibrous membrane underneath the aortic valve is present, perforated by a central opening, or a subvalvular muscular fibrous ring is present;

- Supravalvular aortic stenosis, which appears as a familial or sporadic form;

- Coarctation of the aorta.

Hypertrophic subaortic stenosis is a disease of unknown etiology; more precisely, it probably includes several varieties of varying etiology. Congenital malposition of the mitral leaflet has been thought to be present in some; congenital and familial disease of the myocardium in others; acquired asymmetrical hypertrophy of the septum — perhaps as an unusual form of response to overload (e.g., hypertension) — in still others.

The structural deformity of the aortic valve obstructing outflow from the left ventricle occurs in different forms (Fig. 31–1):

- Congenital fusion of three commissures,

- Congenital deformity with a fused bicuspid valve,

- Unicommissural valve,

- Congenital unequal size of the three cusps with secondary degenerative changes,

- Acquired fusion of commissures between three leaflets,

- Acquired fusion of commissures between leaflets of a bicuspid valve,

- Fibrosis and calcification of leaflets, interfering with their motion.

- Hypoplasia of the aortic annulus.

Congenital *subvalvular aortic stenosis* most frequently occurs in the

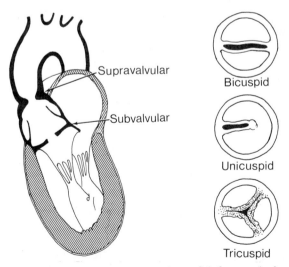

Figure 31–1. Diagrammatic presentation of left ventricular outflow obstructions: Left diagram — supravalvular and subvalvular (fixed) aortic stenosis. Right diagram — three types of valvular (congenital) aortic stenosis.

form of a fibrous diaphragm with a central perforation or a musculofibrous ring—within 1 to 2 cm. underneath normal aortic leaflets.

Supravalvular aortic stenosis involves a coarctation-like structure above the coronary orifices; or the obstruction may involve only the lumen, the outside contour of the aorta remaining normal. This deformity may also involve a general hypoplasia of the aorta. It is occasionally associated with anomalous origins of large aortic branches (particularly brachiocephalic).

Hypertrophic subaortic stenosis does not present a uniform etiological picture, nor is the pathological basis for the obstruction always clear-cut. The most constant finding is left ventricular hypertrophy, with preferential involvement of the septum.

Coarctation of the aorta, presenting itself in the typical form in older children and adults, is almost always of the "adult" variety, i.e., the point of obstruction is beyond the ligamentum arteriosum (Fig. 31–2). It may include in the obstruction the origin of the right subclavian artery. Typically, it is represented by a narrowing, with an hour-glass deformity visible from the outside of the vessel, and with a varying degree of poststenotic dilatation of the aorta beyond the obstruction. Occasionally, longer segments of the aorta are stenotic or even atretic. Typically, adult-type coarctation (postductal) is associated with pronounced enlargement of collateral channels, usually involving intercostal arteries. Infantile (preductal) coarctation may present itself with persistent patency of the ductus arteriosus, in which the lower part of the body is perfused with blood originating in the right side of the heart and ejected via the pulmonary artery system and the duct.

From the pathophysiological standpoint, a significant obstructive lesion in the left side of the circulation involves a stenosis severe enough to produce a pressure gradient across it. Under ordinary circumstances of flow within the arterial circulation, a gradient develops if the area of stenosis is reduced to one-third of the lumen of the vessel or of the aortic orifice. Lesser degrees of stenosis produce no important impediment to flow when the cardiac output is normal, but may

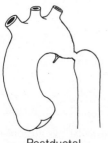

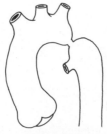

Figure 31–2. Diagrammatic presentation of preductal (infantile) and postductal (adult) coarctation of the aorta.

Postductal   Preductal

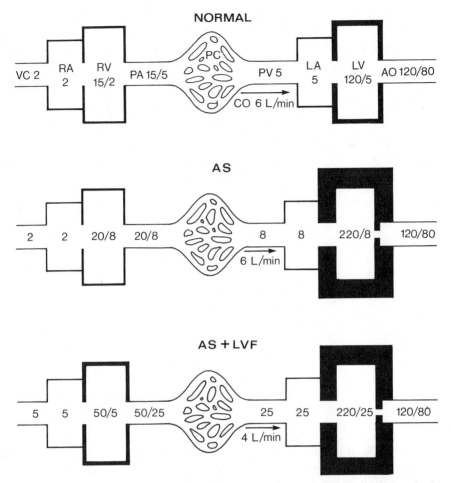

Figure 31-3. Hemodynamic diagram showing the normal circulation *(top),* an example of severe valvular aortic stenosis (AS), compensated *(middle diagram),* and one showing aortic stenosis with left ventricular failure (LVF) *(lower diagram).*

become significant when it rises (e.g., in exercise). The formula depicting relationships of flow through a stenosed orifice (derived from Poiseuille's equation) shows an orifice to be related directly to blood flow through it but inversely to the square root of the pressure gradient across it; hence increase in flow through an obstructed orifice produces greatly exaggerated (squared) increase in pressure gradient. It should also be noted that, as an orifice gradually becomes stenotic, it reaches a critical zone in which laminar flow changes into turbulent flow, giving origin to a murmur which may be perceived even before a pressure gradient appears. Thus, in mild stenosis of the aortic valve or of other structure in the arterial system, murmurs appear before measurable stenosis can be demonstrated.

A stenosis producing murmurs and pressure gradients does not necessarily involve an anatomic reduction of the lumen caused by a small fixed orifice. Gradients and changes in laminar flow are expressions of resistance to outflow in general; such a resistance can be brought about by a temporary narrowing (in hypertrophic subaortic stenosis), or by excessive stiffness of valve leaflets that cannot open under physiological pressure. This latter mechanism is of crucial importance in calcific aortic stenosis of old age for several reasons:

- A heavily calcified valve may appear on inspection to open along all commissures, and yet may be severely stenotic because of its immobility due to stiffness.

- Building up higher pressure (e.g., during exercise) permits a slightly better systolic opening, hence reduces the degree of stenosis.

- Conversely, when systolic pressure in the left ventricle falls, the stenosis automatically increases, since the valve opens even less than with a normal systolic pressure.

- The dependence of the degree of stenosis upon the height of the systolic pressure creates a dangerous vicious circle: onset of cardiac failure may reduce cardiac output, which in turn makes the stenosis more severe, which imposes more overload upon the left ventricle, and so on and on.

Aortic stenosis of significant degree overloads the left ventricle and produces its hypertrophy. As is usual in the case of pressure overload, the resulting hypertrophy is concentric, preserving a small left ventricular cavity until late, when overt cardiac failure develops. All forms of left ventricular outflow obstruction, with the exception of supravalvular stenosis, induce some interference with the coronary arterial perfusion. The following factors may contribute to this:

- The systolic intraventricular pressure is greatly elevated, as is the intramural left ventricular pressure, yet coronary perfusion occurs at the level of aortic pressure, which is much lower (the coronary orifices are beyond the obstruction producing the pressure gradient).

- High velocity jet may induce the Venturi phenomenon, reducing blood flow into the coronary ostia. This coronary deficit may induce clinical manifestations of myocardial ischemia, e.g., anginal pain with effort, and arrhythmias. Although it has not been definitely proved, this mechanism may also contribute to the well-known tendency to sudden death in aortic stenosis.

The pathophysiological basis for syncopal attacks occurring in aortic stenosis is not entirely clarified; multiple factors may contribute to the production of syncope:

- Tachyarrhythmias may be induced by the abovementioned coronary deficit;

- Acute failure of the hypertrophied left ventricle, building up very high systolic pressure, may be abrupt enough to produce syncope as a manifestation of predominant "forward" failure;

- An impaired pressure-regulating mechanism due to altered baroreceptor sensors may be present in aortic stenosis.

In supravalvular aortic stenosis the obstructive lesion is located beyond the origin of the coronary arteries. In it the coronary arterial circulation is subjected to high perfusion pressure; these arteries enlarge appreciably, often reaching unusual caliber. However, high pressure present since birth accelerates the atheromatous process; premature obstructive coronary disease is common.

The effect of the coarctation of the aorta differs from that of the more proximally located obstructive lesions. Here, between the heart and the point of stenosis the entire circulation to the upper part of the body, or most of it, is contained. The resistance to flow is thus dissipated and shared by the arteriolar system of the upper part of the body. The question as to whether the measurable hypertension present in the upper part of the body is the result of the mechanical obstruction to flow or to a humoral renal mechanism has not yet been definitely answered. The answer to this controversy may be that both factors contribute to the pressure elevation. It seems reasonable to assume that in patients with predominant elevation of the systolic pressure the mechanical factor is most important; in those with elevation of diastolic pressure a renal factor is probably involved.

THE CLINICAL ENTITIES

Congenital Valvular Aortic Stenosis

This variety of aortic stenosis is, as a rule, evident since infancy by the early presence of the characteristic ejection systolic murmur.

Natural History. The natural history of all types of valvular aortic stenosis has many similarities, the principal difference being the age at which the symptoms become clinically apparent.

Congenital valvular aortic stenosis occurs, as already mentioned, in various anatomic forms, which produce a wide spectrum of severities of outflow obstruction. The most severe stenosis may cause some deaths in infancy and may present itself as a surgical emergency: given an infant with signs of aortic stenosis who shows evidence of cardiac failure, immediate aortic valvotomy is considered a lifesaving procedure.

Patients with less severe degrees of congenital aortic stenosis may remain asymptomatic in infancy and, often, in early childhood. First symptoms are likely to manifest themselves as exertional chest pain or syncopal attacks (often presyncopal dizziness), also usually related to effort. Effort intolerance due to dyspnea is less common, often because the earlier symptoms usually lead to surgical treatment before heart failure has time to develop. A great many patients with aortic stenosis — even with demonstrated severe obstruction — remain asymptomatic. Congenital aortic stenosis is recognized as the commonest cause of sudden death in childhood and adolescence. It is believed that some patients die suddenly without previous symptoms, though it is difficult to be sure that patients did not have early warning symptoms that they ignored. Sudden death occurs most often during exercise. The incidence of sudden death is probably smaller than was believed in the past, not more than 1 per cent. Patients with milder degree of aortic stenosis may develop symptoms and reach a stage requiring surgical intervention at any time of life. As stated, aortic stenosis has to be considered a progressive lesion. Although it is not definitely known, it seems unlikely that patients with aortic stenosis remain asymptomatic and retain mild aortic valvular obstruction for life in a manner analogous to those with pulmonary stenosis.

The natural history of congenital aortic stenosis after aortic valvotomy varies. It is related first of all to the correctability of the lesion, which ranges from a condition permitting easy freeing of the commissures of a fused tricuspid aortic valve, to totally inoperable hypoplasia of the aortic annulus. In general, an appreciable proportion of patients show after valvotomy residual gradients, indicating incomplete relief of the obstruction. It is also clear that after valvotomy some valves are more prone than others to restenosis. As a consequence, aortic valvotomy should be considered in most patients a palliative operation.

There are relatively few complications occurring in the course of congenital aortic stenosis. Infective endocarditis represents a definite risk, though it probably is less common than in patients with aortic regurgitation. Various arrhythmias may develop but are neither common nor characteristic for this entity.

Diagnosis. The essential features of congenital valvular aortic stenosis include the following:

1. The characteristic ejection systolic murmur is usually located in the second right intercostal space at the sternal border and is well con-

ducted above the clavicle and to the neck. The murmur may also be heard, usually with lesser intensity, at the left sternal border and the apical area. The murmur is characteristically diamond-shaped, crescendo-decrescendo in character, is at least grade IV in intensity, and is accompanied by a thrill. The length of the murmur and the lateness of its peaking reflect upon the severity of the obstruction, in that milder degrees of stenosis produce short, early-peaking murmurs. The loudness of the murmur has some relationship to the severity of stenosis, but it is a crude one. The systolic ejection murmur is a sine qua non of aortic stenosis, with the possible exception of moribund infants in severe cardiac failure.

2.   An ejection sound is characteristically found along the left sternal border, occasionally in the apical area. This sign has high specificity as an indication of valvular obstruction; on careful auscultation it is present in almost every case.

3.   Both components of the second sound are usually audible. Reversed splitting can be found only in severe degrees of aortic stenosis. It is not a specific sign for this condition.

4.   Early diastolic murmur of aortic regurgitation is occasionally present; the degree of aortic regurgitation may then be trivial and the diagnosis of "aortic stenosis" may still be made. It has no discriminating significance regarding point of obstruction.

5.   Gallop sounds occur commonly in all forms of aortic stenosis. An S4 gallop sound is a fairly constant finding of significant aortic stenosis. Though not specific for this disease, it is helpful to rule out trivial degrees of obstruction. S3 gallop may appear late, when cardiac failure ensues.

6.   Arterial pulses may show an anacrotic notch and a slow upstroke. This finding, more often observed in older patients, reflects the severity of aortic obstruction (regardless of the location of the stenosis).

7.   A sustained and forceful apical (left ventricular) impulse is usually present in patients with severe degree of aortic stenosis. This is an important clinical sign demonstrating the presence of significant left ventricular hypertrophy.

8.   The electrocardiogram shows left ventricular hypertrophy in association with significant aortic stenosis. Inasmuch as the voltage criteria for left ventricular hypertrophy overlap with the normal population in children even more than in adults, the electrocardiogram becomes an index of severity of aortic stenosis when ST-T changes begin to appear. The electrocardiogram is often used as a discriminator between trivial and significant aortic stenosis. This approach should be

applied with caution because of the overlap zone between the normal and abnormal.

9. Radiographic examination shows, as a rule, a normal-sized cardiac shadow. The "rounding" of the lower left cardiac border, considered by some as evidence for left ventricular hypertrophy without dilatation, is a finding of low specificity. The most characteristic finding is evidence of dilatation of the ascending aorta (poststenotic dilatation), which may discriminate between valvular aortic stenosis and the subvalvular varieties in which it is not present. It can be detected in plain films in most but not all patients with valvular aortic stenosis.

10. Echocardiographic examination may reveal confirmatory changes of valvular aortic stenosis. Diminished motion of the aortic valve echo has been described, along with evidence for supravalvular dilatation of the aorta. These findings are, however, of low sensitivity: severe valvular aortic stenosis occurs often without showing echocardiographic abnormalities of the aortic leaflets. Echocardiography acquires more sensitivity and specificity in older patients in whom valvular calcifications develop.

11. Carotid pressure tracings may reveal slow upstroke and the presence of an anacrotic notch. Prolongation of the ejection period occurs in severe aortic stenosis, yet this sign is also of low sensitivity.

Invasive studies include cardiac catheterization as the most important method for the determination of severity of aortic stenosis. This requires measurement of transvalvular pressure gradient and of cardiac output. The importance of interpreting the pressure gradient only in the light of the cardiac output cannot be overemphasized, for many errors are being perpetrated by considering the gradient alone: in children with naturally higher-than-average cardiac output, even moderate aortic stenosis may produce very high pressure gradients. Conversely, in the presence of cardiac failure, when the cardiac output is reduced, modest pressure gradients must not be dismissed, for they can still indicate significant degrees of outflow obstruction.

The calculated valve areas for aortic stenosis best reflect the severity of the obstruction:

- 0.3 to 0.5 cm.^{2} for adult size signifies very severe aortic stenosis (0.2 to 0.4 per M.^{2} of body surface area);

- 0.6 to 0.9 (0.4 to 0.6) represents moderately severe aortic stenosis;

- 1.0 to 1.2 (0.6 to 0.8) represents moderate aortic stenosis;

- 1.3 and more (0.8) represents mild aortic stenosis.

Gradient should be measured simultaneously or in a withdrawal tracing; accuracy requires that left ventricular and aortic tracings be measured rather than that of peripheral arterial pressure. Withdrawal records from the left ventricle permit a differentiation of the area of obstruction, i.e., at the valve, below the valve, or above the valve; yet, interpretation of withdrawal curves is subject to errors, so this differentiation should be confirmed by other methods.

Angiocardiography permits an insight into the anatomic type of valvular obstruction. A specially important use of this procedure is to provide means of evaluation of the size of the aortic annulus, and thereby to assess the operability of the lesion (fortunately the inoperable hypoplastic annulus is rare). In cases in which the site of the obstruction is not clear, angiocardiography provides means of differentiation between the various locations of the outflow obstruction from the left ventricle, particularly the identification of supravalvular stenosis.

Differential diagnosis of congenital valvular aortic stenosis in children and young adults involves the following problems:

1. In patients with mild valvular aortic stenosis the following conditions may present differential diagnostic difficulties:

  • innocent ejection murmurs commonly found in children;

  • vascular bruits originating in the great vessels, also commonly found in young patients (usually of no clinical significance);

  • pulmonary stenosis;

  • unusual forms of mitral regurgitation;

  • ventricular septal defect.

2. In severe valvular aortic stenosis the diagnosis can usually be made with ease, but the site of the obstruction may not be readily apparent. This problem has already been discussed in part and will be further elaborated in connection with other forms of left ventricular outflow obstruction.

Treatment. Medical management of patients with congenital valvular aortic stenosis involves the following points:

1. Preventive measures against endocarditis should be observed;

2. Unusually strenuous physical effort should be avoided;

3. The progressive nature of the disease requires careful follow-up, even in asymptomatic patients with mild obstruction.

Surgical treatment is indicated in severe aortic stenosis producing significant symptoms. Except for the rare cases of annular hypoplasia, valvular aortic stenosis is amenable to aortic valvotomy; valve replacement in children and young adults is usually avoided and used only in cases where more conservative surgical treatment is impossible.

Patients with valvular aortic stenosis present a wide range of priorities in terms of surgical treatment. The urgent, often emergency nature of the symptomatic infant with severe aortic stenosis has already been mentioned. In older children and young adults comparable urgency is seldom encountered. Indications for surgical treatment require demonstration of severe aortic stenosis. First priority is given to patients with significant symptoms (syncope, chest pain, effort dyspnea); patients with vague symptoms, questionably related to aortic stenosis (fatigability, abdominal pains, etc.) represent the next priority. Asymptomatic patients with severe aortic stenosis represent a controversial subject. Patients with severe aortic stenosis with advanced electrocardiographic changes of left ventricular hypertrophy are often advised to have valvotomy performed; its justification is fair, in view of the danger of sudden death. However, in older patients, who might require valve replacement, the risk of the operation may well be higher than that of not operating.

"Rheumatic" Valvular Aortic Stenosis

Rheumatic etiology of valvular aortic stenosis can be definitely accepted only in patients who show evidence of coexisting mitral stenosis. Nevertheless, rheumatic fever undoubtedly accounts for some other cases of aortic stenosis appearing in middle age, even if isolated aortic valve disease appears to be present, especially if there is a reliable history of rheumatic carditis. The remainder, probably the majority of cases, represent nonspecific valve disease developing on bicuspid or otherwise malformed aortic valves.

Natural History. More often than not, aortic stenosis is discovered accidentally in asymptomatic subjects in connection with routine checkups or examinations for other reasons. It is basically a progressive disease; the aortic systolic murmur may be of low intensity when first discovered, and unassociated with any other detectable abnormalities. When a fully developed picture of aortic stenosis is present, clinical findings are related to the severity of the obstruction. Occasionally symptoms bring the patient to the physician's attention.

The natural history of adult aortic stenosis can be divided into five stages:

1. Asymptomatic stage;

2. Stage of prefailure symptoms (chest pain, syncope, occasionally milder forms of effort dyspnea);

3. Stage of left ventricular failure;

4. Stage of right ventricular failure;

5. Postoperative stage.

Patients with milder degrees of aortic stenosis are almost always asymptomatic. Prefailure symptoms have been discussed in connection with congenital aortic stenosis. They consist of angina-like exertional chest pain and of syncope or presyncopal attacks of dizziness, also related to effort.

The onset of left ventricular failure may take place in previously asymptomatic patients, or in those who had in the past exhibited chest pain, dizziness, or both. Failure is more apt to appear abruptly in the form of paroxysmal nocturnal dyspnea or pulmonary edema than in the form of gradual onset, starting with increasing effort dyspnea.

The stage of right ventricular failure occurs either sequentially after the patient has shown the earlier stages, or, occasionally, as the first manifestation of cardiac difficulty in the form of fluid accumulation, abdominal fullness, and pain and fatigability.

The risk of sudden death — common to all forms of aortic stenosis — has been mentioned in connection with the congenital variety. One of the critical questions concerning aortic stenosis relates to the significance of the prefailure symptoms (anginal pain, syncope) as precursors of sudden death. The definitive answer to this question is not available. Traditionally, these symptoms are considered ominous, and are often taken as indications for immediate surgery. The danger of these attacks may well be exaggerated. Two older studies dealing with patients in the presurgical era revealed an average survival period of three to four years for patients exhibiting either of these symptoms (with ranges from a few months to 18 years). On the other hand, patients in cardiac failure showed a mean survival period of less than one year. In the absence of more definitive observations, taking under consideration the severity of aortic stenosis and the hemodynamic status of patients suffering from chest pain or syncope, one is justified in giving serious weight to these symptoms but not considering them ominous *per se.*

In contrast, the development of cardiac failure should be considered a very serious turn in the course of the patient's disease. Occasionally, patients may respond to medical therapy and remain controlled for long periods of time; in general, however, it is wise to consider the development of cardiac failure, especially of the congestive phenomena from right ventricular failure, as a danger sign that requires immediate surgical attention.

Among complications of aortic stenosis, infective endocarditis plays a small, but important role, as already mentioned. Other complications are as follows:

- Valve calcification occasionally may lead to calcium embolization.

- Atrial arrhythmias occur occasionally in middle-aged and older patients, though they are rare in comparison with those in mitral valve disease. However, atrial fibrillation may have serious consequences, since the hypertrophied left ventricle needs the "atrial kick" more than a normal ventricle.

- Ventricular arrhythmias as possible results of relative ischemia have been discussed above.

- Patients with long-standing left ventricular hypertrophy may develop irreversible myocardial fibrosis, introducing a "myocardial factor" to the consequences of pure pressure overload.

- Patients first seen in the stage of right ventricular failure may lose some characteristic features of aortic stenosis: the left ventricle dilates—seen as cardiomegaly in the radiograph; reactive pulmonary hypertension occasionally develops with its consequences upon the clinical picture. Even the systolic murmur may become faint or absent.

- Mitral regurgitation may develop as a result of the high left ventricular systolic pressure, producing an apical holosystolic murmur (though seldom dynamically significant).

Following surgical treatment for aortic stenosis the course varies greatly. Valve replacement is almost always necessary in middle-aged and older individuals: the possible consequences of prosthetic valves have been mentioned in Chapter 13. Many patients show dramatic results—symptomatic improvement in patients who show disability prior to the operation is more consistent in aortic stenosis than in mitral stenosis or in the regurgitant lesions. Nevertheless, persistence of cardiac failure is occasionally observed. A specific complication has been reported as occurring after aortic valve replacement, namely, the development of progressive, new obstructive lesions in the main left coronary artery, and possibly proximal right lesions as well. Thus patients who develop anginal pain after the operation need careful and prompt evaluation.

Diagnosis. The diagnostic features of valvular aortic stenosis have been presented in conjunction with congenital aortic stenosis. Only a few additional comments are needed as applicable to this group of patients:

1.   Valve calcifications may appear relatively early in aortic stenosis; they are occasionally found in patients in the third decade of life; their presence is the rule in the fifth decade. The presence of valvular calcification is important confirmatory evidence for valvular aortic stenosis and a valuable differential point from subvalvular or supravalvular stenosis.

2.   With increasing stiffness of the aortic leaflets due to calcification, some physical findings may change: the ejection sound may diminish in intensity and then disappear; the aortic component of the second sound may also become soft or inaudible.

3.   The arterial pulse reflects the severity of aortic stenosis better in adult patients than either in children or in old age. The narrow pulse pressure, slow anacrotic arterial upstroke, and prolonged ventricular ejection are helpful signs of severe aortic stenosis.

4.   Radiographic examination requires fluoroscopic search for the presence of calcification of the aortic valve. The presence of cardiac failure, particularly that involving the right ventricle, produces cardiac enlargement: concentric hypertrophy of the left ventricle that is present in the compensated state changes into enlargement of the left ventricular cavity. Furthermore, the radiographic examination is a valuable aid in the detection of pulmonary vascular congestion, hence confirmatory evidence of left ventricular failure in patients whose principal complaint is dyspnea.

5.   As mentioned, in patients first seen in cardiac failure the systolic murmur may be faint or inaudible.

The *evaluation* of patients with valvular aortic stenosis in the middle age group involves two problems:

- Assessment of severity of left ventricular outflow obstruction by all available means, including cardiac catheterization;

- Interpretation of the patient's symptomatology in the light of the severity of aortic stenosis. Thus, it is necessary to acquire reasonable assurance that chest pain, if present, is not due to coexisting coronary artery disease, that syncope is not related to heart block or carotid artery obstruction, and that dyspnea is not due to obstructive pulmonary disease. The differential diagnosis of the patient's symptoms assumes special importance if aortic stenosis is found to be of only modest severity, in which case a skeptical approach to a causal relationship between aortic stenosis and the patient's symptomatology may be justified. Thus the finding of less than severe aortic stenosis in symptomatic patients may require the performance of coronary arteriography (in some institutions it is routinely performed in all patients in whom cardiac catheterization for aortic stenosis is being done), a pulmonary function panel, and a neurological and cerebro-angiographic examination before surgical treatment is recommended.

Treatment. The treatment of adult aortic stenosis is analogous to that of congenital valvular aortic stenosis of the juvenile patient. Medical therapy is primarily that of prevention and careful serial follow-up. Serious symptoms require surgical considerations; however, the presence of aortic valve calcifications, which greatly increase the likelihood of aortic valve replacement, justifies conservatism in recommending operation, as explained above, particularly if aortic stenosis—even in symptomatic patients—is found to be of only moderate severity.

There are patients with aortic stenosis who develop cardiac failure and become urgent candidates for cardiac surgery, but who either refuse to submit to cardiac surgery or have coexisting conditions that contraindicate the performance of a cardiac operation. In these patients aggressive nonsurgical therapy for cardiac failure should be followed. Experience has shown that some such patients may survive many years.

Senile Calcific Aortic Stenosis

Senile aortic stenosis merges as a continuum with that discussed above. It involves a more slowly developing aortic valve obstruction dependent primarily on stiffening and loss of mobility of the aortic leaflets. This variety is the most typical example of the nonspecific form of valvular disease, related to abnormal flow patterns, presumably initiated by a congenital bicuspid valve or by another minor deformity of the aortic leaflets.

Natural History. Patients with senile calcific aortic stenosis seldom give a history of a known cardiac murmur since childhood. The murmur is usually discovered during an asymptomatic state in middle age. Occasionally it may not be noted until the patient is severely symptomatic. Except for the development of symptoms at a later age, the course of disease is similar to that of the other two types of valvular aortic stenosis, i.e., the appearance of significant symptoms in the prefailure stage in many patients (estimated at about 50 per cent), usually exertional chest pain and syncope or presyncopal dizziness. Left ventricular failure may be the first symptom and, in some cases, the patient appreciates his symptoms only when combined left and right ventricular failure are in evidence. One of the most important features of senile calcific aortic stenosis is the potentially rapid deterioration of patients who have reached the stage of cardiac failure. The dependence of left ventricular ejection upon adequate driving pressure in patients with heavily calcified valves makes the fall of cardiac output particularly undesirable, hence the onset of cardiac failure often produces emergencies that may require immediate surgical intervention. In general, the older age of patients in this type of aortic stenosis increases the likelihood of coexistence of other diseases which may obscure the clinical picture and affect the natural history (sometimes providing contraindications to surgery). Such diseases include ischemic heart disease, pulmonary disease, and hypertension.

Diagnosis. The diagnosis of calcific aortic stenosis has been discussed in the preceding section. Calcification of the valve leaflets affects valve mobility; therefore auscultatory signs generated by valve motion may be absent, namely, ejection sound and aortic closure sound. Another diagnostic feature of this group of patients is the tendency to softer murmurs as compared with younger patients. The combination of the commonly present hyperinflation of the lungs and the lower cardiac output in older patients affects the intensity of the systolic ejection murmur, occasionally reducing the loudness of it to grades I or II; hence the severity of aortic stenosis may be underestimated, or its presence even overlooked. Patients in cardiac failure, when seen for the first time, may present without systolic murmurs, the vibrations being below the auditory threshold.

Other diagnostic features may also be minimized by other coexisting lesions, often of no clinical importance but obscuring the diagnosis of aortic stenosis. Thus, intraventricular conduction defects may make the electrocardiogram less specific; coronary artery calcification may divert the attention to ischemic heart disease, and so on. Loss of elasticity of the large arteries counteracts the effect of aortic stenosis upon the arterial pulse; it widens the pulse pressure and quickens the upstroke.

Evaluation of senile aortic stenosis requires invasive studies as presented above. Patients with anginal pain as a presenting symptom require at least a screening study of the coronary arterial tree, and often selective coronary arteriography. Patients in cardiac failure should have an assessment of left ventricular function by means of ventriculography.

Treatment. The management of aortic stenosis is largely surgical, given a symptomatic patient with an adequate left ventricular function. Valve replacement is virtually always necessary. This operation often reverses symptoms and abolishes cardiac failure dramatically in patients as old as 80 years. Priorities for surgical treatment are as follows:

- Patients with aortic stenosis and congestive failure should be considered surgical emergencies. If seen for the first time, they require invasive evaluation at once and immediate operation as soon as operability is established.

- Patients in left ventricular failure (paroxysmal nocturnal dyspnea, severe effort dyspnea) are urgent candidates. Abrupt and severe onset of left ventricular failure may bring them into the category of emergency, similar to those in right ventricular failure.

- Patients with anginal chest pain are considered candidates for valve replacement; the timing is related to the severity of symptoms and the hemodynamic findings. The relationship between the pain and aortic stenosis should be reasonably well established.

- Patients with syncopal attacks should be considered individually before a surgical decision is made; it is axiomatic that other causes of syncope should be reasonably well ruled out.

- Patients are considered inoperable if severe congestive cardiac failure is present, poor ventricular function is demonstrated by left ventriculography, and the aortic stenosis is found to be of mild or moderate severity. Under similar circumstances, but in the presence of very severe aortic stenosis, the higher risk of operating may be accepted if medical therapy is ineffective.

- Patients with significant aortic stenosis who present themselves with chest pain and are also shown to have a bypassable lesion in a coronary artery may be considered for a combined operation: valve replacement with aortico-coronary bypass. The decision should be arrived at individually and should be considered in the light of the facility and experience of the surgical team available. Conversely, "prophylactic" bypass operations added to aortic valve replacement in patients with mild coronary obstructive lesions are to be discouraged.

Medical therapy is indicated in patients who are unsuitable for the operation or who refuse to undergo surgical treatment. General supportive therapy and conventional management of cardiac failure can be offered to them.

Congenital Fixed Subaortic Stenosis

This is a relatively rare form of left ventricular outflow obstruction. The physiological consequences of the obstruction below the valve are identical with those at the valve; hence the natural history of the lesion is similar to that of valvular congenital aortic stenosis, being primarily determined by the severity of the obstruction. However, the two anatomic forms may differ from each other:

- The subvalvular diaphragmatic form is presumably always nonprogressive; its surgical treatment may be satisfactory and permanent.

- The subvalvular ring (tunnel type) composed of fibromuscular tissue may be progressive; it often presents technical difficulty when surgical relief is sought, and results are often less than satisfactory.

The symptomatology of subaortic stenosis is identical with that of valvular aortic stenosis of comparable severity. However, diagnostic differences may permit its clinical differentiation from valvular stenosis. In subaortic stenosis:

1. The murmur may be located predominantly to the left of the sternum, although its radiation to the neck and above the clavicles is usually preserved.

2. The ejection sound is absent.

3. Poststenotic dilatation of the aorta may be absent.

It should be emphasized that murmurs of aortic regurgitation are found as often as in valvular aortic stenosis, perhaps even more frequently.

Invasive studies may definitely demonstrate subvalvular location of the obstruction. It should be noted, however, that a critical evaluation of the findings is needed to avoid pitfalls:

- The pressure curve upon withdrawal from the left ventricle shows the pressure gradient to be present within the left ventricle and not at the ventricular-aortic junction (i.e., the valve). Yet, if the diaphragm or the ring is separated from the valve by a very narrow chamber, the catheter may not remain in this chamber long enough to record curves with lower systolic pressure, hence the curve may simulate that of valvular stenosis.

- Angiocardiographic studies usually reveal the obstruction to be below the valve; yet a thin diaphragm may be missed in the angiocardiogram.

Treatment of subvalvular stenosis is largely surgical if the severity of the lesion justifies intervention. The somewhat better prospect of long-range results in one variety have already been mentioned.

Hypertrophic Subaortic Stenosis

As already indicated, hypertrophic subaortic stenosis cannot be considered a distinct clinical, physiological, or pathological entity, but rather a pathophysiological disturbance of left ventricular function produced by several different mechanisms. The natural history of this condition is not yet well known, in spite of the fact that several good studies have attempted to review it. The wide variety of factors influencing the course of the disease will require many more studies dealing with larger numbers of cases in order to assess the prognosis of this disease. As stated, at least three varieties of hypertrophic subaortic stenosis are thus far recognized:

• The familial—probably a congenital form;

• The acquired form of asymmetrical septal hypertrophy as an expression of cardiomyopathy;

• The secondary form resulting from left ventricular overload lesions (hypertension, valvular aortic stenosis).

Natural History. The following are the recognized characteristics of this disturbance:

1. It is basically a progressive lesion, though in many patients the progression occurs very slowly, over decades.

2. There is a risk of sudden death, not necessarily related to the severity of the obstruction. In a recent prospective study this risk was estimated at 15 per cent.

3. Symptoms vary greatly and are also not necessarily related to the severity of the disease. Symptomatology increases sharply with age.

4. Responses to medical and surgical therapy are variable.

5. Some observations indicate that patients may eventually develop congestive failure and lose left ventricular outflow obstruction.

The majority of patients are now diagnosed when asymptomatic or mildly symptomatic, in view of the wide awareness of this disease entity. Early, nondisabling symptoms include chest pain, which usually resembles anginal pain, but only occasionally presents itself in the form of typical effort angina. The pain may be nonexertional and more often than in true angina is perceived as an ill-defined apprehension. Dyspnea may develop with exercise or at rest. Dizziness and syncopal attacks are likely to develop at later stages, when chest pain and dyspnea become more pronounced. This combination may produce severe disability. Paroxysmal atrial arrhythmias are common. Those characterized by excessively rapid rates account for some of the syncopal attacks. Congestive failure is rare and, as stated above, may be associated with the loss of signs of left ventricular outflow obstruction.

The proneness to sudden death, mentioned above, represents the principal risk of this disease. Patients occasionally give a history of a relative who died suddenly "of a heart attack," undoubtedly representing an unrecognized case of familial hypertrophic subaortic stenosis.

The response to therapy is as variable as is the symptomatology itself. Medical therapy consisting of beta-adrenergic blocking agents often controls symptoms: milder symptoms may disappear altogether and more severe ones may be alleviated. Some patients, however, fail to respond to medical treatment.

As a rule, surgical procedures are much less dependable in this disease than they are in other forms of left ventricular outflow obstruction. Whether medical or surgical therapy can significantly improve the prognosis by altering the natural history of the disease is not known.

Diagnosis. Hypertrophic subaortic stenosis presents several clinical and laboratory features that are sufficiently characteristic to establish the diagnosis noninvasively with reasonable accuracy:

1. The apical impulse may show a double systolic motion produced by the early systolic percussion wave that produces a bisferiens type of pulse. With the common presence of a presystolic motion, the presence of a triple impulse or a double systolic impulse is an important, moderately specific sign of this condition.

2. Auscultatory findings include a prominent S4 gallop sound and a systolic murmur. The murmur shows a wide variability in loudness, duration, and character: it originates in part at the point of midventricular obstruction (an ejection systolic murmur at the mid-left sternal border often conducted to the supraclavicular area) and results partly from mitral valve incompetence (pansystolic apical murmur or delayed systolic murmur at the apical region). Some patients show only the ejection component, which may be inconspicuous, even intermittent. Some have mitral regurgitant murmurs so typical that the diagnosis of mitral regurgitation is first suggested. Both components of the murmur are increased during the straining period of the Valsalva maneuver and decreased during post-straining bradycardia. They are also accentuated by the administration of amyl nitrite. While demonstration of these changes in the intensity of the systolic murmur are important diagnostic points, they have only moderate specificity; particularly the mitral regurgitant component may fail to show changes in response to the various maneuvers. In a small proportion of patients an S3 gallop sound is present. Early diastolic murmurs of aortic regurgitation are rare (in contrast to other forms of left-sided outflow obstruction).

3. The arterial pulse shows a bisferiens shape; recording of the carotid pulse reveals a characteristic shape with a rapid upstroke leading to an early thin spike, a valley separating the spike ("percussion wave") from the remainder of the pulse wave. It differs from the bisferiens pulse of combined aortic stenosis and regurgitation in that the latter shows a broader initial wave (see also Fig. 4–5).

4. Radiographically, the cardiac shadow is usually normal in size, often smaller than average; the ascending aorta is also normal (a differential point with valvular aortic stenosis).

5. The electrocardiogram shows a wide range of abnormalities; a normal record may be present in milder forms of hypertrophic subaortic stenosis; some evidence of left ventricular hypertrophy (often merely by the voltage criteria) is most often present. In some cases unusual forms of left ventricular hypertrophy may be found, showing deep and wide Q waves in several leads, sometimes mistaken for signs of myocardial infarction. Complexes similar to the Wolff-Parkinson-White syndrome, with short P-R interval and delta waves, are occasionally present. The association with W-P-W syndrome characterized by paroxysmal arrhythmias occurs occasionally.

6. The echocardiogram shows an abnormal systolic anterior motion of the mitral valve which has moderately good specificity. Thickening of the septum is also apparent. Crude quantification of the obstruction may be attempted by noting the distance between the mitral cusps and the septum during systole.

Invasive studies include cardiac catheterization and angiocardiography, both of which establish the diagnosis or confirm the clinical diagnosis of hypertrophic subaortic stenosis.

The essential part of the diagnosis by cardiac catheterization is the demonstration of a systolic pressure gradient between the body of the left ventricular and its subaortic region. This gradient—the expression of outflow resistance due to obstruction—is variable. In the majority of cases with significant hypertrophic subaortic stenosis a moderate gradient (average of 50 mm. Hg) is present at all times. The gradient may be increased during exercise, straining, and following a premature contraction. A highly specific finding is the reduction of the amplitude of systemic arterial pressure pulse in the first beat after a postextrasystolic pause (the phenomenon also exaggerates its pressure gradient). The most consistent way of provoking a latent gradient is infusion of isoproterenol. Additional observations during cardiac catheterization include the recording of the characteristic arterial pressure pulse with the early percussion wave; the left ventricular pressure trace often shows a notch upon its upstroke or a bifid peak as well.

It should be emphasized, in view of the wide range of degrees of hypertrophic subaortic stenosis, that the disease may be present, may even produce symptoms, and yet basal cardiac catheterization study may show normal findings, and only appropriate provocation may establish the diagnosis.

The question of the "catheter entrapment" as the basis for the ventricular pressure gradients has been raised in the past. While this may well be a factor exaggerating the apparent obstruction in patients with overactive hearts and very low end-systolic volume, it in no way detracts from the importance of the syndrome but merely calls for caution in interpretation of pressure gradients in patients who have no other clinical signs suggesting hypertrophic subaortic stenosis.

Angiocardiography is less specific than cardiac catheterization. It is an important confirmatory technique for hypertrophic subaortic stenosis in patients with appreciably severe disease. In milder cases angiographic study may be inconclusive or may even show normal findings. The characteristic feature of this disease is an hourglass deformity of the midportion of the left ventricular cavity developing during systole, produced by a narrowing between the mitral leaflet and the hypertrophied septum.

Evaluation of hypertrophic subaortic stenosis requires a careful step-by-step differentiation of various diagnostic findings. In milder cases, particularly in patients without symptoms, differentiation involves usually innocent cardiac murmurs or trivial mitral regurgitation. It is occasionally stated that the diagnosis of ventricular septal defect may be difficult to separate from that of hypertrophic subaortic stenosis. In fact these two conditions appear unlikely to be confused with each other by experienced clinicians. Because of the uncertain prognosis of hypertrophic subaortic stenosis, a reasonable suspicion of this disease gives justification for a decisive, invasive study, especially if it should be demonstrated in the future that early treatment by beta-adrenergic blockade may postpone the progression of the disease.

In patients with fully developed signs of hypertrophic subaortic stenosis the clinical diagnosis may be established beyond reasonable doubt. Here invasive evaluation may fulfill the role of determining the severity of the obstruction. It should be noted, however, that the changeable nature of the obstruction makes hemodynamic studies less reliable and reproducible than in any other obstructive cardiovascular lesion. Nevertheless, one can make a good case for the value of longitudinal studies: hemodynamic evaluations performed a few years apart showing no change in the severity of the obstruction with comparable provocations may be interpreted as carrying a better outlook than if progression of the process is demonstrated in serial studies. Aggressiveness of therapy may have to vary in each instance.

Treatment. Once the diagnosis of hypertrophic subaortic stenosis is made, it is necessary to outline the plan for the therapy. The objectives of medical and surgical treatment in this condition differ from most other obstructive lesions within the heart inasmuch as the problem is not purely a mechanical one:

- It has been suggested, though not demonstrated, that medical therapy may slow the progress of the disease; hence there is at least some justification for early and prophylactic treatment.

• Some frequently used drugs may exert a paradoxically untoward effect upon this disease.

• Surgical therapy shows inconsistent results.

The drug most effective in the treatment of subaortic hypertrophic stenosis is propranolol. While probably ineffective to reduce the permanent obstruction within the left ventricular cavity, it eliminates or reduces the obstruction that develops with exercise and the various factors temporarily affecting left ventricular performance. Thus, its most effective use can be anticipated in cases with intermittent obstruction. This drug often relieves symptoms dramatically or may merely reduce their severity, but on occasion it is ineffective. The justification for early use of propranolol, even in asymptomatic patients, has already been discussed.

On theoretical grounds, it is deduced that digitalis is harmful and may increase the degree of obstruction, a fact that can be demonstrated in some short-term experiments. Whether this is actually true in the context of the clinical use of digitalis is not clear. Nevertheless, it should be avoided in patients with hypertrophic subaortic stenosis, in spite of the fact that progressive dyspnea with signs of left ventricular hypertrophy provides a powerful temptation to administer digitalis. Similarly, the use of nitroglycerin for angina-like pain should be discouraged.

In general, patients should be carefully followed and instructed to report unusual and new symptoms. Strenuous exercise should be discouraged.

Surgical therapy offers a variety of approaches. The most widely used procedure involves incising the hypertrophied portion of the septal myocardium. More aggressive excision of the septal muscle has been advocated by some. More recently mitral valve replacement by a low-profile prosthesis has been performed, based on the observation that the mitral leaflet is an essential component of the systolic obstacle to outflow from the left ventricle. All these methods have been claimed to produce dramatic successes, but failures have also resulted. Reduction of pressure gradient is usually taken as a yardstick of effectiveness of the operation, but this may be misleading because of the functional nature of the obstruction and the wide variation of the gradient from day to day. While it is true that mitral valve replacement, in the small number of cases in which serial studies are available, most consistently eliminated resting gradient, it is also apparent that the immediate risk and long-range problems associated with valve prosthesis are a high price to pay for the success. In general, one should not lose track of the fact that the basic disease here is not a mechanical obstruction but myocardial disease; hence any form of therapy can be considered only palliative. The risk of surgery—even in consideration of the danger of sudden death—seems justifiable only in severely symptomatic patients unresponsive to medical therapy, or in those with a very high pressure gradient at rest that is consistently present. At present, the lower risk myotomy appears more logical than the more drastic mitral valve replacement.

Supravalvular Aortic Stenosis

This rare disease involves three possible etiological factors or associations:

- Sporadic congenital malformation of the ascending aorta;
- A complex congenital syndrome showing mental retardation and peculiar facial features in addition to supravalvular aortic stenosis, thought to be related to hypercalcemia;
- A familial form without additional features but occasionally associated with other anomalies of the aorta.

Supravalvular aortic stenosis varies in severity, as do other forms of left ventricular outflow obstruction. Milder forms may be difficult to separate from valvular aortic stenosis; more severe forms show some features that are helpful in differential diagnosis.

Natural History. The natural history of supravalvular aortic stenosis is related to the degree of left ventricular hypertrophy; cardiac failure may develop early in life if the obstruction is very severe. There is one basic difference between valvular and supravalvular aortic stenosis: in the latter the obstruction to flow is located *above* the coronary ostia; as a result, the coronary arteries are perfused under very high pressure since birth, and their caliber thus increases, often to giant size. Occasionally tortuous proximal branches of the coronary arteries are visible in the plain chest roentgenogram. Continuous high pressure in the coronary system accelerates the atherosclerotic process and induces premature coronary artery disease. Sudden death may occur from ischemic disease, via a different mechanism than in valvular aortic stenosis.

The *physical findings* of supravalvular aortic stenosis resemble those of valvular aortic stenosis; some features may help differentiate the two:

- An ejection sound is absent in the supravalvular variety;
- The murmur may be located in the first right intercostal space, rather than the second or third;

- A difference in blood pressure between the two arms (higher in the right) may be present.

The electrocardiogram provides no differential features. Radiographic examination reveals as the most important differential feature a small ascending aorta; the possibility of recognizing enlarged coronary arteries has already been mentioned.

Echocardiographic findings have not yet been fully defined in this condition; this technique is likely to provide diagnostic clues in supravalvular aortic stenosis.

Cardiac catheterization requires a withdrawal tracing from the left ventricle into the aorta, showing no gradient at the aortic valve but a pressure differential above the valve, within the ascending aorta. Angiocardiographic studies are the final means of diagnostic confirmation of the diagnosis, by showing the area of constriction within the aorta.

Supravalvular aortic stenosis is more commonly associated with additional malformations of the cardiovascular system than are other forms of left ventricular outflow obstruction. Associated lesions may be intracardiac or — more commonly — vascular. The latter include hypoplasia of some of the brachiocephalic vessels, hypoplasia of the entire aorta, or coarctation of the aorta. Supravalvular stenosis of the pulmonary artery or stenosis of its branches may also be present.

Treatment. The management of this condition is largely surgical, but results have been disappointing. In contrast to coarctation of the aorta, in which permanent cures may be obtained, correction of the supravalvular obstruction, though technically not difficult, may not eliminate the problem; sudden deaths after seemingly successful operations have been reported, presumably from coronary causes; failure to eliminate left ventricular hypertension may be due to general hypoplasia of the aorta in some cases.

Coarctation of the Aorta

Coarctation of the aorta is one of the commonest congenital cardiovascular lesions. It affects the circulation in various ways, depending upon the location of the obstruction and the condition of the ductus arteriosus. The common form of coarctation ("adult form") involves a localized constriction at or beyond the ligamentum arteriosum. The circulation takes basically a normal pathway, although severe constriction favors the development of collateral channels bypassing it, so that the lower part of the body is in part perfused by the brachiocephalic vessels. If the constriction is very severe — occasionally the narrow area may even become atretic — then the entire body may be supplied via channels originating from the aorta above the constriction. A rare form of coarctation is associated with patency of the ductus arteriosus; with the constriction above the duct, the lower part of the body is supplied from the pulmonary artery via the duct; pulmonary hypertension is then almost always present. Survival of such patients into adult age is rare.

Natural History. In the common type of coarctation the great majority of patients remain asymptomatic through childhood, and often through early adulthood as well. A small minority may develop cardiac failure from the pressure overload in infancy. Pediatricians should be aware of cardiac failure in infancy developing without telltale cardiac murmurs of the common congenital intracardiac lesions, and consider coarctation as an important cause, one amenable to surgical cure.

Because of the usual asymptomatic nature of coarctation, this lesion is discovered as a rule on routine examination, by the detection of arterial hypertension. Occasionally murmurs or abnormal radiographic findings lead to case-finding. Symptoms, if present, include tiredness, headaches, and pain in the calves associated with walking. Inasmuch as coarctation of the aorta has been a surgically correctable lesion for some 30 years, its natural history in unoperated patients is not well known.

Hypertension is seldom severe enough to cause cardiac failure in adolescents or in adults. However, certain complications may develop and lead to disastrous consequences:

- Infective endocarditis affecting the aortic valve or endarteritis affecting the site of the coarctation;

- Intracerebral or subarachnoid hemorrhage from rupture of a berry aneurysm in a cerebral artery;

- Rupture or dissection of the aorta (reported most frequently during pregnancy).

A common associated lesion present in coarctation of the aorta is malformation of the aortic valve, usually the bicuspid valve. This association is noted by the pathologist in more than half of the patients with coarctation; clinically detectable disease of the aortic valve is much lower in incidence but nevertheless common.

Surgical repair of the coarctation is nearly a curative operation. Some patients operated upon in infancy or early childhood may redevelop coarctation with growth, thus need reoperation. A rare late consequence of the operation is aneurysm of the aorta distal to the point of the repair. The more important factors affecting the natural history of operated patients are:

- persistent risk of infective endocarditis,

- the fate of aortic valve disease.

While this information is not now available, considering the currently held views of the process leading to calcific aortic stenosis of old age, one may consider patients with "cured" coarctation potential candidates for late aortic stenosis, regardless of whether or not clinically detectable signs of aortic valve disease are present at the time of the operation.

Diagnosis. The diagnosis of coarctation of the aorta may be very easy on clinical grounds; the most important findings are those detected on physical examination:

1. Absent, diminished, or delayed femoral pulses.

2. Palpable enlarged collateral intercostal arteries (in the back of the thorax).

3. Cardiac murmurs: a systolic murmur originating at the site of the coarctation is often heard over both the anterior and posterior thorax. This murmur may override the second sound, and may even acquire the characteristic of a continuous murmur. In addition, deformity of the aortic valve may produce short systolic ejection murmurs at the right second intercostal space, or an early diastolic murmur at the left side of the sternum due to aortic valve incompetence. Aortic valve closure sound is often accentuated in line with arterial hypertension.

4. Hypertension is present in the upper part of the body, most consistently in the right arm. (The left subclavian artery may be at or below the point of constriction, hence the pressure in it may be variable). If pressure can be determined in the lower extremities, a systolic gradient of at least 30 mm. Hg is found. The degree of hypertension in the precoarctation arteries varies; more often than not only a systolic hypertension is present; in children readings of 130 to 150 are commonly found, in adults up to 200. Very severe systolic and diastolic hypertension with levels approaching "malignant" hypertension is rare; its presence suggests additional factors, among which are:

   • Hypoplasia of the aorta in addition to the coarctation;

   • Severe renal involvement;

   • Atypical site of coarctation, e.g., diaphragmatic or abdominal constriction.

5. Electrocardiographic findings are variable; in general, normal tracings are more often found than not. Left ventricular hypertrophy may be present in more severe degrees of hypertension. In infants, findings may be misleading: left ventricular overload may be insufficient to override the physiological right ventricular preponderance, hence the patient may appear to show "right ventricular hypertrophy."

6. Radiographic findings are probably the most specific for diagnosis of coarctation of the aorta; the two principal abnormalities are:

- Notching (scalloping) of the ribs: small indentation upon the lower surface of the ribs produced by tortuous enlarged intercostal arteries participating in the collateral circulation, seen in late childhood and beyond.

- Deformity of the aorta, consisting of a small aortic knob and showing the indentation of the aorta, distal to which is a bulge of poststenotic dilatation of the aorta. This can be seen both in the plain film in the anteroposterior view and also in the right anterior oblique view: the deformity encroaches upon the barium-filled esophagus.

Invasive diagnostic methods offer relatively little new diagnostic information. Differential pressure measurements between arteries originating above and those below the coarctation confirm the clinical diagnosis. Direct aortic pressure tracings can usually be obtained by passing the catheter through the point of obstruction, showing its location as well as the severity as measured by pressure differential. Cardiac study is superfluous, unless significant aortic valve disease is clinically suspected. Angiocardiographic studies outline the narrowing and the adjacent areas of the aorta, often providing helpful information to the surgeon.

Evaluation of patients with suspected coarctation of the aorta provides a challenge to the clinician, who can solve most of the problems without sophisticated diagnostic methods. In the differentiation only occasionally difficulties arise:

- In adults atherosclerosis or saddle embolus may produce absence of femoral pulses.

- Kinks in or below the aortic arch may produce a radiographic picture simulating coarctation ("pseudocoarctation"), but in such cases dynamic effects of the obstruction would be missing.

In general, coarctation of the aorta is one of the few conditions in which invasive studies prior to surgical treatment may be omitted, provided the clinical diagnosis regarding the presence of coarctation is clear-cut, its severity sufficient to justify surgical treatment, and its location in the typical area.

Treatment. The treatment of coarctation is largely surgical. The risk of the operation is small; nevertheless, potential damage to the spine from cessation of the circulation during repair introduces some danger. Consequently the operation should best be handled by an experienced surgical team (even though facilities for open heart surgery are not required). There can be no question that in severe coarctation of the aorta prophylactic surgical correction in asymptomatic patients is fully justified. Some ambivalence may develop regarding the need for surgical therapy in patients with mild coarctation; if the arterial pressure is normal a conservative course of action is probably preferable. The optimal age of the repair is often debated. The older the child, the less likely is the possibility of restenosis; however, this complication is rare in children who undergo repair after the age of five.

Medical treatment should include the usual preventive measures from endocarditis. In patients in whom the operation cannot be performed, medical treatment of hypertension may be indicated. The effectiveness of such therapy can be attested by occasional patients in whom the diagnosis of coarctation of the aorta was missed and who were treated under the mistaken diagnosis of essential hypertension.

Bibliography

Adelman AG, Wigle ED, Ranganathan N, Webb GD, Kidd BSL, Bigelow WG, Silver MD: The clinical course of muscular subaortic stenosis. Ann. Int. Med. 77:515, 1972.

Braunwald E, Goldblatt A, Aygen MM, Rockoff SD, Morrow AG: Congenital aortic stenosis: I. Clinical and hemodynamic findings. Circulation 27:426, 1963.

Braunwald E, Lambrew CT, Rockoff SD, Ross J Jr, Morrow AG: Idiopathic hypertrophic subaortic stenosis. Circulation 30(Suppl. IV):1, 1964.

Campbell M: Natural history of coarctation of the aorta. Brit. Heart J. 32:633, 1970.

Edwards JE: Etiology of calcific aortic stenosis. Circulation 26:817, 1962.

Goodwin JF: Congestive and hypertrophic cardiomyopathies. A decade of study. Lancet 1:731, 1970.

Hancock EW, Fleming PR: Aortic stenosis. Quart. J. Med. 29:209, 1960.

Hancock EW: The ejection sound in aortic stenosis. Amer. J. Med. 40:568, 1966.

Hohn AR, VanPragh S, Moore AAD, Vlad P, Lambert EC: Aortic stenosis. Circulation 32(Suppl. III):4, 1965.

Maron BJ, Humphries JO, Rowe RD, Mellits ED: Prognosis of surgically corrected coarctation of the aorta. Circulation 47:119, 1973.

Myers AR, Willis PW III: Clinical spectrum of supravalvular aortic stenosis. Arch. Int. Med. 118:553, 1966.

Ross J Jr, Braunwald E: Aortic stenosis. Circulation 38(Suppl. V):61, 1968.

Perloff JK: Clinical recognition of aortic stenosis. The physical signs and differential diagnosis of the various forms of obstruction to left ventricular outflow. Prog. Cardiovasc. Dis. 10:323, 1968.

Shah PM, Adelman AG, Wigle ED, Gobel FL, Burchell HB, Hardarson T, Curiel R, dela Clajada C, Oakley CM, Goodwin JF, Yu PN: The natural (and unnatural) course of hypertrophic obstructive cardiomyopathy. A multicenter study. Circ. Res. 35(Suppl. II):179, 1974.

Wood P.: Aortic stenosis. Amer. J. Cardiol. 1:553, 1958.

32

Left Ventricular Inflow Obstruction

Definition. Among conditions interfering with the inflow into the left ventricle, the most important clinical entity is *rheumatic mitral stenosis*. There is only a minute fraction of cases in which other causes of inflow obstruction are present; these include the following:

- Left atrial myxomas propelled in diastole into the left ventricle;

- Nonrheumatic stenotic lesions of the mitral valve secondary to atrial septal defect (Lutembacher's syndrome);

- Congenital mitral stenosis.

In addition to those, some rare congenital lesions produce physiological changes that imitate those of mitral stenosis, even though they do not interfere with left ventricular filling:

- Cor triatriatum (membrane-like obstruction within the left atrium);

- Stenotic lesions of the pulmonary veins (particularly in conjunction with the total anomalous pulmonary venous return).

The discussion in this chapter deals with rheumatic mitral stenosis.

ETIOLOGY

Mitral stenosis is considered a late manifestation of rheumatic damage to the endocardium. Though in chronic mitral stenosis pathological stigmata of rheumatic disease are usually absent, no other mechanism has been demonstrated that can produce the anatomic changes upon the mitral leaflets that are found in mitral stenosis. Doubts have been expressed from time to time regarding alternate causes, particularly in the light of the high percentage of patients with mitral stenosis in whom no evidence of acute rheumatic carditis can be found (more than 40 per cent). Inasmuch as the acute rheumatic process represents a hypersensitivity reaction to streptococcal infection (see Chapter 21), other pathogens, especially viruses, have been suspected as capable of triggering a rheumatic-like reaction. Direct evidence for this, however, has never been presented.

While we assume that the initial effect upon the valve leaflets is rheumatic in origin, no evidence exists that smoldering rheumatic activity is essential as a cause of progression of the obstructive valve lesions years after the initial attack or attacks. Recently doubt has been expressed regarding the continuous rheumatic etiology. As an alternative possibility it is postulated that rheumatic activity causes the initial sealing together of the two mitral leaflets, thereby producing a mild, often hemodynamically and clinically insignificant reduction of the mitral orifice. Later, in a process analogous to that occurring in bicuspid aortic valves, the somewhat smaller mitral orifice alters diastolic flow patterns through the valve, producing turbulence that traumatizes the leaflets, gradually causing their thickening. Thus it may be stated that the rheumatic process produces the initial insult to the valve, upon which a nonspecific, self-perpetuating process may lead to gradual progression of the valvular stenosis. The speed of progression of the nonspecific process is related to the extent of the initial (or repetitive) rheumatic damage and its location; hence, the various clinical patterns of mitral stenosis are discussed in a subsequent section of this chapter.

Congenital mitral stenosis is very rare. It is usually a serious lesion; its varieties may or may not be amenable to surgical treatment. However, untreated patients seldom if ever survive to adult age; therefore discovery of mitral stenosis in an adolescent does not suggest a congenital origin of the lesion but rather early rheumatic disease.

Mitral stenosis associated with atrial septal defect is now considered a nonspecific lesion produced by alteration of the flow patterns in patients with atrial septal defect. Patients with atrial septal defect were once thought to be especially susceptible to rheumatic fever, but this view has now been largely abandoned. Mitral stenosis is at present the commonest valve lesion. It affects women two to three times more often than men.

PATHOLOGY AND PATHOPHYSIOLOGY

Pathologically, three types of mitral stenosis can be recognized (Rusted et al., 1956):

- Commissural type, consisting of fusion of the commissures but without major involvement of the cusps and chordae (Fig 32–1);

- Cuspal type, with primary involvement of the leaflets, leading to thickened and calcified cusps (Fig. 32–1);

- Chordal type, producing fusion of chordae tendineae with their thickening and shortening, thereby interfering with the mobility of the leaflets.

These changes can occur exclusively or, more often, in combination with each other, though one type usually predominates as the cause of valve stenosis.

The production of fully developed mitral stenosis takes many years. The first changes occurring during acute rheumatic carditis consist of small verrucous vegetations developing upon the line of closure of the two leaflets. Some similar lesions may develop upon the chordae tendineae. The valve involved in this process is not stenotic, although minor degrees of incompetence of it may develop. Years afterward the first obstructive lesion may develop by the fusion of the two leaflets at points closest to the papillary muscle — "critical tendon insertion" (Brock, 1952). As a result of this:

- Mild mitral stenosis may develop, though seldom clinically significant;

- Commissures lateral to this area of fusion, at first not attached, lose mobility and gradually may become obliterated.

This process may initiate the commissural and cuspal types of mitral stenosis. The early change — even when obliteration is completed — may not produce significant resistance to flow, because atrioventricular flow normally occurs through the center of the mitral

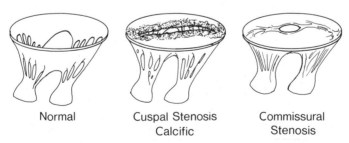

| Normal | Cuspal Stenosis Calcific | Commissural Stenosis |

Figure 32–1. Diagrammatic presentation of cuspal (calcific) and commissural mitral stenosis.

orifice. It may result, however, in turbulent flow, which in turn may produce the following consequences:

- Further fusion of the commissures, now involving parts central to the first point of contact, that may eventually lead to mitral stenosis with a small central orifice ("commissural type");

- As an alternative, no further commissural obliteration may take place, but the leaflets may become thickened, leathery, eventually calcify, and lose mobility to a point where they can no longer open under physiological filling pressures ("cuspal type").

Another route of production of mitral stenosis takes place in patients who from the beginning showed involvement of the chordae in addition to the cuspal involvement. Here the whole mitral valve apparatus may stiffen with a gradual development of an immobile funnel ("chordal type" of mitral stenosis). Chordal involvement interferes not only with the opening but the closure of the mitral valve as well, producing combined mitral stenosis and regurgitation. It will be discussed later in connection with mixed lesions.

The consequences and associated lesions occurring in significant mitral stenosis include the following:

- Left atrial hypertrophy or dilatation or both occur; in long-standing atrial fibrillation resulting from mitral stenosis the atrium may actually become thin; its musculature may show fragmentation and replacement with fibrous tissue;

- Mural thrombi occur frequently in the left atrium—a potential source of systemic emboli;

- Calcification of mitral cusps may extend into the mitral annulus;

- Right ventricular hypertrophy and dilatation may occur as a reflection of higher pressure in the pulmonary circuit;

- In patients with reactive pulmonary hypertension, thickening of the pulmonary arterioles is often found as well as atherosclerotic changes in the pulmonary artery and larger branches.

Pathophysiologically, mitral stenosis produces resistance to left ventricular inflow; this is expressed in terms of a gradient between the left ventricle and the left atrial pressures during diastole. Since the left ventricular workload is normal, left ventricular diastolic pressure remains, as a rule, normal. Thus the direct consequence of mitral stenosis is hypertension within the left atrium, the magnitude of which is related to two factors:

- the severity of mitral stenosis,

- the cardiac output.

At rest, under basal conditions, the left atrial pressure is at its lowest level; during exercise, tachycardia, or stress it rises in proportion to the *squared* increment of the cardiac output. The consequence of left atrial hypertension is pressure elevation within the pulmonary circulation: the pulmonary veins, the pulmonary capillaries, the pulmonary artery, and the right ventricle. If the right ventricle remains competent in response to the hypertensive load, only its systolic pressure rises. Hypertension in the right ventricle and the pulmonary artery is termed

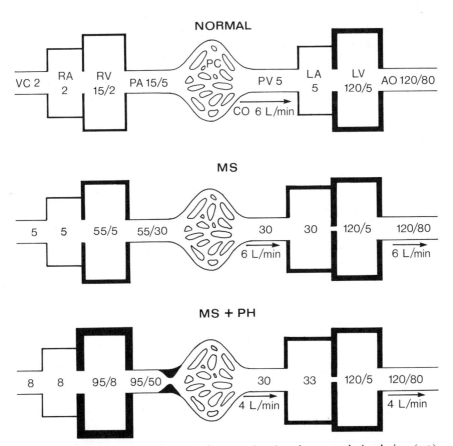

Figure 32-2. Hemodynamic diagram showing the normal circulation (*top*), an example of severe, uncomplicated mitral stenosis (MS) (*middle diagram*), and one of severe mitral stenosis complicated by reactive pulmonary hypertension (PH) (*lower diagram*).

"passive" pulmonary hypertension; it reaches moderate proportions, never being very severe.

The rise of pulmonary capillary pressure produces conditions under which alveolar transudation and pulmonary edema may develop. The gradual increase of left atrial hypertension caused by chronicity and slow progression of the mitral valve stenosis permits adaptive changes to take place, protecting the patient from pulmonary edema. The most important of these adaptive changes is enlargement and enhanced function of the lymphatic system in the lungs, permitting rapid drainage of the excess fluid.

Some patients, thought to have a hyperreactive pulmonary vasculature, respond to elevation of the left atrial pressure in mitral stenosis by intense vasoconstriction of the pulmonary arterioles. It is estimated that about 15 per cent of patients with mitral stenosis show this reaction; it is more common in those with severe mitral stenosis, affecting at least 40 per cent of patients with a mitral valve area under 0.7 per cent. This reactive pulmonary hypertension, superimposed upon the passive pulmonary hypertension, has the following consequences:

- Pulmonary arterial pressure rises very high, often to systemic levels;

- Right ventricular failure, sometimes combined with tricuspid valve incompetence, may develop;

- Cardiac output tends to be lower and rises inadequately during exercise;

- As a consequence of the limitation of cardiac output, pressure in the left atrium and the pulmonary capillaries may be lower than in patients without pulmonary vascular reaction.

It should be emphasized that this increase in pulmonary vascular resistance is largely due to arteriolar constriction, hence is reversible by surgical reduction of left atrial pressure.

NATURAL HISTORY

The time necessary to produce clinically recognizable mitral stenosis elapsing from the initial attack of rheumatic carditis is not definitely known. It is estimated that between 5 and 15 years is necessary to reduce the mitral orifice sufficiently to produce the characteristic auscultatory findings of mitral stenosis. When first recognized, mitral stenosis is usually well tolerated and the patient asymptomatic. Thus, the natural history of mitral stenosis can be divided into the following periods:

1. Latent period (between the attack of carditis and the development of mitral stenosis);

2. The asymptomatic stage;

3. The early symptomatic stage;

4. The stage of severe symptoms;

5. The postoperative stage.

In general, mitral stenosis shows an extraordinary variety of courses with remissions and exacerbations, with changes caused by secondary sequels and complications. An intimate knowledge of all factors is essential for the appropriate evaluation of patients with mitral stenosis, especially when surgical treatment is being considered.

Mitral stenosis is basically a progressive lesion, as was pointed out in the earlier section of this chapter. Yet, progression shows great variability (Fig. 32–3). Once significant mitral stenosis is clinically evident, there are several ways its future course can be determined:

- Mild mitral stenosis may remain stable for decades, sometimes for the duration of life;

- Further progression may be very slow but may proceed at a steady rate;

- Nonprogressive or slowly progressive mitral stenosis may take an abrupt turn, changing into rapidly progressive mitral stenosis in the fifth or sixth decade of life;

- A steadily progressive, accelerated course may bring the patient into a severely disabled state in the second or third decade of life.

In general, symptoms reflect the severity of mitral stenosis, but only in a crude manner. Patients may develop significant symptoms despite the presence of mild mitral stenosis. Conversely, some patients — especially those with slowly progressive mitral stenosis — adapt themselves to the disability to a point that they may be denying symptoms while overt cardiac failure is clinically evident. The principal

Figure 32-3. Natural history of mitral stenosis, illustrating five types (I to IV — functional classes; D — death).
1 — mild nonprogressive
2 — moderate nonprogressive
3 — stable, with rapid late progression
4 — progressive
5 — accelerated

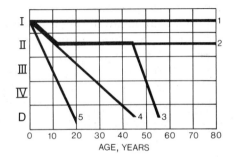

disability-producing symptoms of mitral stenosis are, in order of frequency:

- Effort dyspnea;

- Palpitations, particularly occurring during exercise;

- Paroxysmal dyspnea and pulmonary edema;

- Excessive fatigability.

Chest pain, often considered one of the common findings in mitral stenosis, is a symptom with a doubtful relationship to mitral valve disease. It may represent coincidental ischemic heart disease or nonspecific chest-wall pain, so often encountered in middle-aged women.

Clinical disability develops in about one half of the patients gradually and one half abruptly. The latter group most often develop symptoms in a response to a detectable precipitating factor. Among these factors are the following (in order of frequency):

- onset of atrial fibrillation,

- upper respiratory infection,

- pregnancy,

- overexertion,

- other incidental factors.

Patients who develop clinical disability as a result of a precipitating factor—with or without clinical evidence of overt cardiac failure—may regain their former asymptomatic or mildly symptomatic stage if the precipitating factor is eliminated or brought under control (e.g., restoration of sinus rhythm or control of ventricular rate in atrial fibrillation).

The natural history may be further influenced by other complications: e.g., noncardiac disability from a cerebral embolus.

As mentioned, a proportion of patients with mitral stenosis develop reactive pulmonary hypertension. This may alter the natural history of mitral stenosis: dyspnea, particularly its paroxysmal form, may become less prevalent, while fatigability, related to the low cardiac output, may dominate the clinical picture. Clinical evidence of severe right ventricular overload, often accompanied by tricuspid regurgitation, may also make its appearance.

In recent years it became apparent that there are epidemiological differences in the natural history of rheumatic heart disease in general, and of mitral stenosis in particular. Certain patterns can be recognized:

- In many developing countries in Asia, Africa, and in some South American countries mitral stenosis may take an accelerated course, with a significant proportion of patients becoming severely symptomatic before the age of 20.

- In areas with wider prevalence of rheumatic fever than in this country an intermediate course is observed: the preponderance of disabled patients considered for surgical treatment are found to be in their third or fourth decade.

- In the United States, at present, most patients develop significant disability in the fifth and sixth decades.

While the cause of these wide variations in the natural history is not definitely known, it is surmised that they are related to the prevalence of rheumatic reinfection, which, in turn, is influenced in a negative manner by poverty, crowding, poor hygiene, and inadequate medical care, all of which facilitate repeated streptococcal infections.

The natural history of mitral stenosis, as discussed in the preceding paragraphs, justifies the recognition of some patterns. The following list is a purely arbitrary classification, and it should be noted that some patients may remain in a certain class, while in others that class may represent merely a stage of the disease and transition to another class may occur.

1. *Mild mitral stenosis.* Here all the findings of mitral stenosis may be present: the patient is asymptomatic or mildly symptomatic.

2. *Mitral stenosis with significant symptomatology.* In this group there is usually moderate to severe degree of mitral obstruction with stable or progressive disability, usually due to effort dyspnea.

3. *Mitral stenosis characterized by complicating factors in the foreground.* Here one includes asymptomatic or mildly symptomatic patients with mitral stenosis who become disabled because of a cerebral embolus producing hemiplegia or whose principal problem is a therapy-resistant atrial fibrillation.

4. *Mitral stenosis with reactive pulmonary hypertension.* As stated, this most frequently occurs in association with severe mitral stenosis; its consequences have already been commented upon.

5. *Obscure mitral stenosis.* A certain number of patients do not show the usual physical signs of mitral stenosis and it may masquerade as such other forms of cardiac disease as idiopathic atrial fibrillation, primary pulmonary hypertension, or even congenital heart disease.

COMPLICATIONS OF MITRAL STENOSIS

The commonest complication of mitral stenosis is *atrial fibrillation*. In Wood's series the incidence in patients with severe enough mitral stenosis to require surgical treatment was 45 per cent. It is probably higher at present, for now in most patients the disease takes a slower course and reaches the point of requiring surgery about a decade later than in Wood's cases. Atrial fibrillation is associated with and probably related to the age of the patient and the size of the left atrium. The relationship to the severity of mitral stenosis is less evident.

Often atrial fibrillation develops first in the form of short paroxysms and eventually establishes itself in the permanent form, unless treated effectively. It affects the natural history in two ways: First, the onset of uncontrolled atrial fibrillation often coincides with sudden development of cardiac failure. Second, it may limit effort tolerance by excessive tachycardia during exercise, even in digitalized patients.

Systemic embolization constitutes another serious complication of mitral stenosis and is closely related to atrial fibrillation. Its incidence is about 20 per cent, that is, in one of five patients with mitral stenosis one or more systemic emboli are found. The incidence is high in patients in atrial fibrillation and low in those in sinus rhythm. The question as to whether atrial fibrillation is a prerequisite of the mural thrombus formation—i.e., whether those in sinus rhythm represent patients in whom embolization occurred during an unrecognized paroxysm of atrial fibrillation—has not been answered. The important features of systemic embolization include the following:

- Emboli occur just as often in patients with milder degrees of mitral stenosis, often asymptomatic, as in severely ill ones;

- The highest risk of embolization is at the very onset of atrial fibrillation;

- Emboli tend to be repetitive—i.e., the risk of recurrence is higher than in random patients with mitral stenosis and atrial fibrillation;

- Patients who give a history of systemic embolization often are found to have clean atria at operation; conversely, those with large mural thrombi found at operation do not always give a history of previous embolization.

Systemic embolization may have a devastating effect upon the natural history of mitral stenosis. It is perhaps the commonest cause of serious cerebrovascular accidents in young individuals; though many such accidents are totally or partly reversible, a certain number of patients remain severely disabled with permanent neurological deficits.

Pulmonary embolization is less common than that into the systemic circulation, presumbably because the right atrium does not enlarge in mitral stenosis until very late in the course of the disease. Pulmonary emboli are most likely to occur in seriously ill patients with advanced mitral stenosis.

Respiratory infections occur more commonly in mitral stenosis than in the general population. They constitute one factor among those precipitating cardiac failure.

Left ventricular dysfunction has been considered a common association of mitral stenosis, even though the left ventricle is hemodynamically spared the overload. Early evidence of its existence is rather flimsy. Recently sophisticated left ventricular function tests demonstrated occasional left ventricular malfunction. It is doubtful, however, whether such malfunction — for which there are some reasonable explanations — is of sufficient magnitude to produce clinically significant cardiac failure. The "myocardial factor" is often blamed for unsuccessful results of mitral valve operations. More likely other factors are to be blamed; at present clinically significant left ventricular dysfunction remains as nebulous as ever.

Hemoptysis, a relatively common complication of mitral stenosis, represents hemorrhages from the pulmonary venous system, which is characterized by abnormally high pressure and intercommunicates with the bronchial venous system. The amount of blood expectorated ranges from merely blood-tinged sputum to a life-threatening hemorrhage. Fortunately, severe hemorrhages ("pulmonary apoplexy") are rare, and are estimated to occur in less than 1 per cent of patients with mitral stenosis. The average pulmonary hemorrhage is in the magnitude of 10 to 30 ml. of blood. They tend to be repetitive.

Bacterial endocarditis is a rare complication of pure mitral stenosis, but its probability increases with the presence of an apical systolic murmur, indicating some degree — regardless of how trivial — of mitral regurgitation.

Chronic lung disease is found in association with mitral stenosis probably more commonly than coincidental coexistence of two common diseases would allow. It is particularly significant at present, when older patients are being considered for open heart surgery.

POSTOPERATIVE COURSE

The natural history of operated patients with mitral stenosis depends upon the type of the operation and the anatomic condition of the valve prior to the operation.

Mitral valvotomy, closed or open, can never restore normal conditions. Even in young patients with mitral stenosis, sufficient stiffening of the mitral valve occurs so that even complete surgical separation of the cusps merely causes change from a significant mitral stenosis to a less severe degree of it. Characteristic diastolic murmurs of mitral stenosis almost never disappear completely. Interpretation of symptomatic improvement after the operation has to be interpreted with caution, since significant clinical improvement is occasionally reported by patients who for technical reasons did not obtain effective surgical relief of obstruction at the valve, or who by hemodynamic measurement showed no postoperative improvement. As in many other cardiac disabilities, psychological factors unrelated to the principal disease may profoundly affect the clinical course.

Patients who develop reactive pulmonary hypertension show, after a successful operation, a return of the pulmonary vascular resistance to normal, or at least a significant reduction of it.

In general, postoperative improvement develops gradually over a period of weeks or months. Inasmuch as mitral stenosis is basically a progressive lesion, restenosis in the future is highly probable. The anatomic condition of the valve determines how widely the valve can be open. This and the overall stiffness of the leaflets set the stage of future progression of the obstructive process. Valvotomy seems merely to turn the clock of this progressive disease backward: in favorable cases it may be reset 20 years; in unfavorable, 2 or 3 years, or conditions, by physiological measurements, may even remain unchanged despite the fact that the two leaflets are surgically separated.

Valve replacement provides in principle a more satisfactory relief of the obstruction at the mitral valve, but even this technique does not restore a normal mitral orifice; rather, it is equivalent to mild mitral stenosis. The benefits of this operation are, however, lessened by the higher initial risk and the variety of postoperative problems, as well as uncertainty over the long-range fate of prosthetic valves.

The Final Outcome. Sudden death, which represents a major hazard in aortic stenosis, is uncommon in mitral stenosis. Only exceptionally do emergencies arise in which immediate surgical relief is indicated. Unoperated or unsuccessfully operated patients die of chronic progressive cardiac failure or of one of the abovementioned complications of mitral stenosis. Nonfatal emergencies, which as a rule respond to medical therapy, include acute pulmonary edema, often induced by overexertion or under excitement or excessive salt intake, and sudden cardiac failure produced by uncontrolled atrial fibrillation.

DIAGNOSIS

The diagnostic approach to mitral stenosis requires the analysis of the following aspects of the disease:

1. The presence or absence of mitral stenosis;

2. The quantification of the severity of mitral stenosis;

3. The presence or absence of complicating factors.

Clinical history yields relatively little information which would direct attention to mitral stenosis. The symptoms of this condition have been discussed in the preceding section. Effort dyspnea, paroxysmal dyspnea, palpitations — all are nonspecific symptoms found in most forms of cardiac disease.

There are a few points in the history which, though still of low specificity, may draw the clinician's attention to the possibility of mitral stenosis:

- History of rheumatic fever has to be considered within the context of the fact that, on the one hand, some 40 per cent of patients with mitral stenosis do not give such history (they are assumed to have had subclinical rheumatic carditis), while, on the other hand, many patients with rheumatic fever escape without residua (see Chapter 23).

- Paroxysms of rapid and irregular heart action — atrial fibrillation — occurring in a young subject may make the clinician concentrate upon finding or ruling out mitral stenosis.

- A history of transient cerebral vascular episodes early in life also may suggest the possibility of mitral stenosis, especially if associated with bouts of palpitations.

- A history of hemoptysis should be considered with the possibility of mitral stenosis in mind.

Physical examination represents the most important part of the diagnostic examination, one with a potentially high yield in establishing the presence of mitral stenosis. The auscultatory findings consist of the following triad:

- The apical rumbling diastolic murmur,

- The mitral opening snap,

- The accentuated first heart sound.

The murmur has a high specificity, if present in its full form, i.e., in sinus rhythm extending to and accentuated in the presystolic phase, and in atrial fibrillation, lasting well into the diastole. As already explained, other rumbling diastolic murmurs caused by increased or accelerated flow through the mitral valve are of shorter duration. The only functional murmur of sufficient duration to imitate that of organic mitral stenosis is one associated with aortic regurgitation (Austin Flint); thus, in the presence of aortic regurgitation of significant degree the apical diastolic murmur loses specificity.

The specificity of the mitral opening snap is also very high, provided its recognition is made with certainty (see Chapter 3).

It should be pointed out that in advanced mitral stenosis, when the mitral leaflets stiffen, calcify, and lose mobility, the mitral opening snap and the accentuated first sound lose their diagnostic significance. The opening snap gradually becomes soft and then disappears. The first sound no longer is accentuated and becomes normal in intensity or even softer than average.

When all three auscultatory signs of mitral stenosis are unequivocally present, the diagnosis of mitral stenosis is firmly established. The murmur bears no relationship to the severity of mitral stenosis. However, the position of the opening snap in relation to aortic valve closure reflects the height of left atrial pressure, thus indirectly relating to the severity of the stenosis: the closer the opening to the first component of the second sound, the higher the left atrial pressure—that is, given a normal cardiac output, the more severe mitral stenosis.

While the opening snap and the accentuated first sound are widely

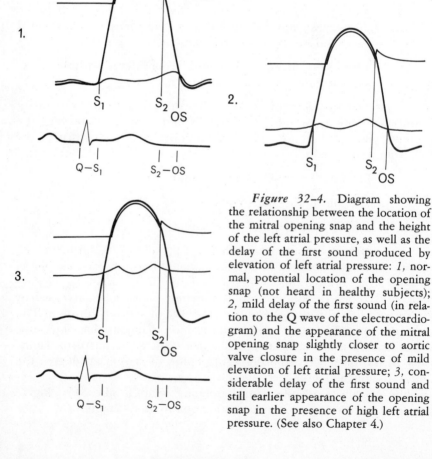

Figure 32–4. Diagram showing the relationship between the location of the mitral opening snap and the height of the left atrial pressure, as well as the delay of the first sound produced by elevation of left atrial pressure: *1*, normal, potential location of the opening snap (not heard in healthy subjects); *2*, mild delay of the first sound (in relation to the Q wave of the electrocardiogram) and the appearance of the mitral opening snap slightly closer to aortic valve closure in the presence of mild elevation of left atrial pressure; *3*, considerable delay of the first sound and still earlier appearance of the opening snap in the presence of high left atrial pressure. (See also Chapter 4.)

heard over the precordium, the diastolic rumble is usually well localized. Errors in evaluation of physical signs are usually in the direction of missing the earmarks of mitral stenosis. If insufficient time is spent to auscultate the apical and periapical area, if the patient is not turned on the left side, or exercised — both maneuvers bring into range subaudible or faint rumbles — the murmur can easily be overlooked. True cases of "silent" mitral stenosis (i.e., with the murmur absent) are occasionally found, but these are mostly advanced cases of mitral stenosis, pulmonary hypertension and severe failure, or patients with coexisting pulmonary disease diminishing overall auscultatory cardiac phenomena.

The opening snap and the accentuated first sound not only may provide some information regarding the severity of mitral stenosis but their presence may also demonstrate mobility of the mitral valve. As stated, when the valve leaflets stiffen excessively and calcify, the first sound becomes softer and the opening snap is reduced in intensity and eventually disappears.

Other auscultatory findings are unremarkable and noncharacteristic unless a complicating factor is present. The most important among these is reactive pulmonary hypertension. When it develops, the following additional signs may be present:

- Pulmonary valve closure becomes accentuated;

- The murmur of pulmonary regurgitation may appear;

- A systolic murmur of tricuspid regurgitation may develop;

- A right-sided S4 gallop sound may appear.

There are no noteworthy findings detectable by palpation and inspection, unless mitral stenosis is severe or complications are present. In severe mitral stenosis, particularly when complicated by reactive pulmonary hypertension, additional evidence for right ventricular hypertrophy and pulmonary hypertension may be obtained as follows:

- Right ventricular (left parasternal) lift is often palpable;

- A prominent *a* wave in the jugular venous pulse may develop;

- Visible and palpable consequences of tricuspid regurgitation may be present (prominent *v* wave of the venous pulse with high venous pressure, pulsating liver).

Electrocardiographic examination. The electrocardiogram presents no specific diagnostic features of mitral stenosis but is often used as a means of confirming the diagnosis and evaluating the increase in severity of the disease. In milder, uncomplicated mitral stenosis the electrocardiogram is often normal. The earliest sign of mitral stenosis may be a bifid P wave with an exaggerated negative component in leads V_1 or V_2 as evidence of left atrial enlargement. The next most common early sign is a modest right axis shift of the limb leads — still within the norm — to about 90°. In severe mitral stenosis, particularly when associated with reactive pulmonary hypertension, evidence of right ventricular hypertrophy appears. This may take the following forms:

- Development of a late R(R') in lead V_1;

- Shift of the frontal plane axis beyond + 90°;

- Development of deep S waves in left precordial leads.

The electrocardiogram is, of course, the principal means of recognition and confirmation of the presence of the commonest complication of mitral stenosis — atrial fibrillation.

Radiographic examination. While not entirely characteristic per se, radiographic examination adds significant diagnostic information that helps interpret clinical findings. The commonest findings in early, uncomplicated mitral stenosis are the following:

- Normal cardiac size or often small overall cardiac size,

- Mild enlargement of the left atrium (primarily detected by backward displacement of the portion of esophagus adjacent to the atrium).

Late radiographic findings may include the following:

- Enlargement of right heart chambers,

- Severe enlargement of the left atrium ("double density" in the right heart border and prominence of the left atrial appendage — middle arc of left border),

- Kerley's B lines in lower lung fields,

- Calcifications in the mitral leaflets.

In the presence of severe pulmonary hypertension reaction, the following findings may be present:

- Generalized cardiomegaly,

- Prominence of the main pulmonary artery,

- Prominence of pulmonary arterial branches.

Phonocardiographic examination may be of assistance in two ways:

1. As a means of identification of uncertain auscultatory findings, e.g., differentiation between mitral opening snap and an S3 gallop

sound, or resolution of the occasional difficulty of distinguishing an S4 gallop sound from a presystolic murmur.

2.   As a means of rough quantification of the severity of mitral stenosis by measuring the distance between the aortic valve closure and the opening snap (given normal cardiac output, trivial mitral stenosis shows the opening snap 0.13 sec. after the aortic valve closure or more; moderate mitral stenosis, 0.09 to 0.12; severe mitral stenosis, 0.06 to 0.08 sec.). Of similar significance is the distance between the Q wave of the electrocardiogram and the onset of the first sound: normal Q-1 interval is 0.08 sec. or less; severe mitral stenosis, 0.12, with corresponding intermediate values.

Echocardiographic examination provides the most important and most specific noninvasive means of evaluation of mitral stenosis. The concordant motion of the two mitral leaflets recorded by ultrasound provides a specific sign of the presence of mitral stenosis; its severity can be roughly estimated by the E-F slope. In addition, the size of the left atrium and of the right ventricle can be estimated by this method. A differentiation of mitral stenosis from left atrial myxoma can be made; the presence of large atrial thrombi can sometimes be detected by echocardiography.

Cardiac catheterization constitutes the means of accurate quantification of mitral stenosis; it permits, furthermore, an evaluation of cardiac performance, particularly its response to exercise; it provides the opportunity to quantify the responses of the pulmonary vasculature to mitral stenosis and to evaluate its effect upon the right ventricular function and the competence of the tricuspid valve.

1.   The Gorlin formula, based on a carefully collected set of data obtained during cardiac catheterization, provides a reasonably good, reproducible estimate of the severity of mitral stenosis. At the present time measurements include direct determination of the gradient across the mitral valve. Originally designed to use an assumed left ventricular diastolic pressure and an indirectly recorded left atrial pressure (pulmonary arterial wedge pressure) — at the time when only right-sided cardiac catheterizations were being performed — this simplified method can still be used in patients with pure mitral stenosis in whom disease of the left ventricle has been ruled out by clinical means.

2.   Evaluation of intracardiac pressure and of the cardiac output at rest and during exercise provides a means of determining how mitral valve obstruction is tolerated by the patient. This evaluation may be of considerable importance in interpretation of clinical symptoms of patients whose clinical history is unreliable, or whose professed disability appears doubtful, or, on the other hand, who may minimize their symptoms.

Angiocardiography supplements cardiac catheterization as a means of definitive evaluation of a patient with mitral stenosis. The important information obtained by angiocardiography is as follows:

1. Evaluation of the mobility of the mitral valve. This is often of crucial importance in presurgical studies: the operability and type of approach often hinges upon this information. This is best determined by injecting the contrast substance into the left atrium (preferably), or into the pulmonary artery.

2. The size of the left atrium can be assessed.

3. Left ventriculogram provides the opportunity to evaluate left ventricular contractility; the presence of mitral regurgitation can be established and crudely quantified; the mobility of the mitral leaflet can be judged, although details of the valve are not as well seen as in left atrial injection.

4. Left atrial thrombi (large) or tumors can be demonstrated.

Differential Points in the Diagnosis. Despite the fact that physical signs of mitral stenosis have an excellent specificity and a fair sensitivity, there are many situations in which diagnostic differentiation may present some difficulties. The following clinical situations exemplify some of the problems:

1. In mild mitral stenosis it may be difficult to prove the existence of cardiac disease. Faint diastolic rumbling murmurs may be difficult to hear: uncertainty may develop over whether an early diastolic sound represents an opening snap. The fact that in such cases the electrocardiogram and the roentgenogram may show normal findings may compound the difficulty. The echocardiogram is the most valuable diagnostic tool in this situation.

2. In severe mitral stenosis, especially complicated by reactive pulmonary hypertension, the differentiation from congenital shunting lesions (particularly atrial septal defect) or from "primary" pulmonary hypertension may be difficult.

3. Patients in chronic atrial fibrillation and in cardiac failure may present diagnostic difficulties, particularly in the older age group. The murmur may be inconspicuous and all the findings nonspecific. Here, the possibility of mitral stenosis has to be given serious consideration with a specific search for radiographic evidence of mitral valve calcification and echocardiographic findings related to abnormal mitral valve motion.

4. Patients with known mitral stenosis may present difficulties in the interpretation of new symptoms, signs, and events. Thus, alertness

for any neurological problems such as "dizziness" is required to consider the possibility of cerebral emboli; hemoptysis may represent a fairly common complication of mitral stenosis but could also signify pulmonary emboli with infarction.

Evaluation. The evaluation of a patient with mitral stenosis should be done with specific objectives in mind. The objectives must be based on knowledge of the natural history of mitral stenosis. The commonly considered questions constituting the basis of the evaluation include the following:

1. Where does the patient fit in over the course of the natural history of mitral stenosis?

2. If disabled, are the patient's symptoms related to mitral stenosis?

3. In view of the variability of the course, could the patient's symptoms be reversed by medical means?

4. If mitral valve surgery is contemplated, are the clinical and hemodynamic causes of disability likely to be reversible?

The objectives of evaluation vary under different clinical situations as exemplified below:

1. In an asymptomatic patient evaluated for mitral stenosis, a definitive diagnosis may be established by physical examination and supported by electrocardiographic and radiographic examinations in the great majority of instances. It is important, however, to include in the evaluation a rough quantification of the degree of mitral stenosis. One should recognize the fact that symptoms may appear late in the course of the disease, and that near-normal electrocardiographic and radiographic findings are still consistent with moderately severe mitral stenosis. Noninvasive quantification of mitral stenosis may be performed by the phonocardiographic measurement of Q-1 and 2-OS intervals (see above) and by echocardiographic measurement of the E-F slope. If significant mitral stenosis is found, the possibility of invasive evaluation should be considered.

The goal of invasive evaluation of mitral stenosis in an asymptomatic patient is to establish a baseline against which future studies would reveal whether or not the disease is progressive and, if so, how rapid its progression takes place. This information may have a decisive bearing on future recommendations regarding surgical treatment. While in many institutions surgical treatment of mitral stenosis is being performed with a minimum of hemodynamic studies, it is believed that invasive serial studies provide information which encourages a more conservative and better selection of patients for operations; furthermore, such studies permit a more reasonable estimation of the risk-benefit ratio for this operation.

2. The patient with moderate symptoms requires evaluation regarding the severity of mitral stenosis but also the establishment of a reasonable relationship between mitral valve disease and the disability. In a middle-aged patient dyspnea may be caused by anxiety and hyperventilation or by coincidental pulmonary disease rather than be related to mitral stenosis. Fluid retention may be due to noncardiac causes. Thus it is essential to direct evaluation toward the establishment of a hemodynamic basis for the disability as well as to evaluate alternate possibilities (e.g., by the performance of pulmonary function tests). Hemodynamic evaluation of cardiac function usually plays a decisive role in consideration of surgical therapy.

3. Patients who are seen for the first time during an emergency (pulmonary edema, onset of atrial fibrillation), should have the diagnosis of mitral stenosis made qualitatively by the simplest means (usually auscultation). Quantification by noninvasive and invasive techniques should be postponed until the factor producing the emergency is brought under control. As stated previously, in mitral stenosis emergencies that are not responsive to medical therapy and that require immediate evaluation for surgery are rare.

4. Patients in whom the diagnosis of mitral stenosis is merely suggested as a possibility require a diagnostic evaluation that includes all available techniques. In dealing with the possibility of a surgically correctable lesion, it is advisable to have a high index of suspicion regarding mitral stenosis in patients with unexplained cardiac failure, chronic atrial fibrillation, and so on. Echocardiography can be used as a screening technique. Complete cardiac catheterization study combined with angiocardiography is then indicated if mitral stenosis is found.

5. The importance of postoperative evaluation of patients with mitral stenosis cannot be overemphasized. After mitral valvotomy, echocardiography may provide a rough index of the attained improvement of mitral valve function. This, however, may not be sufficient. A hemodynamic measurement is justified for the following reasons:

> As a means of documenting and quantifying the improvement attained by the operation (by comparison with a preoperative study);

> • As a baseline study with which future studies will be compared to determine whether or not restenosis has occurred.

Following valve replacement, hemodynamic studies are also justified:

- Improvement here also needs documentation;

- The possibility of damage to the left ventricle needs assessment;

- A baseline study performed postoperatively may permit early detection of valve malfunction.

The optimal time for the performance of postoperative studies is between 6 and 12 months after the operation.

It is axiomatic that patients who fail to improve or who deteriorate after the operation require an evaluation as soon as this fact is recognized.

THERAPY

The objectives and problems involved in therapy of mitral stenosis include the following:

- Management of the asymptomatic patient,

- Management of the symptomatic patient,

- Prevention and management of complications of mitral stenosis,

- Selection and timing of surgical therapy,

- Postoperative management.

The Asymptomatic Patient. In asymptomatic patients active therapy is seldom needed; counseling and preventive measures constitute the basis of therapy.

Prevention of recurrences of rheumatic fever should be a goal in young patients. Although some recommendations include life-long administration of penicillin or equivalent antibiotic prophylaxis, the proneness to recurrences drops considerably with the passage of time from the last known attack and with the aging of the patient. Current views regarding late progression of mitral stenosis also minimize the potential role of rheumatic reinfection. Thus one can question whether reasonable justification exists to extend rheumatic fever prophylaxis beyond the mid-twenties, except, perhaps, for patients who have higher than average exposure to streptococcal infection.

Measures for prevention of endocarditis apply to all forms of valvular heart disease, including mitral stenosis. To be sure, the incidence of infective endocarditis in mitral stenosis is very low; nevertheless, the low risk of antibiotic therapy in connection with dental manipulations is justified even in this condition.

In counseling patients with mitral stenosis, specific regulation regarding activities or alteration of the mode of living is as a rule not needed. Pregnancy is usually well tolerated in mild mitral stenosis. Asymptomatic women in the childbearing age should be carefully evaluated as to the possibility of having severe mitral valve obstruction, in which case the increased risk of pregnancy, the desire to have children, and the option of earlier valvotomy should be reviewed with the patient.

The Symptomatic Patient. In symptomatic patients medical management is related to the basic decision concerning whether or not surgical treatment is contemplated and when. Patients with nonprogressive symptoms of moderate degree seldom need active therapy. Usually they experience reduced effort tolerance resulting from dyspnea in which case symptoms are controlled, often intuitively, by self-limitation on the part of the patient. More severe dyspnea and early signs of fluid accumulation may require diuretic therapy. Digitalis is ineffective if sinus rhythm is present.

Occasionally patients with disabling symptoms or those with overt signs of cardiac failure are, for a variety of reasons, subjected to medical therapy rather than cardiac surgery. Many such patients can be adequately controlled at a reduced level of activities with the aid of sodium restriction and diuretics and, whenever indicated, digitalis.

The common complications of mitral stenosis that require treatment include arrhythmias and thromboembolism. Atrial fibrillation is by far the most frequent sequel to mitral stenosis. While its incidence increases with age, some patients develop a tendency to this arrhythmia early in life. Treatment includes three phases:

1. Treatment and prevention of paroxysms of atrial fibrillation. In some patients atrial fibrillation first appears as brief, self-limited episodes. Oral quinidine taken at the beginning of an episode—in those cases in which the duration of previous spontaneous episodes exceeded two hours—often aborts attacks. If attacks occur at frequent intervals, e.g., several times a month, prophylactic administration of quinidine, and/or propranolol may be tried, provided a tally of attacks shows reasonable evidence that the therapy is effective.

2. Treatment of established atrial fibrillation involves two options: to restore sinus rhythm, or to accept chronic atrial fibrillation and control ventricular rate.

Restoration of sinus rhythm is indicated in patients in whom there is a reasonable prospect that the normal mechanism will be maintained. This is true under the following circumstances:

   • in younger patients,

- in patients without severe left atrial enlargement,
- in patients with recent onset of atrial fibrillation.

Patients who show these three features can be treated first with modest doses of quinidine and, if ineffective, then with direct-current shock therapy. Maintenance antiarrhythmic therapy is advisable after sinus rhythm is reestablished.

Following surgical correction of mitral stenosis, prospects of restoration and maintenance of sinus rhythm improve somewhat, but patients who fulfill the above criteria are still considered the most suitable candidates. One can liberalize somewhat the indications by requiring partial fulfillment of the criteria, but those who have poor scores in all three criteria continue having very poor prospects for conversion to sinus rhythm and in those the risk, time invested, and expense of the therapy may not be justified.

Patients who develop atrial fibrillation for the first time immediately after mitral valve operations (within the first two weeks), on the other hand, are excellent candidates for conversion. Virtually all such patients respond favorably to therapy; many may have the antiarrhythmic drug maintenance discontinued a month or two after conversion and will remain in sinus rhythm.

3. In patients who are to be left in atrial fibrillation, the *control of ventricular rate* is regulated by digitalis or, to a lesser extent, by propranolol. It is necessary to titrate the drug or drugs, using not only the resting ventricular rate but the response to mild exercise as a yardstick of effective therapy. In the great majority of patients this aspect of therapy presents no problems; in a few difficulties arise in that either the rate cannot be reduced at all or with a reasonable resting rate excessive tachycardia develops during exercise, producing disability. Some such patients may present a serious therapeutic problem; occasionally an attempt to restore sinus rhythm may be made to try to overcome the problem even if the patient is a poor candidate by the above-listed criteria.

Management of Thromboembolic Complications. Primarily prophylactic therapy is employed, but occasionally surgical removal of a large peripheral embolus (e.g., saddle embolus in the abdominal aorta) is necessary. The principal — perhaps even the exclusive — etiological factor is atrial fibrillation, which predisposes to mural thrombosis in the left atrium. The combination of mitral stenosis and atrial fibrillation provides a more likely background for systemic embolization than atrial fibrillation without mitral stenosis; nevertheless no definite evidence is available that anticoagulant therapy given in all patients with mitral stenosis and atrial fibrillation reduces significantly the incidence of emboli to the point of balancing the risk of therapy. Given a patient who has thrown a major systemic embolus (unfortunately cerebral embolism is among the commonest), the options then are as follows:

- Effective restoration of sinus rhythm and prevention of recurrent atrial fibrillation,

- Continuous anticoagulant therapy,

- A combination of both methods.

Inasmuch as the risk of systemic embolization is highest at the very inception of atrial fibrillation, total protection of the patient from recurrences would be contingent upon "guaranteed" prevention of even minor paroxysms of atrial fibrillation, which at present is unattainable. Consequently, continuous anticoagulant therapy is the preferable method in most centers, often combined with antiarrhythmic therapy as well.

There is a widespread impression that mitral valve operations prevent recurrences of systemic embolization. Statistics on which this impression is based do not discriminate as to whether mitral stenosis is severe or mild, or whether sinus rhythm after the operation can be successfully maintained or not. One might expect that patients with severe mitral stenosis whose obstruction is effectively relieved will be less prone to form mural thrombi; such patients also constitute better targets for eventual restoration of sinus rhythm. However, the most serious dilemma involves the not too rare cases of mitral stenosis with no symptoms prior to the embolic accident and with demonstrated mild mitral stenosis. In these, more evidence is needed before recommending valvotomy for the sole purpose of prevention of emboli. (Valve replacement in itself provides a potential additional source of systemic embolization, hence should not even be considered in such cases.)

Surgical Selection. Surgical treatment consists of three operations: closed mitral valvotomy, open mitral valvotomy, and mitral valve replacement. Selection of patients depends upon the surgeon's preference and upon the anatomic conditions of the mitral valve. Nevertheless, the risk in the three operations is different and the clinician who decides whether or not the patient should be considered for surgery needs to know the risk of an operation to construct the therapeutic equation (risk vs. benefit) for a given patient. Thus, closed mitral valvotomy with a risk of 3 per cent or less in experienced centers, and with virtually no significant prospect of late untoward sequels of the operation, justifies a more lenient attitude than mitral valve replacement, which has a much higher immediate risk and a host of late complications and risks. Open valvotomy carries only a slightly higher risk than closed valvotomy, a risk primarily related to the occasional complications of total body perfusion (hepatitis, microembolization).

Conditions in which valvotomy offers a favorable prospect of relief of mitral stenosis for varying lengths of time are primarily determined by the mobility and the thickness of the valve. Thin and mobile valves, particularly those with the purely commissural type of mitral stenosis, can be very effectively separated by valvotomy and offer the most lasting results. Given these conditions—and the clinician should be able to obtain a reasonable estimate of these features of the mitral valve—early operations are justified on the basis that the risk is small and the benefits excellent. On the other hand, in patients with stiff, immobile, calcified valves, in whom mitral valve replacement is virtually certain, conservative criteria for the selection for surgery should be established.

The selection of patients for surgical treatment is highly individual and varies from institution to institution. Nevertheless, decisions are only too often made on the basis of incomplete information, on the basis of the principle that mitral stenosis is a surgically treatable disease, or on the basis of the patient's wishes, and more often than not these are unrealistic. Few would deny that patients with severe disability, particularly if they are unable to earn a livelihood or fulfill minimal duties as a housewife, should have surgical treatment of any type that offers improvement, unless a specific contraindication is present. Patients with moderate disability, who show definite clinical progression of symptoms (preferably reinforced by evidence of hemodynamic progression) also constitute good candidates. Marginal candidates include the following:

- Patients with intermittent symptoms (bouts of cardiac failure or acute pulmonary edema), but controlled by medical means;

- Patients with onset of disability related to a specific complication, who have not undergone optimal medical therapy;

- Patients with symptoms related to atrial fibrillation;

- Patients with the principal problem of systemic embolism (see above).

Patients in these categories should be evaluated individually; hemodynamic studies are usually helpful. In such cases a more conservative attitude often pays off: many patients may remain unchanged, leading tolerable lives for years or decades, and may well be better off unoperated.

It should be reemphasized that patients' symptoms need critical evaluation. Inasmuch as in our epidemiological setting many patients with mitral stenosis who come for consideration of surgery are menopausal women, the possibility of misinterpretation of vague, nonspecific symptoms as cardiac disability is a real one. Furthermore coexisting cardiac conditions (ischemic heart disease, hypertension, left ventricular dysfunction) should be searched for, and, if present, their relation to symptoms evaluated.

When is a severely symptomatic patient to be considered inoperable? This question cannot be answered by any specific rules and guidelines. Severe reactive pulmonary hypertension, once considered a contraindication to surgical treatment of mitral stenosis, is no longer in this category: its reversible nature (in contrast to congenital heart disease) has already been mentioned. The presence of elevated pulmonary vascular resistance increases the risk of the operation, but with the present methods of postoperative management the increment of risk is not a great one. One can easily defend the position that "no patient is too ill to have mitral valve surgery performed, provided severe mitral stenosis is the basis of the problem."

In general, selection of patients for surgical treatment should be made with realization that clinical and hemodynamic results of the operation (any type) are best if severe mitral stenosis is present. In patients with lesser degrees of mitral stenosis — even though symptoms are cardiac in origin — the clinical improvement may be disappointing. This is particularly true in middle-aged and elderly patients with chronic atrial fibrillation and moderate mitral stenosis. Here it is probable that mitral stenosis is only one of the factors producing the disability; its relief may not be sufficient to make a discernible change in the patient's condition.

Postsurgical Therapy.   Following mitral valvotomy there are few problems that require special comment. The question of management of atrial fibrillation has been discussed above. Postoperative complications, particularly postcardiotomy syndrome, have been mentioned in Chapter 13. The most important problem in management is that pertaining to patients whose results are disappointing. Here one might consider a study to determine whether the operation was unsuccessful for technical reasons or whether mitral obstruction was not the basis of the patient's symptoms. If the former possibility is true, reoperation for valve replacement may be necessary. In a few instances intraoperative myocardial damage is responsible for bad results.

After mitral replacement alertness to the many problems that may come to light is important. Continuous anticoagulation is widely used in prosthetic ball valves, although technical improvement promises to make this form of therapy superfluous. The important part of the management is a careful follow-up, which not only provides the opportunity to find objective abnormalities but also encourages patients to report some symptoms which they may not consider sufficiently important to consult a physician about, but which may indeed be of great importance.

Bibliography

Bailey GWH, Braniff BA, Hancock EW, Cohn KE: Relation of left atrial pathology to atrial fibrillation in mitral valve disease. Ann. Int. Med., *69*:13, 1968.

Brock, RC: The surgical and pathological anatomy of the mitral valve. Brit. Heart J. *14*:489, 1952.

Dubin A, Cohn KE, March HW, Selzer A: Longitudinal hemodynamic and clinical study of mitral stenosis. Circulation *44*:381, 1971.

Ellis LB, Harken DE: Closed mitral valvuloplasty for mitral stenosis. A twelve-year follow-up study of 1571 patients. New Engl. J. Med. *270*:643, 1964.

Olessen KH: The natural history of 271 patients with mitral stenosis under medical treatment. Brit. Heart J. *24*:349, 1962.

Reeve R, Selzer A, Popper RW, Leeds RF, Gerbode F: Reversibility of pulmonary hypertension following cardiac surgery. Circulation *33*(Suppl. I): 107, 1966.

Reichak N, Shelburne JC, Perloff JK: Clinical aspects of rheumatic valvular disease. Prog. Cardiovasc. Dis. *15*:491, 1973.

Roberts WC, Bulkley BH, Morrow AG: Pathologic anatomy of cardiac valve replacement: a study of 224 necropsy patients. Prog. Cardiovasc. Dis. *15*:539, 1973.

Rowe JC, Bland EF, Sprague HB, White PD: Course of mitral stenosis without surgery. Ten and twenty years perspectives. Ann. Int. Med. *52*:741, 1960.

Rusted IE, Scheifley CH, Edwards JE: Studies of the mitral valve. II. Certain anatomic features of the mitral valve and associated structures in mitral stenosis. Circulation *14*:398, 1956.

Selzer A, Malmborg RO: Some factors influencing changes in pulmonary vascular resistance in mitral valvular disease. Amer. J. Med. *32*:532, 1962.

Selzer A, Cohn KE: Natural history of mitral stenosis. A review. Circulation *45*:878, 1972.

Selzer A, Cohn KE: The "myocardial factor" in valvular heart disease. Cardiovasc. Clinics V: 2, 177, 1973.

Wood P. An appreciation of mitral stenosis. Brit. Med. J. *1*:1051, 1113, 1954.

33

Semilunar Valve Incompetence

Definition. This chapter deals with pulmonary regurgitation and aortic regurgitation. Clinical conditions discussed include those produced by anatomic abnormalities of the two semilunar valves or of the adjacent structures, producing significant valve incompetence. Thus regurgitation through the pulmonary valve occurring in severe pulmonary hypertension or "functional" aortic regurgitation manifested by early diastolic murmurs heard often in patients with systemic hypertension will not be included; aortic regurgitation associated with ventricular septal defect was presented in Chapter 28.

ETIOLOGY

Pulmonary valve incompetence, as seen by the clinician in its "primary" form, is, as a rule, caused by one of two etiological factors:

- Congenital malformation of the pulmonary valve;

- Trauma to the valve at the time of surgical operation.

Aortic regurgitation is produced by a variety of etiological factors:

- Congenital malformation of the aortic valve (most frequently bicuspid valve);

- Rheumatic carditis;

- Infective endocarditis;

- A variety of diseases involving the aortic root: lues, rheumatoid spondylitis, other forms of aortitis, atherosclerotic disease;

- Dissecting aneurysm;

- Trauma: spontaneous rupture of a cusp, surgical injury;

- Marfan's syndrome.

The disease process varies, depending on whether aortic regurgitation develops suddenly or gradually. Those cases with sudden onset are usually combined under the term "acute aortic regurgitation."

PATHOLOGY AND PATHOPHYSIOLOGY

Pulmonary regurgitation of congenital origin is a rare lesion when unassociated with any other malformation. It usually involves hypoplasia of one or more cusps. The postsurgical variety is most often encountered after surgical repair of lesions involving the right ventricular outflow tract or the pulmonary annulus, such as valvular pulmonic stenosis, tetralogy of Fallot, or some of the more complex cardiac malformations. It may be the result of pulmonary valvotomy. Occasionally a hypoplastic pulmonary annulus requires enlargement by means of prosthetic or pericardial "gussets," in which case the diminutive pulmonary valve cannot cover the new, enlarged orifice. In some operations the pulmonary valve may be found to be altogether absent or may be sacrificed at operation.

Aortic regurgitation may be produced by a variety of pathological changes in the aortic leaflets or adjacent tissues. The more important mechanisms producing valve incompetence include the following:

- Deformity of valve leaflets, usually rheumatic, involves, as a rule, a shrinking and foreshortening of the cusps, which cannot completely cover the aortic orifice;

- Dilatation of the aortic ring makes the normal aortic leaflet too small to cover the enlarged orifice; this mechanism is present in the various forms of aortitis and in some cases of Marfan's syndrome;

- Abnormal traction upon the valve resulting from deformity of a nondilated aortic ring occurs in dissecting aneurysm;

- Lack of support of the valve on the ventricular side may cause prolapse of one of the cusps, as occurs in association with the ventricular septal defect (Chapter 28);

- Perforation of cusps after endocarditis.

The pathological consequence of severe aortic regurgitation is hypertrophy and dilatation of the left ventricle (eccentric hypertrophy). Left ventricular hypertrophy reaches sizable proportions in chronic aortic regurgitation: hearts of patients with this lesion are among the heaviest ever encountered (cor bovinum may exceed 1 kg. for an adult patient). Hearts from such patients often show diffuse fibrotic changes, which represent the pathological counterpart for the impaired myocardial contractility that may be present in patients with this lesion.

The aorta is usually dilated above the valve in cases in which the disease originates in the aortic valve (congenital and rheumatic). Aortic disease, as stated previously, may be the cause of aortic regurgitation, especially in cases in which it is acquired later in life.

Pathophysiological effects of *pulmonary valve incompetence* are of relatively little significance. Considering the fact that between the pulmonary artery and the right ventricle there is only a 5 mm. average diastolic pressure gradient, it is easy to see that even a large opening in the pulmonary valve causes regurgitation of modest proportions, which can be easily tolerated by the right ventricle. In some cases right ventricular dilatation and hypertrophy may develop, but the appearance of right ventricular failure is uncommon. The situation is entirely different, however, if the patient has pulmonary arterial hypertension, in which case a serious overload upon the right ventricle may develop and the production of tricuspid regurgitation is common.

Thus, in the congenital variety, pulmonary regurgitation as a rule has little influence upon circulatory dynamics. In postsurgical pulmonary regurgitation its consequences are related to the underlying (usually residual) lesion. It presumably may add to the overload of the principal lesion, thereby aggravating its hemodynamic effect.

The effect of *aortic regurgitation* upon left ventricular performance is related to the magnitude of the reflux. This lesion produces volume overload upon the left ventricle, which ejects not only its usual stroke output, but, in addition, the regurgitant volume of blood. Volume overload constitutes a powerful stimulus to left ventricular hypertrophy and dilatation, as already mentioned.

The physiological consequences of significant aortic regurgitation are as follows:

- Shortened and more abrupt than usual left ventricular ejection, producing rapid upstroke of the arterial pulse;

- Lowered diastolic pressure in the aorta and peripheral arteries, often associated with a significant rise of systolic pressure (both the systolic and diastolic pressure readings by sphygmomanometer are exaggerated, thus the pulse pressure in indirect determination is higher than that obtained by direct reading);

- Left ventricular enlargement with increased end-systolic and end-diastolic volumes;

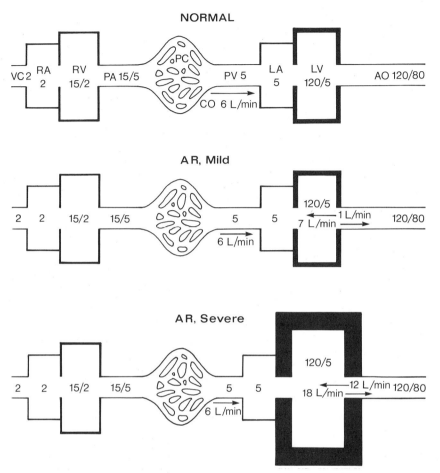

Figure 33-1. Hemodynamic diagram showing the normal circulation (*top*) and two examples of aortic regurgitation (AR): mild aortic regurgitation shows no hemodynamic consequences (*middle diagram*); severe aortic regurgitation, shown here in compensated state, produces severe eccentric left ventricular hypertrophy (*lower diagram*).

- Elevated end-diastolic left ventricular pressure;
- Increased "atrial kick," i.e., left atrial *a* waves;
- Peripheral systemic vasodilatation.

It is not known what constitutes a "significant" or "free" aortic regurgitation to produce the above consequences; the critical dividing line between "mild" and "significant" aortic regurgitation probably varies from individual to individual. It is doubtful whether the regurgitation of a quantity less than that equal to the forward flow would be capable of producing the peripheral effects of "free" aortic regurgitation.

It should be pointed out that the peripheral signs of aortic regurgitation are contingent upon reasonably good function of the left ventricle. In the chain of events producing these changes a normal or near-normal cardiac output is implied. When left ventricular failure ensues and the cardiac output (forward flow) becomes reduced, peripheral vasodilatation may no longer be present and the secondary signs of aortic regurgitation may become minimized.

Inasmuch as the amount of retrograde flow is related to the length of the diastole, tachycardia exerts a favorable effect and bradycardia an unfavorable effect upon aortic regurgitation.

In spite of the commonly found elevation of left ventricular end-diastolic pressure early in the course of aortic regurgitation, clinically significant cardiac failure develops only when the mean diastolic pressure is elevated in the left ventricle and the left atrium. Once this occurs, the usual consequences upon the pulmonary circulation can be observed: the pulmonary capillary pressure becomes elevated, and the mean pulmonary arterial pressure rises, as does the systolic pressure in the right ventricle. At first these changes can be observed during exercise and are temporary, associated with a subnormal rise in cardiac output. Later these abnormalities occur at rest and the basic cardiac output (forward flow) may become abnormally low. Some patients will develop reactive pulmonary hypertension with an abnormally high pulmonary vascular resistance. Right ventricular failure—often associated with tricuspid regurgitation—may develop secondarily to right ventricular overload.

It should be pointed out that the above pathophysiological changes occur in chronic aortic regurgitation, in which left ventricular hypertrophy compensates for the overload for a long time and cardiac failure develops late. In acute aortic regurgitation severe reflux may develop abruptly, overloading a *normal* left ventricle. Here the development of cardiac failure may be instantaneous, or—in less severe cases—at an accelerated pace.

CLINICAL ENTITIES

Pulmonary Regurgitation

Natural History. The natural history of this disease is not well known because of the rarity of its congenital form and the complexity of the surgically produced form. While cases of serious consequences of pulmonary regurgitation have been reported in infancy, the consensus is that older children and adults with isolated incompetence of the pulmonary valve do very well, are mostly asymptomatic, and probably have a normal life expectancy. Occasionally right ventricular enlargement has been reported. Postsurgical pulmonary regurgitation is found in patients who have undergone correction of complex congenital malformations; it is difficult to assess the role of pulmonary reflux in their postoperative suboptimal performance. However, many patients show normal effort tolerance in spite of obvious pulmonary regurgitation, thereby demonstrating that the latter may be consistent with good cardiac function.

Diagnosis. The diagnosis of pulmonary regurgitation rests entirely upon the finding of the characteristic, delayed, decrescendo or diamond-shaped diastolic murmur in the second or third left intercostal space. The unique acoustical quality of this murmur makes diagnosis easy; confusion with left-sided semilunar valve incompetence is unlikely by an experienced diagnostician. A systolic murmur may also be present. The heart sounds are unaffected by this condition. In the congenital form, the chest roentgenogram and the electrocardiogram are usually normal; in the postsurgical form they are related to the residua of the original lesion. Cardiac catheterization shows, as a rule, normal pressure, but the low diastolic pressure in the pulmonary artery may produce identical pressure curves from the pulmonary artery and the right ventricle. Direct angiographic demonstration of pulmonary regurgitation requires injection of the contrast medium into the pulmonary artery.

In an asymptomatic patient with clinical signs of "idiopathic" congenital pulmonary regurgitation invasive studies are not indicated unless strong evidence of an associated cardiac lesion is uncovered.

Treatment. Pulmonary regurgitation requires no special treatment, although appropriate reassurance to the anxious patient is important.

Chronic Aortic Regurgitation

Natural History. The course of aortic regurgitation depends upon many factors, the most important of which are:

- the age of its development,
- magnitude of the reflux,
- individual compensatory mechanisms.

In many patients aortic regurgitation is evident early in life, the etiology being congenital and rheumatic. In contrast to mitral stenosis, aortic regurgitation may develop during the attack of rheumatic carditis, so that the latent period between the attack and the obvious presence of an organic cardiac lesion is omitted. Aortic regurgitation may be progressive, yet, as far as is known (knowledge of the natural history of this lesion is rather scanty), most often it is a stable lesion. Thus, in contrast to mitral stenosis in which clinical symptoms usually reflect increasing severity of the lesion, in aortic regurgitation cardiac enlargement, effort intolerance, and eventually cardiac failure are related to the breakdown of the compensatory mechanisms. As a corollary, it appears probable that mild degrees of aortic regurgitation have an excellent prognosis—perhaps a normal life expectancy—unless new insults (particularly infective endocarditis) produce additional damage to the valve. However, aortic regurgitation developing later in life as a result of diseases of the aortic root is likely to be progressive and its evaluation and prognosis require more caution.

Given a young patient with significant aortic regurgitation (i.e., with pronounced peripheral effects of it), the high probability is that he will be asymptomatic and capable of normal activities, even athletic feats. Patients usually remain asymptomatic, even though they may show electrocardiographic evidence of left ventricular hypertrophy and radiographic evidence of moderate cardiomegaly. If studied hemodynamically, normal findings at rest and normal responses to exercise are the rule. Symptoms are likely to develop in the fourth or, more often, the fifth decade of life. Hemodynamic abnormalities during exercise usually precede the development of clinical disability.

The earliest symptoms are usually nondisabling:

- Palpitations—not related to arrhythmias but rather representing the patient's consciousness of overactivity of the heart and excessive vascular pulsations. This may be perceived as heavy pounding in the thorax, throbbing sensation in the neck, etc.

- Chest pain. Though angina is thought to be common in aortic regurgitation, this is probably a misconception, since the great majority of patients experience nonexertional atypical pain in the left hemithorax; this pain is likely to originate in the chest wall and be related to anxiety or to the effect of the excessive force of cardiac motion. Rarely exertional angina-like pain is observed. An especially unusual form of cardiac pain consists of attacks of substernal pain at rest, often nocturnal, associated with anxiety, tachycardia, and perspiration, promptly relieved by nitroglycerin.

- Fatigability—more often than not this is related to anxiety. The usual hemodynamic basis for fatigability—marked restriction of cardiac output—is not seen in aortic regurgitation until overt cardiac failure is present.

Limitation of activities, when occurring consistently, may be due to exertional dyspnea and may signify reduction of left ventricular performance. As mentioned, hemodynamic abnormalities are always present in the stage of disability; usually there is a considerable degree of cardiomegaly in evidence. Progression of this symptom is variable, but more often than not it is very slow. Only occasionally acute left ventricular failure in the form of pulmonary edema or paroxysmal nocturnal dyspnea takes place in the absence of an obvious provoking factor (e.g., arrhythmia, infection).

After the stage of left ventricular failure the patient is likely to develop right ventricular failure. When this occurs, deterioration may be rapid; response to therapy is often disappointing, although occasionally patients may be controlled by a medical regimen for lengthy periods of time.

Complications. The most serious problem facing the patient with aortic regurgitation is infective endocarditis. This lesion is one with the highest proneness to bacterial infection. Other complications are rare. Arrhythmias are very much less frequent than in mitral valve disease; some patients may have bouts of paroxysmal supraventricular tachycardias; occasionally ventricular ectopy is provoked by the severe hypertrophy of the left ventricle. Atrial fibrillation is rare, but if it occurs it may have a more serious effect upon this lesion, since circulatory efficiency depends so much upon the "atrial kick."

Postsurgical Course. Aortic regurgitation almost always requires valve replacement. Results of this operation depend largely upon the stage in which the operation is performed. Patients whose correction is performed at the time they had significant symptoms show, as a rule, only modest improvement; left ventricular hypertrophy and dilatation seldom regress; residual disability is common. The problems related to sequels and complications after valve replacement were discussed in Chapter 13.

Diagnosis. The goals of diagnostic approaches to aortic regurgitation are as follows:

- The diagnosis of the lesion and its differentiation from similar lesions;

- The quantification of its severity;

- The recognition of its various forms;

- The assessment of its effect upon the circulation.

The clinical history may sometimes provide some information regarding the nature of the disease; the actual symptomatology is nonspecific. On the basis of the background information the following clues may be of some assistance in the overall evaluation of a patient with aortic regurgitation:

- History of acute rheumatic fever only occasionally is of assistance—this subject is presented in connection with mitral stenosis (Chapter 32);

- History of the presence of a heart murmur since an early age may help concentrate upon the chronic forms of this entity;

- Discovery of a murmur after an attack of severe chest pain may draw attention to the possibility of dissecting aneurysm;

- A history or the presence of diseases such as lues, rheumatoid spondylitis, or Reiter's syndrome may reveal the etiology of the lesion.

Physical examination usually reveals findings which are specific enough for aortic regurgitation to make the diagnosis highly likely.

The most characteristic finding is the early diastolic murmur. The murmur (see also Chapter 3) starts with the aortic component of the second sound and continues, with decreasing intensity, into mid- or late diastole. Its most characteristic location is at the lower left sternal border, with maximum intensity in the third, fourth, or fifth intercostal spaces. The murmur is equally well conducted to the apex and to the "aortic" area (right upper sternal border). Atypical locations of the murmur may occur; some murmurs are heard only or predominantly in the apical area, and others are heard only or predominantly at the right sternal border.

Apical early diastolic blowing murmurs have no special diagnostic connotations; however, those present most prominently at the right upper sternal border are often associated with aortic regurgitation caused by diseases of the aortic root (the specificity of this finding is moderate).

The intensity and length of the murmur bears only a very crude relationship to the severity of aortic regurgitation. In general, very faint murmurs more often than not signify mild reflux, but the reverse is not correct. Severe aortic regurgitation is occasionally seen in the presence of very short, faint murmurs. "Silent" aortic regurgitation probably exists, though it is difficult to be sure because of the variability of the aortic diastolic murmurs, which can greatly change in loudness from day to day, and occasionally may be inaudible at certain times.

Associated auscultatory findings include frequently an ejection systolic murmur indistinguishable from that of aortic stenosis. While aortic stenosis and regurgitation often coexist, the murmur occurs sometimes even in the presence of a dilated aortic annulus; "functional" systolic murmurs are usually short and of low intensity—grades 1 to 3 (of 6).

The first heart sound is unremarkable; the second varies from being inaudible to unusually loud. Gallop sounds are commonly present, particularly S3 gallop. Occasionally a systolic ejection sound may be present, especially in the presence of a dilated aortic root.

A common finding in significant aortic regurgitation is a mitral-like apical rumbling diastolic murmur (Austin Flint), thought to be produced by vibration of the medial leaflet of the mitral valve, which in diastole floats between atrioventricular flow and the regurgitant stream.

In significant aortic regurgitation inspection and palpation of the precordium reveals exaggerated precordial motion, often of "rocking" character. The apical impulse is typical of volume overload: sustained and forceful and at the same time overactive. Peripheral signs of aortic regurgitation involve rapid upstroke of the arterial pulse, a widened pulse pressure and a rapid downstroke, usually obliterating the dicrotic notch. These features of the arterial pulse are usually visible as well as palpable: strong and jerky pulsations of the carotid are usually noted, sometimes with nodding of the head synchronous with the pulse. Palpation of the pulses reveals a possible range from merely perceiving rapid upstroke and widening of the pulse pressure to a fully blown collapsing "water-hammer" pulse. Traditional confirmatory signs, such as the Duroziez sign (double femoral souffle) or the capillary pulse are seldom recorded now, since they add no specific diagnostic information. Widened pulse pressure is documented by sphygmomanometer. The abnormally low diastolic pressure is a more important sign of severity of aortic regurgitation than the elevated systolic pressure. As stated, cuff readings show exaggerated values: the diastolic pressure occasionally cannot be determined at all—the Korotkoff sound persisting unchanged with the cuff pressure lowered to 0. Direct pressure measurement seldom shows diastolic pressure lower than 40 mm Hg.

The electrocardiogram shows in patients with aortic regurgitation the pattern of left ventricular hypertrophy. It ranges from a mere increase in QRS voltage to the full picture, including ST-T changes and prolonged QRS duration.

Radiographic examination reveals varying degrees of cardiomegaly primarily due to left ventricular enlargement. The ascending aorta is usually enlarged as well, regardless of whether or not abnormalities within the aortic root caused aortic valve reflux. In contrast to aortic stenosis, left ventricular dilatation is observed early: calcification of the aortic leaflets (in the rheumatic and congenital types of aortic regurgitation) is rare, even in older subjects.

Phonocardiography permits the registration of the auscultatory findings; it is noteworthy, however, that the high frequency diastolic murmur is more difficult to record than to hear. In general, phonocardiography presents no discriminatory diagnostic information.

Echocardiography cannot directly demonstrate aortic regurgitation. It does permit, however, its confirmation indirectly by registering vibratory motion in diastole of the anterior leaflet of the mitral valve (the equivalent of the Austin Flint murmur). Its value is to estimate the size of the left ventricular cavity and its thickness; left ventricular dilatation can be demonstrated with greater sensitivity than by radiography. This feature, furthermore, renders itself well as a means of longitudinal follow-up of patients.

Invasive procedures are of less value in the diagnosis of aortic regurgitation than in other valve lesions. Cardiac catheterization does not present any diagnostic features in this condition except for the shape of the arterial pressure curve (which duplicates information available noninvasively). This procedure is important, however, in the evaluation of the function of the left ventricle, and — when the latter fails — of the responses of the pulmonary circulation.

Angiocardiography demonstrates directly aortic regurgitation with the contrast medium injected into the aortic root. It permits a crude estimation of its severity. The following limitations of this technique should be recognized, however:

- Retrograde opacification of the left ventricular cavity could be misleading, since the density of this opacified chamber depends not only on the quantity of regurgitant contrast substance but on left ventricular capacity (i.e., end-systolic volume) as well.

- Artifactitious retrograde flow may occur with supravalvular aortic injection, partly as a result of injecting the substance during systole with the valve open; consequently, it is hazardous to diagnose mild aortic regurgitation solely on the basis of an angiographic examination.

Throughout the preceding section the various diagnostic signs of aortic regurgitation have been discussed. Aortic regurgitation represents a spectrum: somewhere in the center of it is the dividing line between "mild" and "significant" degrees of it. On the "mild" side of the spectrum one frequently encounters a single finding — the early diastolic blowing murmur; none of the accompanying physical signs are present, and the laboratory data reveal all normal findings. On the other end of the spectrum one can find the classical signs and laboratory findings in their most pronounced form. The center of the spectrum presents, however, considerable diagnostic difficulties in deciding whether aortic regurgitation is of sufficient severity to present a significant threat to the patient's health and life. The discriminating value of the various diagnostic features is estimated as follows:

- Peripheral signs of aortic regurgitation represent the most important differential feature. It should be recognized, however, that factors other than the magnitude of aortic reflux contribute to these signs (e.g., peripheral vasodilatation), hence they may be occasionally misleading. Of the peripheral signs, lowering of the diastolic pressure is usually the earliest sign pointing to significant degree of regurgitation.

- Evidence of left ventricular hypertrophy, by physical examination or electrocardiography, can be taken as evidence of significant left ventricular overload.

- Radiographic evidence of left ventricular enlargement is less reliable: theoretically dilatation of that chamber develops early; yet variability of its normal size and of its responses to overload produces situations in which significant, long-standing aortic regurgitation may be present without radiographic evidence of cardiac enlargement.

- Echocardiographic abnormalities, if present, imply with a reasonable probability that significant regurgitation takes place.

Differential Points in the Diagnosis. The characteristic features of aortic regurgitation usually make the diagnosis relatively easy on clinical grounds; nevertheless, some difficulties in the differential diagnosis may occasionally arise:

1. In mild aortic regurgitation the murmur is of sufficient specificity as to make the diagnosis reasonably certain, even if no confirmatory findings can be obtained.

2. The presence of the apical diastolic rumble may raise the question as to whether aortic regurgitation is the sole lesion or two valves are involved; here echocardiographic examination may be decisive.

3. The presence of wide pulse pressure and rapid rising, or even collapsing, pulses may present occasional difficulties. Other conditions associated with run-off from the arterial system (patent ductus arteriosus, arteriovenous fistula, rupture of the sinus of Valsalva, or other aorticocardiac communications) may present such atypical physical findings as to bring about confusion. Many of the other clinical and laboratory findings in these conditions resemble those of aortic regurgitation; hence the diagnosis may be difficult. Careful auscultation usually, though not always, suggests the correct condition. Angiocardiography is the most valuable differential diagnostic tool.

Evaluation. The objectives of the diagnostic workup are presented in the preceding section. Modes of evaluation of the diagnostic information are presented below:

1. In patients with mild aortic regurgitation—as defined ear-

lier—i.e., those presenting the typical murmur but no other abnormalities, invasive studies should not be performed. In contrast to mitral stenosis, where such studies are often advised even in asymptomatic patients, no significant information can be obtained in aortic regurgitation by cardiac catheterization, while angiocardiography is superfluous, and, as pointed out, may even be misleading.

2. In asymptomatic patients with "significant" rheumatic or congenital aortic regurgitation (i.e., known to be present early in life) invasive evaluation is also considered superfluous. Angiographic quantification of aortic regurgitation is not more reliable than its estimation on the basis of clinical signs (particularly the peripheral effects of the lesion), and it plays a relatively small role in the decision-making process regarding management of the patient. However, should a patient in this category be followed longitudinally by noninvasive techniques and found to have progression of left ventricular hypertrophy or enlargement, then cardiac catheterization with an exercise study may be advisable as a means to recognize early disturbance of left ventricular function.

3. In patients who are symptomatic, it is first necessary to evaluate the symptoms in their relation to aortic regurgitation. If they appear to suggest genuine reduction of effort tolerance, invasive evaluation is in order.

4. Patients severely symptomatic who are candidates for early surgical treatment should have a complete evaluation and a study of both the dynamics and left ventricular contractility.

5. Patients with the onset of aortic regurgitation late in life (older than 40) should be evaluated regarding the etiology of the lesion, if possible. Such patients may also be studied by cardiac catheterization, even if asymptomatic, on the basis that their lesion is likely to be progressive and a baseline hemodynamic study may be of importance in the decision-making process at a later time.

6. Patients in the middle or older age groups who suffer from chest pain which is not clearly "functional" may need a coronary arteriographic study to evaluate the possibility of coexisting coronary artery disease.

Treatment. Active medical therapy in asymptomatic patients with aortic regurgitation is seldom necessary. It is often important to protect patients from overtreatment. Only too often patients with significant aortic regurgitation, still young and asymptomatic, are being treated for "high blood pressure" because of the physiologically overshooting high levels of the systolic arterial pressure, are being unduly restricted, or are sent to cardiovascular surgeons even though they are clearly in class I. Patients probably should be discouraged from undertaking unusually strenuous occupations and from participating in competitive sports. The principal preventive treatment consists of the observance of endocarditis prophylaxis. Those who have chest pain (the submammary type) or palpitations deserve sympathetic reassurance. When the patient develops exercise intolerance, then the choice of medical vs. surgical treatment may have to be made.

Surgical treatment of aortic regurgitation presents the clinician with one of the most perplexing dilemmas, at present insoluble. Unquestionably, valve replacement relieves the mechanical effect of the volume overload. It is furthermore certain that aortic regurgitation, with its powerful stimulus for left ventricular hypertrophy, produces eventually a "point of no return," i.e., irreversible damage to the left ventricular myocardium. In order to prevent myocardial damage valve replacement would have to be done at an early stage, when hypertrophy first starts developing. However, viewing the problem from the standpoint of risk vs. benefit, it is probable, that a 20-year-old patient with free aortic regurgitation, who might appear to be a logical candidate for "prophylactic" valve replacement, has an estimated 90 per cent probability of surviving the next 20 years and remaining in class I—a record that cannot possibly be matched by the surgical alternative, with its definitive operative mortality, the many problems related to valve prosthesis, and the uncertain fate of the valve beyond a few years. A compromise solution might be provided by selecting the point at which the patient begins to show the first clinical symptoms or hemodynamic deterioration as the time when the risk and benefit might balance each other. Yet experience has shown that progression of symptoms to true disability may be years past this point; hence conservative management may have a smaller risk and be preferable up to the development of disability, even if the results of surgery performed then may be suboptimal.

Acute Aortic Regurgitation

Acute aortic regurgitation is most often produced by infective endocarditis and by aortic dissection. Not all patients who develop aortic regurgitation in the course of these two diseases develop the clinical syndrome of acute aortic regurgitation to be described here. Only a sudden development of severe incompetence of the valve has this effect. This happens when perforation of an aortic cusp occurs in infective endocarditis or when a major deformity develops with aortic dissection causing nonclosure of the valve cusps. Rarer causes of acute aortic regurgitation include trauma and spontaneous rupture of an aortic cusp.

Natural History. In very severe degrees of aortic regurgitation the patient may immediately develop congestive cardiac failure, or even go into shock. Alertness to the nature of this condition may be lifesaving, by channeling patients into immediate valve replacement in spite of the active infection (in the case of endocarditis). In less severe degrees of aortic regurgitation the long-drawn out course of chronic aortic regurgitation appears to be telescoped into weeks or months instead of years. Progressive dyspnea, then congestive failure is apt to develop and progress rapidly. In patients with endocarditis, the prognosis and final outcome depend not only on the management of the hemodynamic problem but on the cure of the infections as well.

In dissecting aneurysms, the condition of the aorta as well as condition of the heart determines the prognosis; operations are frequently performed primarily because of the dissection, with valve replacement only a secondary goal.

Diagnosis. Most of the diagnostic features described in the section on chronic aortic regurgitation apply to the acute form. However, some important differences are noteworthy:

1. Abrupt development of aortic regurgitation does not allow time for the appearance of left ventricular hypertrophy and dilatation, for the first few weeks. Consequently, palpatory evidence of left ventricular hypertrophy, its electrocardiographic signs, and radiographic evidence of cardiomegaly are usually absent.

2. Early appearance of cardiac failure minimizes peripheral signs of aortic regurgitation; hence guidelines for the severity of the lesion may be misleading.

3. Tachycardia is commonly present: the murmur of aortic regurgitation may be soft, even inaudible.

4. Cardiac catheterization studies often reveal inordinately elevated left ventricular diastolic pressure. In late diastole aortic and left ventricular pressures may equilibrate and the mitral valve may reclose.

Evaluation. The most important point in acute aortic regurgitation is to be aware of the misleading clinical features in the fulminating forms. Patients with infective endocarditis who go into shock or develop severe cardiac failure should be suspected of having perforated aortic valves, even if no direct evidence for this exists. Immediate invasive studies are necessary with prime emphasis upon evaluation of possible aortic regurgitation and of left ventricular contractility (embolic myocardial infarction may be the alternative diagnosis, or may be an associated feature).

Perforation of the aortic valve with less disastrous consequences usually presents no major diagnostic difficulties. The appearance or the accentuation of the diastolic murmur of aortic regurgitation and the sudden fall in the diastolic arterial pressure easily give away the diagnosis. If medical management successfully keeps the patient in a reasonably good condition, further studies should be postponed until the infection is eliminated. Then, however, invasive evaluation is indicated, inasmuch as a more aggressive attitude toward cardiac surgery is indicated in acute aortic regurgitation.

Treatment. In acute aortic regurgitation due to endocarditis, the choice of therapy must be selected from three possible courses of action:

1. Supportive, nonspecific therapy, or no treatment at all;

2. Aggressive medical therapy;

3. Surgical replacement of the aortic valve.

In patients who tolerate acute aortic regurgitation well, especially if clinical indications are such that the magnitude of the reflux is modest, a "wait and see" attitude may be adopted. While some progression of the lesion during the healing stage may be anticipated, many patients may be left with a benign cardiac valve disease and overall good prognosis.

Patients who show some evidence of intolerance of newly developed valve incompetence should first be subjected to medical therapy. Whether or not they become surgical candidates depends largely upon two factors:

- Their response to treatment;

- Result of the evaluation (in terms of severity of hemodynamic abnormalities).

The possibility that the development of compensatory hypertrophy within weeks from the insult may ameliorate the effects of the valve disease should not be overlooked; hence a conservative course of action initially may be adopted if the patient's condition warrants it.

Early surgical treatment is indicated, in addition to the already mentioned emergencies, in patients who remain in congestive failure without responding satisfactorily to medical therapy.

Patients with acute aortic regurgitation due to aortic dissection present the additional problem of the condition of the aorta. In unstable situations emergency surgical treatment of the aneurysm may have to be performed. One should not overlook the possibility that aortic regurgitation may be produced by mere distortion of the aortic root from the dissection, resulting in faulty coaptation of the cusps. This being the case, restoration of the normal conditions in the aortic root may make the valve competent again without the need for its replacement.

The present tendency for a more conservative approach to aortic dissection with a stable course may make it necessary to focus upon the cardiac response to the valve incompetence. If this is the case, the guidelines applicable to endocarditis can be followed in dissecting aneurysm as well.

Bibliography

Braniff BA, Shumway NE, Harrison DC: Valve replacement in active bacterial endocarditis. New Engl. J. Med. 276:1164, 1967.

Brawley RK, Morrow AG: Direct determination of aortic blood flow in patients with aortic regurgitation: effects of alternation in heart rate, increased ventricular preload and afterload and isoproterenol. Circulation 35:32, 1967.

Gault JH, Covell JW, Braunwald E, Ross J Jr: Left ventricular performance following correction of free aortic regurgitation. Circulation 42:773, 1970.

Goldschlager N, Pfeiffer J, Cohn KE, Popper R, Selzer A: The natural history of aortic regurgitation. A clinical and hemodynamic study. Amer. J. Med. 54:577, 1973.

Gorlin R, Goodale WT: Changing blood pressure in aortic insufficiency. New Engl. J. Med. 255:77, 1956.

Harvey WP, Segal JP, Hufnagel CA: Unusual clinical features associated with serious aortic insufficiency. Ann. Int. Med. 47:27, 1957.

Hegglin R, Schey H, Rothlin M: Aortic insufficiency. Circulation 37 (Suppl. V):77, 1968.

Price BO: Isolated incompetence of the pulmonic valve. Circulation 23:596, 1961.

Rotman M, Morris JJ, Behar VS, Peter RH, Kong Y: Aortic valvular disease: comparison of types and their medical and surgical management. Amer. J. Med. 51:241, 1971.

Tompsett R, Lubarsh GD: Aortic valve perforation in bacterial endocarditis. Circulation 23:622, 1961.

Wigle ED, Labrosse CJ: Sudden, severe aortic insufficiency. Circulation 32:708, 1965.

34

Atrioventricular Valve Incompetence

Definition. Incompetence of the tricuspid valve is a common sequel of systolic overload in the right ventricle. As such, it is a secondary phenomenon, often reversible by treatment. Organic disease of the tricuspid valve very rarely is found as an isolated lesion, but rather constitutes a part of polyvalvular involvement, usually of rheumatic origin. Other causes of tricuspid regurgitation include congenital defects, particularly Ebstein's disease. These conditions will be discussed in the appropriate sections of the book. This chapter thus deals entirely with *mitral regurgitation*, concentrating upon its clinically significant, usually primary forms. Clinical entities involving mitral regurgitation include the following:

1. Rheumatic mitral regurgitation

2. Common nonrheumatic syndromes

   • Isolated rupture of chordae tendineae

   • Midsystolic click and late systolic murmur

   • Postinfarctional mitral regurgitation

3. Rare nonrheumatic syndromes:

   • Congenital mitral regurgitation

   • Postendocarditic mitral regurgitation

   • Cardiac tumors

   • Mitral regurgitation of undetermined etiology

4. Secondary forms of mitral regurgitation

- Hypertrophic subaortic stenosis
- Myocardial disease

ETIOLOGY

Rheumatic fever accounts for less than half of cases of primary or clinically important pure mitral regurgitation. More often than not rheumatic damage to the valve involves some degree of stenosis; pure mitral regurgitation is found in only about 10 per cent of patients with significant mitral valve disease due to rheumatic fever. In some patients predominant mitral stenosis may change into pure regurgitation, the two important causes of such a change being infective endocarditis and surgical trauma during mitral valvotomy.

The etiology of isolated rupture of chordae tendineae is not known. This clinical entity affects mostly men in their fifth to seventh decades of life, only occasionally being related to known trauma. Reviews of consecutive series showed that such causes as mild rheumatic insult or occult infective endocarditis are highly unlikely to play a significant role in the causation of this syndrome. It most likely is the result of an "accidental" tearing of an aging chorda, with secondary stresses producing further chordal rupture.

The symptom-complex of midsystolic click and late systolic murmur affects subjects of all ages without sex preference. It is now clear that this is not a well-defined clinical syndrome; rather, several etiological factors may produce changes in the mitral valve apparatus that cause a late systolic prolapse of a cusp, evidenced by the characteristic auscultatory findings. Among these is a familial form, often but not always related to Marfan's syndrome. Nonfamilial cases of mucoid degeneration of the mitral valve ("floppy valve") constitute another group. Some patients with rheumatic heart disease may show these auscultatory findings. Mitral valve malfunction after myocardial infarction may also induce these findings. Congenital cardiomyopathy has also been found in association with mitral valve prolapse.

Myocardial infarction produces mitral regurgitation by affecting the muscular part of the mitral valve apparatus – the papillary muscles. However, in order to produce significant mitral regurgitation it is necessary to have damage (usually necrosis or fibrosis) to the papillary muscle (usually the posterior) associated with dyskinesia of the free wall of the left ventricular myocardium.

Congenital mitral regurgitation involves several processes to be discussed in the following section. It includes congenital malformation of the mitral valve or other congenital lesions indirectly damaging the mitral valve apparatus.

Endocarditis may change mitral stenosis into mitral regurgitation, as already mentioned, usually by disrupting chordae tendineae. In addition, some patients develop endocarditis on mitral valves which have not been previously known to be abnormal, developing acute mitral regurgitation analogous to acute aortic regurgitation (Chapter 33).

PATHOLOGY

Mitral regurgitation may develop as a result of anatomic changes in any of the three components of the mitral valve apparatus: the cusps, the chordae, and the papillary muscles. Changes in other parts of the left ventricle — the mitral ring, the ventricular wall, and the atrium — may also participate in the pathogenesis of this lesion. In addition, functional incompetence of the valve may be present without structural changes in this apparatus.

Cuspal changes are characteristically of rheumatic etiology. Rheumatic scarring may produce retraction rather than fusion of the leaflets. However, the process almost always involves stiffening of the valve; therefore some resistance to flow, i.e., stenosis, is often associated with it, though not necessarily dynamically significant. Chordal type of rheumatic mitral valve disease may produce pure regurgitation: thickened and shortened chordae interfere with the normal position and closure of the cusps or conversely stretched or torn chordae make one leaflet overshoot the other.

Nonrheumatic involvement of the mitral cusps includes congenital clefts. These should be distinguished from the normal shallow bays present in healthy valves and the exaggerated acquired incisures of the rheumatic valves. Congenital clefts are usually located in the center, more often involve the anterior leaflet, and extend deep into the base of the cusp. Commonly present in association with atrioventricular canal lesions, isolated congenital clefts do occur occasionally and represent a form of congenital mitral regurgitation.

The third type of cuspal disease involves degenerative change of the connective tissue of the cusps, the commonest of which is mucoid degeneration. It produces enlargement and redundancy of the leaflets, which usually results in stretching of the chordae, which in turn permits prolapse of a leaflet leading to regurgitation.

Secondary changes in the cusps may develop in isolated rupture of the chordae tendineae, affecting the prolapsing segment of the leaflet, which fibroses and thickens from the trauma of turbulent flow.

Chordal disease may be primary or secondary. Primary "idiopathic" rupture occurs in otherwise normal mitral valves. No consistent pathological changes have been reported in the ruptured segments of the chordae, although some excessive hyalinization is occasionally seen.

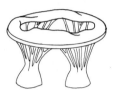

Rheumatic

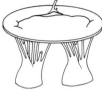

Ruptured Chordae

Figure 34-1. Diagrammatic presentation of four types of mitral regurgitation.

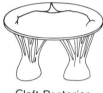

Cleft Posterior
Leaflet

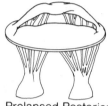

Prolapsed Posterior
Leaflet

Chordae attached to the posterior cusp are involved by spontaneous rupture four to five times as often as anterior cuspal chordae. Rupture usually involves one to three adjacent chordae, most frequently central in location. The rupture occurs close to the edges of the leaflets.

Secondary rupture involves chordae previously involved in disease processes. The cause of initial chordal changes varies: rheumatic disease, infective endocarditis, surgical trauma. Occasionally chordae attached to an infarcted papillary muscle rupture, usually close to that muscle.

Papillary muscle disease leading to mitral regurgitation involves ischemia, necrosis, or fibrosis of the muscle. Rarely one of the heads of the papillary muscle (to which usually two or three chordae are attached) ruptures. A total rupture of the base of the papillary muscle, occasionally seen in patients with acute myocardial infarction, is usually immediately fatal.

Functional mitral regurgitation—malfunction of the valve without organic changes in the mitral valve apparatus proper—involves the following mechanisms:

- Dilatation of the left ventricle produces a wider separation of the papillary muscles, as a result of which chordal traction upon the leaflets is weakened because it occurs at obtuse rather than right angles.

- Dilatation of the left side of the heart may involve the mitral annulus; the enlarged ring does not have sufficient valve tissue to cover it. (This is a much rarer mechanism of mitral regurgitation than hitherto believed.)

- Considerable dilatation of the left atrium may exert abnormal traction upon the posterior leaflet and interfere with its closing function.

Morphological consequence of mitral regurgitation depends upon:

- the severity of the reflux,
- the speed of the development of regurgitation.

In chronic mitral regurgitation, of which the rheumatic variety is the principal representative, left ventricular hypertrophy and dilatation occur. The left atrium is also dilated—less often hypertrophied. The size of the left atrium may reach very large proportions, on the average larger than in mitral stenosis. "Aneurysmal" dilatation of the left atrium is a term used occasionally to designate very large atria holding a liter of blood or more. As in mitral stenosis secondary changes in the pulmonary vasculature and the right heart chambers may develop in patients who reach the stage of cardiac failure.

In acute mitral regurgitation chamber enlargement is, as a rule, not present, even if the reflux is severe. Some forms of mitral regurgitation, particularly that associated with rupture of chordae tendineae, involve high velocity regurgitant jets which often produce white endocardial fibrous patches upon the appropriate areas of the atrial wall ("jet lesions"). Given enough time, the left ventricle hypertrophies.

PATHOPHYSIOLOGY

Mechanisms of Mitral Regurgitation. Competence of the mitral valve is contingent upon the following:

- The presence of large enough leaflets to cover the orifice;
- Good contact and apposition of leaflets without the possibility of overshooting one another;
- Appropriate tightening traction exerted by the chordae.

Even a structurally normal mitral valve apparatus may become incompetent under certain circumstances: In the normal heart a premature contraction ejecting blood from a half-filled ventricle may make the mitral valve incompetent for that beat. Acute ischemia may produce temporary, reversible dyskinesia of the left ventricular wall and for its duration cause mitral regurgitation.

The anatomic bases for the various forms of mitral regurgitation have been presented in the preceding section. To recapitulate, rheumatic disease and congenital valve clefts produce regurgitation resulting from the lack of sufficient valve tissue to cover the orifice; prolapse of the entire valve occurs with stretching of chordae (most frequently seen with mucoid degeneration of the valve). Rupture of chordae — primary or secondary — produces focal prolapse of the portion of the cusp detached from the chordae. Inadequate tightening and traction exerted upon the cusps can be produced by ventricular dilatation, by malfunction of the papillary muscle reinforced by abnormal motion of the free wall of the left ventricles, or by severe dyskinesia of the ventricular wall alone.

It should be pointed out that mitral regurgitation frequently is a self-perpetuating process: left ventricular, left atrial, and occasionally annular dilatation may increase the degree of mitral valve incompetence by mechanisms discussed above.

Pathophysiological Consequences of Mitral Regurgitation. Mitral regurgitation of significant degree produces volume overload of the left ventricle. Comparing incompetence of the mitral valve with that of the aortic valve, it is noteworthy that the latter produces a greater overload for an equivalent quantity of regurgitant volume: in aortic regurgitation all the regurgitant volume has to be re-ejected against the systemic pressure; in mitral regurgitation the excess volume returning from the left atrium to the left ventricle is ejected back into the low impedance left atrial chamber at a much lower energy cost, with only its usual forward output ejected into the aorta. Nevertheless, severe mitral regurgitation overloads the left ventricle, producing its dilatation and hypertrophy. Left ventricular ejection is more rapid than normal, hence in mitral regurgitation the upstroke of the arterial pulse is often steeper and quicker, although the pulse pressure and the level of the diastolic pressure are not altered.

The effect of the retrograde flow upon the left atrium depends upon its size and compliance. In a small, noncompliant atrium, such as one frequently encounters in acute forms of mitral regurgitation, the pressure rises in late systole, producing prominent v waves — often as high as 60 mm. Hg. Conversely, a very large, baggy left atrium of the chronic variety accommodates the regurgitant volume of blood with little or no pressure change; occasionally its mean pressure may be normal in spite of a large volume of reflux.

In general, left atrial pressure is elevated with a crude relationship between the regurgitant volume and the magnitude of its v waves. Left atrial hypertension is transmitted back in a manner analogous to mitral stenosis, producing mild to moderate passive pulmonary hypertension. Patients with hyperreactive pulmonary vasculature develop reactive pulmonary arteriolar constriction and severe pulmonary hypertension. The incidence and magnitude of this reaction in mitral regurgitation is

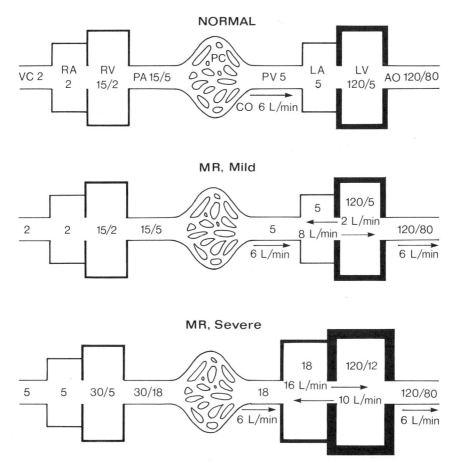

Figure 34-2. Hemodynamic diagram showing the normal circulation (*top*) and two examples of mitral regurgitation (MR): mild mitral regurgitation produces no significant hemodynamic consequences (*middle diagram*); severe mitral regurgitation produces left ventricular hypertrophy and mild pressure elevation in the pulmonary circuit (*lower diagram*).

comparable to that of mitral stenosis. As in the latter, the response of the right ventricle is related to the pulmonary pressure; right ventricular failure with secondary tricuspid regurgitation occurs in patients with pulmonary hypertension. These effects of mitral regurgitation upon the pulmonary circulation and the right side of the heart occur both in acute and chronic mitral regurgitation. As in mitral stenosis they are reversible upon correction of the mitral valve incompetence.

Chronic left ventricular overload occurring in hemodynamically significant mitral regurgitation eventually may lead to left ventricular failure. Cardiac failure in this condition, however, is not as clearly defined as in other lesions overloading the left ventricle, because mitral regurgitation in itself elevates pressures in the left atrium and the pulmonary circulation. Cardiac failure can definitely be diagnosed hemodynamically when the forward cardiac output is reduced and the left ventricular diastolic pressure is consistently elevated.

CLINICAL ENTITIES

Rheumatic Mitral Regurgitation

Natural History. Rheumatic mitral regurgitation differs in some respects from mitral stenosis in its course and prognosis:

- Its presence is evident immediately during the attack of acute carditis, or shortly afterward;

- It is less apt to progress in middle age;

- It affects left ventricular function, hence may produce myocardial failure.

Mild forms of rheumatic mitral regurgitation present themselves as holosystolic apical murmurs without any other detectable abnormalities. Except for the risk of infective endocarditis, patients with this type of mitral regurgitation are likely to remain well, and probably have a normal life expectancy. Some patients with a history of rheumatic carditis have, as a residual lesion, late systolic murmur and midsystolic click—a form of mitral regurgitation to be discussed later.

Moderate degrees of mitral regurgitation produce clinical evidence of left ventricular overload, but its common association with a symptom-free life and its nonprogressive course indicate that the overload may be adequately compensated. As far as information is available, many patients in this category can live useful lives into old age with only occasional instances of deterioration in middle age or late in life.

Severe mitral regurgitation may present serious problems at any age. Occasionally patients develop intractable failure in childhood or adolescence: valve replacement may then be required early in life as a condition for survival. These are unusually severe cases. More often the course parallels that of significant mitral stenosis: patients with moderate disability run a stationary course or may go into cardiac failure at any time. The course involves complicating and secondary factors, such as atrial fibrillation and upper respiratory infections, which may initiate a more symptomatic stage. Cardiomegaly is, as a rule, more profound than in mitral stenosis; giant enlargement of the left atrium is often found; yet patients with this feature do not necessarily have a poorer prognosis than those with smaller hearts.

Symptoms of mitral regurgitation include the following:

- dyspnea of effort,
- paroxysmal nocturnal dyspnea and cough,
- palpitations,
- excessive fatigability.

Patients with atrial fibrillation and large left atrium may reach a point of moderate limitation of activities, but if they can adapt their mode of living to their limitations may go on for years or decades without change. Inasmuch as some patients in this category show disappointing results from surgical valve replacement, consideration should always be given to conservative treatment of patients who show a stable course.

Complications of mitral regurgitation are similar to those of mitral stenosis. *Atrial fibrillation* is more common in mitral regurgitation than in mitral stenosis; the respective incidences have been estimated at 75 and 45 per cent in patients with lesions severe enough to be considered for surgical treatment. The average larger left atrium makes patients with mitral regurgitation even poorer candidates for restoration of sinus rhythm than those with mitral stenosis.

Systemic embolization occurs in patients who are in atrial fibrillation. Its incidence, though, is considerably lower than that in mitral stenosis.

Upper respiratory infections are common and may initiate the development of cardiac failure.

Hemoptysis occurs, but less frequently than in mitral stenosis.

Infective endocarditis is a common complication of mitral regurgitation. If recognized and treated early, the natural history of the cardiac lesion may be unaffected, provided the infection is curable. Endocarditis may, however, exert further damage upon the mitral valve; this can range from the production of more severe mitral regurgitation without any immediate consequences to massive new damage produced by chordal rupture or valve perforation that may require emergency surgical intervention.

Postoperative Course. Rheumatic mitral regurgitation almost always requires valve replacement. Consequently, the postoperative course relates to reversibility of the physiological and clinical sequels of the valve lesion and to the problems associated with valve replacement. In general, surgical results vary considerably: As in mitral stenosis, patients with long-standing atrial fibrillation often show only modest improvement. In some patients spectacular results are achieved. Problems related to valve replacement have been discussed in Chapter 13.

Diagnosis. Diagnostic features of chronic rheumatic mitral regurgitation vary with the severity of the lesion. In mild cases the murmur may be the only abnormality. In severe cases evident signs permit the establishment of the diagnosis as well as a reasonable quantification of the lesion.

Auscultation. The apical holosystolic murmur represents the most specific sign of mitral regurgitation. Typically, the murmur is of low or medium frequency; its maximum intensity is around the apical region, but it is usually widely heard; its directional transmission is preferential toward the axilla and the left subscapular area; conduction to the left sternal border is less pronounced, becoming more a function of its intensity. The loudness of the murmur covers the entire range from grade I to grade VI. There is a mild relationship between the intensity of the murmur and the magnitude of regurgitation, but not enough to represent a significant diagnostic clue. Atypical location and radiation of the murmur are rare; if present, they may overlap with the murmur of mitral regurgitation associated with isolated rupture of chordae tendineae, which will be discussed below.

Given a case of moderately severe or severe mitral regurgitation, the following additional auscultatory findings may be present:

1. The first sound is often of diminished intensity, absent, or overridden by the murmur.

2. An S3 gallop sound is very common.

3. An S4 gallop sound is rare in this form of mitral regurgitation.

4. A decrescendo apical delayed rumbling diastolic murmur, similar to that of mitral stenosis, is heard frequently, usually initiated by the S3 gallop sound. The murmur is short and in sinus rhythm does not extend into presystole.

5. Occasionally a mitral opening snap may be heard. While this finding proves existence of mitral stenosis, the stenotic component may be so trivial that for practical purposes pure mitral regurgitation may be assumed.

6. Pulmonic valve closure sound may be accentuated if pulmonary hypertension develops.

Other physical signs include an overactive, forceful, and sustained apical impulse. An overall rocking motion of the entire precordium can sometimes be observed in severe mitral regurgitation. The ventricular gallop may be perceived as a diastolic apical motion. Severe mitral regurgitation occasionally produces outward systolic motion of the parasternal region. This may be caused by one of two mechanisms:

> • As a right ventricular lift if reactive pulmonary hypertension develops;

- As a transmitted left ventricular pulsation related to the overall exaggerated pulsation.

Parasternal lift due to pulmonary hypertension is more sustained than the briefer transmitted left ventricular motion.

Peripheral signs of mitral regurgitation are few and noncharacteristic. As mentioned, rapid upstroke of the arterial pulse may be present. If reactive pulmonary hypertension develops, signs of right ventricular failure may appear.

Electrocardiographic examination reveals a wide range of findings. The electrocardiogram is often normal for one of two reasons:

- The lesion may be too mild to produce hypertrophy of cardiac chambers;

- Left and right ventricular hypertrophy may cancel each other out in their effects upon the ventricular complexes.

Left atrial enlargement is often present in patients who are in sinus rhythm. Left ventricular hypertrophy occurs as the commonest finding in severe mitral regurgitation. Right ventricular hypertrophy may be present, however, in those who develop severe reactive pulmonary hypertension. Recognizable features of biventricular hypertrophy may also be encountered as an alternative electrocardiographic expression of balanced overload to a normal electrocardiogram.

Radiographic examination. Normal radiographic findings occur in milder cases. Left atrial enlargement, associated with some left ventricular enlargement, is present in moderately severe and in severe mitral regurgitation; the pronounced enlargement of the left atrium in some patients with atrial fibrillation has already been mentioned. Features of pulmonary hypertension and enlargement of right heart chambers are related to the degree of pulmonary pressure elevation. Kerley's B lines are common in patients who have significant elevation of the left atrial pressure. One of the most important features differentiating rheumatic from nonrheumatic mitral regurgitation is the presence of mitral valvular calcifications, which are common in patients 40 years old or older. In some, calcifications occur at younger ages.

Phonocardiographic examination may serve the purpose of identifying some questionable auscultatory findings. The timing of early diastolic sounds and the analysis of the holosystolic murmur may need graphic demonstration.

Echocardiographic findings are of importance in differentiating the varieties of mitral regurgitation. In rheumatic lesions thickened valve leaflets with restricted motion can usually be demonstrated.

Cardiac catheterization fulfills an important role in evaluation and may supply the decisive information needed to select patients for surgical treatment. Yet the range of findings is wide and the interpretation may be difficult. It should be emphasized that the presence of mitral regurgitation or its severity cannot be directly demonstrated by hemodynamic study. The important information gained from the study concerns the response of the pulmonary circulation and the left atrium to the overload of the mitral reflux, and its changes caused by exercise. The most consistent finding is prominent v wave in the left atrial pressure curve. Yet, it has already been pointed out that the size and compliance of the left atrium may exaggerate the v wave in some patients, and completely obliterate it in others.

Angiocardiography permits direct demonstration of mitral regurgitation and its rough quantification. Caution should be applied, however, in interpreting the findings:

- Artifactitious mitral regurgitation may be present with left ventricular injection of the contrast medium if runs of ectopic beats develop after the injection.

- The visualization of the left atrium after left ventricular injection—considered the yardstick of the severity of mitral regurgitation—is related not only to the magnitude of regurgitant volume but also to the size of the receiving left atrium.

Differential Points in the Diagnosis. Diagnosis of rheumatic mitral regurgitation involves the following points:

- differentiation from other cardiac lesions,

- differentiation from nonrheumatic mitral regurgitation,

- diagnosis of "pure" mitral regurgitation, i.e., without significant mitral stenosis.

The principal diagnostic feature of mitral regurgitation is the regurgitant apical systolic murmur. It is holosystolic in the great majority of cases, although—as explained in Chapter 4—it rarely may be early systolic and occasionally late systolic. Considerable discussion has taken place regarding the frequency with which mitral regurgitation may occur without the systolic murmur. Thus far, only two situations have definitely been identified in which this occurs:

- if the patient is in shock,

- in perivalvular leaks around prosthetic mitral valves.

Thus, for ordinary purposes it may be accepted that the regurgitant murmur is a *sine qua non* of mitral regurgitation. Two other conditions may produce regurgitant murmurs occasionally heard in the apical region:

- ventricular septal defect,

- tricuspid regurgitation.

The former has considerable overlap with mitral regurgitation not only in the auscultatory findings but in other clinical manifestations as well. Clinical differentiation, though, is usually but not always possible; sometimes hemodynamic studies have to be performed for that purpose.

Tricuspid regurgitation, as stated, very seldom is found as an isolated lesion. Thus the differentiation between mitral and tricuspid regurgitation may come under consideration in association with another lesion — usually mitral stenosis. Given a patient with clinical features of mitral stenosis and a loud periapical holosystolic murmur, the question may arise whether mitral regurgitation or tricuspid regurgitation is present. Here the respiratory change in intensity of the murmur in tricuspid regurgitation but not in mitral regurgitation usually, though not always, may settle the point.

Given an apical holosystolic murmur characteristic of mitral regurgitation, the question often arises whether this lesion is the principal disease or a more prominent feature of another form of cardiac disease in which mitral regurgitation is either a secondary or an accompanying event. Conditions in which this may occur include the following:

- hypertrophic subaortic stenosis,

- cardiomyopathy,

- congenital lesions of the "endocardial cushion" type,

- more complex congenital malformations which include among other features congenital mitral regurgitation.

The differentiation of rheumatic mitral regurgitation from the various nonrheumatic varieties involves the identification of features suggestive or indicative of rheumatic heart disease. Among those are:

- demonstrated chronicity of the lesion,

- reliable history of rheumatic fever with a "heart murmur" persisting after the attack,

- presence of a mitral opening snap,

- mitral valve calcifications.

Clinical differentiation of pure mitral regurgitation from combined mitral valve disease may be difficult; hemodynamic studies may be necessary. This subject will be discussed in Chapter 35.

Evaluation.   The goals of evaluation of rheumatic mitral regurgitation include the following:

- To estimate the severity of the lesion,

- To observe the progress of the disease,

- To determine relevant information regarding operability.

These points can be investigated in the context of the following clinical settings:

1.   Patients with *mild* mitral regurgitation. Here the characteristic murmur may be the only detectable abnormality. Assuming that the diagnosis is reasonably certain on clinical grounds, invasive studies are not ordinarily indicated. Patients in this category may be followed noninvasively with the aid of electrocardiographic, radiographic, and echocardiographic examinations regarding the possible progression of the lesion.

2.   Patients with *moderate* mitral regurgitation but no disability. Here a crude quantification of the degree of regurgitation may be made from noninvasive studies. The use of cardiac catheterization and angiocardiography is optional: baseline studies are often relevant to longitudinal observations in determining how soon operative treatment should be considered.

3.   Symptomatic patients with *severe* mitral regurgitation are actual or potential surgical candidates. Invasive studies, including angiographic examination, are essential and should include a ventriculogram to determine left ventricular contractility.

Treatment.   Medical therapy of milder cases of mitral regurgitation consists primarily of general counseling regarding vocation and activities, the prevention of endocarditis, and—in youngsters—antistreptococcal prophylaxis.

In symptomatic patients supportive therapy may be needed; those with atrial fibrillation should be treated with digitalis, unless the left atrium is small, in which case restoration of sinus rhythm may be worthwhile. As in mitral stenosis, the onset of cardiac failure should be carefully analyzed regarding its precipitating factor and a trial of medical therapy invoked before surgical approaches are considered.

In view of the fact that surgical therapy consists almost entirely of mitral valve replacement, a more conservative approach is needed than that in patients with mitral stenosis, who might be candidates for mitral valvotomy. Thus, patients with disability which is tolerable and nonprogressive may be better off from the standpoint of the risk-benefit ratio to remain on a medical regimen than to undergo valve replacement. Patients with severe disability, medically nonresponsive cardiac failure, or signs of severe pulmonary hypertension are, of course, prime candidates for surgical treatment. The role of the invasive studies to help make a decision regarding surgical therapy has been mentioned above. Occasionally discrepancies between the patient's symptoms and the detected hemodynamic abnormalities are encountered. For patients who progress to severe disability but who show normal or near-normal hemodynamics, a skeptical approach toward surgical treatment should be taken. However, those who minimize their symptoms but show serious abnormalities may be treated more aggressively.

Nonrheumatic Mitral Regurgitation: Isolated Rupture of Chordae Tendineae

Natural History.   Isolated rupture of chordae tendineae is found, as stated, most frequently in middle-aged and elderly men. Cases of this clinical entity are discovered usually in one of two ways:

- As an incidental finding in an asymptomatic subject,

- In patients who suddenly develop cardiac failure.

Asymptomatic variety of ruptured chordae tendineae most often involves the separation of a single chorda; consequently the mild mitral regurgitation may be evidenced only by the characteristic murmur. In symptomatic patients disability may develop over a period of hours, days, or weeks—seldom months. Onset of effort dyspnea or attack of nocturnal dyspnea, cough, and pulmonary edema commonly represent the initial symptomatology. Chest pain and palpitations are rare. Patients when first seen may give a history of nonpenetrating trauma to the thorax (about 20 per cent). Most have no previous knowledge of cardiac disease, though some knew of a "murmur" in the past, but as a rule such murmurs have been dismissed as unimportant. History of rheumatic fever is very rare, as is history of an infection suggestive of endocarditis.

When first seen, patients with symptoms of left ventricular failure often show signs of congestive failure as well. They may, however, respond to therapy quite well, although they seldom re-establish the normal effort tolerance they had prior to the onset of symptoms.

Complications of this syndrome are rare; atrial fibrillation only exceptionally develops in spite of the fact that the patients' age makes them prone to this arrhythmia. Systemic embolization is virtually unknown. Infective endocarditis constitutes a persistent risk, which is probably eliminated by successful correction.

Though most severely symptomatic patients are treated surgically, occasional patients treated medically improve and persist in a stable state, often acquiring some of the features of "chronic" mitral regurgitation.

The postsurgical course is very impressive in patients who are suitable candidates for a successful plication operation. In those, signs of overload disappear, the murmur usually vanishes, and the operation can be considered a curative one. Those with lesions requiring valve replacement show clinical improvement far beyond those with rheumatic mitral regurgitation, but may develop problems related to prosthetic mitral valves.

Diagnosis. The diagnostic features of this syndrome are often distinctive enough to permit a firm clinical diagnosis. The following features are of importance:

1. The holosystolic murmur (of variable intensity) may be heard equally well at the apical area as along the left sternal border and the right sternal border. The murmur may even be heard best at the right upper sternal border and conducted above the clavicles, thereby imitating the murmur of aortic stenosis. This is even more striking in the fact that the murmur often acquires a crescendo-decrescendo, diamond-shaped quality. Its conduction to the axilla is rare. The radiation of the murmur to the aortic area is caused by partial detachment of the posterior cusp of the mitral valve with a jet of regurgitant blood thrown against the septal wall of the left atrium which is adjacent to the aortic root. This jet may set vibrations which may become palpable as a systolic thrill in the "aortic" area or as a systolic vibration transmitted through the trans-septal needle engaged in the interatrial septum. If the anterior leaflet is partially detached from the chordae, the usual radiation of the murmur to the back of the thorax is retained and occasionally the murmur may be conducted along the spinal column to "the top of the head."

2. An S4 gallop sound is more often found than an S3 gallop sound.

3. The electrocardiogram is usually normal.

4. The roentgenogram shows, as a rule, a normal-sized heart or a modest cardiac enlargement. Mitral valve calcifications are absent. Pulmonary vascular congestion may be present in patients who clinically exhibit left ventricular failure.

5. The phonocardiogram may be helpful in differentiating the diamond-shaped murmur of aortic stenosis from that found in this syndrome by the relationship of the murmur to the first and second sounds (holosystolic vs. ejection).

6. Echocardiographic studies usually show a distinctive systolic motion of the posterior mitral cusp, consistent with its partial prolapse

into the left atrium. If present, this sign is not only highly specific for this syndrome, but also may localize which leaflet is detached—a point of considerable practical importance.

7. Cardiac catheterization shows consistently high v waves in the left atrial pressure trace. Severe pressure abnormalities are often present, but the cardiac output may remain normal or near-normal.

8. Angiocardiographic demonstration of mitral regurgitation is obvious in most patients, but in addition the prolapse of a mitral leaflet can frequently be demonstrated as well.

Evaluation. Patients have to be evaluated for the following purposes:

- To confirm the diagnosis of mitral regurgitation (differentiating from aortic stenosis);

- To assess the severity of the lesion as well as its tolerance by the circulatory system;

- To identify the affected mitral leaflet.

The differentiation between this form of mitral regurgitation and aortic stenosis is often easy, but may present serious difficulties in some cases, namely if the murmur is preferentially well heard in the "aortic" area. Furthermore, in elder individuals the possibility of combined mitral regurgitation and aortic stenosis needs to be considered. When the clinical signs described above and the echocardiogram are inconclusive, it may be necessary to perform cardiac catheterization to establish the presence or absence of a transvalvular gradient across the aortic valve.

Determination of the severity of the lesion is of sufficient importance to require hemodynamic studies. In this acute form of mitral regurgitation the indirect indices—electrocardiographic and radiographic signs so helpful in rheumatic mitral regurgitation—may be misleading, hence direct measurement is of importance to document the significant nature of the lesion to justify surgical considerations. In this respect, the question as to whether one is dealing with the common variety—detachment of the posterior leaflet—or the rare involvement of the anterior leaflet is of considerable prognostic significance. The important differential points here in favor of the posterior leaflet are:

- The clear-cut aortic radiation of the systolic murmur (vs. radiation to the "top of the head" in anterior cusp involvement);

- The echocardiographic findings which can identify the prolapsing leaflet;

- The angiocardiographic findings.

Of these the echocardiogram offers the most specific findings, followed by the radiation of the systolic murmur, and the angiocardiographic findings the lowest specificity.

Treatment. The prognosis of this lesion is favorably affected by the availability of a conservative operation which can restore, often perfectly, the normal function of the mitral valve. The operation consists of plication of the posterior leaflet, which is shortened so that the intact chordae may support the entire leaflet and prevent its prolapse. Long-range follow-up of a series of patients after this operation revealed a consistent restoration of normal cardiac function with most of them losing any evidence of mitral regurgitation. No recurrences were observed. This operation carries a minimal risk—as low as open heart surgery would allow—and presents no known delayed complications. In contrast, involvement of the anterior leaflet permits only occasionally a successful plication: the majority of cases need valve replacement.

The unequal risk and results of the two available operations justify one to take a more aggressive attitude in detachment of the posterior leaflet but a more conservative attitude toward surgical correction of cases with involvement of the anterior leaflet, in which considerations similar to those of rheumatic mitral regurgitation should be adopted.

The Symptom Complex of Midsystolic Click and Late Systolic Murmur

Natural History. Once considered an innocent murmur or an extracardiac noise, the auscultatory findings of a midsystolic click and late systolic murmur have only recently been associated with malfunction of the mitral valve.

Certain facts regarding this set of findings are generally accepted:

1. Midsystolic click—late systolic murmur is caused by a delayed systolic prolapse of the mitral valve and is almost always associated with mild mitral regurgitation of trivial hemodynamic significance.

2. This late systolic prolapse can be produced by various mechanisms and various etiological factors, hence does not constitute a distinct clinical syndrome.

3. In some patients associated findings are present, which are as yet of uncertain relationship to this symptom complex but certainly are not caused by mitral regurgitation. These associated findings may affect the prognosis.

Within this symptom complex, the following subgroups have thus far been identified:

- The syndrome of mucoid degeneration of the mitral valve,

often associated with Marfan's features; when the latter are missing, familial Marfan traits can often be found, in which case mitral valve changes may be considered forme fruste of Marfan's syndrome.

• Another familial form, probably not identical with the first one, shows associated myocardial changes, namely angiocardiographically determined abnormal contraction ring. This may be a special form of cardiomyopathy; its incidence has been thus far highest in children.

• Some patients give a documented history of one or more attacks of rheumatic carditis. In these the results of mild rheumatic damage to the mitral valve may be assumed. Elderly patients have been known to fit this category, suggesting that this may be a stable form of rheumatic mitral valve disease, not a stage in its progression.

• Auscultatory findings of midsystolic click and late systolic murmur developing for the first time after acute myocardial infarction have been noted in patients. They undoubtedly represent a mild form of postinfarctional mitral regurgitation (vide infra).

• Patients who undergo plication of the mitral valve for rupture of chordae tendineae to the posterior leaflets are occasionally left with a late systolic murmur, a minor residual postoperative mitral regurgitation occurring in late systole.

In general, patients with this symptom complex fall into two categories:

• Those with auscultatory findings but no associated signs or symptoms;

• Those with coexisting manifestations of cardiac disease.

Inasmuch as the associated disturbances determine the natural history of this form of mitral regurgitation, the first group—if proved beyond reasonable doubt—can unequivocally be considered as having an innocent and clinically insignificant set of findings.

The associated signs and symptoms include the following:

• Chest pain, usually left submammary pain, not related to exercise;

• Palpitations;

• Arrhythmias, presenting themselves as ectopic ventricular beats, supraventricular beats, tachycardias, or atrial fibrillation;

• Electrocardiographic abnormalities, most commonly consisting of T wave abnormalities in leads II, III and AVF; rarely prolongation of the Q-T interval has been observed;

• Psychotic episodes have been occasionally reported.

The most serious — potentially — of the associated findings are ventricular arrhythmias. They may be aggravated by exercise. Few cases of sudden death have been reported; these are unquestionably related to ventricular fibrillation triggered by an ill-placed premature contraction. Some patients reported sudden death in kin, usually blamed on "heart attacks." However, the ominous nature of this complication should not obscure the fact that this symptom complex is a very common clinical finding, while only a handful of cases of sudden death have been reported, so that the probability of this disaster is very low and the condition may be considered benign even if premature contractions are demonstrated.

Patients exhibiting these auscultatory findings are discovered at any age, from childhood on. While the natural history has not been studied by means of longitudinal follow-up, it is generally assumed that the mitral valve changes are nonprogressive. Only very few cases have been observed in which the late systolic murmur evolved into a holosystolic murmur of more severe mitral regurgitation. It is especially noteworthy that patients with the more serious syndrome of isolated rupture of chordae tendineae as a rule do not have late systolic murmurs at earlier stages: the two conditions seem totally unrelated to each other.

Inasmuch as the mechanical effects of mitral regurgitation are absent, the prognosis is entirely related to possible complications: arrhythmias have already been discussed; the other most important is proneness to infective endocarditis.

Diagnosis. Obviously, the principal diagnostic criteria for this condition are the two auscultatory findings: midsystolic click and late systolic murmur. Each is independent of the other. They are often present together, but only one or the other may be present or one of them may be apparent while the other may have to be elicited by special maneuvers.

The late systolic murmur varies greatly in quality and intensity, and considerable variation may occur in the same patient with changes in body position. Thus soft blowing murmurs may change into grade V or VI musical honks and whoops. At times the midsystolic click is the only consistent finding: a search for the murmur might then reveal its presence, by change in position, by squatting, by assuming a knee-chest position, or by exercise.

Clicks are less specific than murmurs. They originate mostly by tightening of the mitral valve apparatus at the time the valve prolapses, probably in the chordae. However, similar midsystolic clicks could also be extracardiac, and have been observed in pneumothorax and after recovery from pericarditis. Clicks of mitral origin can be multiple. They, too, may not be apparent at first; finding of a late systolic murmur often induces a search for a midsystolic click, which can be found by carefully inching the stethoscope over the precordium, or by having the patient stand up, change the body position, and so on.

As expected, in view of the trivial hemodynamic consequences, other physical signs of mitral regurgitation are as a rule absent.

The radiographic examination reveals normal findings. The electrocardiogram shows in the majority of patients normal tracings; in some the above described nonspecific T wave abnormalities are found. Echocardiogram is the most important confirmatory method of examination: A characteristic late systolic motion of one of the mitral leaflets is found in almost all patients with this condition. This is particularly important in patients who present themselves showing only a midsystolic click.

Cardiac catheterization shows as a rule normal findings. The absence of any significant abnormalities in hemodynamics, even with exercise, makes cardiac catheterization not indicated in this form of mitral regurgitation. Angiocardiographic studies, in which the contrast substance is injected into the left ventricle, often show the late systolic prolapse of a mitral leaflet. Yet the noninvasive demonstration of the prolapse by echocardiography makes angiocardiography also superfluous.

Evaluation. The symptom complex of late systolic murmur–midsystolic click requires a different approach from other forms of mitral regurgitation in terms of evaluation of patients. Severity of the lesion is not at issue; it is almost axiomatic that its effects upon the heart are trivial. Thus the objectives of diagnostic evaluation are as follows:

- To establish the definitive diagnosis in the few cases in which the midsystolic click is the only finding (echocardiography is the method of choice).

- To determine whether mitral regurgitation is a manifestation of wider disturbance or an isolated finding (i.e., connective tissue disorder in Marfan's syndrome, myocardial abnormalities). A corollary of this is the question of its etiology and whether or not there is familial incidence.

- To search for features indicating a potential risk (ventricular ectopic beats, prolonged Q-T interval).

Treatment. This condition need be treated only in a limited way. All patients require prophylactic antiendocarditic therapy. Patients with ventricular ectopic beats may require antiarrhythmic drugs, if:

- Premature beats occur early in diastole;

- Exercise increases their number.

Propranolol appears to be an effective agent in this respect; however, its continuous use is justified only if it can be demonstrated to reduce the number of premature beats. Those with paroxysms of supraventricular tachycardia or atrial fibrillation should be treated in the conventional manner.

Surgical treatment of this form of mitral regurgitation is not indicated, though some thought has been given to the possibility that a redundant, ballooning abnormal mitral valve may traumatize the ventricular wall and produce its irritability, and therefore its removal may be beneficial. This is at present a mere speculation, totally insufficient to justify an operation as serious as mitral valve replacement.

Postinfarctional Mitral Regurgitation

Natural History. Postinfarctional mitral regurgitation differs from most other forms of mitral valve incompetence in that its existence is predicated upon the presence of another serious disease; a significant degree of valvular insufficiency does not develop unless serious myocardial damage is present. Inasmuch as the natural history depends upon the course of both diseases, the significance of mitral regurgitation, from a practical standpoint, depends upon its reversibility under conditions in which improvement might ensue by its elimination. Thus only mitral regurgitation of a degree severe enough to produce significant circulatory overload need be considered here. Trivial degrees — merely apical systolic murmurs present in patients during and after myocardial infarction — are of no practical significance.

The most serious form of postinfarctional mitral regurgitation is rupture of a head of a papillary muscle. In this condition sudden acute myocardial infarction may present an emergency, which — if recognized — may be overcome by surgical valve replacement. The development of mitral regurgitation here manifests itself by the sudden deterioration of the patient's condition — by the appearance of either shock or acute pulmonary edema — coincidental with the appearance of an apical systolic murmur. Occasionally sudden cardiac failure due to rupture of a papillary muscle head appears without the previous evidence of the myocardial infarction — representing either a "silent" infarction or rupture of a previously infarcted fibrotic head of the papillary muscle. Occasionally patients survive this complication of myocardial infarction and make a clinical recovery, but the persistence of chronic congestive failure is the rule.

The commoner form of postinfarctional mitral regurgitation — that due to combined papillary muscle and myocardial malfunction — takes generally a more benign and more gradual course. More often than not clinical evidence of cardiac failure does not appear during the acute stage of myocardial infarction but afterward, when the patient resumes normal activities. The systolic murmur usually is evident during myocardial infarction, but occasionally even its appearance may be delayed beyond the recovery period.

The course of patients varies with the ability of the damaged and overloaded myocardium to perform and the aggressiveness of medical therapy. In addition, the progression of ischemic disease—continuing angina, future myocardial infarction, sudden death—affects the natural history of patients.

Diagnosis. The diagnosis of postinfarctional mitral regurgitation depends primarily on the presence of an apical holosystolic murmur. However, in contrast to other forms of mitral regurgitation, other physical signs as well as electrocardiographic and radiographic findings cannot be helpful in the assessment of the severity of the overload, since the abnormalities present may reflect myocardial damage from the infarction.

The intensity of the murmur may serve as a rough guideline to the severity of mitral regurgitation, but its reliability is poor. In seriously ill patients the mitral systolic murmur may be unduly soft; in shock it may even be absent. Conversely, some factors may exaggerate its intensity, producing loud murmurs in the presence of minor degrees of reflux. Other features of the murmur include occasionally its delayed onset, making it sound more like an ejection murmur. While delayed systolic murmur has been widely thought to be characteristic for postinfarctional mitral regurgitation, in reality one finds this type of murmur only in a minority of patients and, if present, it is likely to occur in milder cases. Thus the holosystolic murmur is the one of clinical importance. The occasional appearance of a late systolic murmur has been mentioned in the preceding section.

Additional physical signs, as stated, are affected both by mitral regurgitation and by myocardial scars—often aneurysms—the two factors overlapping. Thus the low intensity of the first sound, the S3 gallop sound, even the short mid-diastolic rumbling murmur, the excessive precordial motion, the sustained apical impulse—all are non-discriminating in the differentiation. The electrocardiogram usually shows old myocardial infarction, but other patterns, such as left ventricular hypertrophy or conduction defects, may be found. Varying degrees of cardiomegaly with left ventricular enlargement and pulmonary vascular congestion are usually demonstrated by radiography. Echocardiographic studies may show faulty apposition of the mitral leaflets in systole, but the findings are less specific than those in other forms of mitral regurgitation.

Invasive studies include cardiac catheterization, which often shows very prominent v waves produced by mitral regurgitation, by left ventricular failure, or by both. Pulmonary hypertension, passive and reactive, is commonly found, as is left atrial hypertension. Angiocardiography represents the most crucial means of evaluation of mitral regurgitation. These features are of importance:

- the magnitude of regurgitant volume,
- the presence or absence of left ventricular dyskinesia,
- the overall evaluation of left ventricular wall motion.

Evaluation. Postinfarctional mitral regurgitation presents a complication of a more serious disease. Evaluation of the contribution of mitral regurgitation to the patient's disability and symptomatology is of practical importance only when its correction is being contemplated. The overall approach to surgical treatment of complications of ischemic heart disease will be discussed in Chapter 37; it should be emphasized here, however, that only patients with disability unresponsive to medical therapy should be considered potential surgical candidates. The evaluation then should assess not only malfunction of the mitral valve but also the presence of a resectable aneurysm (occasionally also bypassable occlusive coronary disease). Indications for surgical treatment include the following:

1. Demonstration of a severe degree of mitral regurgitation by angiocardiography (recognizing the pitfalls of the technique, mentioned above).

2. Demonstration of a reasonable contractility of the left ventricular wall—even if only the basal portion of the ventricle participates in it.

Treatment. Medical therapy involves aggressive treatment of congestive cardiac failure. The approach to surgical treatment has already been discussed in the preceding sections. It should be mentioned that, in spite of careful selection of cases of mitral valve replacement, surgical results are unpredictable. Some borderline candidates may show spectacular improvement while, on the other hand, patients who appear to be ideal candidates may remain unimproved. It is axiomatic that patients who are in chronic cardiac failure and have severely compromised myocardium offer a higher surgical risk than average candidates for mitral valve replacement.

Other Forms of Mitral Regurgitation

Congenital Mitral Regurgitation. The most important variety of congenital mitral regurgitation, unassociated with other lesions and consistent with survival into adult life, is the isolated valve cleft. Patients usually have murmurs discovered in childhood but not in infancy. The diagnosis of rheumatic heart disease is most frequently carried in such cases. The course varies with the severity of the hemodynamic consequences. Some patients remain asymptomatic and merely show apical pansystolic murmurs. Their diagnosis may be surmised if associated congenital malformations are present or if the murmur happens to be reliably established very early in childhood. More severe degrees of mitral regurgitation resemble the rheumatic variety very closely; even mitral valve calcification may be present — the traumatized valve tissue around the cleft may lead to calcium deposition. The diagnosis is usually made at operation, if the severity of the lesion and its consequences leads to surgical treatment.

Other forms of congenital heart disease involve a number of rare mechanisms, some of which are related to endomyocardial fibrosis (congenital fibroelastosis, anomalous origin of coronary artery).

Postendocarditic Mitral Regurgitation. The risk of infective endocarditis in patients with mitral regurgitation and, to a lesser extent, in those with mitral stenosis has already been discussed. Here a known cardiac lesion may be accentuated by new damage to the valve (particularly perforation of a cusp or rupture of chordae tendineae) or the disease may be changed from primarily mitral stenosis to predominant or pure mitral regurgitation.

However, in addition to these secondary lesions, patients may develop endocarditis on valves which have not previously been known to be affected by disease. Whether the infection sets on intact valves or develops in valves that previously had subclinical disease cannot be determined in most instances.

These patients fall into two categories:

1. Those in whom an obvious attack of endocarditis is present and the mitral valve becomes damaged under observation.

2. Those in whom the infectious process may be overlooked, mitral regurgitation is found without an obvious etiology, but anatomic changes later reveal healed endocarditis.

The first category is clinically important; it requires alertness since sudden destruction of the mitral valve may produce immediate severe cardiac failure in which only a well-timed surgical operation may save the patient's life. While acute mitral regurgitation due to infective endocarditis does not lead to surgical emergencies as often as equivalent damage of the aortic valve, such cases, nevertheless, are not rare.

The clinical features are those of acute mitral regurgitation and resemble most closely those of isolated rupture of the chordae tendineae. Patients with damage to the mitral valve that is not catastrophic may develop symptoms and signs of congestive cardiac failure more slowly. In those initial medical treatment is indicated and a conservative period of observation—aimed at determining whether medical therapy is effective and whether the circulatory system is capable of adapting to the sudden overload—is well justified.

Cardiac tumors may produce the clinical picture of mitral regurgitation; left atrial myxoma which typically produces obstruction of the inflow into the left ventricle, thereby imitating mitral stenosis, occasionally presents itself as pure mitral regurgitation. These findings will be discussed later.

Bibliography

Barlow JB, Bosman CK, Pocock WA, Marchand P: Late systolic murmur and non-ejection ("mid-late") systolic click. Brit. Heart J. *30*:203, 1968.

Burchell HB, Edwards JE: Rheumatic mitral insufficiency. Circulation 7:747, 1953.

Burgess J, Clark R, Kamigaki M, Cohn K: Echocardiographic findings in different types of mitral regurgitation. Circulation *48*:97, 1973.

DeBusk RF, Harrison DC: The clinical syndrome of papillary muscle disease. New Engl. J. Med. *281*:1458, 1969.

Hancock EW, Cohn KE: The syndrome associated with midsystolic click and late systolic murmur. Amer. J. Med. *41*:183, 1966.

Levy NJ, Edwards JE: Anatomy of mitral insufficiency. Prog. Cardiovasc. Dis. 5:119, 1962.

Mittal AK, Langston MF Jr., Cohn KE, Selzer A, Kerth WJ: Combined papillary muscle and left ventricular wall dysfunction as a cause of mitral regurgitation. An experimental study. Circulation *44*:174, 1971.

Perloff JK, Roberts WC: The mitral apparatus: Functional anatomy of mitral regurgitation. Circulation *46*:227, 1972.

Pocock WA, Barlow JB: Etiology and electrocardiographic features of billowing posterior mitral leaflet syndrome. Amer. J. Med. *51*:731, 1971.

Raftery EB, Oakley CM, Goodwin JF: Acute subvalvar mitral insufficiency. Lancet 2:360, 1966.

Selzer A, Kelly JJ Jr, Vannitamby M, Walker P, Gerbode F, Kerth WJ: The syndrome of mitral insufficiency due to isolated rupture of chordae tendineae. Amer. J. Med. *42*:822, 1967.

Selzer A, Kelly JJ Jr, Kerth WJ, Gerbode F: Immediate and long-range results of valvuloplasty for mitral regurgitation due to rupture of chordae tendineae. Circulation *45*(Suppl. I):52, 1971.

Selzer A, Sakai FJ, Popper RW: Protean clinical manifestations of primary tumors of the heart. Amer. J. Med. *52*:9, 1972.

Selzer A, Katayama F: Mitral regurgitation: clinical patterns, pathophysiology and natural history. Medicine *51*:337, 1972.

Silverman ME, Hurst JW: The mitral valve complex, interaction of anatomy, physiology and pathology of the mitral annulus, mitral valve leaflets, chordae tendineae and papillary muscles. Amer. Heart J. 76:399, 1968.

Sweatman T, Selzer A, Kamigaki M, Cohn K: Echocardiographic diagnosis of mitral regurgitation due to rupture of chordae tendineae. Circulation *46*:581, 1972.

35

Combined Valvular Disease

Definition. In the preceding chapters the principal valve lesions were presented. Combinations of valvular diseases occur frequently. The relationships between component lesions in combined valvular disease include the following:

- Structural changes in a valve making it both incompetent and stenotic;

- A common etiological factor affecting two or more valves;

- Secondary incompetence of a valve developing as a consequence of diseases of other valves.

The following combinations of valve lesions occur frequently:

1. Mitral valve disease with stenosis and regurgitation;

2. Aortic valve disease with stenosis and regurgitation;

3. Combination of mitral and aortic disease including stenosis or regurgitation of each valve or both;

4. Disease of left-sided valve or valves combined with organic tricuspid disease;

5. Left-sided valvular disease with secondary tricuspid regurgitation.

ETIOLOGY

Mitral valve disease involving both stenosis and regurgitation is considered to be rheumatic in origin. Bivalvular left-sided disease is also almost always rheumatic in nature, especially if an element of mitral stenosis is apparent. Pure regurgitation of both left-sided valves

579

can be nonrheumatic (e.g., mucoid degeneration of valve cusps) but is rare. A combination of rheumatic mitral valve disease with congenital (i.e., bicuspid) calcific aortic stenosis probably occurs, but is difficult to prove. Organic tricuspid valve disease occurs almost always in combination with left-sided valve lesions and is considered rheumatic in nature. "Functional" tricuspid regurgitation may develop in any form of cardiac disease producing pulmonary hypertension; it is particularly common in mitral lesions and in combined mitral-aortic rheumatic lesions.

PATHOLOGY AND PATHOGENESIS

Mitral valve disease producing stenosis with or without regurgitation consists of a scarring process initiated by rheumatic fever. Involvement of mitral cusps frequently leads to their foreshortening, leaving tissue defect, thereby making the valve incompetent. It has been pointed out in connection with mitral regurgitation that cuspal involvement is more likely to produce combined stenosis and incompetence than either of the two alone.

Aortic valve disease also manifests itself frequently by a combination of regurgitation and stenosis. In contrast to mitral valve disease, cuspal involvement of the aortic valve is not always rheumatic; consequently other scarring processes, e.g., that initiated by a bicuspid aortic valve, may produce combined aortic valve disease. Here, too, shrinkage of valve tissue may make the valve incompetent, whereas stiffness and fusion of the cusps produce obstruction to flow.

Tricuspid valve disease that includes an element of stenosis is usually produced by thickening and fusion of the leaflets secondary to rheumatic involvement. Anatomically it has been estimated to be present in some 10 per cent of rheumatic valvular disease; clinically significant tricuspid stenosis is rarer than that. Pure tricuspid regurgitation is very commonly found in cardiac failure from any cause. The tricuspid ring dilates easily along with dilatation of the right ventricle, and the valve may become too small to close the atrioventricular orifice during systole. A rare disease leading to organic nonrheumatic tricuspid valve disease is scarring of the endocardium caused by the carcinoid syndrome. This process may include pulmonary valve involvement as well.

Pulmonary valve disease is almost always congenital; its coexistence with other valve lesions is exceedingly rare, and if present, is most likely coincidental (except for the already mentioned carcinoid syndrome).

The *hemodynamic* and clinical consequences of combined valve disease relate to the respective contribution of the component lesions. In the majority of cases a single lesion dominates the clinical picture. For example, a patient may show the presence of aortic stenosis and regurgitation combined with mitral stenosis and regurgitation, yet mitral stenosis dominates the picture: the hemodynamic consequences as well as the natural history would then be similar to those of pure mitral stenosis.

Combined mitral valve disease has predictable hemodynamic consequences, since both stenosis and regurgitation of the mitral valve produce similar effects upon the pulmonary circulation and the right side of the heart. The principal contribution of mitral regurgitation is left ventricular overload, which often helps to gauge the severity of mitral valve incompetence in the overall effect of the lesion.

Combined aortic valve disease shows some distinctive features. Inasmuch as aortic stenosis and aortic regurgitation exert opposite effects upon the systemic circulation, as evidenced by the arterial pulses, combined lesions will have an intermediate effect. The arterial pulse in combined aortic disease (with significant degree of stenosis and regurgitation) may be normal, or—more often—has a bisferiens quality. Except for the pulse, the effects of the combined lesion are similar to those of either component lesion alone; left ventricular dilatation occurs earlier in the combined lesion than in pure aortic stenosis.

Tricuspid regurgitation produces an elevation of systemic venous pressure with a prominent venous v wave; in severe cases right atrial pressure becomes "ventricularized"—i.e., identical with right ventricular pressure. In tricuspid stenosis a gradient across the tricuspid valve can be recorded. A prominent a wave is seen in the venous pressure curve and the y descent is slow. In tricuspid disease of significant degree and duration hepatomegaly is common (pulsating liver may be present) and icterus may occur.

CLINICAL PICTURES

Combined Mitral Valve Disease

The *natural history* of mitral stenosis and that of rheumatic mitral regurgitation are very similar. Consequently, combined lesions of the mitral valve present a course not different from that of either lesion alone, comparable in severity. There is no evidence that the two component valve lesions potentiate each other. As in mitral stenosis or in mitral regurgitation alone, patients often remain asymptomatic for many years in spite of hemodynamically significant lesions. When clinical disability develops, they may progress or remain stable. The various complications (atrial fibrillation, systemic embolization, pulmonary hypertension, etc.) occur at rates comparable to those with single mitral valve lesions.

Clinical features combine those of mitral stenosis and mitral regurgitation. Auscultatory findings may provide evidence for the combination of stenosis and regurgitation, yet in the final analysis almost pure stenosis may be found in some cases and almost pure regurgitation in others. The spectrum ranges from cases showing all findings of mitral stenosis with the addition of a holosystolic apical murmur to those presenting physical findings of mitral regurgitation except for longer apical diastolic rumbles and the presence of a mitral opening snap. When it is obvious that significant stenosis and significant regurgitation of the mitral valve coexist, the quantification of the components may not be easy. Often palpatory evidence of left ventricular hypertrophy and exaggerated precordial motion indicate a significant degree of mitral regurgitation.

Noninvasive laboratory procedures may help the differential analysis.

- The electrocardiogram is helpful only if left ventricular hypertrophy points to a significant mitral regurgitation. A "balanced" pattern, or right ventricular hypertrophy may occur in both.

- The echocardiogram provides information regarding the thickness and the motion of mitral leaflets; it helps provide information regarding the severity of stenosis and may show changes caused by mitral regurgitation. Yet this technique cannot quantify the respective contributions of the stenosis and regurgitation of the mitral valve.

- Radiographic demonstration of left ventricular enlargement points to significant mitral regurgitation; other findings are nondiscriminatory in the differentiation.

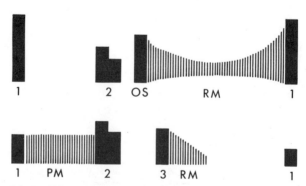

Figure 35-1. Diagrammatic presentation of auscultatory findings in pure mitral stenosis (*upper*), contrasted with that of pure mitral regurgitation (*lower*). Auscultatory components are helpful in determining whether stenosis or regurgitation predominates in mixed lesions. (1, 2, 3 — heart sounds; PM — pansystolic murmur; OS — mitral opening snap; RM — rumbling diastolic murmur).

Cardiac catheterization and angiocardiography serve two purposes: (1) to determine the overall effect of the mitral lesion upon the circulation and cardiac function; (2) to quantify the respective contributions of stenosis and regurgitation as far as possible. Even these techniques provide only a crude estimation of the degree of stenosis and regurgitation. Hemodynamic measurements that can fairly well evaluate the degree of mitral stenosis are not applicable to combined lesions because only the forward flow and not the total flow through the valve can be adequately measured. The shape and size of left atrial v waves only crudely reflect the degree of mitral regurgitation. Angiocardiography with left ventricular injection of the contrast material represents the best way of estimating mitral regurgitation. Theoretically, mitral regurgitation can be quantified by estimating end-systolic and end-diastolic volumes and comparing them with the hemodynamically measured forward flow; however, the frequent presence of atrial fibrillation and the common occurrence of premature contractions following left ventricular injection of the medium may interfere with the accuracy of this measurement. Similarly, dye dilution techniques have proved disappointing in the quantification of mitral regurgitation.

Combined mitral stenosis and regurgitation is treated similarly to mitral regurgitation in that surgical treatment requires valve replacement. Consequently, criteria for the selection of time for operation are similar to those already discussed in Chapters 32 and 34.

Combined Aortic Valve Disease

As in mitral valve disease, combined aortic valve disease involves a spectrum ranging from pure aortic stenosis to pure aortic regurgitation. Patients with predominant aortic stenosis resemble in all respects those with pure aortic stenosis, mild regurgitation playing an insignificant role in the clinical picture and natural history. As aortic regurgitation is found to be more severe, some of the specific features of aortic stenosis become rare. Thus, it is unusual to find syncope or anginal pain in patients with a significant aortic regurgitation combined with aortic stenosis. It appears that aortic regurgitation makes the lesion better tolerated and tends to obliterate the ominous prefailure symptoms with their threat of sudden death.

Diagnostic features of aortic stenosis with regurgitation combine the respective findings of each component lesion. As stated, the arterial pulse is by far the best index of the degree of stenosis or regurgitation. A slow-rising anacrotic pulse — regardless of the intensity of the aortic diastolic murmur — almost always means that predominant aortic stenosis is present; conversely, collapsing arterial pulses point to predominant aortic regurgitation. Bisferiens type pulse indicates a significant degree of stenosis and of regurgitation, but may not be helpful in determining the preponderance of each lesion.

Noninvasive diagnostic methods are less helpful here than in combined mitral lesions. Neither electrocardiography nor echocardiography permits any significant discrimination between the two component lesions.

Cardiac catheterization determines the competence of the left ventricle in response to the overloading lesions. Transaortic gradient indicates the presence of aortic stenosis but, as in mitral valve disease, does not permit the quantification of the severity of aortic stenosis, except in most general terms. Supravalvular aortogram provides means of estimating the degree of aortic regurgitation with limitations already mentioned.

The surgical therapy of combined aortic lesions requires valve replacement. Inasmuch as the natural history of combined aortic disease resembles that of pure aortic regurgitation, criteria for the selection of patients follow more closely those discussed in connection with the latter lesion.

Combined Mitral and Aortic Lesions

Of the four potential lesions—stenosis and regurgitation in each valve—the majority of patients present themselves with either a single lesion or a combined lesion of a single valve predominating and therefore setting the pattern for natural history, course, and treatment. The commonly encountered combinations with a single lesion predominating include the following:

- Mitral stenosis with trivial aortic regurgitation;

- Aortic regurgitation with insignificant mitral valve disease (stenosis or regurgitation or both).

The most important combination of lesions in which significant disease of both valves is present is the coexistence of mitral and aortic stenosis.

From time to time the question is raised, How does a lesion of one valve affect the other valve? Opinions have been expressed to the effect that disease of two valves is less well tolerated than comparable disease of single valves or, on the other hand, that disease of one valve may protect the heart from the ravages of the disease of the other valve. Neither of these views has more to it than speculation, for it is impossible to make comparison with the great number of factors at issue and with a variability of the effect of each factor. Thus, one is safest in adopting the view that the course and natural history of combined lesions of the two left-sided valves are similar to those of the more severe of the lesions that can be identified.

The diagnostic approach to bivalvular lesions has two objectives:

- The recognition of all component lesions;

- The assessment of which lesion or lesions are the predominant ones, therefore the pacesetter.

Auscultatory findings only occasionally present difficulties. Inasmuch as each of the four valve lesions has its characteristic murmur, their recognition may be easy. Certainly there is little overlap between the diastolic murmurs of aortic regurgitation and those of mitral stenosis. The two systolic murmurs may be confused with each other, but in most cases their coexistence can be recognized. The specific difficulties include the following:

- In severe aortic regurgitation an apical diastolic murmur may be an Austin-Flint murmur or may be due to organic mitral stenosis;

- In severe, combined aortic and mitral stenosis a murmur of one of the two lesions may be faint, so as to be missed.

Among auscultatory findings other than murmurs the mitral opening snap represents an important clinical finding pointing to organic mitral stenosis (e.g., in aortic regurgitation), even though its presence does not provide information regarding the significant nature of mitral stenosis.

The electrocardiogram can be helpful only in showing right-sided preponderance or balanced patterns, both of which suggest an important contribution of mitral valve disease. Roentgenographic examination may be of diagnostic aid in showing calcification in both valves (which does not prove, however, significant involvement of a calcified valve). The most important noninvasive diagnostic tool is echocardiography, especially if the mitral lesion is clinically the less evident one. The presence of mitral stenosis can be established by echocardiography beyond reasonable doubt, and its severity roughly estimated.

Cardiac catheterization and angiocardiography remain the most important diagnostic techniques in analyzing the respective valvular disease. Guidelines for the analysis of the findings have been presented in an earlier section of this chapter.

In considering surgical treatment, the following points are worthy of mention:

1. Even though the difference is not great, replacement of two valves carries a higher immediate risk and higher probability of late complications and failure.

2.   Because of the above, trivial lesions (e.g., mild aortic regurgitation in severe mitral valve disease) are better left alone than treated surgically, especially since some claims that repair of mitral lesions makes aortic disease more serious have not been substantiated.

3.   The progression of stenotic lesions of the two valves may occur at different rates. One sees not infrequently mitral stenosis requiring operation with minimal aortic disease. If a mitral valve operation is then performed, one can find years later that aortic stenosis outweighs mitral disease in severity. However, since progression of valvular disease is not inevitable, prophylactic aortic valve replacement is not indicated.

Tricuspid Stenosis

As mentioned, tricuspid stenosis is almost always rheumatic and occurs in association with other valvular involvement. Tricuspid stenosis of high degree is rare; it is as a rule milder than the other accompanying valve lesions. As a consequence, the natural history of tricuspid stenosis is almost impossible to assess; perhaps the only indications that mild or moderate degree of tricuspid stenosis may adversely affect the circulation are observations dealing with patients who have undergone mitral valve operation, in whom the tricuspid valve stenosis was either overlooked or considered unimportant and therefore left alone and whose postoperative course has been unsatisfactory. Such observations merely imply but do not prove the adverse effect of tricuspid stenosis because of the associated other factors. It is furthermore true that tricuspid stenosis almost always is associated with incompetence of the tricuspid valve; this in itself exerts an unfavorable influence upon the course of the disease.

The diagnosis of tricuspid stenosis is based upon the following features:

1.   A mid-diastolic murmur audible around the xiphoid area, increasing in intensity during inspiration, may be present. Its absence does not rule out tricuspid stenosis; furthermore, this murmur frequently blends with that of concomitant mitral stenosis.

2.   A holosystolic murmur of associated tricuspid regurgitation, also showing respiratory variation, may be present.

3.   Tricuspid opening snap is rarely heard; if present it constitutes an important sign of tricuspid stenosis.

4.   If sinus rhythm is present (in the minority of cases) a giant a wave can be seen in the jugular venous pulse. The v wave is usually exaggerated and shows a slow y descent.

5. Right atrial P waves (tall, pointed) may be present in the electrocardiogram.

6. Considerable enlargement of the right atrium may be present in the roentgenogram.

7. Echocardiographic criteria have not been definitely established. The tricuspid valve is usually visible in the echocardiogram and its motion can be expected to be normal.

8. Cardiac catheterization reveals abnormalities of the right atrial pulse tracing: tall *a* wave (if present), slow *y* descent. Direct demonstration of a gradient across the tricuspid valve is the most reliable evidence of tricuspid stenosis. Inasmuch as many patients suffer from chronic atrial fibrillation and have low cardiac output, great care should be exercised to detect the gradient — often a small one. Double-lumen catheters with simultaneous tracing on both sides of the tricuspid valve are helpful; pressure recording should be made throughout several respiratory cycles.

Treatment of tricuspid stenosis is surgical, although indications for operation have not been firmly established. Since it is an additional lesion in the presence of a more serious one, evaluation of surgical success is exceedingly difficult. Surgical approaches include tricuspid valvotomy and tricuspid valve replacement. Not enough is known about results of operation to consider tricuspid valve surgery ever as the prime target for the operation. When the overall disability provides an indication to operation for disease of other valves, one might consider the addition of tricuspid valve surgery in patients whose right-sided hemodynamics are seriously deranged.

Tricuspid Regurgitation

Incompetence of the tricuspid valve is most frequently encountered as a secondary phenomenon, and then it is often transient. The diagnosis of tricuspid regurgitation is based upon the holosystolic murmur and the prominent *v* wave or a ventricularized systolic wave in the right atrial pulse. While a certain overlap occurs between right ventricular failure with and without tricuspid regurgitation, it may be assumed that very tall *v* waves with rapid *y* descent and ventricularized systolic right atrial waves demonstrate tricuspid regurgitation. Accepting these theses, it is necessary to recognize that the systolic murmur is present only in the minority of cases with tricuspid regurgitation. The overlap between right ventricular failure — usually caused by systolic overloading of the right ventricle (i.e., pulmonary hypertension) — and tricuspid regurgitation makes it virtually impossible to assess the adverse effect of tricuspid valve incompetence upon cardiac performance. Certain clinical observations, however, are pertinent.

1.   It has been known for a long time that patients with tricuspid regurgitation (or right ventricular failure or both) are less dyspneic and do not display orthopnea as compared with those with a compensated right ventricular overload and a competent tricuspid valve.

2.   Chronic tricuspid regurgitation, as stated, predisposes to hepatic malfunction. Either spontaneously or, more often, in response to bilirubin loading (pulmonary infarcts, postcardiac surgery), icterus develops with considerable frequency.

The diagnosis of tricuspid regurgitation is based on the cardiac murmur and the abnormalities of venous pulse. The murmur is holosystolic, present usually at the lower left sternal border, near the xiphoid area, and increases in intensity with inspiration. Laboratory findings, such as electrocardiography, roentgenography, and echocardiography, add little to the diagnosis. Cardiac catheterization merely records the atrial pulse better, confirming the bedside observation.

When detected, tricuspid regurgitation should first be considered from the standpoint of permanency vs. reversibility. Onset of cardiac failure is frequently associated with evidence of tricuspid regurgitation, which in these circumstances regresses within a day or two in response to therapy. Rheumatic polyvalvular disease, when associated with tricuspid regurgitation, tends to be permanent.

Treatment of tricuspid regurgitation overlaps with treatment of right ventricular failure. As in tricuspid stenosis, surgical therapy—in this case tricuspid valve replacement—is never indicated for this lesion alone, and therefore comes under consideration only when tricuspid regurgitation is a concomitant lesion in rheumatic polyvalvular disease in which the condition of another valve justifies surgical consideration.

Given a patient with mitral valve disease or combined mitral and aortic valve disease who needs open heart surgery and who shows evidence of tricuspid regurgitation, the question often comes up whether or not tricuspid valve replacement is indicated along with that of the other valves. The answer to this question is not clear. On the one hand, successful mitral valve surgery which reverses pulmonary hypertension often produces complete disappearance of tricuspid regurgitation. On the other hand, some such patients do not do well in spite of successful mitral valve surgery, in which case one often regrets that the tricuspid valve was not replaced, even though one can never be sure that suboptimal surgical results were caused by persistent tricuspid regurgitation. Those patients in whom the tricuspid valve has been replaced may also show striking successes in some cases but failures in others.

With so many factors at play, it is impossible to solve this problem by any type of controlled study and it has to be handled "by ear." Perhaps a good compromise might be suggested in that all patients with rheumatic polyvalvular disease who show evidence of tricuspid regurgitation should undergo intensive medical therapy in the hospital to determine whether any improvement in the function of the right ventricle and reduction of tricuspid valve incompetence can be accomplished. If a trial period of therapy is totally unsuccessful, then tricuspid valve replacement should be considered. On the other hand, even modest success in response to medical therapy might suggest that further improvement might be anticipated without tricuspid valve replacement.

Bibliography

Hansing CE, Rowe GG: Tricuspid insufficiency: a study of hemodynamics and pathogenesis. Circulation *45*:793, 1972.

Perloff JK, Harvey WP: The clinical recognition of tricuspid stenosis. Circulation *22*:346, 1960.

Reichek N, Shelburn JC, Perloff JK: Clinical aspects of rheumatic valvular disease. Progr. Cardiovasc. Dis. *15*:491, 1973.

Salazar E, Levine HD: Rheumatic tricuspid regurgitation. The spectrum. Amer. J. Med. *33*:111, 1962.

Shine KI, DeSanctis RW, Sanders CA, Austen WG: Combined aortic and mitral incompetence. Clinical features and surgical management. Amer. Heart J. *76*:728, 1968.

36

Ischemic Heart Disease — Anginal Syndromes

Ischemic heart disease is arbitrarily divided and presented in three chapters which roughly correspond to stages of the disease, though admittedly the stages neither consistently develop in each patient nor follow in a specific sequence. These stages are:

- Inter nittent reversible ischemia,
- Acute myocardial infarction,
- Chronic cardiac failure from myocardial damage.

This chapter, dealing with intermittent ischemia, provides an overview of the disease process and contains an overall discussion of its natural history.

Definitions. "Angina pectoris" is the traditional term for intermittent chest pain, usually of short duration, not associated with acute myocardial infarction. Its commonest form is that provoked by exercise or excitement and relieved by rest. Longer attacks occurring without apparent exciting factors have been in the past designated by various names, none of which has been widely accepted: "coronary insufficiency," "coronary failure," "angina decubitus," etc. The present tendency of referring to such attacks as "preinfarction angina" utilizes a term that is probably no better than its predecessors, for it has been amply demonstrated that only a small portion of such attacks lead to myocardial infarction.

Today, when independent means of recognizing ischemia and coronary disease are available, it is apparent that anginal pain is not the

590

only clinical manifestation of reversible myocardial ischemia. Ischemic myocardium may be present in patients who exhibit the following:

- no symptoms at all,

- anginal pain,

- anginal equivalents (dyspnea, dizziness, apprehension),

- arrhythmias.

ETIOLOGY

Atherosclerosis accounts for the great majority of cases of intermittent myocardial ischemia. Other causes include some functional disturbances of coronary perfusion, such as that occurring in aortic stenosis (see Chapter 31), coronary arterial spasm, and rare congenital lesions affecting the coronary circulation.

The etiology of atherosclerosis in general, and coronary involvement in particular, is discussed in Chapter 21. Some of the following discussion amplifies and recapitulates the earlier presentation.

Occlusive coronary artery disease represents an active process, not merely the aging of the arterial wall. The risk factors listed in Chapter 21 contribute to the formation of occlusive disease, especially in its accelerated forms, i.e., affecting young subjects:

1.   Patterns of lipid metabolism play an important role in coronary atherogenesis:

- Severe hereditary hyperlipoproteinemias;

- Alimentary hyperlipidemia, thought to bring the average serum cholesterol level of the population of Western countries above 200 mg/100 ml.—much higher than that of infants;

- Abnormal lipid metabolism, leading in some patients to deposition of cholesterol upon arterial walls in the presence of low or normal cholesterol blood levels.

2.   Carbohydrate metabolism may play a contributory role in atherogenesis, as exemplified by premature coronary disease in diabetics as well as the frequent findings of abnormal glucose tolerance curves in young patients with ischemic heart disease.

3.   Hypertension accelerates coronary disease; there may be a straight line relationship between the level of blood pressure and the incidence of coronary atherosclerosis.

4.   Tobacco is also a well demonstrated risk factor.

5.   Stress is thought to play a role in atherogenesis; difficulties in measuring and defining stress make this factor a hypothetical one.

6.   Hereditary factors other than the presence of hyperlipoproteinemia play an important role in the causation of ischemic heart disease; hence the importance of family history.

7.   Lack of exercise as a factor in atherogenesis is a subject of controversy.

The major factor in the development of atherosclerotic occlusive disease of the coronary arteries is age: the older the patient the less important are the definable risk factors. The peak of frequency of clinical manifestations of ischemic heart disease occurs in men in their forties and fifties and in women in the postmenopausal period. The growing impression of an increasing incidence of premature coronary disease in young men is probably correct, although better methods of recognition and wider cognizance of this disease at present make the comparison with its incidence of 20 or 30 years ago inaccurate.

PATHOLOGY

Since the basic disease process is occlusion of arterial lumina, the principal process involves the intima of the coronary arteries. The fundamental lesion of the disease is the atherosclerotic plaque. Basically a product of a focal disease, plaque is initiated by the deposition of lipid-filled macrophages in the intima. Later the lipid material is deposited outside the cells, producing crystallization, fibrosis, and, frequently, calcification of the plaque. Progression of the occlusive process may take place either gradually, by growth of the plaque, or abruptly, either by rupture of a plaque or by a subintimal hemorrhage. The role of thrombosis in occlusion is discussed in Chapter 22.

The location of atherosclerotic plaques varies, but as a rule they most frequently affect larger branches of the coronary arteries. Proximal location of the plaques is more common than distal, and there is some preferential location at bifurcation of arteries.

The pathological consequences of occluding plaques are only discernible if irreversible ischemia follows. The typical sequel is represented by myocardial infarction (see Chapter 22). However, in patients who do not have clinically recognizable myocardial infarction, less concentrated permanent damage to the myocardium is often found in the form of scattered or disseminated focal fibrosis or necrosis. Thus it appears probable that some anginal attacks may leave behind irreversible myocardial scars too small to be detected by any known clinical means. This is probably the basis for the more diffuse forms of ischemic myocardial disease to be discussed in the following chapter.

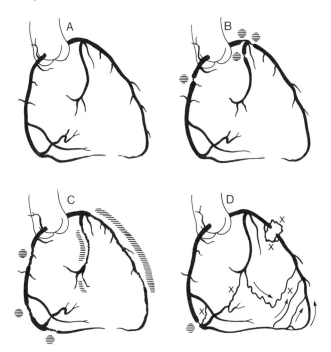

Figure 36-1. Semidiagrammatic presentation of the arteriographic image of the coronary circulation, illustrating various types of coronary artery disease:
A, Normal coronary tree;
B, Proximal severe stenosis (indicated by striped circles); the main left coronary artery and all three branches show obstructing lesions;
C, Diffuse, tubular three-vessel disease extending into the periphery;
D, Complete occlusion of left anterior descending artery; stenotic lesion in the distal right coronary artery; illustration of various types of collateral vessels (x).

Information obtained from *coronary arteriography* greatly reinforced the knowledge of pathological details regarding the distribution of occlusive coronary artery disease. Previously obtainable only by complex techniques of postmortem injection, unsuitable for routine pathological examination, the broad spectrum of the variations of normal and diseased coronary arteries unfolded. The concept of "dominance" of the right or left coronary artery was reinforced, illustrating its effect upon the natural history of ischemic heart disease. It became clear that the speed of progression of occlusive plaques varies greatly; some are stable or slowly progressive, while others progress at a rapid pace. (Not to be confused with the abovementioned are acute changes in the coronary arteries, e.g., thrombosis.) Local predisposing factors can be recognized, such as the development of lesions in the main left coronary artery in patients with prosthetic aortic valves, or the accelerated progression of lesions in arteries in which a bypass graft was implanted distal to the lesion. The role of collateral vessels has been defined, showing that occluded arteries can be revascularized by nature by connections from other larger coronary arteries, or by many small "bridging" collaterals.

PATHOPHYSIOLOGY

Ischemic heart disease is the consequence of inadequate blood supply to the working myocardium. This "coronary deficit" may be relative, involving a temporary disproportion between supply and demand, or absolute, with total inability to perfuse an area of the myocardium, leading to its necrosis.

The coronary flow is governed by several factors:

1. Perfusion pressure in the aorta;

2. Overall coronary arteriolar resistance;

3. Local regulation by means of regional changes in arteriolar resistance;

4. The adverse effects of run-off areas and steals (e.g., coronary arteriovenous fistulae, coronary-pulmonary artery communications).

The very high myocardial oxygen demands are met not only by adequate coronary perfusion but also by the highest tissue extraction of oxygen from the blood in the body. The coronary arteriovenous oxygen difference is very high, coronary venous blood being about 30 per cent saturated as against the saturation of mixed venous blood of 75 per cent. This means, however, that there is little reserve oxygen available in the blood and any increase in oxygen demands has to be met by a corresponding increase in coronary flow, which is governed by a sensitive autoregulatory mechanism, with local myocardial hypoxia acting as the most powerful coronary vasodilator.

Ischemia — disproportion between oxygen supply and demand — can be caused either by increased demand or by lowered supply of coronary blood. The following factors may contribute to such disproportion affecting the entire heart:

1. Increased oxygen demand:

    • exercise,

    • stress (rise in systemic pressure, catecholamine release),

    • increased cardiac rate.

2. Decreased oxygen supply:

    • lowered arterial pressure,

    • anemia,

- abnormal hemoglobin dissociation,

- coronary run-off.

These factors are seldom severe enough to produce lasting ischemia of the entire heart, in which case fatal cardiac failure could ensue. They play an important role, however, in further reducing the oxygen supply from an area in which the local blood flow is actually or potentially impaired. Thus these factors profoundly affect the course of focal coronary arterial disease due to atherosclerosis.

An atherosclerotic plaque developing in the lumen of a coronary artery does not produce impediment to blood flow until there is significant resistance to flow, evident by a pressure gradient across the point of obstruction, which under conditions of normal flow develops when the lumen is reduced to about 33 per cent of its original size. Beyond this point of obstruction the pressure gradient facilitates immediate collateral flow from the available small intercoronary branches; furthermore, it stimulates the growth of these collaterals which, given time, may grow into large vessels that can completely take over the blood supply even if the original plaque progresses to total closure of the affected branch.

A malperfused area may continue to provide sufficient oxygen to the affected myocardium to perform minimal functions. However, any of the above listed factors that would increase the demand or lower the supply of coronary blood flow might cross the threshold between potential and actual ischemia, producing its clinical manifestations. It follows, furthermore, that ischemia due to disproportion between the blood supply and the demand, if of sufficient duration, may produce myocardial death — infarction — without complete occlusion of the affected vessel (see also Chapter 22).

The question of coronary spasm has been widely debated for many years as a possible cause of myocardial ischemia. In the past, coronary arterial spasm was often suggested as an explanation for attacks of chest pain at rest. This subject was for a long time looked upon with skepticism, or rejected outright by some, until recently, when significant evidence in favor of coronary arterial spasm came to light. While it is still presumed to represent a rare and unusual mechanism of myocardial ischemia, it is clear that occasionally arterial spasm may produce severe ischemic episodes — not only inducing anginal pain but provoking serious arrhythmias as well. Spasm appears to affect large vessels, usually the right coronary artery or primary branches of the left, which are either completely free of occlusive disease or have mild, dynamically insignificant focal lesions within their lumen.

The pathophysiological consequences of temporary myocardial ischemia include the following:

- Abnormal, paradoxical wall motion of the affected part of the myocardium;

- Evidence of cardiac failure—if a sufficiently large portion of the myocardium becomes ischemic (elevated left atrial and left ventricular diastolic pressure);

- Electrical instability, often inducing arrhythmias.

NATURAL HISTORY OF ISCHEMIC HEART DISEASE

In oversimplified terms the clinical manifestations of ischemic heart disease can be placed in the following stages:

- Asymptomatic stage,

- Stage of stable angina,

- Stage of unstable angina,

- Myocardial infarction,

- Chronic "pump" failure,

- Death.

These stages do not occur sequentially; the course can be one of changing from one stage into another in either direction, often bypassing some. This can be exemplified by citing some possible courses:

1. Asymptomatic patients may develop stable angina, unstable angina, acute myocardial infarction, sudden death, or—directly—chronic cardiac failure.

2. Patients with stable angina may progress into unstable angina, leading to myocardial infarction, or may directly develop myocardial infarction which may result in death.

3. Patients with either stable or unstable angina may gradually lose symptoms, and eventually recover, showing no detectable ischemia.

4. Following acute myocardial infarction, the patient may die, may recover for an indefinite period, may develop cardiac failure, or may re-enter the stage of chronic (stable or unstable) angina and repeat the cycle in the future.

In spite of certain as yet unexplained variations and exceptions, the course of ischemic heart disease reflects, in general, the anatomic progression of the disease and the individual's adaptation to it. The dominant factors in the natural history are the following:

1. The speed of development of obstructive intra-arterial coronary lesions and their progression;

2. The location of the lesions and their number;

3. The capabilities for the development of effective coronary collaterals.

As stated, coronary arteriography has demonstrated that some arterial plaques remain unchanged for long periods of time, while others may be rapidly progressive. Pathologists have recognized "burned-out" plaques as contrasted with active plaques. Yet this most crucial information cannot as yet be recognized during life.

The relationship between the location of the lesion and the course of ischemic heart disease can be judged on the basis of some arteriographic clinical correlations. The normal variability of the arterial blood supply to the various regions of the myocardium is considerable—the guidelines are only general. Lesions in the main left coronary artery and its left anterior descending branch are believed to be the most precarious. Progressive occlusion of either often induces massive myocardial infarction or sudden death. Lesions in the left circumflex branch and the right coronary artery (even if it is dominant) are less likely to produce the disastrous consequences of occlusion. While the effectiveness of the collateral circulation has been challenged from time to time, there appears to be little justification for doubting the major compensatory function of collateral channels, given enough time for their growth and development. One need only cite cases with a congenital origin of the left coronary artery from the pulmonary artery, in which the entire heart is supplied by the right coronary artery and the anomalous left can be ligated with impunity—even with improvement—it being a vessel for a coronary steal.

The relationship between clinical symptoms and the severity of ischemic heart disease is generally good, though many exceptions can be found.

Stable angina with good effort tolerance is usually considered a benign condition. It presumably indicates a nonprogressive process, or a slowly progressive one compensated by collateral circulation. More rapid progression of coronary disease may be manifested by acceleration of angina, namely:

- Provocation of chest pain by progressively lower levels of exercise;

- Development of attacks in response to factors other than exercise (e.g., excitement);

- Appearance of pain at rest;

- Nocturnal attacks;

- Longer duration of attacks and less predictable relief by rest or nitroglycerin.

Such accelerated angina seems a reasonable indication that obstructive coronary disease is progressive—sometimes beyond the capabilities of compensatory mechanisms. Before reaching this conclusion it is necessary, however, to rule out some general factors governing coronary blood supply and demand that may have developed to account for the change.

The reverse phenomenon to acceleration of angina—decrescendo type of angina—develops occasionally. This may mean increase in effort tolerance—pain occurring only with more and more strenuous exercise and sometimes disappearing altogether—or retrogression of the various forms of accelerated angina with return to a stable, milder form. This may be produced:

- by spontaneous remission (presumably effective development of collaterals),

- in response to various forms of medical treatment,

- following acute myocardial infarction (sometimes subclinical).

There are clinical situations in which the severity of the disease appears to be out of proportion to the clinical symptomatology. Some patients are shown to have severe three-vessel disease yet clinically are asymptomatic. Patients may die suddenly with advanced coronary disease, allegedly without warning symptoms prior to the fatal attack. Asymptomatic serious ischemia—detected by stress tests or by monitoring devices—is also found at times. At present not enough critically conducted studies are available to indicate whether these are isolated instances or common occurrences. The possibility of patients ignoring or denying symptoms needs to be considered in the interpretation of these discrepancies. The present evidence favors the interpretation that the clinical course reasonably well reflects the severity and the progression of occlusive coronary artery disease and that major inconsistencies are infrequently present.

While the cardinal symptom of myocardial ischemia is chest pain, the features of which are described in detail in Chapter 2, it is necessary to recapitulate the clinical aspects of chronic ischemic heart disease, as it affects the natural history of this condition:

1.   Typical chest pain—both in location on the thorax and in its relation to exciting factors –is most frequently present. A firm clinical diagnosis can be based on the clinical history alone, if this symptom is present.

2.   Atypical chest pain may present confusing pictures. However, as stated in Chapter 2, a careful history may still retrieve important fea-

tures from many patients, using "atypical" pain as a guide to the progress of the disease.

3. Pain equivalents include "pressure," "burning," "difficulty in breathing," and other unusual sensations about the thorax, neck, or arms.

4. Truly painless ischemia occurs — as shown during stress tests and patient monitoring. The patient may perceive two sequels to ischemia and report them if carefully questioned:

- Left ventricular failure, producing dyspnea (as contrasted with "difficulty in breathing" because of tightness in the chest) or weakness;

- Arrhythmias, producing palpitations, "pounding," or syncopal attacks.

The typical course of ischemic heart disease involves anginal attacks occurring in response to the increased workload of exercise. As mentioned, progression of the anginal syndrome leads to attacks which may occur with other provoking factors — e.g., excitement — or at rest, without any known precipitating events. There are, however, variants of attacks of myocardial ischemia in which anginal pain occurs only at rest (often only at night), in spite of the fact that the patient performs strenuous work that undoubtedly taxes his coronary blood supply. An electrocardiogram taken during an attack of this type may show the usual evidence of ischemia — S-T segment depression — but occasionally may show S-T segment elevation instead. These attacks are often referred to as Prinzmetal's type of angina, though they were reported before Prinzmetal's article appeared (see Bibliography).

A great deal of recent discussion concerns the use of the term and the definition of "preinfarction angina." This term acknowledges the fact that acute myocardial infarction is frequently preceded by unstable angina, progressing in a crescendo manner into the attack initiating the infarct. Yet, the variability of attacks of pain preceding myocardial infarction is sufficiently great to question the validity of any pattern in predicting an impending infarction. Furthermore, two recent studies indicated that patients hospitalized for "preinfarction angina" "cool off" without developing myocardial infarction in 80 to 90 per cent of cases (Fulton et al., 1972; Krauss et al., 1972).

The introduction of effective surgical treatment of ischemic heart disease brought into focus the question as to what is the prognosis of patients with ischemic heart disease in relation to the clinical and coronary arteriographic findings. Studies of the natural history of coronary artery disease have approached the subject from various viewpoints and have reached widely divergent conclusions. Certain tentative impressions are presented here; they will be further evaluated in connection with surgical therapy of angina:

1.   Stable angina, as stated, offers generally a good prognosis.

2.   Crescendo (unstable) angina often, though not always, indicates progression of coronary artery disease but, as mentioned, does not reliably predict myocardial infarction or sudden death.

3.   Two clinical signs imply that ischemia is of unusual severity and may be caused by a precarious change in the coronary circulation:

   • Pronounced displacement of the S-T segment of the electrocardiogram (greater than 2 mm.) in tracings recorded during attacks;

   • Serious ventricular arrhythmias recorded during attacks (multiform ventricular ectopic beats, bouts of ventricular tachycardia, paroxysms of ventricular fibrillation).

4.   Occlusive disease in the coronary arteries demonstrated by coronary arteriography appears to be of prognostic significance in that single-vessel disease is associated with a benign course, the mortality being only slightly higher than in age-matched general population. Three-vessel disease carries a high risk of dying, with a less than 50 per cent probability of surviving 5 years. Two-vessel disease has a prognosis intermediate between one- and three-vessel disease.

The *postsurgical course* of ischemic heart disease is not yet well enough known to make meaningful comments. Patients who were selected for aortico-coronary bypass operations and showed an uncomplicated course are usually symptomatically improved, often totally asymptomatic. Whether their life is prolonged and myocardial infarction avoided is not yet known. Their prognosis depends largely upon two factors:

   • Progression of occlusive coronary disease in arteries other than those affected by the bypass operation;

   • The fate of the bypass graft.

Because of the great variability and often unpredictable changes in the course of ischemic heart disease, on the one hand, and the benign nature of many forms of coronary disease, on the other hand, it will take a long time and very critically designed studies to answer this question in an authoritative manner.

DIAGNOSIS

The goals of the diagnostic approaches to chronic ischemic heart disease include the following:

1.   The analysis of pain suspected as being ischemic to determine the following:

- Whether it is cardiac or non-cardiac in origin;

- Whether it is caused by reversible ischemia or produces myocardial damage;

- Whether it can be used as a guideline to estimate the severity of the patient's disease.

2.   The detection of ischemic heart disease with atypical features;

3.   The evaluation of myocardial function;

4.   The evaluation of the anatomic details of occlusive coronary disease.

In order to fulfill these goals it may be necessary to go through the entire chain of diagnostic procedures, up to and including coronary arteriography. Since the latter is an invasive procedure with an appreciable risk to the patient, this diagnostic step is indicated only if the results of the study are likely to materially change the management of the patient.

The *clinical history* is the fundamental part of the diagnostic approach to ischemic heart disease, as has been repeatedly stated. On the basis of a history a definitive diagnosis can be established; in some cases the diagnosis is firm enough to outweigh the negative results of most other tests. The characteristic features of anginal pain are presented in Chapter 2. Other symptoms are mentioned above.

Physical examination varies in its contribution to the diagnosis. Given a patient with chronic angina who has never had myocardial infarction, examination of the heart is frequently unremarkable. An S4 gallop sound is often detected in patients with ischemic heart disease; yet this finding in subjects over the age of 40 may occur without evidence of cardiac disease and therefore has a low specificity. If the opportunity presents itself to examine the patient while he experiences chest pain, the following findings may support the diagnosis of angina:

- development of an S3 gallop sound during pain,

- development of an apical systolic murmur,

- development of an abnormal systolic precordial pulsation,

- development of arrhythmias.

Additional information obtained during examination includes the detection of possible risk factors (hypertension, evidence of hyperlipidemia), and in later stages of the disease signs of cardiac failure and some of the postinfarctional complications.

Radiography as a rule shows normal cardiovascular shadows unless late stage disease and cardiac failure are present. A sign of some value, yet of low specificity, is the presence of calcification of the coronary arteries.

Electrocardiography more often than not shows a normal resting tracing unless myocardial damage is already present. The value of electrocardiography lies in the following special procedures:

- serial tracings in patients with chest pain of sufficient severity to arouse suspicion of myocardial infarction,

- stress testing,

- monitoring over long periods of time,

- electrocardiograms taken during an anginal attack.

Stress testing has been discussed in Chapter 5; treadmill tests are more frequently used now than the two-step test. Valid results can be anticipated if the following indications are followed:

- The resting electrocardiogram is normal or, at least, a precordial lead with an upright QRS complex and normal ST-T is present;

- The patient is not on digitalis.

Stress tests should not be performed in patients who have frequent prolonged attacks of chest pain at rest ("preinfarction angina") or immediately after recovery from a myocardial infarction.

Monitoring of patients suspected of having ischemic heart disease is indicated in those who suffer from frequent attacks of pain at rest. The following techniques can be used:

- conventional bedside monitoring,

- telemetric in-hospital monitoring, giving patients mobility in the ward,

- continuous recording on 8 to 24 hour tapes.

The objective of monitoring is to find any of the following:

- S-T segment depression,

- S-T segment elevation,

- serious arrhythmias.

If any of these findings is detected it is important to determine its relationship to chest pain or other symptoms. Significant findings are as follows: (see also above)

- 1 mm. or more S-T segment deviation,

- ventricular ectopic beats appearing in salvos, runs of tachy-cardia, ventricular fibrillation.

Cardiac catheterization provides little direct diagnostic information; nevertheless it may be useful in the fulfillment of special objectives:

- As a means of evaluating cardiac function; multivessel coronary disease may impair cardiac function, providing abnormal hemodynamic findings, especially during exercise;

- As a means of provoking anginal attacks by atrial pacing, or making observations during spontaneous attacks.

Anginal attacks often produce prompt evidence of left ventricular failure with elevation of left ventricular diastolic and left atrial pressures. Reduction of cardiac output may also take place. These changes are reversed by nitroglycerin. Atrial pacing is an alternate form of stress testing. Patients whose electrocardiograms are abnormal, therefore unsuitable for the production of ischemic electrocardiographic changes during exercise, are particularly suitable candidates for atrial pacing. The reproduction of chest pain, especially when supported by the appearance of hemodynamic abnormalities, may provide conclusive evidence that the attacks are anginal in nature.

Coronary arteriography represents the "ultimate" in the diagnosis of ischemic heart disease. While there can be no question that coronary arteriography has revolutionized the diagnosis and understanding of ischemic heart disease, the pendulum of enthusiasm may have swung beyond the point of reasonableness, for the risk of this test is surely not justified in everyone in whom there is any suspicion of ischemic heart disease, as some advocate. The prime indication for coronary arteriography is to determine the feasibility of bypass surgery; this will be discussed later. Only occasionally coronary arteriograms are indicated in patients in whom surgical treatment appears unlikely. Among such problems are patients who carry the diagnosis of ischemic heart disease and claim to be totally disabled by it. Even if the diagnosis of noncardiac pain is firmly established by other means, the performance of coronary arteriography may be necessary to provide authoritative proof. Another situation arises occasionally in connection with asymptomatic subjects with suspicious abnormalities (e.g., abnormal electrocardiograms) whose livelihood may be jeopardized by the uncertainty of suspected cardiac disease (e.g., airline pilots).

Evaluation. When facing a patient suspected of having ischemic heart disease, the physician has to make certain basic decisions in answer to the following questions:

1. How definite should the diagnosis be made and by what means?

2. How reliable a diagnosis can be arrived at, given the facilities of the patient's primary physician?

3. At what point need a local consultant be brought in?

4. When is hospital evaluation needed?

5. When is referral to a cardiac center indicated?

In many cases the establishment of a definitive diagnosis is easily within the reach of the patient's primary physician. If the patient produces a classical history of effort angina, if the effort tolerance is good, if symptoms do not interfere with the patient's occupation and reasonable recreational activities, the decision not to proceed with further studies is well taken. Simple confirmation of the diagnosis — e.g., by a two-step test or, if easily available, by a treadmill test — might then be considered the frosting on the cake. The task facing the physician then is the initiation of therapy.

Patients with stable angina at a more advanced level — e.g., restricting some of the patient's ordinary activities — may be left at the same point in diagnosis as the previous case; here more aggressive therapy may be indicated.

Patients with atypical features, in whom the clinical diagnosis is uncertain, need further investigation. Here, background information may be helpful — risk factors, family history. Noninvasive studies should be performed, but referral to a cardiac center for coronary arteriography does not automatically follow, unless serious disability is present so that surgical treatment might be contemplated if coronary disease is found. In nondisabling atypical cases whose symptoms are nonprogressive, a tentative diagnosis based on probabilities is preferable.

Patients with progressive symptomalogy require a great deal of thought and careful consideration. As stated, progressive symptoms imply progression of the disease; alertness regarding possible surgical indications is now in order. Evaluation of such patients should depend upon careful assessment of the progression. Patients who first develop symptoms are obviously progressive, their level of angina increasing from 0 to level X. Yet, if such patients level off with nondisabling angina of effort, a conservative attitude is justified. When progression of the symptoms consists of gradual reduction of effort tolerance, the speed and consistency of the increase in symptoms need careful review. It is important, for example, to rule out the possibility that an extraneous factor may have increased myocardial demands (intercurrent illness, development of hypertension, cold weather, change in therapy, etc.), thereby increasing the probability that progression is real and spontaneous. The effect of medical therapy needs also to come into consideration: The patient may be given more active treatment, which may reverse the progression, in which case the urgency may no longer be present.

There are clinical symptoms that require prompt decisions — often immediate referral to a cardiac center. These include the following:

- Consistent development of angina at rest and nocturnal attacks;

- Prolonged attacks of pain, no longer responsive to nitroglycerin;

- Attacks suggestive of left ventricular failure;

- Attacks suggestive of serious arrhythmias.

The presence of the above symptoms often leads — as the first step in the evaluation — to hospitalization of the patient for continuous monitoring. Monitoring facilities are available in most community hospitals; nevertheless, even though the diagnosis can be supported by monitoring, it is advisable not to lose time for that but to refer the patient immediately to a major cardiac center where full diagnostic and surgical facilities are available because of the potential life-threatening emergencies that could arise. Such emergencies requiring instant intervention will be discussed in connection with surgical therapy.

The evaluation of asymptomatic patients may pose difficult dilemmas. Patients in the following categories come under consideration:

- Those who had an uncomplicated myocardial infarction and made a complete recovery;

- Those who never had symptoms but have electrocardiographic abnormalities strongly suggestive of ischemic heart disease;

- Those found to have electrocardiographic evidence of ischemia on stress tests without experiencing symptoms.

The purpose of proceeding with invasive studies in such patients would be the localization of the lesion, with consideration of prophylactic operations in the presence of serious disease. This can be justified at present in only very exceptional cases, as will be discussed below; hence these findings do not constitute accepted indications for invasive procedures.

THERAPY

Ischemic heart disease represents the most serious health problem affecting Western civilization. As a consequence of its wide prevalence, its treatment has to be approached from the broadest possible stand-point. Thus, the overall objectives of therapy can be summarized as follows:

1. The prevention of atherosclerosis in subjects prone to it;

2. Reversal or arrest of existing atherosclerotic process;

3. When indicated, surgical bypassing of life-threatening or severely disabling occlusive lesions;

4. Prevention of sequels and complications of coronary disease;

5. Relief of symptoms.

Primary prevention of atherosclerosis should ideally be applied to the entire population. Broad educational campaigns to that effect are still in infancy. However, on an individual basis prevention of athero-sclerosis might be attempted in subjects with a high risk of acquiring this disease; those with strong family history of premature coronary dis-ease, with familial hyperlipidemias, diabetes, and so on. Measures should logically start in childhood and include the following:

- Avoidance of obesity;

- Consistent exercise programs;

- Diet low in saturated fats;

- Avoidance of tobacco;

- Early identification and control of hypertension.

In patients who are known to have ischemic heart disease a basic plan to arrest (or reverse) the atherosclerotic process should be at-tempted over and above any other therapeutic measures. This is done by the best possible control of risk factors:

1. *Reduction of serum lipids.* This can be approached by diet and drugs. The basic dietary treatment consists of the substitution of polyunsaturated fats for regular fats, with an overall reduction of fats. Some forms of hyperlipidemias require other modification of diet, such as reduction in the amount of consumed carbohydrates (in type IV hyperlipidemia). This may be supplemented by the administration of clofibrate or cholestyramine. The former interferes with cholesterol metabolism and reduces serum triglycerides and to a lesser extent cholesterol blood levels, particularly in patients with hypercholestere-mia and hypertriglyceridemia. The latter is an exchange resin interfer-ing with fat absorption in the diet. A more drastic measure with a simi-lar effect is a surgical bowel shunting operation reducing food absorption in the jejunum. The choice of the therapeutic methods for lipid control has to be individually decided upon. Dietary treatment requires good motivation on the part of the patient. Drug therapy

produces untoward symptoms in many patients. Bowel surgery should be reserved only for extreme cases.

2. *Elimination of tobacco.* The effect of smoking upon the progression of atherosclerosis is reasonably well established; encouragement to have the patient give up smoking is always highly desirable from broader aspects than coronary disease, but is so often unsuccessful.

3. *Control of blood pressure.* The current aggressive approach to even modest blood pressure elevation may have as a major objective better control of this risk factor even in individuals without known ischemic heart disease. Certainly in those who have coronary artery disease great care should be exercised that the level of blood pressure is under the best possible control.

4. *Weight control.* Even though obesity is not a proven risk factor it has many undesirable effects that would justify stringent measures for its control. Among these are the mechanical load upon the circulation of excess body weight, the tendency to increase hyperglycemia, and its possible effect upon fat metabolism.

5. *Control of stress.* Stress is assumed though not proven to be a risk factor. Yet, not enough is known about the effects of stress elimination to come out for strong recommendation to eliminate all stressful occupations. Inasmuch as stress is often the price for success in life, both the physician and the patient have to weigh the consequences of giving up competitive jobs in favor of ones with low responsibilities. Nevertheless, patients with ischemic heart disease might be encouraged to have reasonable working habits, devote weekends to rest or recreation, and arrange for suitable vacations at regular intervals.

6. *Exercise.* While lack of exercise is only a qualified risk factor for the production of ischemic heart disease, physical fitness has been shown to have a favorable effect at least upon the symptomatic aspects of ischemic heart disease. A physical reconditioning program is discussed in Chapter 12. It occupies an intermediate place between reduction of a risk factor and active therapy.

Symptomatic therapy involves a variety of measures, medical and surgical. The effectiveness of all such measures is difficult to evaluate. Anginal pain and possibly other clinical manifestations of ischemia are influenced by many factors, including the psychogenic. While suggestion undoubtedly plays an important role in reduction of symptoms in response to effective therapeutic measures, psychogenic and neurogenic influences may on occasion actually produce changes in the myocardial oxygen supply-demand ratio by affecting blood pressure, catecholamine excretion, and other regulatory mechanisms. Thus, the evaluation of effectiveness of symptomatic treatment of ischemic heart disease is often difficult even in controlled studies because placebos may be very effective, obliterating the difference between pharmacologically active and inert forms of therapy.

In designing symptomatic therapy for patients with ischemic heart disease, those with stable effort angina represent the best target. Many patients can control anginal attacks without drug therapy, by eliminating those forms of exercise that are likely to induce attacks or by avoiding contributory factors (walking in cold weather or after meals). The next step in active therapy is the use of nitroglycerin. Its use at the very inception of the attack, or prophylactically before an attack-provoking activity is initiated, may be very effective and render the patient asymptomatic. More disabling angina may require the use of long-acting nitrates and propranolol—both of which are discussed in Chapter 12.

Typical anginal attacks, including those occurring at rest and during sleep, may or may not respond to nitroglycerin and other antianginal drugs. Occasionally some provoking factors can be identified and eliminated: arrhythmias and latent cardiac failure with nocturnal fluid retention. Here, antiarrhythmic drugs and diuretics might bring relief where other drugs fail.

When rapidly progressive angina is present, including attacks at rest, patients may be hospitalized. The purpose of this includes the following:

- Bed rest seems to stop the progression of symptoms in some patients;

- Electrocardiographic monitoring may provide important additional information;

- If the patient has "preinfarction angina" and is prone to develop acute myocardial infarction the high-risk "prehospital" stage of infarction will be eliminated;

- Out of the patients in this category some surgical candidates may be selected—occasionally even for emergency treatment.

Surgical therapy has generated great emotional appeal and continues to be the center of a wide controversy regarding the aggressiveness with which a surgical approach should be sought. The history of the various surgical procedures recommended throughout the past several decades as effective treatment of coronary disease demonstrated that great enthusiasm and energy have been invested in procedures totally unproved, based on poor theoretical considerations, and later shown to be ineffective. In spite of the fact that the mammary artery implantation into the myocardium (Vineberg procedure) still has some advocates, it is generally agreed by most students of the subject that direct revascularization by means of an aortico-coronary bypass or an equivalent operation is the first surgical procedure both sound theoretically and with demonstrated effectiveness. This very fact led to exaggerated claims, namely to the effect that the operation basically changes the natural history of ischemic heart disease and that it consistently prevents the development of myocardial infarction or sudden death. Accepting such claims uncritically, some institutions are advocating the use of this operation purely for prophylactic purposes.

The pros and cons of the bypass operation can be summarized as follows:

1. The bypass operation can be performed without difficulty; the immediate risk in good cardiac-surgical units is very low (1 to 5 per cent).

2. Revascularization is immediately available; the flow through the anastomosis is large enough to provide adequate blood supply to the myocardium via alternate channels.

3. Symptomatic relief occurs more consistently than after previous operations and can be supported by objective means (e.g., stress test reversal).

4. In individual cases, if critical lesions located proximally in large coronary branches are present prior to the operation, it is reasonable to assume that myocardial infarction and sudden death may be prevented.

On the negative side:

1. While the mortality of the bypass operation and that of the preliminary coronary arteriography are low, each of these procedures causes some nonfatal serious complications: myocardial infarction (some "impending" but others affecting areas in which they might not have occurred, were it not for the procedures), strokes, diffuse myocardial damage, etc. The rate of intraoperative myocardial infarction varies from 10 to 20 per cent.

2. Closure of the bypass channel occurs consistently: two-year figures show closure rates between 15 and 30 per cent. The long-range fate of the anastomosis is not known.

3. Good evidence is now available that the narrowed areas in the coronary arteries proximal to the bypass (the ones which are being bypassed) may completely close within months after the operation. Comparison between bypassed and non-bypassed vessels shows definitely that providing an alternate flow channel to the artery accelerates closure of the lesions. Thus, considering that some plaques were "burned out" and nonprogressive and may never have progressed,

were it not for the bypass, one has to accept the thesis that some patients are made worse by the operation: those in whom the natural channel closes and the bypass subsequently becomes obliterated.

4. Ancillary considerations regarding coronary artery surgery should include the cost and the time loss in connection with the operation in patients who were not seriously disabled.

Considering the overall therapeutic principle—risk balanced by benefit—the following principles can be listed as a means of selecting patients for the aortico-coronary bypass operation (by the same token, patients in whom coronary arteriography is indicated).

1. Clinical considerations:

   a. Patients with disabling angina, inadequately controllable by a good medical regimen, may be candidates for coronary bypass.

   b. Patients with accelerating angina may be considered for bypass.

   c. Also, patients suspected of suffering from premature, rapidly progressive coronary atherosclerosis: young individuals with progressive angina, even if not disabling; those with more than one myocardial infarction at a young age.

   d. Patients with "preinfarction angina" are studied and operated on in some institutions; this is still experimental. At this time one can justify emergency study and revascularization (if found suitable) in patients who show signs of higher than average risk—very pronounced S-T segment deviation at rest, malignant arrhythmias.

   e. In some institutions bypass operations are thought to reverse ischemia at the time when the patient appears to be developing an acute myocardial infarction. This is only practicable in patients in whom myocardial infarction develops as a complication of coronary arteriography, for the operation would not be considered effective unless performed within 2 to 4 hours after the *known* onset of the infarction. Preliminary information (as yet inconclusive) suggests that this is the critical time during which revascularization might reverse the myocardial damage.

   f. Patients whose clinical problem is cardiac failure, but who do not suffer from anginal attacks, should not be considered for bypass surgery.

2. Anatomic considerations (after coronary arteriography):

a. Obstructive lesions to be bypassed should be severe, involving certainly no less than 70 per cent of the lumen.

b. Proximal lesions with good run-off in peripheral parts of the vessels should be the prime, if not the only, targets for the operation.

c. Anastomosis to secondary and tertiary branches on the periphery appear to have a poor prospect of good function and their use can be questioned.

d. High priority should be given to the "precarious" lesions, namely those affecting the main left coronary artery and the proximal part of its anterior descending branch. Solitary lesions of the right coronary artery and those in the left circumflex branch are considered less likely to have serious consequences. The fact that lesions affecting one artery are associated with a good prognosis was already discussed. Unless an especially precarious lesion is present, operations for single-vessel disease are questionable.

e. Totally occluded arteries with good collateral flow may represent benign, stable lesions. They should never be considered the sole reason for aortico-coronary surgery.

f. Good myocardial contractility should be demonstrated by left ventriculography; in the presence of a poorly contracting left ventricle the risk of the operation has been shown to be greatly increased. Operations under such circumstances should be performed only in life-threatening situations.

It should be pointed out that these guidelines are largely conjectural and speculative. Only controlled randomized study of aortico-coronary bypass operations can provide definitive information. While some such studies are being initiated, it remains to be seen whether a sufficient number of randomized cases will be available to supply meaningful figures.

At present, the strongest indication for surgery is the presence of severe clinical disability. This constitutes a justifiable reason for the operation per se—other potential benefits are merely a free dividend. Operations of prophylactic nature—some of which are listed above—are based on speculation and should still be considered tentative.

Postsurgical therapy can be summarized as follows:

In the immediate postoperative period alertness for complications, particularly myocardial infarction, is of great importance. Patients who sustained an intraoperative myocardial infarction should have incorporated in their postoperative therapeutic regimen therapy for myocardial infarction.

Aggressive further therapy aimed at risk factors should be instituted because the operation has no influence upon the basic occlusive coronary disease.

Treatment of ischemic chest pain, if it persists after the operation, follows the pattern described above.

Delayed onset of pain needs evaluation that usually includes coronary arteriography: it may signify graft closure or progression of the disease in areas other than the operated one. Repeat surgical therapy often has to be considered in cases of graft closure, particularly if serious disability recurs after a period of symptom-free existence.

Bibliography

Dunkman WB, Perloff JK, Kastor JA, Shelburne JC: Medical perspectives in coronary artery surgery—a caveat. Ann. Int. Med. *81*:817, 1974.

Epstein SE, Richmond DR, Goldstein RE, Beiser G, Rosing DR, Glancy DL, Reis RL, Stinson ER: Angina pectoris: Pathophysiology, evaluation and treatment. Ann. Int. Med. *75*:263, 1971.

Frank CW, Weinblatte E, Shapiro S: Angina pectoris in men. Prognostic significance of selected medical factors. Circulation *47*:509, 1973.

Fulton M, Duncan B, Lutz W, Morrison SL, Donald KW, Kerr F, Kirby BJ, Julian DG, Oliver MF: Natural history of unstable angina. Lancet *1*:860, 1972.

Goldschlager N, Sakai FJ, Cohn KE, Selzer A: Hemodynamic abnormalities in patients with coronary artery disease and their relationship to intermittent ischemic episodes. Amer. Heart J. *80*:610, 1970.

Hultgren HN, Miyagawa M, Buck W, Angell WW: Ischemic myocardial injury during coronary artery surgery. Amer. Heart J. *82*:624, 1971.

Kannel WB, Feinleib M: Natural history of angina pectoris in the Framingham study. Amer. J. Cardiol. *29*:154, 1972.

Krauss, KR, Hutter AM, DeSanctis RW: Acute coronary insufficiency: course and follow-up. Arch. Int. Med. *129*:809, 1972.

McNeer JF, Starmer CP, Bartel AG, Behar VS, Kong Y, Peter RH, Rosatti RA: The nature and treatment selection in coronary artery disease: Experience with medical and surgical treatment. Circulation *49*:606, 1974.

Oliva PB, Potts DE, Plus RG: Coronary arterial spasm in Prinzmetal's angina documented by coronary arteriography. New Engl. J. Med. *283*:745, 1973.

Prinzmetal M, Kannamer R, Merliss R, Wada T, Bor N: Angina pectoris: I. A variant form of angina pectoris. Amer. J. Med. *27*:375, 1959.

Reeves TJ, Oberman A, Jones WB, Sheffield LT: Natural history of angina pectoris. Amer. J. Cardiol. *33*:423, 1974.

Scherf S, Cohen J: "Variant" angina pectoris. Circulation *49*:787, 1974.

Vlodaver Z, Neufeld HN, Edwards JE: Pathology of angina pectoris. Circulation *46*:1048, 1972.

37

Ischemic Heart Disease: Late Sequelae

Definition. In the preceding chapter the ischemic aspects of coronary artery disease were presented. As a result of ischemic injury, large or small, cardiac function may be affected in a chronic manner, not merely as the immediate result of the ischemia. In this chronic category the following conditions can be included:

1. Sequelae of focal myocardial damage from infarction:

   a. Dyskinesia,

   b. Akinesia,

   c. Hypokinesia,

   d. Ventricular aneurysm.

2. Diffuse myocardial injury — usually after multiple infarcts.

3. Ischemic "cardiomyopathy" — diffuse discrete myocardial injury without known myocardial infarction.

4. Complications of myocardial infarction producing chronic cardiac overload:

   a. Mitral regurgitation,

   b. Perforation of ventricular septum.

PATHOLOGY AND PATHOPHYSIOLOGY

Chronic myocardial disease associated with coronary artery disease involves the replacement of myocardial fibers with fibrous tissue.

613

Fibrosis develops as a late sequel to ischemic necrosis. The following forms of fibrosis can be found in patients with ischemic myocardial disease:

- Fibrosis due to healed myocardial infarction involving a mixture of normal myofibrils and fibrous tissue in the infarcted area. This may produce diminished or absent contractility of the affected segment of the left ventricle (akinesia, hypokinesia, dyskinesia).

- Fibrosis resulting from transmural myocardial infarction uniformly affecting a left ventricular segment. Here aneurysm of the left ventricle is present if the fibrous area bulges out; if it retains its shape, merely representing a thinned out area, it may function as a dyskinetic segment. Long-standing aneurysms may eventually develop calcification in their walls and frequently contain mural thrombi.

- Disseminated fibrosis may not be well visible on inspection of the heart. Fibrous tissue may or may not be visible on sectioning the left ventricular wall; microscopic sections may show scattered fibrous tissue not unlike that in chronic myocarditis.

- Mitral regurgitation produced by ischemic heart disease has been discussed in Chapter 34. It involves separation of one of the heads of the papillary muscle or—more often—involvement of a papillary muscle (usually the posterior) in the infarction. However, significant mitral regurgitation that produces left ventricular overload involves, in addition to infarction of the papillary muscle, also extensive fibrosis of the free wall of the left ventricle, often in the form of an aneurysm.

- Septal perforation is caused by myocardial infarction involving the ventricular septum. It usually is located in the apical area. Chronic acquired ventricular septal defect caused by septal perforation often takes the form of a fibrous scar in the ventricular septum with one or more perforating holes. In order to be consistent with survival, these holes have to be small, as a rule less than 1 cm. in diameter.

Secondary changes found in patients with chronic cardiac failure due to ischemic heart disease include the following:

- Work hypertrophy of the healthy left ventricular myocardium (except in the diffuse "cardiomyopathy" form);

- Sequels to pulmonary hypertension produced by chronic left ventricular failure—right ventricular hypertrophy.

Pathophysiological sequels to myocardial involvement include the usual chain of events of chronic cardiac failure, as described in Chapter 14. As a rule, cardiac enlargement with increased end-systolic and end-diastolic volume is present; the hemodynamic abnormalities vary greatly. There are cases of gross cardiac aneurysms in which surprisingly good hemodynamic function is preserved for long periods of time.

NATURAL HISTORY

The essential pathophysiological abnormality here is pump failure; hence clinical symptoms include dyspnea on effort, other forms of dyspnea, weakness, and fluid accumulation, with the related symptomatology. Chest pain due to myocardial ischemia may coexist with pump failure but will not be considered here. The clinical course of patients who develop cardiac failure from ischemic heart disease shows a considerable variation:

1. Patients may develop cardiac failure during the acute stage of myocardial infarction:

- Following recovery, failure may spontaneously subside;

- Following recovery, failure may be easily controlled by appropriate medication with minimal disability or none at all;

- The patient may remain in chronic cardiac failure with significant limitations, in spite of optimal medical therapy;

- The patients may remain in, or lapse into, intractable cardiac failure.

2. Patients — with or without evidence of cardiac failure during the acute stage of myocardial infarction — may proceed with a satisfactory clinical recovery but gradually lapse into failure upon resumption of ordinary activities, usually within a few weeks after the infarction, occasionally later than that.

3. Patients may gradually and insidiously develop cardiac failure, often, but not always, without clinically evident myocardial infarction, or without temporal relationship to a known infarction.

The variability of the course of patients with ischemic pump failure applies to all the forms of myocardial damage, including the mechanical complications (large ventricular aneurysms, mitral regurgitation, and septal perforation), except for the last category (insidious onset of cardiac failure), which is most often encountered in "ischemic cardiomyopathy."

The subsequent course and prognosis of patients in chronic cardiac failure with ischemic cardiac disease are related to the following factors:

1. The stability of myocardial damage—patients who had recovered after massive myocardial infarction which produced cardiac failure and who do not develop new myocardial damage may remain indefinitely in the various categories listed above:

- latent cardiac failure,

- controlled cardiac failure,

- poorly controlled cardiac failure.

Those with intractable cardiac failure are likely to develop some complications (often a thromboembolic complication) and die—unless surgical palliation is feasible.

2. The presence of myocardial ischemia—patients with anginal attacks in addition to cardiac failure have two independent variables influencing their course: progression of ischemia and progression or consequences of myocardial disease.

3. Development of new myocardial insults—either further myocardial infarcts or subtle ischemic destruction of the myocardium.

Complications may alter the course of patients with ischemic pump failure. They are mostly those accompanying cardiac failure in general, including pulmonary infarcts, pulmonary infections, chronic atrial arrhythmias, conduction disturbances, etc. While the overall course of ventricular aneurysms overlaps in all respects with that of other forms of ischemic myocardial damage, certain specific complications should be mentioned in connection with ventricular aneurysms:

- Ventricular rupture is exceedingly rare in chronic aneurysms; the occasional cases with cardiac rupture show, as a rule, the tear occurring through a new area of necrosis (often clinically unsuspected).

- Systemic embolization occurs in ventricular aneurysms inasmuch as larger aneurysms commonly have mural thrombi. At one time thought to be a common risk in ventricular aneurysms, it is a relatively rare complication, considering that angiocardiography has increased the recognition of true ventricular aneurysms many times over those identified in the past by plain radiography and fluoroscopy.

- Occasionally ventricular aneurysms are associated with intractable ventricular arrhythmias.

DIAGNOSIS

Clinical examination of patients with ischemic heart disease should always include a careful questioning for the more subtle manifestations of cardiac failure. Traditionally, the principal effort is concentrated upon eliciting as accurate an accounting of ischemic chest pain as possible. The presence of effort dyspnea (occasionally an anginal equivalent, as explained in Chapter 36) needs to be evaluated in regard to decreasing left ventricular competence. Nocturnal attacks of dyspnea or cough, unexplained weight gain, epigastric discomfort, undue fatigability — all these require careful evaluation.

Physical findings may reveal significant abnormalities that fall into four categories:

- The presence of abnormal cardiac motion: diffuse periapical pulsations, pulsations of areas separated from the apical impulse;

- Signs of left ventricular failure: S3 gallop sound, pulsus alternans, pulmonary rales;

- Signs of right ventricular failure: abnormal jugular venous pulse and evidence of systemic venous congestion (hepatomegaly, edema, serous effusions);

- Signs of complications: mitral regurgitation or ventricular septal perforation. Holosystolic murmur occurs in both; its location is frequently apical in septal perforation as well as in mitral regurgitation.

Electrocardiography as a rule adds little to the evaluation of cardiac function. There is virtually no relationship between the magnitude of electrocardiographic postinfarctional abnormalities and cardiac performance. Only one sign bears a relationship to the subject under discussion, though not necessarily to cardiac function: the presence of persistent S-T segment elevation is a sign of ventricular aneurysm - this sign is of medium specificity.

Radiography may fail to provide specific signs for the presence of cardiac failure. Occasionally an unusual increase in the size of the pulmonary artery or the presence of pulmonary vascular congestion or bilateral pleural effusions may provide radiological clues to that effect. Cardiac enlargement common to all forms of cardiac failure is usually present; however, in ischemic pump failure the degree of cardiac enlargement is, on the average, less pronounced than in cardiac failure produced by other etiological mechanisms. Radiography is helpful in the recognition of cardiac aneurysms which may be further explored by fluoroscopic examination. However, only a fraction of aneurysms can be diagnosed without the more reliable contrast techniques. In septal perforation increased pulmonary vascularity may be present in the radiograph, yet it may be difficult to differentiate it from passive pulmonary congestion.

Systolic time intervals recorded with the aid of the phonocardiogram show abnormal values in the ischemic type of cardiac failure. However, the discriminatory value of these measurements in individual cases is limited, and they are more suitable as a means of following the progress of a case.

Echocardiographic demonstration of impaired left ventricular wall motion serves as a simple means of confirming akinesia or dyskinesia. Dilatation of the left ventricular cavity corroborates the fact that serious myocardial damage has resulted from myocardial infarction. Nevertheless, this information is of only inferential significance and does not directly relate to left ventricular performance. Furthermore, only portions of the posterior and septal walls are explorable by echocardiography; hence this technique cannot rule out the presence of abnormal wall motion in other areas.

Cardiac catheterization is the most elaborate and accurate test serving to evaluate cardiac performance. Measurements of intracardiac pressures and of cardiac output, including the changes produced by exercise, should be considered a standard procedure in all cases in which invasive studies are indicated. To be sure, discrepancies between hemodynamic performance and clinical performance occur: some patients with gross hemodynamic abnormalities—even at rest—may still have the capability of leading a useful, if not very active, life. This discrepancy has been discussed in connection with other forms of cardiac disease, particularly valvular heart disease. In general, results of hemodynamic study permit a good evaluation of the patient's symptomatology and, furthermore, provide a good baseline against which future studies may be compared as a means of establishing the progression of disease vs. failure to progress.

Additional information obtained by cardiac catheterization includes:

- Direct demonstration of septal perforation by means of an oxygen step-up in blood samples obtained from the right ventricle;

- Indirect demonstration of mitral regurgitation by the presence of tall v waves in left atrial or pulmonary arterial wedge pressure tracings.

Angiocardiography is the most important diagnostic procedure in the evaluation of sequels to ischemic heart disease. While results of angiocardiography do not necessarily have direct bearing upon the presence and the degree of cardiac failure, the information permits the identification of localization of abnormally contracting myocardium. The following play an important diagnostic role in angiocardiography:

- Demonstration of dyskinesia, akinesia, hypokinesia, or cardiac aneurysms;
- Overall left ventricular contractility;
- Demonstration of mitral regurgitation;
- Demonstration of septal perforation.

An important objective of angiographic examination of the left ventricle is the determination of the resectability of aneurysms. Here the determinant factors are:

- The size of the aneurysm,
- The amount of myocardium that is contracting normally,
- The localization of the aneurysm.

In addition to the qualitative aspects of the left ventriculogram, quantification of the end-systolic and end-diastolic volume can be made, as well as a semiquantitative estimation of the magnitude of mitral reflux. It should be pointed out, in connection with qualitative or quantitative determination of left ventricular performance by left ventriculography, that some caution should be applied to the results. It is well recognized that temporary left ventricular malfunction develops during ischemia; should the patient develop myocardial ischemia — with or without an anginal attack — about the time the injection of the contrast medium is done, the ventriculogram may reflect not the basal performance of the left ventricle but one under temporarily depressed conditions. Comparisons of left ventricular contractility under varying circumstances should not be accepted completely at face value.

Evaluation. The diagnostic evaluation of a patient with ischemic heart disease should always include some insight into cardiac performance — during basal conditions as well as during ischemic attacks. In order to proceed with such evaluation all diagnostic means listed in the preceding section are available. It is important, however, to define how far along this list it is necessary to proceed: particularly, whether or not studies available only in specialized centers should be done and whether or not the risk of invasive tests is indicated and, if so, how extensive an invasive evaluation is needed in each instance. The objectives of diagnostic evaluation can be summarized as follows:

1. Identification of patients with latent (subclinical) malfunction of the left ventricle;

2. Evaluation of the degree of pump failure in patients with clinical disability due to failure of the left ventricle or both ventricles;

3. Evaluation of left ventricular contractility in patients considered for aortico-coronary bypass operations;

4. Evaluation of possible candidates for aneurysmectomy;

5. Evaluation of possible candidates for mitral valve replacement;

6. Evaluation of possible candidates for septal repair.

The above objectives presuppose that the basic diagnosis of ischemic heart disease is firmly established. This is a reasonable assumption in the great majority of cases, for most patients in this category have a past (or present) history of clear-cut angina or myocardial infarction or both. One only needs to assess the possibility that ischemic heart disease may be superimposed upon another chronic cardiac disease involving and overloading the left ventricle, in which case the latter, or a combination of both, may be responsible for the pump failure. Among the other diseases one can mention:

- hypertension,

- aortic valve disease,

- mitral valve disease,

- cardiomyopathy.

When reasonable differentiation leads to the conclusion that ischemic heart disease is the only significant factor, then the evaluation should proceed along the line of identifying potential surgical candidates, in whom more elaborate studies are needed.

In considering the surgical aspects of pump failure in ischemic heart disease, two points should be emphasized:

1. Surgical treatment, though theoretically remedial and not palliative, is of only partial help in improving cardiac performance, since serious myocardial damage and the potentially dangerous ischemic aspect of the disease are still left after the operation.

2. It is difficult to predict to what extent, if any, patients will be helped by the operation. For example, resection of large aneurysms, mitral valve replacement, and elimination of interventricular shunts may still leave the patient with severe pump failure. Significant clinical improvement often ensues after a cardiac operation but it must be remembered that a critical dividing line may exist between intractable failure and disease controllable by medical therapy. Thus the patient may be taken by the operation across this critical line to a point when he can function comfortably, even though his cardiac function may still be grossly abnormal.

Because of the above considerations it is clear that prophylactic operations cannot be considered to be based on rational indications. The mere presence of a ventricular aneurysm in a patient who has few symptoms should not be considered a reason to place him in a surgical category and assure the resectability of the aneurysm.

Thus, given a patient with latent cardiac failure or controlled cardiac failure after myocardial infarction, a simple clinical evaluation should suffice. Noninvasive methods can be used as indices to study objectively the effectiveness of therapy and the progress of the disease. In some laboratories where reproducible hemodynamic studies are being performed daily, a case can be made for the performance of right heart catheterization in order to quantify cardiac performance. The information may be valuable from the prognostic standpoint and used as a baseline for comparison later in the course of the disease. Even though invasive, the risk of such study is negligible and may be outweighed by the diagnostic benefit.

Patients in overt cardiac failure who are disabled despite medical therapy can be considered potential surgical candidates. The clinical selection should be made individually, selecting for invasive study patients with a high probability of being found to be good surgical candidates. Among those are the following:

1. Patients with a reasonable probability of having a localized ventricular aneurysm (electrocardiographic evidence, discrete bulge in the plain roentgenogram);

2. Patients with a modest degree of cardiomegaly;

3. Patients with postinfarctional mitral regurgitation, in whom clinical evidence favors severe mitral reflux;

4. Patients with perforation of the ventricular septum showing increased pulmonary vascularity in the radiograph.

On the other hand, the following patients are *a priori* unlikely candidates for successful surgery:

1. Those with documented multiple myocardial infarcts in the past, particularly if several areas of the myocardium are involved electrocardiographically;

2. Those with disability from anginal attacks in addition to pump failure;

3. Patients with gross cardiac enlargement and a low intensity apical systolic murmur.

The evaluation of potential surgical candidates should include a complete hemodynamic evaluation by means of a right heart catheterization, left ventriculography (biplane cineangiography, or two injections in two views, represents the most widely used approach), and usually coronary arteriography. While revascularization procedures are not necessarily combined with aneurysmectomy or other surgical procedures, the advantages of knowing the extent of the coronary artery disease, as well as the importance of recognizing the possibility of some crucial collateral channels running over an aneurysm, justify the additional risk of the combined procedure.

THERAPY

The objectives of therapy in patients with pump failure due to ischemic heart disease include the following:

1. Continuation of basic therapy of ischemic heart disease;

2. Designation of a plan that permits the best possible function of the impaired pump, i.e., the least clinical disability;

3. Enhancement of cardiac performance by surgical therapy in carefully selected patients.

Patients suffering from myocardial damage produced by ischemic heart disease fall into two categories:

- Those with a continuing progressive occlusive coronary artery disease,

- Those with arrested coronary disease.

In the former category the stage of pump failure may be a short episode between myocardial infarction or may present itself as a competition between effort angina and effort dyspnea as to which is the more disabling factor. The presence of cardiac failure, of variable degree, may here be merely an addition to the natural history of coronary disease as outlined in Chapter 36. The second category occurs quite frequently. It represents the group of patients who were struck by myocardial infarction as a single insult. The majority of such patients return to normal activities and remain well, often for years or decades. The minority are left with a damaged myocardium, but the initiating occlusive coronary disease has ceased to be a problem.

Treatment of manifestations of ischemic disease—including management of the risk factors, as outlined above—is imperative in patients in the first category, along with control of cardiac failure.

In designing a plan for patients showing signs and symptoms of pump failure, it is first necessary to assess the severity and permanency of the disability. As stated in the section on natural history, some patients with overt cardiac failure during infarction regain good compensation after recovery and remain well; some do not develop evidence of failure until they have resumed active lives after convalescence from myocardial infarction. Cardiac failure developing insidiously may be progressive or may remain stable at any stage. Thus, after the assessment is made concerning which category the patient is placed into, the responses to medical therapy should be evaluated. Only after these two steps have been taken is one justified in advising the patient regarding his long-range plans: resumption of gainful activity, full responsibility vs. change in position, retraining for a less strenuous (or stressful) occupation. Regulation of recreational activities and travel should also be considered in the light of the actual and potential disability.

The actual treatment consists of conventional therapy for congestive cardiac failure: digitalis, diuretics, dietary restriction, regulation of activities.

Surgical therapy involves, in theory, three approaches:

- Revascularization by means of bypass operations,

- Enhancement of myocardial contractility,

- Reduction of overload.

Revascularization procedures have been discussed in Chapter 36. It was pointed out that poor myocardial function increases the risk of bypass operations so that it is considered a relative contraindication for this type of surgery. It follows that most patients with overt pump failure would fall into this category. The question was raised early in the history of coronary bypass surgery as to whether poorly functioning myocardium may not show better performance after revascularization. This can obviously apply only to ischemia and not to permanent fibrotic changes in the myocardium. Even though some studies showed improved myocardial contractility after revascularization, more convincing evidence is now available that such improvement is rare — perhaps applicable only to those whose preoperative studies were performed in severely ischemic states ("preinfarction angina"). Thus bypass surgery is not indicated for the primary purpose of enhancement of myocardial contractility.

Patients who suffer from both severe angina and pump failure are, as already stated, not good candidates for bypass surgery. Yet, given a situation where a study is performed and a very precarious lesion is found — e.g., severe obstructing lesion of the main left coronary artery — the higher risk of the operation may be acceptable.

Similar considerations occur in patients who are to undergo operations for aneurysmectomy, mitral valve operation, or septal repair. The demonstration of an especially precarious obstructive coronary lesion may lead to the decision to add a revascularization procedure to the principal operation even if the patient does not have active ischemic symptoms.

The prime indication for aneurysmectomy is the presence of cardiac failure unresponsive to medical therapy. In addition, there are rare patients in whom persistent ventricular arrhythmias may be life-threatening but who are unaffected by antiarrhythmic treatment. Experience has shown that aneurysmectomy may entirely eliminate the proneness to arrhythmias, and this constitutes an additional indication for aneurysmectomy. (Aneurysmectomy during acute myocardial infarction for intractable arrhythmias has been mentioned in Chapter 22.) Occasional arguments to the effect that aneurysmectomy may be justifiable for the prevention of systemic emboli from mural thrombi are not supported by data showing a favorable risk-benefit ratio. Presently available information suggests that the risk of serious emboli is too small to balance the surgical mortality.

From the standpoint of surgical feasibility and prospects for clinical improvement, the prime candidates for aneurysmectomy are patients with apical aneurysms. Even large apical aneurysms leave, as a rule, important portions of the left ventricular musculature, including the papillary muscles, intact. As already indicated, the principal conditions for a favorable case are:

- Vigorous contractility of the nonaneurysmal part of the ventricle;

- Absence of gross enlargement of the entire left ventricular cavity;

- Noninvolvement of the papillary muscle in the aneurysm;

- Absence of important collateral channels across the subepicardial portion of the aneurysm.

Indications for mitral valve replacement include primarily the demonstration of severe mitral regurgitation. Inasmuch as the goal of the operation is reduction of overload, at least a 3+ mitral regurgitation (upon the scale of 4+) may constitute a significant increase in workload to provide good probability of improvement. The presence of mitral regurgitation is frequently combined with major damage to the free wall of the left ventricle; consequently aneurysms commonly coexist with mitral regurgitation. Patients should thus be investigated from the standpoint of resectable aneurysms, which — if found — should be removed at the time of valve replacement.

Indications for the repair of septal perforation follow the same guidelines as those for mitral regurgitation: large shunt and a search for a coexisting aneurysm.

Bibliography

Davis RW, Ebert PA: Ventricular aneurysm: A clinical pathological correlation. Amer. J. Cardiol. *29*:1, 1972.

Herman MV, Heinle RA, Klein MD, Gorlin R: Localized disorders in myocardial contraction. Asynergy and its role in congestive heart failure. New Engl. J. Med. *277*:222, 1967.

Jacobs JJ, Feingenbaum H, Corya BC, Phillips JF: Detection of left ventricular asynergy by echocardiography. Circulation *48*:263, 1973.

Selzer A, Gerbode F, Kerth WJ: Clinical, hemodynamic and surgical considerations of rupture of the ventricular septum after myocardial infarction. Amer. Heart J. *78*:598, 1969.

Selzer A, Katayama F: Mitral regurgitations: Clinical patterns, pathophysiology and natural history: VII. Postinfarctional mitral regurgitation. Medicine *51*:350, 1972.

38

Cardiomyopathies

Definition. The term "cardiomyopathy" is usually applied to a heterogeneous group of conditions in which involvement of the myocardium is the principal abnormality. There are a great many classifications of cardiomyopathy, mostly because of the varied clinical and pathological manifestations and the many unanswered questions regarding the etiological factors. Another major difficulty in this field is the inability to establish a firm clinical diagnosis by means other than the exclusion of other cardiac diseases. (Myocardial biopsy, which may establish a firm pathological diagnosis, is not yet considered safe or conclusive enough to become a widely accepted procedure.)

Once thought of as a rare form of cardiac disease, cardiomyopathy is now encountered frequently, though its incidence is below that of ischemic and valvular forms of cardiac disease and possibly congenital heart disease as well. Classifications of cardiomyopathy customarily list several etiological factors responsible for the myocardial insult. However, the "idiopathic" form—that of unknown etiology—accounts for the vast preponderance of cases in the Western countries, perhaps as high as 90 per cent, so that more specific forms of it are relatively rare. Not included in this discussion is the obstructive form of cardiomyopathy, in which the principal problem is obstruction of the outflow from the left ventricle and which has been discussed in Chapter 31.

ETIOLOGY

As stated, the commonest form of cardiomyopathy is one with an unknown etiology. The remainder fall into two categories:

- those with a known etiological factor,

- those subject to controversy as to whether the etiological factor is the sole cause or merely a contributory factor.

The principal etiological factors recognized as causes of cardiomyopathy are:

1. Viral infection — usually the chronic stage after acute myocarditis.

2. Infiltrative or degenerative diseases: hemochromatosis, amyloidosis, sickle cell disease, sarcoidosis, glycogen storage disease, carcinomatosis, etc.

3. Toxic: beer-drinkers' disease (cobalt contamination),? alcoholic.

4. Nutritional; beriberi heart disease, ? tropical cardiomyopathy.

Those forms of cardiomyopathy in which an etiological factor may or may not be the sole cause are:

- alcoholic cardiomyopathy,

- peripartum cardiomyopathy.

Among the forms of cardiomyopathy of unknown etiology, one can separate the true idiopathic form — that of congestive failure developing without known cause, usually in middle-aged subjects — and various forms that offer distinctive patterns by their clinical course, their pathological findings, or their association with other disease:

- congenital endomyocardial fibrosis (fibroelastosis),

- familial cardiomyopathy,

- tropical obliterative cardiomyopathy,

- adult fibroelastosis (possibly a nontropical form of the former),

- idiopathic cardiac hypertrophy,

- cardiomyopathy associated with various forms of muscular dystrophy.

PATHOLOGY

Gross pathology includes in the great majority of cases of cardiomyopathy two principal features:

- hypertrophy of the heart — mostly of the left ventricle,

- dilatation and "flabbiness" of the heart.

Special forms of cardiomyopathy may be recognized by some additional features:

- white thickening of the ventricular endocardium,

- various infiltrative processes.

Mural thrombi commonly are found in cardiomyopathic hearts, and are usually located in the ventricles. It is important that the presence of coronary atherosclerosis of significant degree be ruled out before the diagnosis of cardiomyopathy is made.

Microscopic sections reveal hypertrophy of myocardial fibers with or without fibrosis, which can be patchy or disseminated. Only occasionally are cellular infiltrates found.

PATHOPHYSIOLOGY

From the standpoint of pathophysiology three basic mechanisms participate in this disease process:

1. Primary dilatation of the left ventricle with inability to maintain an adequate cardiac output (primary pump failure).

2. Primary cardiac hypertrophy producing decreased cardiac compliance — eventually causing resistance to diastolic filling of a ventricle.

3. Endocardial restriction due to fibrosis, interfering with the diastolic filling in a manner similar to that of constrictive pericarditis.

The fourth mechanism — resistance to left ventricular outflow — was discussed elsewhere (Chapter 31).

Hemodynamic abnormalities in primary pump failure ("congestive cardiomyopathy") present themselves as low-output cardiac failure. Left ventricular failure is the principal feature, with elevated filling pressures and decreased cardiac output. Passive pulmonary hypertension, then right ventricular failure follow. It is probable, though not definitely established, that reactive pulmonary hypertension is rare.

In the hypertrophic (nonobstructive) form of cardiomyopathy the decreased left ventricular compliance is shown by higher filling pressures. Thus the pressure-volume curve may be normal but shifted to a higher pressure level. The cardiac function may remain normal for varying periods of time. When decompensation ensues, the usual chain of hemodynamic events takes place, including further elevation of diastolic pressure, reduction of cardiac output, pulmonary hypertension, and right ventricular failure. Eventually marked dilatation of the heart may develop and the difference between congestive cardiomyopathy and hypertrophic cardiomyopathy becomes obliterated. These same late changes may occur in patients with the obstructive type of hypertrophic cardiomyopathy.

In the restrictive type of cardiomyopathy elevation of atrial pressure in both sides of the circulation develops early. Hemodynamic abnormalities become indistinguishable from those of constrictive pericarditis, namely the M-shaped right atrial pressure curve and the early diastolic dip with a late diastolic plateau found in right ventricular (less often in left ventricular) pressure curves. Right ventricular pressure measurements may show a disproportionate elevation of diastolic pressure in relation to its systolic pressure level.

NATURAL HISTORY

The natural history of cardiomyopathies is not yet fully known. Most information dates back to times when only more advanced cases were recognized and the various forms had not yet been identified, hence the general impression that cardiomyopathy presents itself as a rapidly progressive, unrelenting cardiac failure.

In general, the course of cardiomyopathy is related to its clinical type and pathophysiological pattern, on the one hand, and to the rapidity with which the pathological process progresses (or possibly regresses in response to specific therapy) on the other hand.

In hypertrophic cardiomyopathy one can expect the most benign course. With or without outflow obstruction, the hypertrophic form of cardiomyopathy by definition represents a prefailure stage of the disease. Judging from the obstructive variety, which is as a rule earlier identified clinically, patients may remain in a stable condition for many years. Not enough cases have been followed carefully to know the mode and speed with which congestive phenomena develop.

In congestive cardiomyopathy cardiac failure is clinically evident early. The usual sequence — namely left ventricular failure occurring first, followed by right ventricular failure — seems to predominate. Many patients present themselves with symptoms of cardiac failure; therefore the duration of the asymptomatic stage is not known. (There can be no question that many patients do not have hypertrophy at all, hence myocardial dilatation and failure occur first.) Occasionally, unusual findings bring the attention of the physician to the possibility that he may be dealing with early cardiomyopathy before significant symptoms develop. Such findings include electrocardiographic abnormalities, cardiac enlargement, and arrhythmias — for which there are no other causes. Yet at this stage the difficulty of establishing the diagnosis is obvious.

When florid cardiac failure ensues the responses to therapy vary.

Some patients respond to treatment well—they may be controlled by a medical regimen to a point of resuming an active life, sometimes for many years. Sooner or later, however, they become refractory to medical therapy. The stage of intractable cardiac failure develops in which therapy has little to offer to the patient. In other patients the disease progresses rapidly, shows little response to therapy, and follows a generally malignant course.

Patients with restrictive forms of cardiomyopathy are, as a rule, sicker than those with the congestive form. This may of course be due to their earlier recognition, since the initial appearance of congestive phenomena tends to bring them to the attention of the physician. Here the clinical picture is, as stated, similar to that of constrictive pericarditis, often producing ascites, hepatomegaly, and edema. Dyspnea may be minimal or altogether absent; the patient may become aware of edema and abdominal fullness as the first symptom. Even though the clinical course may be protracted for months or years, the response to medical therapy is usually poor.

The general *symptomatology* of cardiomyopathies is variable. Most patients present themselves with dyspnea of effort or its paroxysmal varieties. Weakness and fatigability are also common, in line with the frequency with which very low cardiac output is present. Anginal type chest pain occurs; some series place its incidence as high as 10 per cent of cases. Some symptoms are related to the complications of cardiomyopathy.

Complications of cardiomyopathies vary with the specific forms as well as the pathophysiological patterns:

- Sudden death is relatively rare. It is known to occur unexpectedly in seemingly well patients with obstructive cardiomyopathy, and possibly in the nonobstructive hypertrophic variety as well. Some patients present a history of relatives dying suddenly without previous knowledge of cardiac disease, obviously representing familial incidence of hypertrophic cardiomyopathy.

- Systemic embolization may occur in all forms of congestive cardiomyopathy. It is considered especially common (but still affecting only a small fraction of cases) in nutritional cardiomyopathy (beriberi), in alcoholic cardiomyopathy, and in the peripartum variety.

- Atrial arrhythmias—chronic flutter or fibrillation—occur commonly, especially in alcoholic cardiomyopathy.

- Ventricular arrhythmias occur occasionally, but are not as frequently encountered as in acute myocarditis.

- Conduction disturbances involving the peripheral portion of the conducting system are very common — bundle-branch block represents a frequent electrocardiographic abnormality. Higher blocks, including complete heart block, occur occasionally and may lead to the Stokes-Adams type of syncope. They are thought to occur preferentially in congenital forms, especially in fibroelastosis.

- Pulmonary emboli are common in the congestive type — a frequent sequel to low cardiac output from any cause.

- Mitral regurgitation occurs commonly in conditions associated with left ventricular enlargement; hence the presence of an apical systolic murmur is not unusual. Severe mitral regurgitation, however, is much less common in cardiomyopathy than is ischemic heart disease. Its most frequent appearance is in fibroelastosis.

CLINICAL PATTERNS

While the etiological factors and the pathophysiological varieties of cardiomyopathies have been described in the preceding sections, a few comments on the types of cardiomyopathy that may represent specific clinical syndromes are in order. Among those are the following:

- *Alcoholic cardiomyopathy.* It is generally agreed that alcoholic cardiomyopathy is not the result of dietary deficiency, except under unusual circumstances. Two schools of thought propose alcohol as the toxic agent damaging the myocardium (experimental evidence and electron microscopic studies support this principle) — directly, on the one hand, while, on the other hand, alcohol is seen as a precipitating agent in the multifactorial origin of cardiomyopathy or in susceptible individuals. Alcoholic cardiomyopathy may take a protracted course over many years; arrhythmias and systemic embolization are relatively common.

- *Peripartum cardiomyopathy.* This may be a specific disease associated with pregnancy or may be a form of latent cardiomyopathy brought to the surface during the stress of pregnancy. It occurs in late pregancy or in the postpartum period. Sudden onset of cardiac failure occurs; the response to therapy is often gratifying: few women die acutely. It has been suggested that the long-range prognosis is favorable in women who retain small hearts or show only a mild degree of cardiomegaly. Those with gross cardiomegaly may remain in failure, with a large proportion of them running a downhill course within months or years.

DIAGNOSIS

Clinical examination. Because of the broadly nonspecific nature of cardiomyopathy the history is not likely to provide many clues directing attention toward this diagnosis. The past history, family history, and background history are more likely to yield pertinent information than can be obtained from the symptomatology of the present illness.

Physical examination may show—as expected—a broad range of findings:

- Left ventricular hypertrophy may be suggested by a forceful and protracted apical impulse.

- Abnormal precordial motion (including diastolic pulsation) may be present in patients with cardiac failure.

- Gallop sounds—both S3 and S4—are commonly found; reversed splitting of the second sound may be perceived, particularly if left bundle branch block is present.

- Apical holosystolic murmurs signifying mitral valve incompetence are relatively common.

- Arterial pulses show wide variation: small pulses in advanced cardiac failure may be present; rapid pulses are occasionally seen in hyperkinetic states; pulsus alternans may be present.

- Venous pulse may show evidence of increased venous pressure with or without evidence of tricuspid regurgitation.

- Signs of systemic venous congestion—hepatomegaly, ascites, anasarca—are often present, as mentioned, particularly in the restrictive type of cardiomyopathy.

Radiographic examination as a rule shows cardiomegaly. The cardiovascular shadow shows no characteristic abnormalities, only generalized cardiac enlargement. Pulmonary vascular congestion and pleural effusion are often present.

Electrocardiographic findings include the following:

- intraventricular conduction defects, of which complete left bundle branch block is the commonest;

- left ventricular hypertrophy;

- nonspecific T wave abnormalities;

- infarct-like Q wave abnormalities;

- a variety of arrhythmias;

- complete AV block.

Echocardiographic examination reveals no characteristic findings. One can usually detect the presence of a large left ventricular cavity or enlargement of both ventricles. Poor contractility of the ventricular wall can also be detected. Although no systematic studies have been conducted in this respect, it is possible that echocardiographic findings may represent a valuable method of detecting early cardiomyopathy, if decreased amplitude of ventricular contraction combined with electrocardiographic abnormalities is found in asymptomatic patients.

Cardiac catheterization cannot provide any information that would confirm a clinical diagnosis of cardiomyopathy. Nevertheless, it fulfills an important diagnostic role, particularly in ruling out alternate diagnoses. Hemodynamic abnormalities include a broad range, as already mentioned, from a normal performance in the presence of elevated filling pressures to grossly abnormal patterns identical with those of constrictive pericarditis. Cardiac catheterization, in addition to being an aid in differential diagnosis, provides the means of assessing the left ventricular function, thus permitting some rough insight into the prognosis and a means of determining whether the disease is progressive or not, as well as of recognizing the speed of possible change.

Angiocardiography serves a function similar to that of cardiac catheterization. The most important differentiation is that from ischemic heart disease. The basic difference between the two is localized and segmental malfunction of the left ventricular myocardium in ischemic disease and the generally poor contractility in cardiomyopathy. Yet the overlap is considerable. "Cardiomyopathic" types of ischemic heart disease are angiocardiographically indistinguishable from other forms of cardiomyopathy, while segmental malcontraction of the left ventricle is occasionally seen in cardiomyopathy. The question is often considered whether coronary arteriography should be routinely performed as a means of settling this difficult differential diagnosis. Considering the fact that the risk of coronary arteriography is to some extent increased in seriously ill patients, this additional risk is not warranted unless practical information — particularly that pertaining to future management of the patient — is likely to result from the examination. This is seldom the case in patients with the differential diagnosis under consideration, so that coronary arteriography is indicated only under exceptional circumstances.

Evaluation. The objectives of diagnostic evaluation are as follows:

1. The establishment of a firm (or reasonable) diagnosis of cardiomyopathy and the exclusion of other curable or correctable forms of cardiac disease.

2. The assessment of the degree of myocardial involvement and an estimation of the progressive nature of the disease.

3. A search for known factors in the etiology, with special reference to the rare instances of finding those amenable to specific therapy.

As in the other forms of cardiac disease evaluation of patients revolves around the question, When are specialized studies and invasive procedures indicated? In cardiomyopathy this question is even more difficult to answer than in many other cardiac conditions. It has been emphasized throughout the discussion that cardiomyopathy does not have any characteristic features to establish a positive diagnosis by any known means short of biopsy. The exception to this is, of course, hypertrophic obstructive cardiomyopathy, which has been discussed in Chapter 23. Thus, being an exclusion diagnosis, the differential diagnosis has to be even more exhaustive than in other cardiac diseases.

Given an asymptomatic patient or one with minor symptomatology in whom the possibility of cardiomyopathy is suggested by abnormal electrocardiographic findings, by cardiomegaly, and so on, further studies have little to contribute to the diagnosis. Echocardiographic demonstration of impaired cardiac wall contractility is, as stated, a simple and valuable means of firming up the possibility. The only valid indication for invasive studies in such patients is the presence of a positive sign suggesting an alternative possibility, e.g., a cardiac murmur.

In patients who have varying degrees of disability and in whom no other basis for cardiac failure can be found a complete evaluation is indicated. While the value of echocardiography in screening out some diseases that may come up in differential diagnosis—e.g., atypical mitral stenosis, cardiac myxoma—is unquestionable, it is nevertheless important to investigate all possibilities, in view of the generally hopeless nature of cardiomyopathy, and at the same time to evaluate the hemodynamic condition of the patient.

The differential diagnosis of cardiomyopathy involves virtually every other form of cardiac disease. Ischemic heart disease presents the most difficulty, as already discussed. Atypical valvular heart disease, "burned out" hypertension, congenital heart disease, pulmonary disease, pericardial disease—all may present diagnostic difficulties. Because of the wide variety of conditions that need to be excluded when accepting the diagnosis of cardiomyopathy, it is important that the cardiac catheterization and angiocardiographic team have a complete grasp of all the clinical problems that may even remotely point in the direction of another condition.

In the evaluation of the degree of cardiac involvement and the progression of the disease, the initial study is an important part of the overall evaluation. A carefully designed study of cardiac performance, including the response to exercise, will constitute the baseline material for a longitudinal study. A follow-up study may be indicated when the patient shows clinical deterioration, if he fails to respond to therapy, or if new signs and symptoms appear. Usually the follow-up study need only include a right-sided cardiac catheterization without angiocardiographic follow-up examination.

THERAPY

Basically, the treatment of cardiomyopathy has little to offer to the patient in terms of reversing the nature of the disease or arresting its progress. Specific therapy can be considered only under unusual circumstances in rare cases. Among these are:

- Correction of nutritional deficiencies in beriberi heart disease;

- Reversal of alcoholic cardiomyopathy after discontinuing the use of alcohol;

- Steroid therapy in cardiomyopathy caused by immune mechanisms (e.g., in systemic lupus erythematosus);

- Removal of iron storages by bleeding patients with hemochromatosis.

It should be emphasized that many of these conditions are reversible more in theory than in practice. The cardiac damage often reaches a point of no return, in which case even the removal of the etiological agent is of no avail. Nevertheless, occasional successes in these conditions are being reported from time to time, usually in isolated cases.

In the great majority of patients cardiac therapy has the following objectives:

1. Control of cardiac failure;

2. Maintenance of the optimal mode of living for a patient;

3. Treatment and prevention of complications.

In treating cardiac failure conventional means are being used. As a rule patients are less apt to respond to therapy than in many other forms of cardiac disease. Digitalis is poorly tolerated and awareness of digitalis toxicity should be high. Reduction of activities and sodium restriction in the diet may be more effective than diuretic therapy. Long periods of bed rest have been recommended with claims of dramatic successes. It is theoretically possible to postulate a reversible element in some of the myocardial processes comprising cardiomyopathies, given as complete protection from overload as possible. Yet, the impracticability of subjecting patients to a year of absolute bed rest limits the usefulness of this treatment and at the same time does not permit studies of adequate series to test the consistency of the effectiveness of prolonged rest.

Perhaps the important challenge in the therapy of cardiomyopathy—one to which the answer is not available—is how to treat patients when detected in the early stages of the disease. Should one permit patients to perform to the limit of their tolerance or restrict them? If they happen to be of sedentary habits would physical conditioning be an advantage or a detriment in regard to the progress of their disease?

Complications of cardiomyopathy are neither frequent enough nor consistent enough to recommend specific prophylactic therapy. Thus treatment is limited to the management of existing complications and to the prevention of recurrences. Patients who have shown evidence of systemic embolization may benefit from the chronic use of anticoagulants. Those in atrial fibrillation of recent origin may be converted to sinus rhythm by quinidine or electroshock; if successful, quinidine maintenance therapy is indicated for indefinite periods of time. If conversion is unsuccessful or atrial fibrillation recurs, digitalis control of ventricular rate is indicated. Other arrhythmias are treated as necessary. Complete heart block usually requires pacemaker insertion because of the proneness to syncope.

Surgical treatment has little to offer to patients short of cardiac transplantation. However, in very rare instances secondary mitral regurgitation may become very severe, particularly in patients with endocardiac fibroelastosis. Valve replacement has been performed in isolated cases—in some the relief of overload has produced satisfactory remission of the entire process.

Bibliography

Brigden WW, Robinson JF: Alcoholic heart disease. Brit. Med. J. 2:1283, 1964.
Buja LM, Khoi NB, Roberts WC: Clinically significant cardiac amyloidosis. Amer. J. Cardiol. 26:394, 1970.
Davies NJP, Ball JD: The pathology of endomyocardial fibrosis in Uganda. Brit. Heart J. 17:337, 1955.
Demakis JE, Rahimtoola SH, Sutton GC, Meadows WR, Szanto PB, Tobin JR, Gunnar RM: Natural course of peripartum cardiomyopathy. Circulation 44:1053, 1971.
Fowler NO, Gueron M, Rowlands DT Jr: Primary myocardial disease. Circulation 23: 493, 1961.
Fowler NO: Classification and differential diagnosis of the cardiomyopathies. Prog. Cardiovasc. Dis. 7:1, 1964.
Goodwin JF, Oakley CM: The cardiomyopathies. Brit. Heart J. 34:545, 1972.
Goodwin JF: Treatment of cardiomyopathies. Amer. J. Cardiol. 32:341, 1973.
Mattingly TW: Changing concepts of myocardial disease. J.A.M.A. 191:33, 1965.
Perloff JK: The cardiomyopathies—current perspectives. Circulation 44:942, 1971.
Segal JP, Harvey WP: Diagnosis and treatment of primary myocardial disease. Circulation 32:857, 1965.

39

Hypertensive Cardiovascular Disease

Definition. Hypertension represents a state in which the systemic arterial pressure is abnormally high. It is thus not a disease, not even a syndrome—merely a clinical finding. Elevated systemic pressure can be a temporary finding or a permanent finding. Permanent elevation of arterial pressure may be a primary manifestation of a disease state or a secondary phenomenon. In either case hypertension, once established, takes its own course and produces certain consequences that are no longer related to the initiating mechanism which led to elevation of the blood pressure. Thus the term hypertensive cardiovascular disease connotes clinical conditions in which hypertension plays a key part.

Hypertensive cardiovascular disease encompasses the following conditions:

1. Essential hypertension—a disease of unknown cause.

2. Hypertension of known origin in which elevation of blood pressure is the principal manifestation of disease as in the following:

   • renovascular hypertension,

   • pheochromocytoma,

   • primary aldosteronism.

3. Hypertension of known origin in which elevation of blood pressure is one of several problems:

   • glomerulonephritis,

- pyelonephritis,

- polycystic kidneys,

- coarctation of the aorta,

- Cushing's syndrome,

- collagen vascular disease.

One of the more important decisions facing the clinician is the determination in an individual case of the answer to the question, When is hypertension (a disease) present? Arbitrary levels of the upper limit of normal blood pressure are usually set at 150/90, yet the significance of such figures is limited by the variability of blood pressure from moment to moment as well as by the variations related to age and sex. Ideally, basal levels of blood pressure need to be determined. Under ordinary circumstances, only casual readings are usually obtained. The physician's office, the outpatient clinic, the hospital—those are settings in which unusual tension may be present, potentially raising the systemic pressure above the individual's norm. The various techniques of obtaining more reliable readings of blood pressure and the difficulty of their interpretation will be discussed later in the section on diagnosis.

Another difficulty and controversy concerning the problem of hypertension involves the concept of "malignant hypertension." Once a subject of heated arguments as to whether it is a different disease or merely a stage of hypertensive disease in general, malignant hypertension today is widely believed to represent merely an accelerated progression of the sequels of hypertension, produced by its unusual severity.

PATHOGENESIS AND ETIOLOGICAL FACTORS

Hypertensive cardiovascular disease does not represent a distinct clinical entity; hence one cannot discuss its etiology in the ordinary sense. Rather, the various mechanisms that can lead to permanent elevation of blood pressure will be discussed in the light of various initiating and causative factors as well as some background influences.

The systemic blood pressure is maintained at its relatively high level under normal conditions in healthy subjects by the arteriolar resistance according to the following formula:

$$\text{Pressure (mean)} = \text{cardiac output (flow)} \times \text{resistance}$$

It follows that the arteriolar resistance has to vary constantly and inversely with the change in cardiac output. Thus, if during exercise cardiac output increases threefold, an almost equivalent fall in arteriolar resistance has to occur simultaneously since the arterial pressure shows only small variation. This effective regulatory mechanism occurs largely by means of the barostatic sensors within the aorta and the carotids and appropriate reflexes. This homeostatic mechanism is set at a certain level. In addition, swings of blood pressure occur — mostly via changes in arteriolar resistance — by means of various neurogenic and humoral influences, mostly mediated via the autonomic nervous system. In hypertension temporary swings occur first, then more frequently and at an exaggerated pace, and eventually the whole barostatic mechanism is reset at a higher level. Persistent hypertension may develop as a result of an increase either in cardiac output or in arteriolar resistance: in the great majority of cases the latter factor is solely responsible for the pressure elevation. High cardiac output has been demonstrated only in the early stages of hypertension, usually when the hypertension is still labile.

Several mechanisms, occurring independently of each other or in combination (often causally related), are capable of resetting the barostatic mechanism at a hypertensive level. Restoration of a normal setting is possible in most cases, either by the removal of the causative factor or by appropriate drug therapy.

Among the mechanisms the following play an important role:

1. The angiotensin-renin axis — a humoral mechanism initiated in the kidneys and implicated in renovascular hypertension; this probably participates also in the production of other forms of renal hypertension, and is considered by some to be a contributory agent in at least some cases of essential hypertension. For four decades, since the classical experiments of Goldblatt, it has been known that obstruction in the path of arterial circulation to the kidney produces hypertension via a humoral mechanism. What is usually referred to as an "ischemic kidney" but perhaps better termed a "malperfused kidney" (it is difficult to accept the concept of ischemia in the same sense as in "myocardial ischemia" when dealing with the kidney — an organ that has the most wasteful oxygen supply in the body) produces a pressure-increasing substance, presumably angiotensin or its derivatives. This leads to hypertension, its severity related to the extent of the renal circulatory disturbance. Both experimentally and in humans, this mechanism has been shown to operate; its reversibility is demonstrated whenever normal renal circulation can be restored.

2. Catecholamines — primarily norepinephrine — are operating in hypertension produced by pheochromocytoma.

3. Aldosterone is the most important hormone producing hypertension associated with primary or secondary hyperfunction of the adrenal cortex.

4. Neurogenic factors, as mentioned, play the essential role in the regulatory mechanism of blood pressure and are largely responsible for the swings and overshoots of arterial pressure. Suspected by some to play a major causative role in some cases of hypertension, their contribution to this disease is not well understood.

5. Changes in blood volume, usually secondary to other mechanisms, may play an important role in the causation of hypertension, e.g., in acute glomerulonephritis.

6. Electrolyte imbalance—particularly involving sodium—also mostly a secondary factor, may assume a significant role in hypertension. The regulation of sodium intake is a mechanism of increasing or reducing blood pressure.

7. Mechanical factors operate in coarctation of the aorta. Here the resistance to blood flow is a major contributory factor in maintaining hypertension in the upper part of the body (see Chapter 31).

Among the etiological factors affecting hypertension, heredity is by far the most important one. Pickering advances the view that hypertension represents merely a normal variant—i.e., the segment of the normal population contained at the very upper end of the frequency distribution curve of blood pressure, genetically determined and perpetuated. It becomes a "disease" because, once blood pressure is elevated, a chain of events is unleashed that adversely affects the circulatory system. Other factors, such as race and nutrition, have also been implicated. In some races—particularly among Blacks—hypertension tends to take a more serious clinical course. Pregnancy is an important precipitating factor, sometimes bringing hypertension into an overt state.

The hemodynamic abnormalities in hypertension are restricted to the elevation of the systemic arterial pressure. As stated, cardiac output may be abnormally high, but usually it is normal and high pressure is maintained by persistent elevation of arteriolar resistance. The increase in systemic arterial pressure, if unchecked, produces overloading of the left ventricle and may lead to its failure, with all its further consequences.

PATHOLOGY

Pathological changes associated with hypertension include those causing hypertension and those resulting from hypertension. The principal condition is a functional one, without a pathological basis.

In essential hypertension the cause of the disease is not known; thus in the largest group of cases pathological changes appear late; the current trend of early commencement of therapy often makes hypertension a curable or controllable disease—consequently pathological changes are altogether prevented.

The consequences of hypertension show up in the "target organs," which include the arteries and arterioles, the heart, the kidneys, and the brain.

The arterial system presents three sets of changes:

- the effects of prolonged spasm,

- acceleration of atherosclerosis,

- special complications.

The arterioles are the prime targets of prolonged spasm. The early changes resulting there include thickening of the media; with longer duration and increased severity of hypertension ("malignant hypertension") proliferation and vacuolization of the intima take place, eventually leading to obliteration of many arterioles.

The evidence for the acceleration of the atherosclerotic process in hypertensive subjects is convincing. The areas most vulnerable to the acceleration of atherosclerosis are the kidneys, the heart, and the brain. Renal changes are most characteristic, leading to "nephrosclerosis," which may appear early and has raised the question as to whether such renal changes represent the effect or the cause of hypertension.

Among complications resulting from severe hypertension are the following:

- dissecting aneurysms of the aorta,

- hemorrhages in various areas,

- infarcts of organs.

The heart shows pure work hypertrophy similar to that produced by other cases of pressure overload (e.g., aortic stenosis). Concentric hypertrophy is present until late stages when cardiac failure appears, at which time dilatation of the left ventricle appears. The consequences of accelerated atherosclerosis include the usual manifestations of coronary artery disease.

Cerebral changes include hemorrhages, which can affect extracerebral arteries (subarachnoid hemorrhages) or intracerebral arteries, and cerebral infarcts.

NATURAL HISTORY

The course of hypertension is influenced by the following:

1. The severity and duration of hypertension,

2. Effectiveness of therapy,

3. Development of irreversible sequels and complications,

4. The effects of associated diseases.

Wide variations of blood pressure make the evaluation of the severity, even the existence, of hypertensive disease difficult. Practical means of approaching this problem will be discussed in a later section of this chapter. Measurement of blood pressure and its longitudinal follow-up have such low reliability that it is necessary to rely primarily upon the consequences of hypertension, i.e., its effects upon the target organs.

Recently it has been suggested (Laragh, 1972) that essential hypertension may occur in the form of a predominantly vasoconstrictive condition ("high renin") or predominantly as a hypervolemic state ("low renin"), the former carrying a poorer prognosis than the latter. This concept requires confirmation and has not yet been universally accepted.

The effect of therapy upon the natural history of hypertension depends upon several factors:

- Whether surgical cure is available (totally reversible forms include pheochromocytoma, coarctation of the aorta, aldosterone-secreting tumors, and some forms of renovascular hypertension);

- Whether medical (antihypertensive) therapy is applied to an optimal extent and is adhered to by the patient;

- Whether at the time of initiation of therapy irreversible damage to organs was already present (renal insufficiency, severe cardiac hypertrophy).

The two most important late sequels of long-standing and severe hypertension are, as mentioned, renal damage and failure and left ventricular hypertrophy resulting in cardiac failure. Severe vascular disease is best observed by the changes in the ocular fundi, which have been classified by Keith and Wagner in four grades. Complications of hypertension include two major categories:

- Periodic exacerbation of the severity of hypertension, as exemplified by hypertensive encephalopathy;

- The effect of hypertension upon atherosclerotic disease, enhancing and accelerating its severity and leading to cardiac and cerebral occlusive vascular disease.

Among associated diseases affecting the course of hypertension the principal problem involves conditions in which hypertension is a symptom of diseases which have their own effect upon the patient's health, e.g., primary renal disease, Cushing's syndrome, and others, as listed previously.

GENERAL SYMPTOMATOLOGY OF HYPERTENSION

Hypertension produces few symptoms directly related to the elevation of arterial pressure. Headaches are traditionally considered characteristic of hypertension, yet their relationship to the latter is uncertain, and their occurrence is variable. Only in the most severe forms of hypertension—malignant hypertension—are disabling headaches found with a degree of frequency. Patients occasionally are aware of the increased throbbing in the head and neck, particularly at night. Some may refer to this phenomenon as "palpitations."

VARIETIES OF HYPERTENSION

Essential hypertension accounts for the great majority of cases of hypertension. Representing hypertension of unknown etiology, essential hypertension has always served as a "wastebasket" which in the distant past included all forms of hypertension not related to *overt* renal disease and from which, one by one, all presently recognized forms of hypertension were separated. At present "essential hypertension" represents a term applied most widely to benign hypertension of undetermined etiology. The most remarkable feature of essential hypertension is the wide variability of its effect upon end-organs. Some patients—particularly postmenopausal women—may have persistent hypertension for decades untreated, without showing any critical ill effects, even presenting normal electrocardiograms. Other patients who present modest elevation of arterial pressure may show early evidence of left ventricular hypertrophy. While it is logical to assume that the former group of patients may represent those who carry mostly normotensive arterial pressure levels but are subject to severe hypertensive overshoots (particularly at the time their pressure is being recorded), this benign course may be related to other, as yet unidentified, factors.

Malignant hypertension differs from other forms of hypertension in its unusual severity. As already indicated, it was once a subject of controversy as to whether it represents a different disease or merely a stage or phase of hypertension. It is now clearly demonstrated that clinical features of malignant hypertension may be found in severe hypertension produced by some known factors as well as in those of unknown origin. Thus not only may "essential" hypertension acquire malignant features but also renovascular hypertension, that produced by pheochromocytoma, pyelonephritis, or even coarctation of the aorta. Experimentally, features characteristic of malignant hypertension may be reproduced by a more severe derangement of renal blood flow than that producing benign hypertension. The clinical features of malignant hypertension include the following:

- Persistent elevation of diastolic pressure, usually above 120 mm. Hg;

- Advanced changes in the ocular fundi (K-W grade III or IV);

- Evidence of progressive renal failure;

- Presence of severe left ventricular hypertrophy;

- Central nervous system changes with susceptibility to attacks of encephalopathy.

The presence of malignant hypertension with its accelerated progression naturally makes the prognosis guarded. Yet aggressive therapy still is capable of reversing or at least preventing the progression of the process, unless irreversible renal failure is already present.

Renal vascular hypertension encompasses a variety of unrelated conditions in which a disturbance of renal arterial circulation can be found without primary involvement of the renal parenchyma. These include:

- Congenital disturbances of the renal arterial circulation;

- Stenosis of a renal artery by a plaque, fibromuscular hyperplasia, thrombosis, or embolism;

- Arteritis involving the renal arteries;

- External compression (e.g., by tumor) of a renal artery.

The extent and severity of hypertension are related roughly to the degree of the derangement of renal arterial circulation, thus encompassing a range from mild to malignant hypertension. The principal factor in the natural history of renovascular hypertension is its reversibility and curability by a surgical correction of the circulatory disturbance. Inasmuch as the cause and effect between the renovascular lesion and hypertension cannot always be definitely determined, it is occasionally necessary to revise the diagnosis from renovascular to essential hypertension if the successful surgical correction of a renal arterial lesion produces no relief of hypertension. When a renal vascular lesion cannot be identified, the course of the disease is identical to that of essential hypertension, being largely related to the severity of pressure elevation.

Renal parenchymatous disease, associated with arterial hypertension, includes the following conditions:

- acute glomerulonephritis,
- chronic glomerulonephritis,
- pyelonephritis,
- polycystic kidneys,
- obstructive uropathy.

Most of these conditions represent chronic renal diseases and hypertension is merely one of the features. There are, however, some instances of reversible hypertension:

- Acute glomerulonephritis, as a rule, permits a fall of arterial pressure to normotensive levels with the cessation of the acute process.

- Pyelonephritis under rare circumstances may affect one kidney only. Basically a disseminated bilateral process, unilateral pyelonephritis almost always involves secondary infection in a congenitally malformed kidney. In some such cases hypertension may be reversible after nephrectomy.

- Obstructive uropathy is seldom associated with significant elevation of arterial pressure, but if it is, hypertension is reversible upon relief of the obstruction.

In general, glomerulonephritis tends to be associated with moderate elevation of arterial pressure; such elevation may play a secondary role in the natural history of the disease. In pyelonephritis hypertension may become severe and acquire features of the malignant form.

Pheochromocytoma occupies a unique position among diseases associated with hypertension in that hypertension is its principal effect (except in the small fraction of cases—less than 10 per cent—of malignant pheochromocytoma). Pheochromocytoma presents characteristic symptomatology. Basically, it appears in the form of two varieties:

- That associated with persistent hypertension,
- That associated with paroxysmal hypertension.

The former, less often encountered, may appear as benign or malignant hypertension, according to its severity, yet may show unusual variation of pressure and episodic symptomatology. The latter may be associated with normotensive levels of arterial pressure under all circumstances except during paroxysms of severe hypertension. The cause of hypertension is the overproduction of catecholamines: norepinephrine in sustained hypertension and epinephrine in paroxysmal hypertension.

Symptoms of pheochromocytoma consist of attacks of anxiety, headaches, excessive perspiration, palpitations, and occasionally dyspnea or pulmonary edema. Extreme elevation of arterial pressure may be encountered during attacks. Such attacks may be life-threatening since they may lead to acute left ventricular failure, cerebral hemorrhage, or fatal arrhythmias.

The unpredictability of the course of pheochromocytoma and the resulting poorer prognosis compared with other forms of hypertension make it imperative to search for this form of hypertension in all patients, even though its incidence is very small (less than 0.5 per cent of hypertensive subjects). The approach to the investigation of pheochromocytoma is presented later in this chapter.

Aldosterone tumors produce hypertension by means of hypersecretion of aldosterone. They overlap and merge with idiopathic ("primary") hyperaldosteronism, which may be associated with hyperplasia of the adrenal cortex or may have no anatomic basis. The course of hypertension produced by hyperaldosteronism is that of severe hypertension, indistinguishable from any other form of it. Reversibility of hypertension is demonstrated in patients with aldosterone-producing adenomas; those with partial or total adrenalectomy for other forms of hyperaldosteronism have not responded with consistent improvement.

COMPLICATIONS

Complications of hypertensive cardiovascular disease fall into two categories:

- Those related to undue rises of arterial pressure;

- Those in which hypertension facilitates vascular accidents.

In the former category two principal complications are:

- Hypertensive encephalopathy, a condition associated with a temporary rise of arterial pressure, producing convulsions, headache, coma, or a variety of neurological signs and symptoms. This is a temporary condition, the cerebral manifestations of which are assumed to be related to cerebral vascular spasms; it may be fatal or may recede; prompt medical therapy effectively protects patients from the more serious consequences of it.

- Acute pulmonary edema represents the sudden intolerable overload upon the left ventricle from a hypertensive crisis.

Here, too, fatal outcome may be prevented by prompt medical intervention.

The second category of complications includes the following:

- Cerebral hemorrhage — which may be intracerebral or subarachnoid;

- Dissecting aneurysm;

- Acute myocardial infarction;

- Cerebral thrombosis;

- Various hemorrhages (epistaxis, hematemesis, etc.).

DIAGNOSTIC EVALUATION

Hypertension is not a disease but a clinical sign accessible to a simple determination as to its presence or absence at any given moment. Consequently the diagnostic evaluation revolves around the significance of the elevation of arterial pressure, when it is found. Thus, given a hypertensive arterial pressure reading in a subject, the objectives of further steps to be undertaken involve the following:

1. To determine whether the pressure elevation represents a temporary overshoot or a persistent state;

2. To determine the consequences of the hypertension upon the patient's target organs;

3. To search for the possible presence of unusual causes of hypertension which would alter therapeutic approaches or the prognosis.

The first objective is often the most difficult one. The overlap between the normotensive population with casual, innocent pressure overshoots and the hypertensive population is so broad and the reliable means of their separation are so few that only tentative differentiation is possible in many cases. In approaching the problem the full realization of the following points is necessary:

- The great minute-to-minute variability of arterial pressure makes it advisable to have each determination of arterial pressure consist of three or more readings, including those recorded in both arms.

- Apprehension is an important cause of hypertensive overshoots: observing the patient for signs of apprehension (tachycardia, sweating) may help with the decision to discard certain readings.

- Initial examination of a patient by a physician seen for the first time tends to produce exaggerated hypertensive pressure levels; such readings should never be considered a baseline for any kind of observations.

The most commonly accepted upper figure for the normal range of arterial pressure for adults is 145/90. Obviously this is an arbitrary level which cannot be taken literally as a firm "cut-off point." Abnormal pressure levels above these values are considered likely to represent hypertension if one of the following methods of arterial pressure measurement is fulfilled:

1.   Abnormally high arterial pressures are obtained representing the lowest reading of each of at least three determinations at separate times in patients who do not show obvious apprehension during the measurement.

2.   The use of Smirk's "basal pressure" reading: the patient reports to an office or outpatient clinic in the morning for a two-hour (or longer) session during which time blood pressure is recorded at frequent intervals by a nurse or assistant. The early readings, usually higher, are considered the "casual" pressure readings, which then become lower, often reaching a plateau at the basal pressure level for this subject.

3.   Patients with appropriate intelligence and adequate home facilities are instructed to take their blood pressure (or have a family member take it) at intervals on various occasions to try to find a reproducible lowest level of "basal" arterial pressure.

Obviously the separation between hypertensives and benign "overshooters" is arbitrary and based merely on probability. No simple methods are available of recording continuously patients' arterial pressure in a manner analogous to continuous recording of cardiac rhythm. Apparatus suitable for recording arterial pressure without the patient's knowledge is complex and applicable mostly to special research projects; even then it is of limited use. Simple portable semiautomatic pressure recording apparatuses have yielded important information but have the disadvantage of the patient's having to inflate the cuff periodically. Some patients become anxious each time the pressure cuff is inflated, which may account for falsely high pressure readings.

Apprehension makes the error in the selection of true "hypertensives" largely in the direction of false-positives. Rarely, however — as the semiautomatic pressure recorder has demonstrated — prolonged hypertensive periods during daily activities occur in patients whose casual pressure readings may be close to normal levels.

The most certain evidence of the presence of significant hypertension is involvement of the target organs. As mentioned, these include:

- cardiac involvement,

- vascular involvement,

- renal involvement,

- cerebral involvement.

The presence of left ventricular hypertrophy and of vascular disease (particularly evident in ocular changes) directly relates to hypertension; their specificity as the index of hypertensive disease is good. Disturbances of renal function and atherosclerotic disease involving the heart (i.e., myocardial infarction) or the brain represent only indirect support for the diagnosis of hypertension: renal disease may be the cause as well as the result of hypertension; coronary artery disease and cerebral vascular disease may exist without hypertension.

"Routine" Evaluation of Hypertension

History provides little significant information; as mentioned, hypertensive patients are basically asymptomatic: symptoms, if present, are nonspecific in nature. Among symptoms commonly associated with hypertension are headaches, nocturia, fatigability, and transient cerebral symptoms. Of particular importance in the evaluation of hypertensive patients are:

- Family history;

- History of severe neurological disturbances (convulsive seizures, diplopia, syncope) in patients with severe (malignant) hypertension which could represent hypertensive encephalopathy.

Physical examination — other than blood pressure reading — should concentrate upon the more specific signs of target organ involvement:

- Evidence of left ventricular hypertrophy (forceful and sustained apical impulse, S4 gallop sound in younger patients; in later stages signs of left ventricular failure may be present: S3 gallop sound, pulmonary rales, pulsus alternans);

- Funduscopic examination: grades II to IV fundal changes (grade I change is nonspecific).

Physical examination may also provide information regarding special forms of hypertension: auscultation may reveal renal arterial bruits; absent pedal pulses in younger patient may direct attention to the possibility of coarctation of the aorta. The presence of abdominal masses may be pertinent to the diagnosis.

Radiographic examination usually adds little to the diagnosis of hypertension. Cardiac enlargement is likely to develop late, when cardiac failure is clinically already evident. Unfolding of the aorta is frequently found in hypertensive patients; yet, except in young individuals, this finding may be produced by atherosclerosis and is therefore of low specificity. Characteristic signs associated with coarctation of the aorta have been mentioned in Chapter 31.

Electrocardiographic examination may well be the most important laboratory aid to the diagnosis of cardiac involvement in hypertension, especially when no other evidence of cardiac disease can be detected. While the specificity and sensitivity of electrocardiographic changes produced by left ventricular hypertrophy undoubtedly could occasionally confuse the picture in borderline cases, it is nevertheless clear that unmistakable evidence of left ventricular hypertrophy is an important indication of severity of hypertension and can be used as a baseline in evaluation of successes of therapy. Similarly, the presence of an entirely normal electrocardiogram in a patient with long-standing history of hypertension represents a reassuring sign regarding the nature of the disease. Patients with hypertensive disease may also show other electrocardiographic abnormalities, which, however, are of low specificity. Among these are:

- Intraventricular conduction defects,
- Residuals from myocardial infarction,
- T wave abnormalities,
- Evidence of left atrial enlargement.

Other laboratory tests pertinent to hypertension include urinalysis (hematuria, albuminuria, and cylindruria are of low specificity but yield some important information) and determination of blood urea nitrogen and serum creatinine, as well as creatinine clearance test.

INVESTIGATION OF SPECIAL FORMS OF HYPERTENSION

A group of diseases marked by elevated arterial pressure are listed previously. Those in which the cause is correctable and hypertension reversible are of special interest and importance to the clinician.

Renovascular hypertension involves primarily conditions in which there is identifiable obstruction within the renal arterial system. From the clinical standpoint the most important subgroup are cases with unilateral renal arterial stenosis. Diagnostic tools available to identify this form of hypertension include the following:

- Physical examination may reveal vascular bruits over the abdomen;

- Timed excretory urograms often show delayed opacification of the affected kidney;

- Radioisotope scanning of the kidneys may also show delay on the stenotic side;

- Split renal function tests may show water and sodium excretion very considerably reduced on the side of the malperfused kidney;

- Renin assay in samples of blood collected from each renal vein may show higher renin content in the malperfused kidney;

- Renal arteriogram provides the most accurate means of establishing the presence of obstructive arterial lesions.

As seen, except for the renal arteriogram, all tests are based on observing a difference between various findings when assessing each kidney separately, and therefore are slanted toward unilateral renal arterial obstructing lesions. The first three of the above tests are considered screening procedures. Their sensitivity and specificity is within the medium range and results cannot be considered definitive. Their role is to identify the patients in whom further studies are indicated. Split renal function test has considerable sensitivity: renal malperfusion profoundly affects excretory kidney functions, producing changes of great magnitude. Yet, technical considerations and the difficulty of collecting ureteral specimens in totality, as well as the "invasiveness" of the test, make it suitable for clinical use only in institutions with large-scale experience in this procedure.

The two crucial tests are renin assay and renal arteriogram. Both are invasive, require hospitalization, and are obviously unsuited for mass performance. Even these tests have to be interpreted with caution. Renin assay is relatively new: the full range of its specificity is not yet known. The renal arteriogram is subject to the same error of interpretation as the coronary arteriogram; the difficulty of judging the degree of stenosis makes it hazardous to assume cause-and-effect relationship between a given lesion and hypertension unless the arterial obstruction is very severe. Thus there is an indecisive intermediate zone of renal arterial stenosis in patients who have hypertension.

Other unilateral renal lesions. Unilateral nephrectomy was once a popular procedure in patients with severe hypertension; however, critical appraisal of the results indicated that only in a small proportion of such cases could the improvement be really attributed to the operation.

At present only in a small number of patients can one suspect such a relationship, yet a search for those is justified. These include:

- Congenitally malformed kidney with superimposed pyelonephritis;

- Severe unilateral uropathy;

- Unusual vascular lesions: infarcts, aneurysms, venous thrombosis.

The relationship between these lesions and hypertension can be considered only tentative, yet in a hypertensive patient nephrectomy may be indicated provided that the healthy kidney has normal function and the affected kidney poor function.

The diagnostic approach to this group consists of excretory urography as the initial procedure with urological work-up to follow. Renin assays may help confirm the role of the affected kidney in the cause of hypertension.

Pheochromocytoma is a rare tumor, yet its curability makes it important to consider it in our evaluation of the hypertensive patient. The following diagnostic approaches apply to this condition:

- Awareness of the unusual symptomatology: patients with variable hypertension who show attacks of apprehension, headaches, perspiration, palpitations, and occasionally anginal pain should be suspected; however, pheochromocytoma may manifest itself as sustained severe hypertension without any special features.

- Physical examination may show some features resembling those of hyperthyroidism (excessive perspiration, tachycardia, tremor); however the examination is often negative.

- Laboratory studies may show glycosuria, hyperglycemia, and high basal metabolic rate.

- The principal diagnostic test for pheochromocytoma is determination of urinary catecholamines; the most widely used procedure is measurement of urinary vanylmandelic acid (a derivative of epinephrine and norepinephrine). Direct measurement of the two latter catecholamines is preferred in some laboratories: although it is a more complex determination, it gives fewer false-positive results.

- In patients with sustained hypertension phentolamine administration may be used as a diagnostic test. The basis for this test is the alpha-adrenergic blocking effect of this agent, thus counteracting the vasoconstricting effects of the excess catecholamines. A fall in arterial pressure is expected in response to phentolamine in pheochromocytoma but not in other forms of hypertension. This test has to be applied with great caution because of the untoward reaction that may develop in patients with and without pheochromocytoma.

- In patients with normal arterial pressure but with a tendency to periodic hypertension (including hypertensive attacks) the histamine provocation test has been used for some three decades. In this test, histamine may initiate a hypertensive attack in patients with pheochromocytoma but has no effect or reduces blood pressure in normal subjects. The test is not without some risk and is not as widely used now as it was in the past.

- Patients with chemical or pharmacological evidence pointing to pheochromocytoma are then investigated in an attempt to locate the tumor. Obviously of variable usefulness because of the wide range in sizes and locations of the tumor, radiographic examination is of only positive significance (i.e., negative test does not rule out tumor). Plain chest and abdominal films only rarely may show evidence of a tumor, namely, when calcifications in it are present. Excretory urograms may show distortion of calyces, indirectly suggesting the presence of a tumor. In experienced hands, retroperitoneal air injection and aortographic studies may be performed in a search for tumors in that area. Failure to find a tumor in patients with high probability of pheochromocytoma requires surgical exploration.

Aldosterone-excreting tumors represent a form of hypertension related to hypersecretion of aldosterone and overlap with primary aldosteronism caused by adrenal hyperplasia. The former is reversible after removal of the adenoma (usually adrenalectomy); the latter seldom responds to adrenalectomy. The diagnostic clues helpful in arousing suspicion for this syndrome include the following:

- Fatigability and muscular weakness may be present;

- Low serum potassium is usually found and is further accentuated by sodium loading;

- Decreased plasma renin assay may be found;

- Aldosterone excretion in the urine may be increased;

- Glucose tolerance may be lowered.

As a rule these findings, especially potassium loss, are more pronounced in adenoma than in adrenal hyperplasia. The differentiation between the two, however, in individual cases is virtually impossible, and exploratory operation is needed to detect and remove an adenoma of the adrenal cortex.

Coarctation of the aorta has already been discussed (see Chapter 31). The principal means of not overlooking this curable form of hypertension are to measure routinely blood pressure in the legs in all hypertensive patients, especially in young ones, and to pay special attention to chest roentgenograms regarding the characteristic indentation of the descending aorta and the possibility of rib notching.

"WORK-UP" OF HYPERTENSIVE PATIENTS

The question frequently arises as to how far one should proceed with the various diagnostic methods of evaluation of a patient in whom elevation of arterial pressure is first discovered. On the theory that curable forms of hypertension—regardless how rare—should never be overlooked, one could make a case for going "all the way" in every patient. However, the expense and discomfort to the patient and the risk of invasive procedures are unacceptable to the general hypertensive population, and evaluation must be made on a selective basis. Guidelines for high-priority patients in whom extensive investigation is indicated include the following:

1. Patients with unusually severe degrees of diastolic hypertension (with or without "malignant" features);

2. Young patients with sustained hypertension;

3. Patients showing unusual clinical features of hypertension;

4. Patients in whom there is documented evidence of sudden onset of severe hypertension or its rapid progression.

Low-priority patients include elderly individuals with mild or moderate hypertension, women with postmenopausal hypertension, and patients with labile hypertension.

Within these arbitrary groups there is obviously a wide variability as well as an overlap between them. Certain screening techniques are indicated in most patients, especially the tests that can be performed on an outpatient basis, such as timed excretory urograms. In general, progressive work-up includes the performance of noninvasive techniques first, before invasive methods are used. In seriously ill patients in whom the suggestion of a surgically correctable hypertension is uncovered and subsequently tests are inconclusive, surgical exploration may have to be performed.

THERAPY

Treatment of hypertension includes two approaches:

1. Surgical treatment of reversible forms of hypertension in which a permanent cure can be accomplished by an operation;

2. Medical control of hypertension—a life-long task for the physician and the patient.

The former is applicable to only a minute fraction of cases; it can be considered successful only after a prolonged follow-up period demonstrates beyond doubt the permanency of normotensive levels of arterial pressure. The need for careful postoperative evaluation is best exemplified by the wide discrepancy between the many claims of cure of hypertension following unilateral nephrectomy or renal arterial revascularization and the small number of such cases accepted by critical observers as successfully cured.

Thus true surgical cure of hypertension represents the ideal treatment fulfilling the objective of complete elimination of a disease. The great majority of cases, however, require more modest therapeutic objectives, which include the following:

- Maintenance of the arterial pressure within the normal range, or at the lowest attainable level above it;

- Elimination of all reversible sequels of hypertension upon the target organs, their partial regression, or at least their arrest.

- Treatment of complications of hypertension.

The initiation of antihypertensive therapy should be looked upon as a major therapeutic step that should not be undertaken without careful consideration of the risk-benefit relationship. The following points need to be considered:

1. Patients with hypertensive disease are basically asymptomatic; hence therapy has no relationship to the patient's well-being (a point that may affect the patient's motivation to follow medical advice).

2. This form of therapy permits direct assessment of its effectiveness; while a highly desirable feature of treatment, it also compels careful and continuous monitoring of its effectiveness.

3. The variability of blood pressure and the difficulty of determining which patients have hypertensive disease and which are merely pressure hyperreactors makes it necessary to set arbitrary standards for the selection of patients. Inevitably certain patients with hypertensive disease may be left out of therapy while normotensive patients may be included.

In discussing therapy of hypertension it should be pointed out that the subject of treatment of patients without symptoms and without evidence of organic sequels to hypertension is still a matter of controversy. Yet the prevailing view today is that this largely prophylactic therapy is indicated, since the benefit most likely outweighs the risk. The following arguments can be cited in support of this:

- Epidemiological studies show a sharp increase in mortality and morbidity from cardiovascular disease with rise in diastolic pressure in the general population, especially in males.

- Experience in large hypertensive clinics indicates that control of arterial pressure at normal levels is possible in virtually all patients with hypertension by appropriate drug therapy.

- A large study (Veterans Administration Cooperative Study) demonstrated the effectiveness of antihypertensive therapy in reducing morbidity from cardiovascular complications.

- Given appropriate monitoring, the known risk of antihypertensive drugs given over a long period of time is very small.

Patients who show ill effects of hypertensive disease show convincing and overt benefits from antihypertensive therapy:

- "Malignant" hypertension, which when untreated may result in death in a period of a few months, can be successfully arrested or even reversed.

- Target-organ evidences of hypertensive disease—left ventricular hypertrophy and abnormalities in the ocular fundi—can be reversed by antihypertensive therapy.

Selection of Patients for Antihypertensive Therapy

It is seen from the foregoing discussion that hypertensive disease involves in general two classes of patients:

1. Those with evidence of damage produced by hypertension,

2. Those in whom elevated arterial pressure is the only abnormality.

In the first group antihypertensive therapy is mandatory. In the second group treatment depends upon the individual judgment of the clinician. In it a system of priorities should be established with a number of points to be considered. Antihypertensive therapy is most recommended for the following categories of patients:

1.   Patients with persistently high diastolic pressure levels in most or all pressure determinations;

2.   Patients with a strong family history of hypertension;

3.   Patients with clinical evidence of atherosclerotic disease: anginal syndrome, past myocardial infarction, cerebral vascular disease, peripheral vascular disease;

4.   Patients considered high risks for coronary disease: those with a family history of coronary disease, and with hyperlipidemias;

5.   Younger patients should be given higher priority than older ones, other factors being equal;

6.   Patients who fully comprehend the implications of life-long antihypertensive therapy and are likely to be motivated to follow through with it should be given priority over those whose intelligence or habits makes them less likely to comply with instruction.

In addition to the question of whom to treat among patients whose only abnormality is elevated arterial pressure, a second question requires consideration: namely, how aggressive should the therapy be? Given a hypertensive patient who does not respond satisfactorily to simpler antihypertensive agents, should one proceed to drugs that have more profound effects upon some physiological functions and may have undesirable side effects and some risk attached to them? Here, again, careful consideration of all factors should be given, setting priorities on a much stricter level than in the initial selection for therapy.

Antihypertensive Drugs

Thiazides are widely used diuretic agents in the treatment of hypertension. Diuretics enhance sodium elimination, reduce blood volume and may decrease cardiac output, thereby reducing arterial pressure.

Long-term use of thiazides produces a modest reduction of arterial pressure, possibly partly by a decrease in systemic arteriolar resistance. This group of drugs often suffices as the only agent in mild, labile hypertension. Untoward effects of thiazide administration include the following:

- Hyperuricemia, which may induce gout in susceptible patients;

- Hypokalemia, which should be monitored and, if present, corrected by potassium supplementation;

- Hyperglycemia, which may bring latent diabetes into an overt state.

Reserpine is the most widely used alkaloid of the derivatives of rauwolfia. It affects both the central nervous system and the peripheral neurotransmission within the autonomic nervous system. The antihypertensive action of reserpine is most likely related to its catecholamine-depleting action, thereby decreasing peripheral resistance and reducing cardiac output. Untoward effects of reserpine include the following:

- Depression that may lead to suicidal tendencies;

- Gastrointestinal disturbances;

- Nasal congestion and stuffiness;

- Mild negative inotropic action due to catecholamine depression (caution is indicated in patients who may have compromised cardiac function).

Hydralazine occupies a special place among antihypertensive drugs in that it reduces systemic arteriolar resistance while increasing cardiac output and cardiac rate. Untoward effects of this drug include the following:

- Increase in cardiac workload, undesirable in patients who have or are approaching cardiac failure or who suffer anginal attacks;

- Headaches;

- Anorexia and nausea;

- Nasal congestion;

- Possibility of developing systemic lupus erythematosus after prolonged use.

Methyldopa is thought to produce its antihypertensive effect by producing a false neurotransmitter, thereby interfering with the synthesis of norepinephrine and reducing peripheral resistance. Its side effects include:

- Gastrointestinal disturbances;

- Somnolence (which often can be overcome if treatment is continued);

- Postural hypotension may develop;

- Hepatic damage may develop after prolonged use.

Guanethedine exerts its antihypertensive effect by its action on postganglionic nerve endings in that it depletes norepinephrine stores, thereby reducing peripheral arteriolar resistance; its effect upon the heart is that of reducing cardiac rate and cardiac output. The side effects include:

- Postural hypotension;

- Gastrointestinal disturbances;

- Muscular weakness;

- Accentuation of latent cardiac failure (e.g., fluid retention);

- Sexual impotence in males.

Ganglionic blocking agents (pentolinium or mecamylamine) produce autonomic blockade: their antihypertensive effects are combined with some serious consequences of the blockade, such as paralytic ileus, absence of salivation, blurred vision, and others. Their chronic administration is now rare, reserved only for patients with severe hypertension who do not respond to any other drugs or drug combinations.

Diazoxide is the most recently introduced antihypertensive drug. Related to thiazides but without diuretic action, this agent is a quick-acting drug, effective only by intravenous administration. Its principal use is the immediate reduction of a hypertensive overshoot in various hypertensive crises.

Propranolol, the presently available beta-adrenergic blocking agent, is used widely in arrhythmias and in patients with ischemic heart disease. In hypertension it is thought to work primarily by reducing cardiac output via its negative inotropic action. It exerts a synergistic effect in combination with other antihypertensive agents, and therefore finds use in combined drug therapy of hypertension.

Antihypertensive Treatment

When the initial decision is made that antihypertensive therapy is indicated, the following further points need consideration:

- The patient's awareness of possible side effects of drugs;

- Means of monitoring the effectiveness of therapy;

- Periodic checks of the overall progress of the disease;

- Periodic checks of possible undesirable effects of drugs upon various organ functions.

The overall planning for drug therapy should be based upon the principle of selecting the most innocuous drugs or drug combination consistent with acceptable results.

In milder cases of hypertension treatment is usually started by the administration of thiazides alone or in combination with small doses of reserpine (0.25 mg.). Hydralazine or methyldopa is next added to the combination. As an adjunct to the therapy, mild restriction of dietary sodium may be recommended (about 5 gm. of sodium per 24 hours).

In severe hypertension the addition of guanethedine to the various combinations of the milder agents is usually the first step. The use of ganglionic blocking agents is indicated only when careful experimentation with various drug combinations in different dosages is reliably shown to be ineffective.

The means of monitoring the results vary. Patients with the appropriate facilities may take their own pressures at home and prepare charts for review. Visits to the physician's office or an outpatient clinic at variable intervals is the more commonly used means of monitoring. Pressure should always be checked repeatedly and measurements made in recumbent and standing positions as well as in the sitting position. When the therapy is initiated drugs should be administered one at a time with individual dose adjustment. Failure to show satisfactory response is usually presumed to demonstrate ineffectiveness of a drug or drug dosage. Yet, one must not overlook the possibility that the patient may neglect to take the medication.

Periodic checks of the progress of the disease and of the drug side effects require careful physical examinations at intervals, with special reference to the heart and the ocular fundi, electrocardiographic and roentgenographic examinations of the heart, and regular checks of the following:

- Serum potassium,

- Blood uric acid,

- Blood urea nitrogen and creatinine,

- Complete blood counts,

- Hepatic function tests,

- L.E. cell preparation in patients who are taking hydralazine.

In setting the objective of how low a casual reading of blood pressure should be considered desirable, it is necessary to view each patient in the context of his pretreatment level as well as other circumstances. Younger patients should be treated more aggressively, aiming at lower pressure levels. Older patients, especially those with evidence of cerebrovascular disease, should be treated more cautiously, with more modest objectives in view of the possibility, even though remote, of precipitating cerebral thrombosis by a too pronounced fall in arterial pressure.

Patients with malignant hypertension require the most aggressive approach. A controversy as to whether patients who already have seriously compromised renal function may be made worse by a fall in blood pressure is not entirely resolved, but the preponderance of evidence points to a favorable effect of antihypertensive therapy even in this group of patients.

Treatment of Complications and Sequels of Hypertension

Hypertensive encephalopathy represents a medical emergency and requires immediate hospitalization and aggressive therapy. When the diagnosis is definitely established and such conditions as intracerebral thrombosis or hemorrhage ruled out, the patient is given an antihypertensive agent parenterally:

- Reserpine
- Trimethaphan-arfonad (ganglionic blocking agent, not suitable for chronic use),
- Guanethedine,
- Methyldopa,
- Hydralazine,
- Diazoxide.

The choice of the antihypertensive agent depends upon the severity of the hypertensive crisis and the overall urgency of the situation. Reserpine and hydralazine may be started in milder cases, while trimethaphan, diazoxide, or guanethedine can be used in more urgent ones. Once the pressure is brought to a satisfactory level, oral therapy is immediately instituted and regulated to maintain the patient at a mildly hypertensive or normotensive level.

Acute reduction of arterial pressure is also essential by the strongest available means in patients who show such complications of hypertension as intracerebral hemorrhage, bleeding from another source, or aortic dissection. Arfonad is the most frequently used effective agent for such emergencies.

Cardiac failure due to hypertensive disease is treated in a conventional manner, except that in patients who maintain high arterial pressure the use of an antihypertensive agent becomes an important adjunct in relieving cardiac overload. This may become of particular importance in acute left ventricular failure manifested as pulmonary edema.

Bibliography

Biglieri EG, Stockigt JR, Schamberlan M: Adrenal mineralocorticoids causing hypertension. Amer. J. Med. *52*:623, 1972.

Cohn JN, Blood pressure and cardiac performance. Amer. J. Med. *55*:351, 1973.

Fries ED: Age, race, sex and other indices of risk in hypertension. Amer. J. Med. *55*:275, 1973.

Hunt JC, Strong CG: Renovascular hypertension: mechanism, natural history, treatment. Amer. J. Cardiol. *32*:562, 1973.

Koch-Weser J: Hypertensive emergencies. New Engl. J. Med. *290*:211, 1974.

Laragh JH, Baer L, Brunner HR, Buhler FR, Sealey JE, Caughan ED Jr: Renin, angiotensin and aldosterone system in pathogenesis and management of hypertensive vascular disease. Amer. J. Med. *52*:633, 1972.

Lauper NT, Tyce GM, Sheps SG, Carney JA: Pheochromocytoma: fine structural, biochemical and clinical observations. Amer. J. Cardiol. *30*:197, 1972.

Page IH: Arterial hypertension in retrospect. Circ. Res. *34*:133, 1974.

Page LB, Sidd JJ: Medical management of primary hypertension. New Engl. J. Med. *287*:960, 1018, 1074, 1972.

Pickering G: Hyperpiesia: high blood pressure without evident cause: essential hypertension. Brit. Med. J. *2*:959, 1965.

Pickering G: Hypertension: definition, natural histories and consequences. Amer. J. Med. *52*:570, 1972.

Smirk FH: Casual and basal blood pressure. IV. Their relationship to the supplemental pressure with a note on statistical implications. Brit. Heart J. *6*:176, 1944.

Smirk FH: The prognosis of untreated and of treated hypertension and advantages of early treatment. Amer. Heart J. *83*:825, 1972.

Sokolow M, Perloff D: The prognosis of essential hypertension treated conservatively. Circulation *23*:697, 1961.

Veterans Administration Cooperative Study Group on Antihypertensive Agents (Freis ED, Chairman): Effects of treatment on morbidity in hypertension. I. Results in patients with diastolic blood pressures averaging 115 to 129 mm. Hg. J.A.M.A. *202*:1028, 1967. II. Results in patients with diastolic blood pressures averaging 90 to 114 mm. Hg. J.A.M.A. *213*:1143, 1970.

40

Pulmonary Heart Disease

Definition. The term "pulmonary heart disease" is used in its connotation of abnormalities within the pulmonary circulation and their effect upon the heart. In practical terms, the common denominator of pulmonary heart disease is pulmonary hypertension. Inasmuch as pulmonary hypertension plays a significant role in many, if not most, forms of cardiac disease, the discussion here will concentrate upon those conditions in which the pulmonary vasculature is preferentially affected, even though some recapitulation of previously discussed forms of pulmonary hypertension will be included.

Principal conditions covered in this chapter are the following:

- Heart disease secondary to chronic lung disease,

- Thromboembolic diseases of the pulmonary circulation,

- Primary pulmonary hypertension,

- Other forms of pulmonary hypertension.

PATHOLOGY

Clinically evident pulmonary hypertension may or may not be associated with organic changes in the pulmonary arterioles. Temporary increases in pressure in the pulmonary circuit and early pulmonary hypertension may be entirely due to arteriolar spasm. However, once pulmonary hypertension is established, changes in pulmonary arterioles can usually be found: some of them may be the consequence of increased pulmonary arteriolar spasm. On the other hand, certain changes may actually be the cause of pulmonary hypertension. Heath and Edwards proposed a classification of pulmonary vascular disease with six grades of severity, ranging from mere thickening of the arteriolar wall (grade I) to severe obliterative arteritis, resembling changes in systemic arterioles occurring in malignant hypertension, in which the arterioles often contain organized thrombi (grade VI). Inasmuch as a crucial issue in pulmonary hypertension is its reversibility (in cases in which its cause may be eliminated), these authors suggested that grades I to III of arteriolar changes are reversible, while grades IV to VI are not.

These arteriolar changes are nonspecific, i.e., they develop in response to various causes of pulmonary hypertension (left atrial hypertension, large shunt, "obligatory" congenital pulmonary hypertension) as well as in primary pulmonary hypertension. The form of pulmonary hypertension associated with chronic miliary pulmonary embolization from peripheral veins overlaps with other forms of pulmonary hypertension: embolic thrombi, once organized, become indistinguishable from those found in grades V and VI of pulmonary vascular disease (nonembolic).

A common consequence of pulmonary hypertension is atherosclerosis of the major pulmonary arteries. As a rule, even patients with severe systemic atherosclerosis are spared from atheroma in the large pulmonary arteries, but preferential atheromatous changes develop in patients with severe pulmonary hypertension, demonstrating once again that abnormally high pressure enhances the atheromatous process in general.

The consequence of pulmonary hypertension is hypertrophy of the right ventricle, which represents an expression of the increased workload imposed upon that chamber.

PATHOPHYSIOLOGY

The pulmonary circulation differs from the systemic circulation in the following important respects:

1. The entire output of the right ventricle (equal to that of the left ventricle) is ejected into a single organ.

2. The resistance within the pulmonary circuit is very low—about one-sixth of that in the systemic circuit; consequently, the perfusion pressure is low.

3. The autonomic nervous system exerts, under normal conditions, no control over pulmonary arteriolar resistance.

4. The pulmonary capillary bed has vast reserves, only about a quarter of it being perfused under resting conditions. Thus, when cardiac output increases, new capillary channels open up, thereby lowering resistance to flow and preventing rise in pressure. Consequently, a fourfold increase in cardiac output (e.g., during exercise) is possible without any increase in pulmonary perfusion pressure.

5. The low arteriolar resistance makes the pressure gradient across the lungs a small one; elevation of pressure in the left atrium and in the pulmonary veins is thus transmitted passively to the pulmonary arterial circulation, not being protected by the high arteriolar resistance which in the systemic circulation effectively separates the arterial from the capillary and venous circulations.

As a consequence of these differences, the mechanism of pulmonary hypertension is not uniform as it is in systemic circulation but, rather, it may be produced by a variety of causes:

- Pulmonary hypertension may be due to pulmonary arteriolar spasm and/or disease — a mechanism analogous to systemic hypertension.

- Pulmonary hypertension may be caused by passive transmission of high left atrial pressure onto the pulmonary arterial circuit ("passive pulmonary circulation").

- Pulmonary hypertension may be produced by increased pulmonary blood flow ("hyperkinetic or hyperdynamic pulmonary hypertension").

- Pulmonary hypertension may be caused by reduction of the pulmonary vascular capacity (massive pulmonary embolism, pneumonectomy, emphysema — the two latter being only contributory factors).

Pulmonary arteriolar constriction resulting in pressure elevation in the pulmonary artery occurs consistently only in response to one stimulus — hypoxia. Either in high altitude or in any form of alveolar hypoventilation there is a predictable (though variable in different subjects) pulmonary hypertensive response. There is another effective stimulus for pulmonary arteriolar constriction, but this develops only in subjects with hyperreactive pulmonary vasculature: rise in left atrial pressure.

Thus, clinical conditions in which pulmonary hypertension may be present involve the following mechanisms:

- In normal subjects pulmonary hypertension may develop in altitudes above 10,000 feet. Abnormal pressure first is observed during exercise, then may occur at rest as well.

- Very strenuous exercise in normal subjects with cardiac output increased more than four times the resting level may produce transient pulmonary hypertension.

- In congenital heart disease with large interventricular or aortico-pulmonary communications "obligatory" pulmonary hypertension at systemic pressure levels is maintained by increased pulmonary arteriolar resistance and by increased pulmonary flow in variable combinations of these two contributing factors (see Chapters 28, 29).

• In congenital heart disease with other left-to-right shunts pulmonary hypertension develops in only a small proportion (about 15 per cent) of patients in whom high pulmonary flow provokes pulmonary vascular disease (see Chapters 27–29).

• In mitral valve disease with chronic severe elevation of left atrial pressure passive pulmonary hypertension predominates. Some hyper-reactors develop, in addition, pulmonary arteriolar spasm, leading to more severe pressure elevation owing to a combination of passive plus reactive pulmonary hypertension (see Chapter 32). Similar conditions may develop in patients with left ventricular failure from any cause.

• In chronic lung disease hypoxia is the primary factor producing pulmonary hypertension. The elimination of pulmonary capillary space in pulmonary emphysema plays a less important role, but may cause rises of arterial pressure during exercise.

• Alveolar hypoventilation leading to pulmonary hypertension may develop in Pickwickian syndrome or in various neuromuscular disorders affecting respiratory muscles.

• In pulmonary embolism mechanical obstruction involving more than two-thirds of the pulmonary arterial cross-section produces pulmonary hypertension. The problem of a lesser vascular obstruction associated with reflex pulmonary arteriolar constriction has long been suspected but never proven; it remains doubtful as a factor.

• In primary pulmonary hypertension endarteritis of the small pulmonary vessels is responsible for the pressure elevation.

As indicated in the preceding section on pathology, pulmonary hypertension is reversible except in the advanced forms of pulmonary vascular disease. These occur almost exclusively in some patients with congenital heart disease with large shunts and in primary pulmonary hypertension. All other conditions may be assumed to be associated with potentially reversible pulmonary hypertension.

CLINICAL ENTITIES

Chronic Cor Pulmonale

The term "chronic cor pulmonale" is traditionally applied to the cardiac consequences of those noncardiac diseases within the thorax which produce pulmonary hypertension and the resulting right ventricular overload and failure. They can be divided arbitrarily into two classes:

1. Those in which cor pulmonale appears late in the course of an otherwise serious respiratory disease;

2. Those in which its appearance is prominent early and may dominate the clinical picture.

In the first category chronic obstructive lung disease is the most important entity; in the second, hypoventilation syndromes (Pickwickian syndrome, neuromuscular diseases) and thoracic deformities may be included.

Inasmuch as the common denominator of cor pulmonale is significant pulmonary hypertension, identification of this condition depends upon the ease or difficulty with which pulmonary hypertension may be diagnosed. Granting that the only reliable way of estimating pulmonary arterial pressure is its direct measurement by means of cardiac catheterization, its indirect recognition is based upon the following clinical features:

1. Left parasternal lift—the sustained forceful pulsation of the hypertrophied right ventricle;

2. Accentuation of the pulmonic valve closure sound, occasionally producing a booming, seemingly single, second sound that may be palpated as "diastolic shock" at the upper left sternal border;

3. Occasionally the diastolic murmur of secondary ("functional") pulmonary valve incompetence may be heard;

4. Chest roentgenogram may show exaggerated prominence of the main pulmonary artery segment and its principal branches;

5. The electrocardiogram may show the entire spectrum of right atrial and right ventricular hypertrophy;

6. The echocardiogram may show dilatation of the right ventricular cavity.

The specificity of these clinical signs—when present together—is very high and the diagnosis of pulmonary hypertension may be established with considerable confidence. The entire set of findings connotes, of course, an appreciable severity of pulmonary hypertension. In milder degrees of it only some of the findings may be present, in which case the specificity of the diagnosis is lowered. In general the sensitivity of these findings is relatively low; this is particularly true in chronic cor pulmonale for two reasons:

- Degree of pulmonary hypertension is usually modest;

- Some of the findings may be masked by lung disease.

The *natural history* of chronic cor pulmonale depends upon two principal factors:

- The course and prognosis of the underlying lung disease;

- Reversibility of the factor producing pulmonary hypertension — hypoxia.

From the standpoint of cardiac manifestations, two clinical patterns can be distinguished; it should be understood, of course, that they represent the end-portions of a spectrum and overlap often occurs. The two patterns are:

1. Patients with predominant pulmonary emphysema who are capable of compensating the ventilatory impairment by hyperventilating and who may show normal or near-normal arterial oxygen tension and normal or lowered carbon dioxide tension ("pink puffers"). In these cases pulmonary hypertension is a late, often terminal event with poor prognosis, usually incapable of responding to therapy.

2. Patients with an important element of bronchial constriction and bronchial infection often show hypoxia, the resulting pulmonary hypertension, and cardiac failure early ("blue bloaters"). Here, pulmonary hypertension and its sequelae may appear episodically and reverse themselves in response to intensive therapy of the infection and bronchospasm.

In chronic obstructive lung disease the *diagnosis* of cor pulmonale is difficult. Symptoms are almost entirely dominated by those produced by respiratory disease — dyspnea. Identifying signs of pulmonary hypertension may be obscured or minimized by the thoracic hyperinflation:

- Palpatory and auscultatory signs are almost impossible to perceive.

- Roentgenographic signs are minimized by the usually small size of the heart and its more vertical position within the thorax.

- Electrocardiographic findings may also be misleading; some abnormalities produced by the rotation of the cardiac position overlap with those of right ventricular hypertrophy.

Of the diagnostic features of pulmonary hypertension the electrocardiogram is probably the most valuable in spite of its low sensitivity.

The presence of P-pulmonale (tall, "gothic" P-waves) may be the first evidence of pulmonary hypertension. In patients with chronic obstructive lung disease a superior frontal plane QRS axis (-15 to $-60°$) is often present — presumably related to the position of the heart within the thorax. This may reduce the sensitivity of the electrocardiogram for the detection of right ventricular hypertrophy, which may become evident mainly by the exaggerated depth of the S wave in the left precordial leads (V_5).

The recognition of cardiac failure — the serious sequel to pulmonary hypertension — also presents a diagnostic difficulty. It is particularly easy to make a false-positive diagnosis of right ventricular failure in patients with emphysema. Here the hyperinflation of the thorax and the use of accessory respiratory muscles may produce distention of the external jugular veins without underlying elevation of central venous pressure; low position of the diaphragm may displace the liver downward, imitating hepatomegaly; ankle edema commonly occurs in such patients from venous stasis and obstruction to venous return. Thus the clinical signs of right ventricular failure have to be evaluated with particular care in cor pulmonale.

Pulmonary hypertension leads to isolated right ventricular failure. Yet a long-standing controversy exists regarding occasional patients who show evidence of left ventricular failure as well, as to whether the left ventricle is damaged by the cor pulmonale or fails as a result of some other associated cardiac disease. Still unresolved, this debate is of relatively little practical significance, inasmuch as the management of the patient does not differ in relation to the presence or absence of left ventricular failure or its precise nature.

The *therapy* of cor pulmonale complicating obstructive lung disease involves two stages:

1. Treatment of hypoxia and the attainment of the highest possible oxygen tension;

2. Conventional therapy of congestive cardiac failure.

As already mentioned, some types of obstructive pulmonary disease are amenable to a satisfactory control of the hypoxia, while others are not. It is important to review critically all possible reversible factors, for this form of therapy carries a much greater promise than treatment of cardiac failure.

Cor pulmonale due to *conditions other than chronic obstructive pulmonary disease* is much rarer. The following are brief statements of the problems involved:

• The Pickwickian syndrome is rare but has aroused considerable interest. It involves primary alveolar hypoventilation occurring in very obese individuals. Pulmonary hypertension and right ventricular failure — often complicated by polycythemia — appear early and dominate the clinical picture. Spectacular reversals of cardiac disease have been reported in patients in whom sufficient weight reduction could be accomplished to eliminate hypoventilation.

• Hypoventilation occurring in various neuromuscular disorders involving respiratory muscles is similar to the above condition in its effect upon the circulation. Here the prognosis and management are entirely contingent upon the nature of the neurological condition.

• Kyphoscoliotic heart disease involves the effects of severe thoracic deformities upon the circulation. The involvement of the heart in patients with kyphoscoliosis is probably greatly overrated; the diagnosis of cor pulmonale is often based upon radiographic and electrocardiographic abnormalities, both of which may represent some malposition and distortion of the heart rather than increased workload. Nevertheless, atelectasis and perfusion-ventilation imbalance occur in some patients, with resulting hypoxia; thus the background for pulmonary hypertension may be present occasionally.

Primary Pulmonary Hypertension

This is a rare condition, which—according to the most widely prevailing view—incorporates at least two etiological entities:

• Pulmonary hypertension of unknown origin, possibly due to congenitally hyperreactive pulmonary vasculature;

• Pulmonary hypertension produced by chronic showers of small emboli, occluding small branches of the pulmonary arteries.

The second of these two entities is thought to be on the increase in recent years. The possibility that its higher incidence is linked to the wide use of birth control estrogen substances is very suggestive, though perhaps not yet conclusively proven.

Clinically the two entities may be indistinguishable, unless pulmonary embolization includes, in addition to the showers of miliary emboli, major emboli that periodically produce pulmonary infarcts. This occurs in the minority of patients suspected of having the embolic variety of pulmonary hypertension. The natural history is that of slowly decreasing effort tolerance due to exertional dyspnea, excessive tiredness, or both. Chest pain, imitating ischemic pain, may also be present. Syncopal attacks may occur—their incidence is as high as 40 per cent in some series.

The course of primary pulmonary hypertension is that of a gradually progressive disease. The speed of progression varies widely, but in the majority of cases it is slow — in terms of months or years. Pulmonary hypertension is rarely diagnosed in the asymptomatic stage. Thus it may be assumed that a long asymptomatic course precedes the development of symptoms. Eventually patients lapse into right ventricular failure with peripheral cyanosis, fluid accumulation, and often total disability. Therapy is seldom effective beyond temporarily controlling cardiac failure.

The clinical *diagnosis* of primary pulmonary hypertension is relatively easy. It affects most frequently younger subjects, and all clinical signs of pulmonary hypertension listed above are usually evident. In the evaluation of patients, however, it is important to rule out secondary forms of pulmonary hypertension. Most of these have been discussed in earlier chapters. The following conditions may offer special difficulties in differential diagnosis:

- Mitral stenosis with severe reactive pulmonary hypertension (if severe enough, pulmonary hypertension may obliterate any clinical features of mitral stenosis);

- Congenital heart disease with intracardiac shunts;

- Rare instances of chronic pulmonary hypertension due to embolic or thrombotic occlusion of main pulmonary arterial branches.

Background information is often helpful in the clinical evaluation. Idiopathic pulmonary hypertension may be familial, or there may be cases of congenital heart disease in the family. Primary pulmonary vascular disease may have been latent in patients with congenital heart disease and intracardiac shunts (e.g., atrial septal defects) with normal pulmonary vascular resistance. Patients may have had the defect surgically repaired, and yet may develop pulmonary hypertension later in life. The appearance of pulmonary hypertension in young women — especially those taking birth control pills — shifts the weight of responsibility toward the embolic form.

The performance of cardiac catheterization and angiocardiographic studies in patients suspected of having pulmonary hypertension is justified for the purpose of confirming the clinical diagnosis and eliminating the abovementioned other possible causes of pulmonary hypertension. In "primary pulmonary hypertension" pulmonary arterial pressures are, as a rule, greatly elevated, often at systemic levels. Left atrial pressure is expected to be normal. The finding of a right-to-left shunt at the atrial level does not disprove the diagnosis in favor of congenital heart disease: simple patency of the foramen ovale, often present in normal subjects, may become an important pathway of a right-to-left shunt when pressure rises on the right side, especially since right atrial dilatation may stretch the foramen wide open.

Treatment of primary pulmonary hypertension is virtually ineffective. There is no known way of reversing pulmonary vascular disease. Anticoagulant therapy has been recommended as a means of checking the progression of the disease. Its use can be questioned on the following accounts:

- In idiopathic pulmonary hypertension it was suggested that anticoagulant therapy may be of value because thrombi are part of the pathological process involved in endarteritis (apart from the embolic variety). Yet, it is highly questionable whether anticoagulant therapy would ever influence this process.

- In patients with pulmonary hypertension in whom embolic origin is suspected, anticoagulant therapy is used because the theoretical reasoning behind its use is sound (prevention of phlebothrombosis or of its extension and propagation). Yet, once the severity of pulmonary hypertension is established, the disease is likely to continue its unfavorable progress, regardless of whether further emboli are or are not forthcoming. Thus anticoagulant therapy may have a delaying effect upon the natural history of the disease but, in the absence of controlled studies, even this possibility represents a hypothesis rather than an established fact.

The only other means of treatment of patients is the conventional therapy of congestive cardiac failure when it develops. Responses are, as a rule, poor; control of failure is more difficult here than in the common forms of congestive failure secondary to left ventricular lesions.

Pulmonary Embolism and Acute Cor Pulmonale

Acute cor pulmonale represents the clinical syndrome associated with an acute overload of the right ventricle. With the exception of rare cases of high altitude pulmonary edema to which this term might be applicable, it is virtually synonymous with pulmonary embolism severe enough to impose resistance to blood flow into the lungs.

As already indicated, significant right ventricular overload occurs only when the pulmonary arterial tree is reduced to less than one-third of its cross-sectional area. This may occur either as a massive pulmonary embolism blocking most of the principal pulmonary arteries, or a shower of multiple emboli simultaneously occluding enough smaller branches to produce the necessary reduction of the total lumen. The first possibility is by far the commoner one.

The problem of pulmonary embolism in general represents a continuum, which can be arbitrarily divided into three segments:

- Massive pulmonary embolism, producing acute cor pulmonale;

- Smaller pulmonary emboli, producing pulmonary infarcts;

- Chronic repetitive pulmonary embolization, producing chronic cor pulmonale.

The third segment of this problem was already discussed in the preceding section. The first two will be combined in joint discussion.

Phlebothrombosis.   The principal source of emboli to the pulmonary circulation are thrombi in the venous system. Only a very small fraction of pulmonary emboli are thought to originate in the right side of the, heart. The great majority of emboli originate in the region drained by the inferior vena cava, with the leg veins and pelvic veins representing the most important source.

Intravascular clotting takes place only under abnormal conditions. The predisposing factors include the following:

1. General:

- low cardiac output,

- inactivity,

- hypercoagulable states.

2. Local:

- pregnancy,

- trauma,

- abnormality of venous wall,

- varicose veins.

Thus, high-risk candidates for pulmonary embolism include the following:

- patients in congestive cardiac failure,

- patients on bed rest from any cause,

- subjects remaining motionless for prolonged periods of time (e.g., sitting during long airplane rides),

- patients with extremities in a cast, or in a body cast,

- patients recovering from pelvic or prostatic operations,

- patients with abdominal or pelvic tumors,

- patients with varicose veins,

- patients with thrombophlebitis, cellulitis, or infections.

As a general rule, clinically inapparent phlebothrombosis represents a more common source of pulmonary emboli than obvious thrombophlebitis.

Pulmonary Infarction. It is generally believed that only a small proportion of pulmonary emboli produce pulmonary infarcts. Both experimental evidence and clinical implications point to the fact that most emboli from the venous system are lysed in the heart or pulmonary arterial system without any harm to the patient. One can cite in support of this probability the extreme rarity of pulmonary infarcts as a complication of right-sided cardiac catheterization, during which unquestionably large numbers of thrombi are introduced into the pulmonary circulation. It is also well recognized that only a small number of actual pulmonary infarcts are clinically diagnosed. This is particularly true in patients who are in cardiac failure: many cases of pulmonary infarction detected at necropsy were previously clinically unsuspected.

From the standpoint of its natural history, a pulmonary infarct is an exceedingly benign clinical entity which has no significant cardiac or pulmonary sequelae and produces but a few days of mild discomfort to the patient. Yet the presence of a pulmonary infarct provides the warning that a potentially fatal pulmonary embolism may be threatening the patient: pulmonary infarction proves the existence of venous thrombosis capable of generating embolism. Thus pulmonary infarction is a condition of potential rather than actual seriousness.

The diagnosis of pulmonary infarction is based on clinical and laboratory findings which develop with a variable frequency and have a low specificity and sensitivity. A combination of findings often makes the diagnosis reasonably well established — in typical cases virtually certain. However, in the majority of cases the diagnosis is merely suggestive, tentative, and often impossible to make beyond a mere suspicion.

Clinical signs include the following:

- chest pain, most commonly of the pleural type with a definite relationship to respiration,

- rarely, dyspnea,

- hemoptysis,

- finding of a pleural friction rub,

- fever.

Radiographic findings include the following:

- small or medium-sized wedge-shaped pulmonary consolidation,

- "disk" areas of atelectasis,

- small pleural effusions.

Other laboratory studies include the following:

- Mild to moderate elevation of serum lactic acid dehydrogenase without elevation of glutamic-oxalacetic transaminase;

- Radioisotope scanning of the lung may reveal nonperfused areas;

- Serum bilirubin may be elevated;

- Arterial oxygen tension is usually reduced.

Evaluation of patients suspected of presenting a pulmonary infarct has to be done with great care. A great deal may be at stake: a life-threatening condition may be present, if the probability of pulmonary infarct is high; yet, treatment usually involves a period of anticoagulation with the resulting inconvenience and risk to the patient. It is, therefore, important to come up with a best probability of the correct diagnosis rather than to take the easy road of "giving the patient the benefit of the doubt" by accepting every vaguely suspicious sign as evidence in favor of the infarct.

In approaching the diagnosis one should first establish a reasonable probability of the existence of a source of emboli, recognizing, however, that such a source may occasionally not be detectable. This involves:

- Consideration of predisposing factors (see above);

- Direct evidence for venous thrombosis (thrombophlebitis, unilateral edema of legs, positive Homans' sign, etc.).

Weighing the clinical importance of the various features and laboratory findings, it is necessary to consider each in the light of the possibility of alternative causes; the following differential points are noteworthy:

- Clinical signs can be mimicked by almost any type of pulmonary disease (particularly infection) or by pleurisy;

- Hemoptysis is more often produced by venous bleeding (in pulmonary venous hypertension associated with many forms of cardiac disease) or by pulmonary capillary hemorrhages;

- A characteristic radiographic finding of a wedge-shaped shadow is rare; the more usual findings are nonspecific;

- Radioisotope scanning is of reduced value in the presence of clinically evident atelectasis, pulmonary consolidation, pleural effusion, or in patients with bullous emphysema.

Massive Pulmonary Embolism. This is usually defined as one involving detectable overload of the right ventricle, i.e., producing pulmonary hypertension. More often than not massive pulmonary embolism is *not* associated with pulmonary infarct, so that there is relatively little overlap between this condition and pulmonary infarction. Both, however, originate in the same source. Acute cor pulmonale is not too often preceded by smaller emboli causing pulmonary infarct; it is tempting to consider this as evidence of effective therapy after pulmonary infarct had been recognized. This supposition is, however, by no means proved. The clinical picture of acute cor pulmonale due to pulmonary embolism depends upon the gravity of the situation. The smallest emboli producing acute overload, barely diagnosable, take a benign course if not followed by a further catastrophe; larger ones may produce more alarming symptomatology or even sudden death.

Symptomatology of acute cor pulmonale includes the following features:

- Sudden onset—usually dramatic;

- Chest pain, often similar to that of acute myocardial infarction;

- Onset of weakness with clinical features of shock;

- Air-hunger—rapid and deep breathing without evident cause.

Less typical cases have more gradual onset and only some of the above features. Perhaps the most valuable clinical sign of those listed is the hyperventilation if it is possible to rule out its neurotic form.

Clinical signs consist of evidence of right ventricular failure:

- Pulsation of veins above the clavicle in the sitting position—particularly a prominent *a* wave;

- The pulmonary valve closure sound may be accentuated, though this is variable;

- Auscultation of the lungs may reveal signs of bronchospasm (wheezing).

The electrocardiogram is probably the most crucial diagnostic test for acute cor pulmonale, and may show the following changes:

- Appearance of prominent, peaked P waves (P-pulmonale);

- Sudden development of right bundle branch block;

- Rightward axis shift—often manifested by the development of S waves in lead 1 and Q waves in lead 3. (A differentiation from inferior myocardial infarction may present a problem from the electrocardiographic standpoint.);

- T wave inversion in leads V_1 to V_3 may occur.

Greater magnitude of electrocardiographic changes increases the specificity of the diagnosis. The roentgenogram is of little help except in differentiation from pneumothorax, mediastinal emphysema and — sometimes — from aortic dissection. Other laboratory tests as a rule fail to show any significant discriminatory findings. Often time does not even permit the performance of many tests: the reasonable clinical suspicion of acute cor pulmonale imposes upon the clinician the most crucial decision — is it necessary to perform immediately an invasive diagnostic study?

The purpose of the invasive study is:

- To confirm the diagnosis of massive pulmonary embolism;

- To determine the feasibility of embolectomy.

The simplest approach to hemodynamic evaluation is the bedside method, using a flow-directed balloon catheter. Measurement of pulmonary arterial pressure and pulmonary arterial wedge (indirect left atrial) pressure can supply strong evidence in favor of massive pulmonary embolism. The positive findings include:

- Moderate pulmonary arterial hypertension (systolic pressures above 60 mm. Hg are unusual in acute right ventricular overload);

- Normal, or near-normal, left atrial pressure.

This combinatiom of findings supports the clinical diagnosis under question, but is not specific for it: the possibility of having detected previously unknown chronic pulmonary hypertension should be considered.

In addition to pressure measurements, blood sampling for the determination of arteriovenous oxygen difference is of importance. The wider the arteriovenous difference, i.e., the lower the cardiac output, the greater urgency exists to consider aggressive therapy, thus providing the indication for pulmonary arteriography. This procedure has to be performed in the laboratory and carries a higher risk than a bedside hemodynamic study. It offers, however, the final diagnostic confirmation of the diagnosis and, in addition, permits a localization of embolic thrombi, providing the decisive presurgical information.

The decision as to when to intervene by emergency angiocardiography has to be made individually. A key issue is the availability of a surgical team ready to follow with an immediate embolectomy, if indicated. The performance of the diagnostic study in an institution not equipped with surgical facilities, with the thought of later transporting the patient to a surgical unit, is to be discouraged. Patients suspected of having massive pulmonary embolism should be immediately taken to a complete cardiac center. Patients in shock represent high priority among those to be studied, although if shock responds promptly to medical measures the diagnostic study may be, under some circumstances, deferred. The final judgment often depends upon the experience of the diagnostic and surgical unit in handling this type of cardiac emergency. This is a life-threatening condition with a high risk involved in the performance of the test as well as in waiting things out.

Treatment of pulmonary embolism involves several considerations:

1. Prophylactic therapy in patients considered at high risk for phlebothrombosis is indicated in many situatioms. Present-day routine includes early ambulation after operation, early sitting after acute myocardial infarction, and institution of passive and active exercises in all patients expected to be immobilized but especially in those with high proneness to intravascular thrombosis. All these measures serve the purpose of the prevention of phlebothrombosis. More aggressive therapy with anticoagulant drugs for patients who never had pulmonary embolism but are candidates for it — including those with acute myocardial infarction — has often been advocated, but the benefits of this prophylactic therapy have not yet been demonstrated to outweigh the risks. At present only in selected cases with specially recognized high risks of thrombosis is such therapy recommended. The recently introduced low-dose heparin therapy given prophylactically to patients undergoing various surgical procedures carries a smaller risk and the possibility of significantly reducing the incidence of thrombosis. This is a promising approach to the problem but it is as yet too soon to advocate its routine application.

2. The institution of anticoagulation therapy in patients with clinical evidence of venous thrombosis, but who have no evidence of pulmonary infarct or embolus, is a matter of individual judgment. In this category are patients with thrombophlebitis or with evidence of noninflammatory leg vein thrombosis. Since no "hard data" are available as to whether the risk-benefit ratio of anticoagulant therapy makes it justifiable, the clinician should decide in each individual case whether or not intervention is indicated. Routine anticoagulation treatment in patients with thrombophlebitis is not considered standard therapy in most institutions.

3. Treatment of pulmonary infarcts involves no remedial therapy for the infarct but prophylactic anticoagulant therapy directed at prevention of further extension of phlebothrombosis. Patients, as a

rule, are hospitalized and kept under observation. Therapy involves the following considerations:

- How firm is the diagnosis of pulmonary infarction?

- Is there one infarct or more?

- Is there a tentative source of emboli evident?

- How strong are the predisposing factors in this patient?

- Is there a known precipitating factor (e.g., pulmonary infarct after a plane or train trip)?

These considerations should influence the clinician as to the need for anticoagulant therapy and its priority in the overall management of the patient.

Prophylactic anticoagulant therapy instituted in conditions discussed above involves the use of heparin or coumarin derivatives, or both. The optimal time limit for the continuation of anticoagulant therapy is not definitely known. Arbitrarily a period of 6 weeks to 3 months is used as a time after which the risk of pulmonary embolization may recede. Should a patient, however, suffer from repeated pulmonary infarcts, especially a patient with recurrent thrombophlebitis, anticoagulant therapy may have to be continued indefinitely.

In addition to anticoagulant therapy, the question of surgical interruption of venous channels presumably carrying emboli may come under consideration. This is justified in patients with repeated emboli, especially if they occur in spite of an anticoagulant regimen, or in some patients with massive pulmonary embolism (see above). Available methods include ligation of veins up to the level of the inferior vena cava or the insertion of umbrella-like gadgets which are thought to prevent the passage of emboli from the legs. While inferior caval ligation in many patients is well tolerated (occasionally difficult-to-control edema develops), the effectiveness of caval ligation or mechanical partition is not foolproof since large collateral channels connecting with the azygos system form, and the emboli may travel via the detour.

Treatment of acute cor pulmonale confronts the clinician with a serious dilemma, as already stated. If the patient can weather the cardiac overload, embolic thrombi will almost certainly lyse or shrink and organize, thus restoring a normal pulmonary circulation. A serious, life-threatening emergency, acute cor pulmonale is not a condition leading ordinarily to a chronic state. Consequently, the goals of therapy are as follows:

- To support the circulation during the critical time of overload if the probabilities point toward a favorable outcome;

- To remove surgically the pulmonary thrombi if unfavorable outcome is suggested;

- To remove pulmonary thrombi by lysis;

- To prevent the release of further emboli from the peripheral venous system.

The support of the circulation in patients with acute cor pulmonale consists merely of nonspecific treatment of hypotension and shock. Therapy may be minimal if the patient maintains good vital signs and never reaches the stage of shock. When present, shock should be treated individually by monitoring the various circulatory, respiratory, and renal functions and attempting to correct the detected abnormalities. The possibility of using extracorporeal support may be considered, although if this is necessary, surgical removal of the embolus takes precedence. In cases in which angiocardiography shows embolic thrombi located outside the reach of surgical approaches, aggressive nonsurgical support is the only available method of therapy. The question of inferior caval ligation performed as an emergency procedure is considered in patients in whom a more gradual onset of cor pulmonale suggests repeated emboli larger than a single massive embolus. The precariousness of the situation in acute cor pulmonale and the great variability in its clinical picture do not permit any evaluation of the respective results of the various forms of therapy, which become a matter of individual judgment or, perhaps more accurately, guesswork.

Recently extensive trials have been conducted with thrombolytic substances in acute cor pulmonale. Two such substances are now available, though as yet only for experimental trial: urokinase and streptokinase — both thrombolytic enzymes thought to play a role in spontaneous thrombolysis. A recently reported cooperative study using urokinase showed favorable results of thrombolytic therapy in acute cor pulmonale. However, the results in treated cases, though statistically better than those managed by other means, were nevertheless only slightly more favorable than controls — for a very serious disease this represents a modest therapeutic advance.

Bibliography

Conn WW: Operative therapy of venous thromboembolism. Mod. Concepts Cardiovasc. Dis. 43:71, 1974.

Dalen JE, Banas JS Jr, Brooks HL, Evans GL, Paraskos JA, Dexter L: Resolution rate of acute pulmonary embolism in man. New Engl. J. Med. 280:1194, 1969.

Edwards JE: Pulmonary hypertension of cardiac and pulmonary origin. Progr. Cardiovasc. Dis. 9:205, 1966.

Evans TO, van der Reis L, Selzer A: Circulatory effects of chronic pulmonary emphysema. Amer. Heart J. 66:741, 1963.

Kuida H, Dammin GJ, Haynes FW, Rapaport E, Dexter L: Primary pulmonary hypertension. Amer. J. Med. 23:166, 1957.

Oakley CM, Goodwin JF: The current status of pulmonary embolism and pulmonary vascular disease in relation to pulmonary hypertension. Progr. Cardiovasc. Dis. 9:495, 1967.

Oakley CM, Goodwin JF: Current clinical aspects of cor pulmonale. Amer. J. Cardiol. 20:842, 1967.

Owen WR, Thomas WA, Castleman B, Bland BF: Unrecognized emboli to lungs with subsequent cor pulmonale. New Engl. J. Med. 249:919, 1953.

Sasahara AA, Sidd JJ, Tremblay G, Leland OS Jr: Cardiopulmonary consequences of acute pulmonary embolic disease. Progr. Cardiovasc. Dis. 9:259, 1966.

Wessler S, Yin ET: Theory and practices of minidose heparin in surgical patients: A status report. Circulation 47:671, 1973.

41

Chronic Pericardial Disease

Definition. The great majority of cases of clinically significant chronic pericardial disease are of inflammatory origin. Included are patients in whom there is interference with circulatory dynamics, namely inflow resistance into the heart. The term "constrictive pericarditis" is applied to such cases. Localized pericardial adhesions – including those in the region of caval orifices, once thought to be of clinical importance – play little part in the production of signs and symptoms of pericardial disease.

Inasmuch as acute pericarditis (Chapter 25) represents a well-defined clinical entity, patients who progress into a subacute stage are usually included along with chronic cases whenever evidence of constriction is present. They represent a combination of effusion and pericardial thickening.

Diseases of the pericardium other than constrictive pericarditis include scar tissue from trauma (either direct or that produced by radiation) and the formation of pericardial tumors – most commonly mesothelioma. While pericardial involvement in the course of the various collagen vascular systemic diseases is common, constrictive pericarditis produced by such diseases is rare.

ETIOLOGY

Traditionally, tuberculosis was thought to be the principal etiological factor in chronic constrictive pericarditis. Still accounting for some cases, it is now considered a less important etiological factor in the Western countries. However, in patients first seen in late stages of constrictive pericarditis, neither clinical nor pathological findings are likely to reveal the etiological basis of this disease. Occasionally a reliable history of acute tuberculous pericarditis is present or obvious tuberculosis

682

is found elsewhere, in which case tuberculous etiology may be considered demonstrated.

Another recognized etiological factor is mediastinitis; patients with mediastinal infection occasionally develop constrictive pericarditis.

Many patients develop pericardial constriction without previous known disease, in which case the origin cannot be determined. Once thought to be rare, pericardial constriction developing as an aftermath of acute viral pericarditis is now recognized as an occasional occurrence.

Rarely, constrictive pericarditis is an aftermath of pericardial involvement in rheumatoid arthritis. However, constriction developing after repeated attacks of pericarditis of the hypersensitivity type (postcardiotomy syndrome, Dressler's syndrome) is very unusual. Similarly, rheumatic pericarditis does not produce chronic pericardial constriction.

While mediastinitis is recognized as a cause of pericardial constriction, it should be emphasized that pericardial manipulation at the time of cardiac operations seldom, if ever, produces constrictive pericarditis. Dense pericardial scars are often found at repeat operations as residuals from earlier surgery, yet they apparently do not produce the generalized pericardial "envelope" that represents the prerequisite for constriction and thus are physiologically insignificant.

PATHOLOGY

Significant interference with cardiac function is produced by dense generalized pericardial thickening or by pericardial calcifications. Dense fibrous tissue may involve the parietal pericardium, the visceral pericardium, or thickening of a combined two-layer pericardium grown together with obliteration of the pericardial cavity.

In patients in the subacute stage varying amounts of pericardial fluid may be present. The fluid may be inside the thickened parietal pericardium or outside the constricting layer of the thick visceral pericardium ("effusive constrictive pericarditis").

In patients with long-standing severe pericardial involvement the disease extends into the myocardium: superficial layers of the epicardium show fibrosis; surgical removal of the fibrous pericardium may thus be impossible without damage to the epicardium.

While tuberculosis is no longer a common etiological factor producing constrictive pericarditis, it is nevertheless an important initiating disease. Yet only occasionally can characteristic anatomic features of tuberculosis be found: in many patients with tuberculous chronic pericarditis only nonspecific scar tissue can be demonstrated.

PATHOPHYSIOLOGY

The prerequisite of pericardial constriction is a thick fibrous envelope that does not permit the full diastolic expansion of cardiac ventricles, thereby interfering with ventricular filling. The following dynamic consequences develop as a result of this:

- Late diastolic pressure in the ventricles is elevated (typically ventricular pressure falls normally but in late diastole rises and levels off as a plateau).

- Atrial pressures rise correspondingly.

- Ventricular diastolic and atrial pressures are elevated to the same degree on both sides of the heart, being constricted within a single rigid sac.

- Pulmonary arterial systolic pressure is only mildly (passively) elevated: the right ventricle does not decompensate from work overload, but its diastolic pressure is mechanically elevated; hence the diastolic right ventricular pressure is elevated out of proportion to the modest systolic pressure rise.

- The consequences of the severe elevation of right atrial pressure include ascites and edema of unusual prominence.

NATURAL HISTORY

Patients with constrictive pericarditis come to the physician's attention in three ways:

- Those with a well-recognized acute pericarditis who develop pericardial constriction either in continuity with the acute stage or after a latent period;

- Those with an insidious onset of a disease appearing to be chronic from the beginning;

- Asymptomatic patients found by radiography to have pericardial calcification.

In the first group the most typical cases are those with tuberculous pericarditis who may enter a subacute stage — still with pericardial effusion but already showing some evidence of constriction — then eventually lapse into the chronic stage. Antituberculous therapy may check the process but is not always effective.

In viral pericarditis patients often have two or three recurrences of acute pericarditis months apart and eventually may show signs of mild hemodynamic residual abnormalities when recovering. These may clear or persist, but eventually typical constriction may appear.

Radiation pericarditis develops within a few months after extensive radiation to the thorax (usually for treatment of mediastinal neoplasms). It may take the form of constrictive pericarditis or that of the subacute effusive-constrictive variety.

The symptomatology of constrictive pericarditis varies: some patients have no symptoms but become aware of abdominal enlargement and ankle edema. Dyspnea and weakness with fatigability may be present in some. As a rule symptoms and signs develop slowly and gradually, followed by a clinical course that may be stable, with little or no progression taking place for long periods of time. Medical therapy directed at fluid retention is not as effective as in congestive cardiac failure, yet it may control to some extent the congestive manifestations and permit the patient to remain in a stationary state in relative comfort. In patients with tuberculous pericarditis the chronic stage (as opposed to the subacute pericarditis) seldom responds to antituberculous therapy.

Results of surgical decortication of the pericardium include the entire spectrum, from dramatic improvement approaching cure of the disease to a complete failure to improve the condition. Results may depend upon the surgical skill, experience, and the technique used, but more often are related to an inability to remove the thickened visceral pericardium without damaging the myocardium at the same time.

The postoperative course of patients who have obtained significant immediate benefit from the operation is often satisfactory and lasting, but occasionally recurrence of the constriction may be observed.

Complications of constrictive pericarditis are few. Atrial arrhythmias, including atrial fibrillation, may develop, though this occurs less often than in patients with myocardial failure of equivalent degree. Patients with an advanced degree of constriction not amenable to surgical treatment show the various complications similar to those of intractable cardiac failure, mostly related to stasis and low cardiac output (e.g., thrombotic and thromboembolic phenomena).

DIAGNOSIS

The principal diagnostic goal in constrictive pericarditis is to establish the diagnosis of pericardial disease as responsible for congestive phenomena and to evaluate the degree of abnormalities.

Clinical findings reveal the preferential presence of right-sided congestive phenomena:

- Symptomatology is noncharacteristic, as pointed out.

- Elevated venous pressure with an easily visible venous jugular pulse is the sine qua non for the diagnosis of pericardial constriction.

- Kussmaul's sign — inspiratory increase in venous pressure, visible as an increased prominence of the jugular venous pulse — is commonly present.

- Tachycardia and narrow pulse pressure are often present.

- Pulsus paradoxus is occasionally present (less often than in acute tamponade).

- Auscultatory findings reveal as the only abnormality a loud, low-frequency early diastolic sound — diastolic knock — which is related to the sudden deceleration of the blood reaching the maximum distensibility of the restricted ventricle.

- Ascites and hepatomegaly are prominent, often dominating the clinical picture.

- Peripheral cyanosis may be present.

- Severe edema of lower extremities is often present.

Electrocardiographic findings are not characteristic per se; however, low voltage and flattened or inverted T waves are frequently seen in constrictive pericarditis. The presence of specific electrocardiographic abnormalities, such as residual changes from myocardial infarction or hypertrophy of a ventricle, are important signs *against* constrictive pericarditis. Atrial fibrillation may be present.

Radiographic findings include as the most important finding the absence of significant cardiomegaly. As a rule, the smaller the heart in a patient with systemic venous congestive phenomena, the better the case in favor of constrictive pericarditis. The presence of calcium in the pericardium is the most important other radiographic abnormality, though, of course, it is only present in some cases of constrictive pericarditis. It should be mentioned, however, that the specificity of pericardial calcification, although high, is not 100 per cent: nonconstricting pericardial calcifications may be present in a patient who happens to have some other form of cardiac disease.

Fluoroscopic examination often reveals low amplitude of pulsation of cardiac borders. This, however, is a rather unreliable sign, particularly if tachycardia is present or in cases with cardiac enlargement.

Echocardiography plays an important role in the diagnosis of pericardial disease. In constrictive pericarditis the presence of pericardial fluid can be reliably demonstrated by the echocardiogram. This is of particular importance in subacute stages of pericarditis.

Cardiac catheterization is of considerable importance in the diagnosis of constrictive pericarditis. However, the overlap with some forms of myocardial disease is such that a definitive diagnosis cannot be made — merely a high probability suggested. The following findings, based on hemodynamic consequences of pericardial constriction already discussed, play a diagnostic role:

- Severe elevation of right atrial pressure is present.

- Corresponding elevation of right ventricular pressure and end-diastolic pressure is present with the right ventricular pressure tracing showing the "square root" sign (early diastolic dip followed by plateau-like end-diastolic elevation).

- Right ventricular systolic pressure is only mildly elevated.

- Left ventricular diastolic and left atrial pressures are elevated to an extent and manner identical with right-sided pressure rises.

In subacute pericarditis pressure measurements during pericardial paracentesis provide important information regarding the location of the constriction. In effusive-constrictive pericarditis intracardiac pressure shows little change after paracentesis. In contrast, subacute pericarditis with thickening of the parietal pericardium produces a tamponade-like effect, and abnormalities may disappear after paracentesis.

Angiocardiography fulfills a relatively lesser role in the diagnosis of constrictive pericarditis. Thickening of the pericardium may be demonstrated, but unless the thickness is very pronounced or unless pericardial fluid is present as well, an overlap with normal findings makes this sign relatively unreliable.

Other laboratory procedures are of some aid in throwing light upon specific problems:

- In subacute pericarditis examination of the pericardial fluid may provide etiological clues.

- If tumor is suspected percardial biopsy may be indicated.

- Tuberculin skin tests are of limited value but may be of practical assistance in subacute cases.

- Liver function tests should be performed in patients with pronounced hepatomegaly.

In the evaluation of patients suspected of having pericardial constriction it is important to recognize the fact that congestive phenomena caused by myocardial failure overlap with pericarditis in almost all clinical and laboratory findings. Thus only a combination of findings may provide the clues necessary to consider pericarditis. Although none is fully specific, the following clinical findings are emphasized as providing high probability of pericardial constriction:

1. Reliable history of acute pericarditis or development of congestive phenomena in continuation with acute and subacute pericarditis;

2. Small, normal-shaped heart on the roentgenogram;

3. Pericardial calcification, particularly a partial or total calcific shell enveloping the heart;

4. Identity of pressure levels in the two atria with the "square root" sign in right ventricular pressure tracing and the absence of pulmonary hypertension.

Conditions in which differentiation is necessary include the following:

- Myocarditis or cardiomyopathy,

- Ischemic heart disease with myocardial damage,

- Cirrhosis of the liver (to which there is only superficial resemblance).

The first two of these conditions may have elements of "restrictive" disturbance of cardiac function, rather than straight pump failure. In cardiomyopathy some specific forms associated with myocardial infiltration (e.g., amyloidosis) are most likely to imitate pericardial constriction.

Evaluation of patients usually includes all means of study—noninvasive and invasive. A certain proportion of patients may have inconclusive findings. In the presence of a severe degree of congestion it may be necessary to perform an exploratory thoracotomy as the ultimate means of differentiation; the reversibility of pericardial constriction must be considered against the irreversibility of cardiomyopathy.

THERAPY

Inasmuch as the hemodynamic abnormalities produced by constrictive pericarditis are of a mechanical nature and do not involve myocardial malfunction, surgical relief of the constriction is the only effective method of dealing with this problem.

The success of pericardectomy relates to many factors, the most important of which is the anatomic condition of the thickened pericardium. The most favorable conditions for surgical therapy exist if the operation is performed in the subacute stage, particularly if the parietal pericardium is involved and some pericardial fluid still present. Factors unfavorably influencing the chances of success are the presence of dense fibrous scar tissue engulfing the visceral pericardium and evidence of heavy calcification.

It is clear that unless the entire pericardium can be stripped from the heart the outcome in terms of relief of the constriction is uncertain. The risks of the operation involve the following considerations:

- Risk of death, varying from 10 to 25 per cent;

- Risk of aggravating congestion by damaging the epicardial layer of the myocardium;

- Failure to improve after pericardectomy.

In view of these considerations indications for surgical therapy should be based on definite clinical disability in which major benefits could be expected in the clinical rehabilitation of the patient. Those patients who show signs of peripheral systemic congestion but retain reasonable effort capacity should not be considered surgical candidates. The stability of the process may be established in such cases, i.e., the maximum scarring process may have already occurred so that patients may remain permanently at a certain stage without ever showing deterioration.

As an adjunct to surgical therapy in patients with tuberculous pericarditis (in the subacute stage) antituberculous therapy is indicated. The question as to whether the operation should be deferred until this therapy is completed is as yet unsettled: in patients with unquestionable evidence of constriction—even with effusion still present—early operation may be advisable in view of the fact that the prognosis is better in early operations and the risk of the operation minimized.

In patients who do not come to surgery, or in those who underwent pericardectomy but remain unimproved, conventional management of congestive phenomena is indicated. Diuretic therapy, sodium restriction, and reduction of activities may be of some help to the patient but, as stated, are less likely to be effective here than in cases with myocardial failure. Digitalis is of little use, even though the possibility of some additional myocardial malfunction may be present (from involvement of the epicardial layer), unless it is used for the control of the ventricular rate in complicating atrial fibrillation.

Bibliography

Cohn KE, Stewart JR, Fajardo LF, Hancock EW: Heart disease following radiation. Medicine *46*:281, 1967.

Conti CR, Friesinger GC: Chronic constrictive pericarditis. Clinical and laboratory findings in 11 cases. Johns Hopkins Med. J. *120*:262, 1967.

Hancock EW: Subacute effusive-constrictive pericarditis. Circulation 43:183, 1971.

Howard EJ, Maier HC: Constrictive pericarditis following acute Coxsackie viral pericarditis. Amer. Heart J. 74:247, 1968.

Lange RL, Botticelli JT, Tsagaris TJ, Walker JA, Gani M, Bustamante RA: Diagnostic signs in compressive cardiac disorders: constrictive pericarditis, pericardial effusion and tamponade. Circulation 33:763, 1966.

Robertson R, Arnold CR: Constrictive pericarditis with particular reference to etiology. Circulation 26:525, 1962.

Wood P: Chronic constrictive pericarditis. Amer. J. Cardiol. 7:48, 1961.

42

Rarer Forms of
Heart Disease

In this chapter several congenital and acquired forms of cardiac disease, not necessarily related to each other, are discussed. They are less commonly encountered than most of those presented in earlier chapters, yet occur often enough to be included by the clinician among diagnostic possibilities to be considered in patients with heart disease.

CONGENITAL LESIONS

Transposition Syndromes

Transposition of the great arteries represents a common form of congenital heart disease. Yet most of these are instances of complete transposition, in which only occasionally survival beyond infancy is possible, even with the aid of presently available surgical means of correction.

Transposition of the great arteries is the result of embryological errors which may lead to a number of complex congenital malformations. From the practical standpoint three varieties are of sufficient clinical importance that the clinician should have at least a passing knowledge of problems involved:

- complete transposition of the great arteries,

- partial transposition of the great arteries,

- corrected transposition of the great arteries.

Complete Transposition of the Great Arteries. An abnormal division of the primitive arterial trunk into the two great arteries results in their altered position, with the aorta located anteriorly and the pulmonary artery posteriorly. If this is the sole abnormality, the aorta then connects with the right ventricle and the pulmonary artery with the left ventricle. The blood returning to the heart from the systemic circulation via the caval system is ejected by the right ventricle into the aorta, hence is directed, unoxygenated, back into the systemic circulation. Pulmonary venous blood is ejected into the pulmonary artery and returns, fully oxygenated, back to the lungs. Obviously life cannot exist under such circumstances unless some mixing of the two bloods is possible. Survival is thus contingent on the ameliorating effects of such shunting lesions as atrial septal defect, ventricular septal defect, and patent ductus arteriosus, present singly or in combination. The most favorable conditions for survival are the following:

- When a large interatrial communication is present (not only patent foramen ovale);

- If the infant happens to have associated pulmonary stenosis.

As a rule deep cyanosis is present; occasionally blood mixing is so effective that hypoxia is relatively mild and only minimal cyanosis is present. The overall outlook and prognosis in untreated infants is influenced not only by the hypoxia but also by cardiac failure caused by the overload resulting from abnormal circulatory pathways.

The natural history of transposition was drastically changed—at least to a point where many infants can be protected from early death—by the introduction of surgical palliative procedures and particularly by the introduction of septostomy that can be performed during cardiac catheterization. This procedure consists of the introduction of an inflatable balloon catheter via the foramen ovale into the left atrium and retraction of the inflated balloon for the purpose of tearing the atrial septum and enlarging the interatrial communication. Other palliative operations include a shunting procedure (Blalock-Hanlon) in severely cyanotic infants or pulmonary arterial banding in those with very large pulmonary flow producing cardiac failure. A definitive procedure—the Mustard operation or its modification—is based on the principle of reversing the venous return in a manner that pulmonary venous blood would be ejected into the aorta and caval blood into the pulmonary artery. This operation can be performed in children who survive infancy. While it offers correction of the principal physiological circulatory derangement, the long-range effect of the operation is not yet known. The success of the operation and the overall prognosis are enhanced if:

- Pulmonary stenosis is present;

- The ventricular septum is closed.

The *diagnosis* of complete transposition is based on a complete hemodynamic-angiocardiographic evaluation. The difficulty of obtaining the complete diagnosis — not only of the presence of complete transposition but also of all the associated lesions — is considerable; such studies represent a major challenge for the pediatric cardiologist; their discussion is beyond the scope of this book. The suspicion for the presence of complete transposition in infants (also in the rare instance of survivors later in life) should be aroused when the following findings are noted:

- severe cyanosis since birth,

- cardiomegaly,

- increased pulmonary vasculature,

- early onset of cardiac failure.

Partial Transposition of the Great Arteries. This involves incomplete malrotation of the great arteries. Out of the spectrum of possible combinations two clinical syndromes are recognized:

1. The Bing-Taussig syndrome,

2. Double-outlet right ventricle.

Bing-Taussig anomaly consists of a large, equilibrating ventricular septal defect with the pulmonary artery partially transposed to the left, straddling over the defect, while the aorta is completely transposed, arising from the right ventricle. Clinically this syndrome resembles the cyanotic form of large ventricular septal defect, except for the early onset of cyanosis. The diagnosis has to be established by hemodynamic-angiocardiographic evaluation. The overall outlook here is not unfavorable; survival to adulthood and beyond is common. No completely satisfactory surgical correction is available.

The double-outlet right ventricle consists of a normally positioned pulmonary artery and dextroposition of the aorta, which originates completely from the right ventricle. The two ventricles are connected by means of a large septal defect. As in the preceding lesion the dominating abnormality here is the large ventricular septal defect with its obligatory pulmonary hypertension. Streamlining frequently permits left ventricular blood to be preferentially ejected into the malpositioned aorta, hence cyanosis may be mild or absent. This lesion is often misdiagnosed as a simple ventricular septal defect, even after an angiographic study, unless considerable attention is paid to details of the position of the great vessels. Recently echocardiography has established itself as a useful tool in differentiating between plain ventricular septal defect and the double-outlet right ventricle. In spite of dextroposition of the aorta it is often possible to perform surgical correction by extending the septal patch in a manner that brings the aorta in communication with the left ventricle, particularly in the infracristal type of ventricular septal defect.

Corrected Transposition of the Great Arteries. Though rarer than complete transposition at birth, this is by far the most important clinical lesion for the clinician dealing with older children and adults. The developmental defect here is similar to that of complete transposition, in that the great vessels are malrotated, the pulmonary artery posteriorly and medially and the aorta anteriorly and laterally. However, in contrast to the latter lesion, the two ventricles are also inverted, so that the right ventricle, located more posteriorly, connects with the pulmonary artery, while the left ventricle, located more anteriorly, connects with the aorta. The ventricular inversion produces structural reversal of the ventricles: the anatomic right ventricle, with its tricuspid valve, now operates on the left side, while the anatomic left ventricle, with the mitral valve, functions on the right side.

Physiologically, the flow of blood proceeds along normal pathways, so that theoretically a normal circulation may be expected. However, the anatomic abnormality produces the following sequels:

1. Direct consequences of the altered structure:

   • Disturbances of the atrioventricular conduction,

   • Lessened capability of the tricuspid valve to withstand systemic pressure.

2. Frequent association of other congenital defects:

   • Ventricular septal defect,

   • Pulmonary stenosis,

   • Downward displacement of the tricuspid valve (left-sided Ebstein anomaly),

   • Aortic stenosis.

These lesions are most commonly associated with corrected transposition; however, any type of congenital cardiac lesion or any combination of lesions may be present.

The presence of corrected transposition without any sequels or associated lesions is likely to escape attention in spite of the fact that radiological and electrocardiographic clues could separate such patients from the general population. Thus the problem of corrected transposition revolves around the following points:

1. The presence of commoner congenital cardiac lesions that may be associated with atypical features and confusing clinical pictures;

2.   Disturbances of cardiac rhythm in young subjects without obvious congenital heart disease;

3.   Development of nonrheumatic mitral regurgitation early in life.

Clinical features of corrected transposition include the following:

- Roentgenographic findings: narrower and atypical shadows of the great vessels;

- Electrocardiographic features: absence of Q waves in left precordial leads and presence of Q waves in right precordial leads (usually QR complex in lead V_1). First degree AV block is very common; complete AV block may be present.

Each of these features has only a fair specificity and sensitivity. It is estimated that in proven cases of corrected transposition these signs occur in between 50 and 75 per cent of patients. However, if all the features are present, the probability of finding corrected transposition is appropriately increased.

The frequent association of corrected transposition with disturbances of AV conduction justifies a high index of suspicion for the presence of this abnormality in all patients with congenital complete AV block.

In addition to conduction disturbances, other arrhythmias occur more frequently in patients with corrected transposition than in the general population. Wolff-Parkinson-White syndrome is reported in some patients along with the resulting tachyarrhythmias. Other atrial and ventricular arrhythmias have also been frequently observed.

The practical significance of "silent" corrected transposition (i.e., not associated with any significant sequel or abnormality) lies in the potential difficulty that may arise if the patient acquires some form of cardiac disease:

- Technical difficulties in entering the pulmonary artery during cardiac catheterization may interfere with the performance of a hemodynamic study.

- Abnormal course of the coronary arteries may bring about diagnostic difficulties and lead to misinterpretations in patients who develop ischemic heart disease.

When corrected transposition is associated with other congenital defects, the clinical features may be confusing, especially the auscultatory findings: murmurs or aortic or pulmonary stenosis may be present in unusual locations; the two components of the second sound may be confused with each other. Diagnostic evaluation is made more difficult by the already mentioned frequent inability to enter the pulmonary artery. Nevertheless, a combination of cardiac catheterization and angio-cardiography usually permits the establishment of the correct diagnosis of the other defects as well as the corrected transposition.

Corrected transposition may be of major prognostic importance in patients requiring cardiac surgery, especially if ventriculotomy has to be performed (in ventricular septal defect). The anomalous course of the coronary arteries makes ventriculotomy difficult and the possibility of injury to the coronary arteries increased, hence the overall risk of surgical correction higher. This fact often forces a more conservative assessment of operability of patients with corrected transposition and associated congenital lesions in whom, by usual standards, cardiac operations would seem indicated.

Ebstein's Anomaly

The essential congenital malformation of Ebstein's anomaly is a downward displacement of the tricuspid valve. Instead of arising from the tricuspid ring, one or two of the three cusps arise from the wall of the right ventricle, attached to the musculature of its free wall between the ring and the apex of the right ventricle. The extent of the anomaly relates to the distance of the attachment of the cusp from the tricuspid ring: milder cases come off close to the ring, severe ones closer to the apex. Thus part or all of the inflow tract of the right ventricle is func-tionally incorporated into the right atrium, being proximal to the tricuspid valve. Associated with the anatomic malformation may be an atrial septal defect; if one is not present, the foramen ovale often fails to close in the postnatal period, providing a channel for the right-to-left shunt that usually constitutes a part of the Ebstein anomaly.

The pathophysiological consequence of this anomaly is a reduced flow into the lung and a right-to-left shunt into the left atrium. The small capacity of the right ventricle—consisting mostly or only of the noncompliant outflow tract—usually accompanied by regurgitation of the abnormal tricuspid valve, directs caval blood to the left side. Yet, right ventricular pressures and pulmonary arterial pressures are nor-mal or lower than normal.

The wide variability of the anatomic abnormality of the tricuspid valve regarding its size and point of attachment, as well as the re-sponses of the right-sided circulation to it, account for the broad spec-trum of the *natural history* of this syndrome. The most constant feature of it is hypoxia and cyanosis. Deeply cyanotic infants may get into dif-ficulty early in life; with mild cyanosis the prognosis may be very good, consistent even with longevity. The symptomatology associated with Ebstein's anomaly consists of effort intolerance due to dyspnea or ex-cessive fatigability. Tendency to arrhythmias may be present, account-ing for the well-publicized risk of dying during cardiac catheterization.

Clinical features of Ebstein's anomaly are as follows:

- Cyanosis (with clubbing of digits) is usually, though not uniformly, present, showing a wide range in degree.

- Auscultatory findings consist of S3 and S4 gallop sounds (quadruple rhythm is very common); murmurs are occasionally present and are noncharacteristic.

- Radiographic findings include an enlarged, globular heart with normal or diminished pulmonary vascularity.

- Electrocardiogram usually shows signs of right atrial hypertrophy and intraventricular conduction defects, often bizarre and atypical. Wolff-Parkinson-White syndrome is occasionally present in association with Ebstein's anomaly.

- Cardiac catheterization may reveal normal right-sided pressure and a right-to-left shunt via a patent foramen ovale or an atrial septal defect. Signs of tricuspid regurgitation and of right ventricular failure may be present. Electrograms from areas of the right heart in which right atrial pressures are recorded may indicate ventricular potential, thereby providing "atrialization" of the inflow tract of the right ventricle.

- Angiocardiographic studies often show the position of the tricuspid valve directly demonstrating its malattachment.

The *diagnosis* of Ebstein's anomaly may be very easy. When the above features are present in more characteristic form, a firm clinical diagnosis may be done noninvasively. Cardiac catheterization and angiographic study provide then only the frosting on the cake, though they are often necessary to establish the diagnosis beyond doubt and rule out other or associated lesions. The once widely held belief that cardiac catheterization is hazardous in this syndrome has been only partly confirmed in the recent more extensive experience of many centers. Differentiation involves the following conditions:

- In milder cases Ebstein's anomaly may have to be separated from some borderline findings in healthy subjects.

- If the presence of cardiac disease is unquestionable, such conditions as atrial septal defect, mild pulmonary stenosis, and tetralogy of Fallot come into consideration.

- Occasionally acquired valvular heart disease (e.g., mitral stenosis or regurgitation) may overlap with Ebstein's anomaly.

Treatment of this syndrome ranges from none to surgical correction. Ideally, the placement of a prosthetic valve in the tricuspid ring and closure of the atrial septal defect or the foramen ovale may establish anatomic conditions close to normal. This operation is occasionally performed with clinical improvement. Yet, the benign course in many patients with Ebstein's anomaly—the commonly observed stable, nonprogressive course well into the adult life—makes indications for surgical treatment difficult. Uncertainty regarding the long-range fate of a prosthetic tricuspid valve should be considered as a good reason for conservatism and the restriction of surgical therapy to severely symptomatic patients. Furthermore, a collected series of cases (Watson, 1974) indicates unacceptably high risk of surgical treatment of this lesion. At present, only in the most severe, desperate cases can one make a good argument for surgical repair.

Anomalous Pulmonary Venous Return

This group of malformations involves abnormal drainage of the pulmonary veins, which connect with the right atrium, thus directing fully oxygenated blood back to the lungs. It involves the following:

- Total anomalous pulmonary venous return, in which all pulmonary venous blood is mixed with caval blood;

- Partial anomalous pulmonary venous return, with some pulmonary veins connecting normally with the left atrium and some draining abnormally into the caval system. This usually involves abnormal drainage from one pulmonary lobe or one lung and is associated with an atrial septal defect (see Chapter 27).

Total anomalous pulmonary venous return occurs in three principal varieties:

1. Pulmonary veins connect with a persistent left superior vena cava, which carries pulmonary venous blood to the left innominate vein, then to the right superior vena cava and the right atrium.

2. Pulmonary veins drain into the coronary sinus and hence to the right atrium.

3. Pulmonary veins drain via a subdiaphragmatic connection to the portal vein system.

In total anomalous pulmonary venous return there is obligatory patency of the foramen ovale or presence of an atrial septal defect. Mixed blood, containing deoxygenated caval blood and fully oxygenated pulmonary venous blood together, enters the right atrium, therein dividing into the portion directed to the left atrium for the systemic circulation and the portion directed to the lungs. Obviously, blood ejected into the aorta and that ejected to the pulmonary artery have the same content of oxygen. The degree of oxygen desaturation—hence the degree of cyanosis—is related to the respective proportions of the mixture of oxygenated and deoxygenated blood. Thus, the larger the pulmonary blood flow, the more favorable conditions exist regarding oxygenation of arterial blood.

A common complication of total anomalous pulmonary venous return is pulmonary hypertension, which may be hyperkinetic (from increased pulmonary flow alone) or vasoreactive or due to a combination of both factors. Reactive pulmonary hypertension may be initiated and perpetuated by the elevated pulmonary venous pressure which may develop because of the resistance to flow though the circuitous route as well as because of the presence of abnormal narrowing within the venous pathways. This is particularly common in the subdiaphragmatic variety, draining into the portal system.

The clinical course of total anomalous pulmonary venous return shows wide variation. In infancy the presence of large pulmonary flow and of pulmonary hypertension may introduce serious risk to survival, which may require a palliative procedure such as pulmonary arterial banding. The natural history of this lesion is analogous to that of shunting lesions, e.g., the ventricular septal defect, in which serious circulatory disturbances may develop in the postnatal period, but once they are overcome—or if they have never occurred—the course can take a benign turn. Many patients with total anomalous pulmonary venous return who have large pulmonary flow, but not to the extent of an excessive circulatory overload, may have very little hypoxia and virtually no visible cyanosis and may masquerade as a simple atrial septal defect. Such patients reach adult life without difficulty and tend to run the course similar to that of those with an atrial septal defect with a large shunt.

The clinical symptomatology is rather variable: cyanotic patients may have symptoms related to hypoxia and polycythemia. Noncyanotic patients may have few symptoms, such as mild limitation of activities due to dyspnea and excessive fatigability. Arrhythmias occur commonly as a complication of this lesion.

Clinical findings resemble those of an atrial septal defect; there are no distinctive signs except, occasionally, venous hum-like continuous murmurs. Other signs include fixed splitting of the second sound, pulmonary ejection murmur, and early diastolic flow murmurs. The electrocardiogram usually shows right-sided conduction defect, thereby also overlapping with the atrial septal defect. However, the radiographic findings usually present a characteristic picture in pulmonary venous return draining to the left superior vena cava. Here the abnormal upper mediastinal shadow ("figure of eight") may make the diagnosis obvious. In other forms of anomalous drainage, the radiographic findings are less characteristic.

Cardiac catheterization and angiographic studies provide the definitive diagnosis. Cardiac catheterization permits the evaluation of the pulmonary blood flow and pressure; the presence of arterial hypoxia is established. The most characteristic finding is the identity of oxygen saturations of samples obtained from the pulmonary artery and the aorta—both receiving blood from the same mixture. This finding alone, however, cannot be considered proof for the existence of total anomalous venous return, for it is possible to have good mixing of blood in large atrial septal defects (such as a single atrium). Angiography permits the tracing of the course of the pulmonary vein, especially when the injection of the contrast medium is done in each pulmonary artery separately.

Treatment of total anomalous pulmonary venous return depends upon the anatomic feasibility of surgical correction. Patients with supradiaphragmatic types of pulmonary venous drainage are often subject to complete correction by connecting the pulmonary veins with the left atrium. This is performed with a relatively low risk. With simultaneous closure of the atrial septal defect or the foramen ovale, normal anatomic conditions can be established. If no pulmonary hypertension was present, physiological conditions can also approach the norm. As already mentioned, cardiac failure in infancy with very large pulmonary flow may necessitate surgical intervention before the optimal time for corrective surgery, in which case a palliative banding of the pulmonary artery may be performed with reasonable prospect of success.

Other Lesions with Complete Arteriovenous Blood Mixing

In addition to total anomalous pulmonary venous return there are three other congenital lesions in which complete mixing of oxygenated and nonoxygenated blood may occur, and in which survival to adult age is possible. These are:

- Persistent truncus arteriosus.
- Trilocular heart (three-chambered heart),
- Tricuspid atresia.

Persistent Truncus Arteriosus.   In this lesion the primitive trunk fails to divide into two great arteries. Thus a single large arterial trunk emerges from the heart, straddling both ventricles over a large ventricular septal defect. The common trunk gives up two pulmonary arteries which supply the lungs in a conventional manner. These two pulmonary arteries may arise from the sides of the trunk or from its posterior portion. Not to be confused with persistent truncus arteriosus is the so called "pseudotruncus," which merely represents the extreme end of the spectrum of tetralogy of Fallot (see Chapter 30), with complete closure of the pulmonary outflow tract (pulmonary atresia). Here, the large single vessel is the aorta; the pulmonary blood flow arises entirely via collaterals from the bronchial arteries and/or the duct.

In persistent truncus arteriosus the completely mixed oxygenated and deoxygenated blood enters both the systemic and pulmonary circulation. As in the totally anomalous pulmonary venous return, the saturation of the arterial blood is always reduced, though to a variable degree, depending upon the respective contribution of the pulmonary venous and caval blood to the mixture. As in the former lesion, the larger the pulmonary blood flow, the richer this mixture in oxygenated blood, hence the closer arterial saturation is to normal. In addition to causing arterial oxygen desaturation, persistent truncus arteriosus perfuses the pulmonary circulation with blood under systemic pressure, hence there is obligatory pulmonary hypertension. Pulmonary hypertension is maintained by increased pulmonary resistance and increased pulmonary flow. When the former predominates, more cyanosis is present; when the latter is prevalent, cyanosis is minimized.

The course of persistent truncus arteriosus resembles that of a large ventricular septal defect: in infancy serious circulatory derangement may develop and many patients succumb early in life. Yet, some not only survive through infancy but live into adult life.

The diagnosis of persistent truncus arteriosus is based primarily on angiocardiographic findings. Clinical findings are noncharacteristic. A loud single second sound may be present as well as an ejection sound. Murmurs are often absent, and if present are noncharacteristic. Radiographic and electrocardiographic findings, too, do not have distinctive diagnostic features.

Until recently persistent truncus arteriosus was an inoperable lesion, except for some palliative pulmonary arterial banding in selected patients with excessive pulmonary flow but without pulmonary vascular disease. Recently corrective operations have been successfully performed in patients who survive beyond infancy and in whom no pulmonary vascular disease is present. Closure of the ventricular septal defect is combined with reconstruction of a pulmonary arterial system hooked into the right ventricle. Long-range fate of children with this operation is not known.

Trilocular Heart. This involves a heart consisting of three chambers; it therefore includes a single atrium or a single ventricle.

Single atrium can be considered the extreme end of the spectrum of atrial septal defect. Except for the fact that free mixing occurs in the large defect, the clinical features and the course of the disease are identical with those of large atrial septal defect. The usual physiological conditions lead to large pulmonary blood flow with low pulmonary vascular resistance. Thus, even with mixing, cyanosis may be minimal or absent. Surgical correction of a single atrium is possible—it is technically only slightly more complex than the repair of a large atrial septal defect by means of patches; results are good, re-establishing a near normal circulatory status.

Single ventricle represents, in contrast to the former lesion, a very complex malformation. As explained in Chapter 28, the largest ventricular septal defects reach the size of about 3 cm. in diameter; there is thus no gradual transition between a large ventricular septal defect and a complete absence of the ventricular septum. The latter is embryologically and anatomically an entirely different malformation, one which almost never occurs as an isolated lesion but as a rule is combined with other defects. Thus, the single ventricle does not represent a combination of two equal and normal ventricles minus the septum between them but rather a case in which one ventricle—the right (usually) or the left (occasionally)—is rudimentary or hypoplastic. Combined with this defect usually is hypoplasia of one of the great arteries or obstruction of the orifice leading to it. Transposition of the great arteries also occurs commonly in association with a single ventricle.

Inasmuch as a large ventricular septal defect—even though it interrupts only a portion of the ventricular septum—causes the ventricles to work as a single pump, single ventricle physiologically exerts the same effect, except for providing a better opportunity for mixing of oxygenated and deoxygenated bloods. Yet the pathophysiology and the resulting course and natural history are influenced more by the associated lesions.

Thus, from the clinical standpoint, one is dealing with complex congenital malformations that include a single ventricle. Some combinations are more favorable and permit survival beyond infancy, even to adult age. Such patients may show varying degrees of cyanosis, and some may be only mildly cyanotic. Clinical findings vary to a sufficient degree that not even suggestive diagnostic features can be predicted. The diagnosis depends entirely upon hemodynamic-angiocardiographic examination. It should be pointed out that such studies have to be performed with great care and meticulous technique, for the differentiation of a single ventricle from a large ventricular septal defect may be difficult, and both can be associated with other cardiac malformations.

Surgical correction of a single ventricle is not possible. Palliative operations are available under special circumstances: excessive pulmonary flow without pulmonary vascular resistance can be reduced by pulmonary arterial banding; severe pulmonary stenosis with low pulmonary blood flow can be favorably influenced by a shunting operation.

Tricuspid Atresia. This lesion involves absence of a communication between the right atrium and the right ventricle; as a result all the blood enters the left atrium. The oxygenated and deoxygenated blood is mixed in the left atrium and the left ventricle and is then redirected to the right ventricle and the pulmonary circulation via a ventricular septal defect and also ejected into the aorta. The prognosis of tricuspid atresia depends upon the size of the pulmonary arterial system: as in the other mixing lesion, the degree of unsaturation of blood entering both circuits is related to the magnitude of pulmonary flow. Although it is basically a severely cyanotic lesion, children occasionally may show mild or even subliminal cyanosis.

The course of tricuspid atresia resembles more that of other severely cyanotic lesions: severe tetralogy of Fallot, pulmonary stenosis with patent foramen ovale, and transposition of the great arteries. Cyanotic attacks, severe polycythemia, and a tendency to thrombotic complications are more common than cardiac failure. Children with less favorable anatomic conditions do not survive infancy; however, enough children live into childhood, adolescence, or even adulthood to make this lesion one to be considered among cyanotic congenital cardiac malformations.

The characteristic feature of tricuspid atresia—one which gives it an almost unique position—is the presence of left ventricular hypertrophy. This may be evident on clinical examination and is characteristic as the electrocardiographic feature. Cardiac catheterization and angiocardiographic studies establish the diagnosis with reasonable certainty.

Complete correction of tricuspid atresia is not possible; however, successful palliation that can prolong the life of patients and carry them into adulthood is available in the form of the various shunting operations.

ACQUIRED LESIONS

Cardiac Tumors

Secondary tumors—metastatic or invasive—outnumber primary tumors of the heart many times. Yet primary cardiac tumors provide a diagnostic challenge to the clinician by imitating some common forms of cardiac disease and by the fact that they may represent a curable form of cardiac disease.

Metastatic tumors usually appear late in the course of malignant disease, and the presence of this condition is suspected on other grounds. Tumors invading the heart by contiguity or spread from other thoracic organs are more likely to affect the heart at a time when the overall diagnosis may not yet be evident. Invasion of the pericardium is common and the following two features may direct the attention to cardiac involvement by a tumor (though the specificity is very low):

- Pericardial effusion, particularly when yielding sanguineous fluid;

- Persistent atrial arrhythmias—flutter or fibrillation.

Other possible clues for the presence of secondary tumors include the occasional production of conduction disturbances (e.g., complete AV block) and sudden, unexplained cardiac failure. Tumors in the thorax may obstruct caval flow, hence imitate systemic venous congestion.

Primary tumors of the heart involve the following principal varieties:

- Solid tumors, usually intramural;

- Endocardial tumors, usually pedunculated myxomas;

- Pericardial tumors.

Solid tumors include benign neoplasms, such as rhabdomyoma, leiomyoma, teratoma, etc., or malignant ones, such as rhabdomyosarcoma and mesothelioma. Their clinical manifestations depend upon their location and size. The following consequences of tumor invasion of the myocardium may occur:

- Obstructive phenomena, imitating inflow or outflow resistance to a ventricle;

- Development of cardiac failure;

- Production of arrhythmias.

Myxoma is the commonest primary tumor of the heart, accounting for more than half of cases. Its unique clinical features and its complete curability makes it an important clinical entity in spite of its relative rarity.

Myxoma is a gelatinous, pedunculated, often lobulated tumor growing to the size of an orange. Its commonest location is the left atrium, with occasional occurrence in the right atrium, right ventricle, and left ventricle, in that order of frequency. It produces three groups of clinical manifestations:

1. Obstructive—most commonly masquerading as stenosis of one of the cardiac orifices;

2. Embolic — causing major, often disastrous embolic episodes, particularly significant in left-sided tumors;

3. General systemic — producing fever, malaise, and other signs suggestive of a chronic or subacute illness.

The obstructive manifestations show considerable variability. They are due to the great mobility of the tumor, which, as a rule, is attached to the atrial or ventricular wall (usually the septum) by means of the thin peduncle. The mass moves with the flow of blood producing the following consequences:

- In left atrial myxoma — masquerading as mitral stenosis, or mitral regurgitation, or a combination of both;

- In right atrial myxoma — tricuspid stenosis and/or regurgitation, possibly with right-to-left shunting through a foramen ovale;

- In left ventricular myxoma — outflow obstruction (subaortic stenosis);

- In right ventricular myxoma — signs of pulmonary stenosis, rarely, pulmonary regurgitation.

Systemic emboli occur characteristically in left atrial myxoma, causing major cerebral accidents as well as occlusive episodes in other organs and in the extremities.

Systemic manifestations are subject to wide variability; often none are present, but in some cases they dominate the clinical picture long before any more specific clues become apparent. The triad of fever, malaise, and anemia often produces the clinical picture resembling infective endocarditis.

The natural history of cardiac myxomas is often related to the predominance of the clinical manifestations in terms of permitting the early diagnosis and the surgical cure. Untreated, patients develop progressively serious consequences of the obstructive mass, with cardiac failure intervening rapidly in view of the progressive nature of this disease and in contrast to the more static course of rheumatic and other etiological forms of valvular disease. Pulmonary hypertension is particularly common and may be severe. Systemic disease — the nature of which is usually not entirely clear — may lead to irreversible secondary consequences, such as myocarditis, which could even nullify the success of the total removal of the tumor. Emboli may produce disabling hemiplegia or a fatal episode (e.g., coronary embolism).

The varying symptomatology of myxomas as well as the varying speed of their growth make the course of this condition totally unpredictable. Certain clinical symptoms have been traditionally associated with myxomas, such as syncope or marked changes in the presence or intensity of cardiac murmurs. These have been observed in patients with myxoma, yet larger series now available show that they occur only occasionally, have low specificity, and are of little diagnostic help.

The diagnosis of myxoma requires a high index of suspicion in patients with some unusual manifestations of cardiac disease. Furthermore, patients should be screened for the remote possibility of myxoma even in the presence of typical manifestations of such diseases as mitral stenosis or mitral regurgitation. The following features may be of importance in arousing suspicion of myxoma:

- Murmurs of mitral stenosis without an opening snap of the mitral valve but with a dull, low-frequency diastolic sound (tumor plop);

- Sudden appearance and rapid progression of mitral stenosis;

- Showers of systemic emboli in patients who are in sinus rhythm;

- Infective endocarditis-like illness with persistently negative blood culture, unresponsive to antibiotic therapy.

Conventional laboratory tests are usually of little help in the diagnosis. Electrocardiographic and roentgenographic findings usually are those expected in association with the respective obstructive manifestation, i.e., mitral stenosis, subaortic stenosis, etc. Anemia has already been mentioned—it is present in about 50 per cent of patients with myxoma. Patients may show, along with anemia, marked elevation of erythrocyte sedimentation rate and the presence of abnormal serum proteins. Occasionally the diagnosis can be made by examination of the tissue removed during embolectomy. The most important noninvasive test showing myxoma with high specificity is the echocardiogram, which can demonstrate an intracavitary movable mass. The final diagnosis is made by selective cineangiocardiography, which usually demonstrates the tumor, its position, size, and motion.

In the differential diagnosis valvular heart disease is the principal group of lesions to be considered in conjunction with myxomas. It should be remembered that the majority of patients with left atrial myxoma show signs and symptoms indistinguishable from those of rheumatic mitral stenosis; hence the need for screening examinations. This is of considerable practical importance because an operation is indicated early in myxoma, with a patient asymptomatic, which is not the case in mitral stenosis.

In patients with systemic manifestations of myxoma most frequently confusion is with infective endocarditis and with collagen systemic diseases. Here, again, the difference in the therapy and the prognosis makes it imperative to rule out myxoma, regardless of how remote the possibility might appear.

The therapy of myxoma is surgical. Removal of the tumor requires open heart surgery, but it represents a simple operation, usually yielding a complete cure. Complete resection of the pedicle may ensure against recurrences.

Traumatic Lesions of the Heart

Trauma to the thorax involving the heart occurs in the following forms:

- Penetrating wounds,

- Nonpenetrating trauma,

- Other forms of trauma.

Penetrating trauma represents most often a surgical condition requiring early surgical intervention. The common forms of penetrating trauma are stab wounds and shot wounds. Injury to the heart includes the following:

- Pericardial injury, resulting in pericarditis, usually purulent;

- Myocardial injury, which may produce rupture and hemopericardium;

- Endocardial injury, in which damage to the valves is of major importance;

- Injury to the coronary arteries with its various consequences related to ischemia or hemopericardium;

- Injury to the great vessels.

Nonpenetrating trauma includes direct blow to the thorax, compression of the thorax (included in "steering wheel injury"), and the effects of sudden deceleration. The effects of such injury may be immediately detectable or may occur after a latent period. The effects of nonpenetrating injuries are often very difficult to assess as to their relationship to cardiac symptoms and their permanence. Many of the most perplexing medicolegal problems are related to nonpenetrating trauma. It is obvious that a great many forms of cardiac disease can be initiated by the anatomic damage produced by the trauma. Among those in which the causal relationship to trauma appears reasonably well established (provided the appropriate temporal relationship exists) are:

- Perforation of the myocardium with hemopericardium,

- Perforation of the cardiac septum (usually interventricular),

- Sudden appearance of valvular incompetence (rupture of chordae tendineae of the mitral valve or ruptured aortic cusp).

Conditions in which a causal relationship between nonpenetrating trauma and the onset of a cardiac lesion is probable (with the range of probability from slight to high) include the following:

- Acute myocardial infarction,

- Onset of anginal syndrome,

- Onset of cardiac failure,

- Cardiac contusion—often a vague concept with nonspecific symptomatology and nondiagnostic electrocardiographic abnormalities.

The most difficult task is to accept or reject the effect of trauma as an aggravating factor in pre-existing cardiac disease:

- Accentuation of cardiac failure,

- Progression of ischemic symptoms,

- Appearance of new electrocardiographic abnormalities.

Other forms of trauma to the heart include the following:

- That produced during cardiac catheterization (see Chapter 8);

- That resulting from cardiac surgery (see Chapter 13);

- Electrical injury—occasionally resulting from faulty medical apparatus—producing serious arrhythmias, rarely burns;

- Radiation injury, producing perimyocarditis.

High-Output States

Two decades ago, early in the hemodynamic era, the concept of "high-output state" and "high-output failure" attained great popularity. It is apparent now that their significance has been overestimated. Some conditions are no longer considered in this group, their original inclusion having been brought about by inexact technique of measurements. In some, high output is present, but its effect upon the circulation is no longer considered of sufficient importance to produce a clinical entity. (See also discussion in Chapter 14.)

It is probable that elevated cardiac output imposes an overload upon the circulation which is relatively well tolerated. In congenital heart disease with intracardiac shunts, appreciable increases of cardiac output occur in one or the other side of the heart and are well tolerated. It follows that elevated cardiac output is more likely to be a contributory or additive factor in patients who already have some circulatory disturbance than to act as the sole agent producing cardiac disease. Among high-output states the following deserve mention:

Anemia. Patients with less than 10 gm. of hemoglobin require a higher cardiac output to compensate for their reduced oxygen-carrying capacity. Only in very severe degrees of anemia is the magnitude of the increase in cardiac output sufficient to overload the circulatory system. The clinical manifestations of this hypercirculatory state include warm skin, bounding pulses with widened pulse pressure, and cardiac systolic murmurs of the ejection variety. Development of cardiac failure as a result of anemia—even severe anemia—in patients without previous manifestations of cardiac disease is very unusual, though occasionally sudden anemia may produce acute pulmonary edema. Sickle-cell disease may affect the heart more profoundly than other true forms of anemia, not only because of its chronicity and severity but also because of the tendency of abnormal erythrocytes to occlude small blood vessels. Pulmonary hypertension may result from it.

Hyperthyroidism. Whether "thyrotoxic heart disease" represents an important clinical entity has been and still is to some extent subject to controversy. Basically a high-output state due to increased metabolic needs of the body, the direct hormonal influence upon circulatory regulation makes hyperthyroidism a condition having a more profound effect upon the heart than other hypercirculatory states. Yet the importance of hyperthyroidism lies primarily in overloading the circulation of patients with other forms of heart disease, thus often providing a reversible contributory factor. Young individuals with thyrotoxicosis show the florid clinical picture of high-output state but seldom develop signs of intolerance of the load in the form of overt cardiac failure. Hyperthyroidism has unique features distinguishing it from other forms of high-output states; it predisposes to serious and often persistent, treatment-resistant atrial arrhythmias, particularly atrial fibrillation. This effect may be independent of the hypercirculatory state, and associated with only minor clinical manifestations of thyroid hyperfunction. The search for "occult hyperthyroidism" in patients with tachycardias or arrhythmias is well known—perhaps overemphasized in view of the very small yield of documented cases of occult hyperthyroidism. Nevertheless, both occult and overt hyperthyroidism are important because of their therapeutic implications. The easy availability of reliable thyroid function tests at the present time makes the diagnosis relatively easy. Treatment of thyroid hyperfunction may eliminate its untoward effects upon the heart.

Arteriovenous Fistulae. These represent perhaps the only form of high-output state in which cardiac failure is frequently produced by the overload alone. Here, very large volumes of blood flow through the fistulae of large sizes, increasing the output of both ventricles often to levels four to six times the normal output. In addition to the signs of high-output state, the "run-off" from the arterial system into the low-pressure venous system produces collapsing peripheral arterial pulses with lowered diastolic pressure similar to those of aortic regurgitation of severe degree. Inasmuch as arteriovenous fistulae can be locally detected by palpation and auscultation, a search for this condition is indicated in all patients with collapsing arterial pulses without obvious aortic regurgitation. A great many peripheral fistulae, though not all (depending on the location and the type of the connection), are surgically correctable. The effects of cardiac overload—including cardiac failure when present—are as a rule completely reversible.

Beriberi Heart Disease. This condition represents the effect of severe thiamine deficiency upon the myocardium. Basically a disease of the developing countries, it is nevertheless seen occasionally in our setting, particularly in subjects combining poor dietary habits with excessive alcoholic intake. It occurs basically in two forms:

- Acute beriberi heart disease, representing a high-output state;

- Chronic beriberi heart disease, representing a form of chronic cardiomyopathy and leading to low-output failure.

The second variety of beriberi heart disease is more commonly encountered in the United States; the true high-output form of thiamine deficiency is rare here. When encountered, it is manifested by reduction of effort capacity due to dyspnea in the presence of clinical signs of a hypercirculatory state. The acute form responds to thiamine therapy but not the chronic form (its relationship to thiamine deficiency is doubted by some, in the first place).

Cor Pulmonale. This had been considered a "high-output state" leading to high-output failure as a result of some early studies. This concept has now been reliably disproved and there is no longer justification to place chronic pulmonary disease in this category.

Idiopathic High-Output State. Occasional patients show elevated resting cardiac output with its higher-than-average rise during exercise, and no etiological factors can be found. The interpretation of such findings is exceedingly difficult. The possibility of undue anxiety during the hemodynamic study is hard to rule out. One may, furthermore, consider this finding the upper end of the normal hemodynamic spectrum. Perhaps—as suspected by some in the etiology of systemic hypertension—subjects at the upper end of the normal distribution curve of cardiac output may find themselves at a disadvantage, sometimes becoming definitely abnormal. Authentic cases in this category are rare but do exist. They overlap with the simple anxiety neurosis ("neurocirculatory asthenia"), probably also with milder cases of hypertrophic subaortic stenosis, and with normal subjects who have a high sympathetic drive.

Bibliography

Bornham-Carter RE, Capriles M, Noe Y: Total anomalous pulmonary venous return. Brit. Heart J. *31*:45, 1969.

Burroughs JT, Edwards JE: Total anomalous pulmonary venous connection. Amer. Heart J. *59*:913, 1960.

Campbell M: Tricuspid atresia and its prognosis with or without surgical treatment. Brit. Heart J. *23*:699, 1961.

Genton E, Blount SG Jr: The spectrum of Ebstein's anomaly. Amer. Heart J. *73*:395, 1967.

Kumar AE, Fyler DC, Miettinen OS, Nadas AS: Ebstein's anomaly: clinical profile and natural history. Amer. J. Cardiol. *28*:84, 1971.

Leonard JJ, deGroot WJ: The thyroid state and the cardiovascular system. Mod. Concepts Cardiovasc. Dis. *38*:23, 1969.

Muenster JJ, Graettinger JS, Campbell JA: Correlation of clinical and hemodynamic findings in patients with systemic arteriovenous fistulas. Circulation *20*:1079, 1959.

Neufeld HN, DuShane JW, Wood EH, Kirklin JW, Edwards JE: Origin of both great vessels from the right ventricle. Circulation *23*:399, 1961.

Noonan JA, Nadas AS, Rudolph AM, Harris GBC: Transposition of the great vessels: a correlation of clinical, physiological and autopsy data. New Engl. J. Med. *263*:592, 637, 668, 739, 1960.

Liebman J, Cullum L, Belloc NB: Natural history of transposition of great vessels. Anatomy and birth and death characteristics. Circulation *40*:237, 1969.

Lindsay J Jr, Meshel JC, Patterson RH: The cardiovascular manifestations of sickle cell disease. Arch. Int. Med. *133*:643, 1974.

Parmley LF, Manion WC, Mattingly TW: Nonpenetrating traumatic injury of the heart. Circulation *18*:371, 1958.

Rahimtoola SH, Ongley PA, Swan HJC: The hemodynamics of common (or single) ventricle. Circulation *34*:14, 1966.

Selzer A, Sakai FJ, Popper WR: Protean clinical manifestations of primary tumors of the heart. Amer. J. Med. *52*:9, 1972.

Taussig HB, Bing RJ: Complete transposition of the aorta and a laevoposition of the pulmonary artery. Amer. Heart J. *37*:551, 1949.

Van Praagh R, Van Praagh S: The anatomy of common aortico-pulmonary trunk and its embryonic implications. Amer. J. Cardiol. *16*:406, 1965.

Van Praagh R, Van Praagh S, Vlad P, Keith JD: Diagnosis of the anatomic types of single or common ventricle. Amer. J. Cardiol. *15*:345, 1965.

Watson H: Natural history of Ebstein's anomaly of tricuspid valve in childhood and adolescence. An international cooperative study of 505 cases. Brit. Heart J. *36*:417, 1974.

43

Diseases of the Aorta

CONGENITAL DISEASES OF THE AORTA

Among congenital malformations affecting the aorta, those producing obstruction and cardiac overload have already been discussed. These are:

- Coarctation of the aorta,

- Supravalvular aortic stenosis.

Other malformations involve a number of variants of the origin of the four brachiocephalic vessels from the aortic arch. There are two abnormalities of the aortic arch which may produce symptoms:

- Abnormal right subclavian artery, originating proximal to the left subclavian artery, compressing the esophagus by its passage behind it;

- A true "vascular ring" produced by a double aortic arch or related malformations constricting both the trachea and the esophagus.

These lesions may cause dysphagia and stridor varying from mild to that requiring early surgical treatment. They can be recognized by plain radiography assisted by contrast esophagograms and, if necessary, outlined in more detail by an angiographic aortic arch study. Surgical treatment is guided by the severity of symptoms.

Among the many other anomalies of the thoracic aorta, the right-sided aortic arch is worthy of mention. Occasionally occurring as an isolated malformation, it is most often found in combination with other congenital defects, particularly those associated with large ventricular septal defect (e.g., tetralogy of Fallot) or with transposition syndromes.

This anomaly of the arch is of no direct clinical significance. It may, however, present some confusing pictures in radiographic examinations and in angiocardiography; furthermore, it is of importance in terms of the surgical technique in children requiring palliative operation for cyanotic congenital lesions.

Another noteworthy congenital abnormality of the aorta is the aneurysm of a sinus of Valsalva. Inasmuch as this lesion can be either congenital or acquired, it will be included in the following discussion of aneurysm in general.

DISSECTING ANEURYSM OF THE AORTA

Dissecting aneurysm of the aorta represents a clinical entity, the recognition of which is of great importance. Once thought to be a single pathological entity — Erdheim's cystic medial necrosis — it is now considered a nonspecific "accident" separating the layers of the aorta from each other by a hematoma.

While cystic medial necrosis is an important cause of dissecting aneurysms, it is not the commonest cause of it. This condition ranges from a severe form associated with generalized connective tissue disease, occurring in Marfan's syndrome, to a milder forme fruste occurring in association with atherosclerotic changes in the aorta, particularly in patients with systemic hypertension. It has also been shown that dilatation of the aorta from any cause predisposes to dissection.

Thus the etiological and predisposing factors in the production of aortic dissection include the following:

- Medial cystic necrosis in association with Marfan's syndrome;

- Other forms of medial cystic necrosis;

- Atherosclerotic ectasia or aneurysm of the aorta;

- Systemic hypertension;

- Trauma, nonpenetrating, to the thorax;

- Surgical trauma — particularly in connection with various cardiovascular operations;

- Coarctation of the aorta — particularly during pregnancy.

Pathological changes include the separation of the intima from the adventitia by a hematoma, which may represent either a thrombus or liquid blood circulating through a false lumen ("double-barrel aorta"). Intimal tears providing the place of entry of the blood into the false lumen and its exit are usually found, though not in all cases. The possibility of dissection initiated by rupture of the vasa vasorum in the media without actual communication with the aortic lumen has been postulated by some but is probably very rare. More likely the tear may be missed in the aortic intima, which often shows gross atherosclerotic abnormalities.

Dissecting aneurysms are usually classified according to the degree of involvement of the aorta. The commonest form (type I) is that initiated in the aortic root and extending beyond the aortic arch—often as far as the abdominal aorta (estimated at more than 50 per cent of cases). The next commonest form (type III) is located beyond the aortic arch, with the aorta intact up to the exit of the left subclavian artery, and involving part or most of the descending aorta. The rarest form (type II), estimated at 10 to 15 per cent, is supravalvular dissection terminating proximal to the aortic arch.

The *natural history* of aortic dissection is unpredictable. Basically an extremely serious disease that can cause death within a short time by perforating into the pericardium or thoracic cavity, it can also take a very benign course in some cases—occasionally it is discovered accidentally on routine examinations. The course obviously is related to two factors:

1. Condition of the aortic wall outside the false lumen,

2. Extent of the involvement of the dissection and its sequels.

The initiation of the dissection is usually signaled by an attack of pain. It ranges from mild pain that may be dismissed by the patient and forgotten altogether to a sudden catastrophic event, which either permits a clear-cut diagnosis of dissecting aneurysm or limits the diagnosis to the differentiation between it and myocardial infarction. The quality of pain overlaps with that of acute myocardial infarction, but it may show some differences that give it a certain specificity:

- The pain is more often described as tearing rather than constricting in quality;

- It often starts substernally, but may radiate upward and then to the upper dorsal spinal region; the radiation may show sequential changes in location rather than simultaneous involvement of all areas;

- The pain, if severe, often starts very abruptly, without prodromals, with maximum intensity attained at onset (unlike myocardial infarction).

Symptoms other than pain are entirely related to the secondary sequels of the dissection. These include the following:

- Hemopericardium produced by seepage into the pericardium (as contrasted with a full-fledged, immediately fatal rupture into the pericardium) that may produce signs and symptoms of tamponade;

- Production of aortic regurgitation, if severe, may induce acute pulmonary edema;

- Acute myocardial infarction may be induced by dissection into a coronary artery; though rare, this is an extremely important point to consider in diagnosis and recognize the possible coexistence of both dissecting aneurysm and myocardial infarction;

- Cerebral symptoms produced by dissecting occlusion of cerebral arteries;

- Symptoms due to dissecting occlusion of any other arterial region (extremities, abdominal organs, renal arteries).

The *diagnosis* of dissecting aneurysm depends upon the presence of identifiable clinical and laboratory signs, thus ranging from one that is immediately obvious to one that cannot be established at all.

The following diagnostic features contribute to the identification of aortic dissection:

- The pain may show features described above; when present in its most typical form it has a moderately high specificity.

- Development of acute aortic regurgitation is a very specific sign, provided that reasonable assurance is present that no aortic regurgitation existed before the onset of pain; this is even more significant if an appropriate drop in the diastolic arterial pressure is noted.

- Disappearance of one or more peripheral pulses (brachial, carotid, femoral, etc.) is a sign of high specificity.

- In patients with systemic hypertension, the onset of severe chest pain associated with a shock-like clinical picture but without pronounced fall in arterial pressure is considered a differential point in favor of aortic dissection and against myocardial infarction. The value of this sign is probably exaggerated.

- Radiographic appearance of the widening of the shadow of the ascending aorta is a very important clinical sign. Its specificity, however, is dependent upon the availability of good control films taken prior to the attack, and upon the quality and reliability of the chest films. (Often portable films are the only ones available; they may exaggerate various portions of the cardiovascular shadow.)

- The absence of acute ischemic changes in the electrocardiogram carries some weight in the differential diagnosis, but error may occur in both directions. (S-T changes due to acute overload may develop in aortic dissection; early ischemic changes may be missing in acute myocardial infarction.)

- Echocardiography has been shown to be of some aid in the diagnosis in some cases, especially if the dissection is present just above the aortic valves: a double shadow of the aortic wall may be detected. This, however, has to be taken with considerable caution because of the possibility of a false-positive finding.

The definitive diagnosis depends upon contrast visualization of the aorta and demonstration of a double lumen. Selective aortography—even in the acute stage of aortic dissection—carries a risk only slightly higher than routine aortography, provided an experienced team of angiocardiographers performs the study. If such facility is not available but emergency evaluation is necessary, large-bolus intravenous angiocardiography often provides opacification of the aorta well enough to show the aneurysm.

Angiocardiography—obviously the most crucial test available—cannot be considered as reliable in aortic dissection as in many other forms of cardiovascular disease. In a positive sense it can establish the diagnosis beyond any doubt; however, a negative picture may not rule out the presence of aortic dissection. The possibility of poor communication or intermittent communication between the true and the false lumen, the formation of thrombus between aortic layers, and other factors may either present the appearance of a normal aortic lumen or suggest the presence of an ordinary (nondissecting) aneurysm.

Therapy of aortic dissection offers three choices:

- Immediate surgical treatment,

- Delayed operation after a period of medical treatment,

- Exclusively medical therapy.

Dissecting aneurysm carries an unpredictable outlook: studies reporting results of medical or surgical treatment vary in their respective successes. The validity of the statistical figures is difficult to accept at face value, inasmuch as none of the reports deals with controlled studies. Consequently, the choice of therapy is still largely dependent upon individual preferences and on the experience of the team treating the patient.

Medical therapy has as its objective the reduction of arterial pressure to the lowest level consistent with adequate organ perfusion (brain, kidney, heart). The usual systolic pressure level to aim at lies between 90 and 100 mm. Hg. This may be reinforced by the use of drugs decreasing the force of ventricular contraction (dp/dt). As a result of this therapy it is believed (though not proved) that the risk of further dissection as well as that of outside rupture is minimized.

The drugs administered for medical therapy include the following, used, as a rule, in some combinations:

- Trimethaphan (Arfonad) — as a ganglionic blocking agent;

- Reserpine and guanethedine — as catecholamine-depleting drugs;

- Propranolol — as a negative inotropic agent;

- Alpha-methyldopa and thiazides — as hypotensive agents.

Surgical therapy includes not only the actual repair and replacement of the dissected aorta but, if indicated, repair or replacement of an incompetent aortic valve.

Aortic dissection of types I and II — those involving the ascending aorta — are more precarious: they may lead to fatal pericardial tamponade and may induce cardiac failure by causing acute severe aortic regurgitation. The additional risk of external rupture applies to all three varieties of dissection.

In approaching the therapy of a patient in whom the diagnosis of aortic dissection is definite or highly probable, the following questions should be considered:

1. What is the probable duration of the dissection? As stated, aortic dissection is occasionally encountered after a delay, or even as a chronic state. In general, the longer the duration, the stronger the reason to pursue only medical therapy.

2. If acute and of recent origin, is there a sign that the dissection may be progressing? Such signs include progressive dilatation of the aorta in the radiograph or delayed development of a secondary involvement (aortic regurgitation, disappearance of pulses). Progression of the dissection is an urgent indication for early surgery.

3. Is there evidence of cardiac involvement? Two bedside signs are of crucial importance:

- Elevation of venous pressure with paradoxical pulse — as evidence for tamponade — is the most serious sign suggesting immediate intervention.

- Development of aortic regurgitation, when associated with cardiac failure, is a less precarious but still an ominous sign shifting the weight toward early surgical intervention.

4. Is there evidence for impending or actual shock? If there is poor organ perfusion *not* caused by the drugs used, especially if persistent chest pain is present, surgical consideration may be indicated.

In general, management of aortic dissection is one of the most difficult tasks facing the cardiologist and cardiovascular surgeon. The high risk of therapy—positive or negative—makes it imperative that the patient be handled as early as possible in an experienced cardiac center. Thus, the mere suspicion of dissecting aneurysm in a patient who is in a community hospital justifies immediate transfer to a center.

AORTITIS AND ANEURYSMS OF THE AORTIC ROOT

In contrast to dissecting aneurysm, which represents a specific separation of the layers of the aortic wall, aortitis and aortic aneurysms include a wide variety of conditions affecting the first portion of the aorta, and these conditions differ etiologically and pathologically. Basically three morphological forms of diseases of the aortic root can be distinguished:

- Saccular aneurysm of a portion of the aorta or the entire ascending aorta;
- Fusiform aneurysm, usually involving larger segments of the aorta;
- Aortic ectasia due to aortitis or atherosclerosis.

The etiological factors contributing or causing these conditions include the following:

- Congenital aneurysm (especially that of the sinus of Valsalva),
- Atherosclerotic aortic ectasia or aneurysm,
- Syphilitic aortitis,
- Aortitis associated with rheumatoid spondylitis,
- Other forms of aortitis (e.g., giant cell variety),
- Mycotic aneurysms,
- Traumatic aneurysms,
- Postsurgical aneurysms.

Pathology of this group of diseases varies considerably. As stated above, *aortic ectasia* usually involves inflammatory or degenerative changes in the aorta with uniform distribution. The aortic root retains its original shape but is much wider than normally; there may be continuation of a dilated aorta into the arch and beyond, or the aorta may gradually narrow to a normal diameter. With aortic ectasia there is associated, in most cases, widening of the aortic ring, producing incompetence of the aortic valve.

Saccular aneurysm is a localized dilatation of the aorta; it may be a "blow-out" of a portion of the aortic wall in an area with damaged media or actual rupture of the aortic wall with a false aneurysm, the wall of which is formed by the adventitia with periaortic tissue. False aneurysm is particularly common as a consequence of microorganisms — mycotic aneurysms. A special form of saccular aneurysm is *aneurysm of the sinus of Valsalva.* Initiated most frequently by congenital weakness of one of the sinuses (most often that above the right coronary aortic cusp), it may gradually progress and extend into the heart. Often associated with a congenital ventricular septal defect, such aneurysms may extend and rupture into the right ventricle, the right atrium, and, less commonly, into the left ventricle.

Fusiform aneurysm represents an intermediate condition between saccular aneurysms and generalized aortic ectasia. It is a spindle-shaped localized dilatation of the aorta.

Symptoms of aortic aneurysms are virtually nonexistent. Large saccular aneurysms eroding neighboring structures, e.g., the sternum, are now virtually never encountered, even though at one time, with the prevalence of syphilitic aortitis, they were commonplace. The only clinically significant sequel of diseases of the aortic root is aortic regurgitation. Chest pain is rare.

The clinical diagnosis of aortitis or aortic aneurysms can only be suspected in the presence of suddenly developing aortic regurgitation. The diagnosis is based on radiographic appearance of the ascending aorta. Here, as in aortic dissection, comparison with old films is of great diagnostic importance. Even though large saccular aneurysms may produce pathognomonic radiographic appearances, less typical aneurysms overlap with simple tortuosity of the ascending aorta, a common finding in older subjects with atherosclerotic aortas or in hypertensives.

Angiographic studies permit delineation of the aortic disease. These are more reliable than aortography in dissecting aneurysm, inasmuch as the objective of the study is merely the outline of the aortic lumen. Nevertheless, a differentiation between ordinary aneurysm and dissecting aneurysm may be difficult in some cases.

There is no medical therapy for aortic aneurysms. The choices lie between no therapy at all and surgical excision of the aneurysm. The exception to this rule is, of course, the sequel of aortic aneurysm, namely aortic regurgitation or — rarely in aneurysms of the sinus of Valsalva — the consequence of intracardiac shunts.

In conditions in which the etiological factors are theoretically amenable to treatment—e.g., syphilis, aortitis, mycotic aneurysms—one is tempted to institute vigorous specific therapy. However, it is doubtful whether such therapy would actually influence the course of an aneurysm (or aortitis) which is already on its own "collision course," independently of its originating factor.

Since the only objective of surgical resection of the aneurysm is the prevention of its rupture, indications for surgical therapy are not well defined. As in dissecting aneurysms, the skill and experience of the surgical unit often determines the aggressiveness in recommending aneurysmectomy. If respectable mortality, based on reasonably large series, can be demonstrated, a good case can be made for the routine resection of aneurysms. Surgical attack upon the aortic valves has already been discussed. Closure of perforated sinus of Valsalva represents a relatively simple form of open heart operation. In some patients a complete elimination of cardiac overload may be accomplished. Occasionally, however, residual aortic regurgitation (produced by the distortion of the aortic ring from the aneurysm) may perpetuate cardiac difficulty, making the operation virtually ineffective.

AORTIC ARCH SYNDROME (PULSELESS DISEASE, TAKAYASU'S SYNDROME)

This entity was relatively recently described and involves most often young or middle-aged Japanese women, although other races and age groups have also been affected by the disease. It represents a form of arteritis preferentially located in the aortic arch. Its etiology is unknown though it is surmised that it may belong to the group of autoimmune diseases, perhaps with some kinship to polyarteritis.

The pathological features of this entity consist of extensive aortitis within the arch of the aorta producing occlusive involvement of some or all brachiocephalic arteries.

The natural history and clinical manifestations are related entirely to the occlusive process affecting the brachiocephalic vessels and to the speed of the progression of this occlusion. Cerebral circulation is affected more profoundly than that to the upper extremities; hence the symptomatology is predominantly neurologic. Various transient attacks resembling ischemic attacks occur at first, often followed by permanent signs; these include visual disturbances, disturbances of speech and locomotion, and hemiplegia. Temporary manifestations may be related to position or changes in blood pressure. Less commonly, intermittent weakness ("claudication") of the arms and hand may be present.

The course of the disease is progressive and prognosis unfavorable. Survival is usually reported in terms of a few years; the cerebral deficit dominates the picture.

The diagnosis is based on the demonstration of occlusive processes involving the brachiocephalic arteries. Thus, systolic vascular bruits or, occasionally, continuous murmurs may be present over the upper outlet from the thorax. Differences in arterial pressure between the two arms, as well as lowered blood pressure in the arms compared with that in the legs, may eventually develop ("reversed coarctation"). At a later stage pulses may completely disappear.

Diagnostic evaluation includes selective aortography which permits the outline of details of the aortic arch involvement.

Therapy of the aortic arch syndrome has little to offer. Anticoagulant therapy and steroid therapy have been tried, but no evidence exists of their effectiveness. Surgical bypass operations have also been performed with some success. The feasibility, safety, and permanency of surgical therapy are as yet to be determined.

Bibliography

Anagnostopoulos CE, Prabhakar MJS, Kittle CF: Aortic dissection and dissecting aneurysm. Amer. J. Cardiol. *30*:263, 1972.

Barker NW, Edwards JE: Primary arteritis of aortic arch. Circulation *11*:486, 1955.

Blieden LC, Edwards JE: Anomalies of the thoracic aorta: pathological consideration. Progr. Cardiovasc. Dis. *16*:25, 1973.

Edwards JG, Burchell HB: The pathological anatomy of deficiencies between the aortic root and the heart, including aortic sinus aneurysms. Thorax *12*:125, 1957.

Gross RE, Neuhauser EBD: Compression of the trachea and esophagus by vascular anomalies. Surgical therapy in 40 cases. Pediatrics 7:69, 1951.

Lindsay J Jr, Hurst JW: Clinical features and prognosis of dissecting aneurysm of the aorta. A re-appraisal. Circulation *35*:880, 1967.

McKusick VA: The cardiovascular aspects of Marfan's syndrome, a hereditable disorder of connective tissue. Circulation *11*:321, 1955.

Nakao K, Ikeda M, Kimata S, Niitami H, Miyahara M, Ishimi Z, Hashiba H, Takeda Y, Ozawa T, Matsushita S, Kuramochi M: Takayasu arteritis: clinical report of 84 cases and immunological studies in 7 cases. Circulation *35*:1141, 1967.

Wheat MW Jr: Treatment of dissecting aneurysm of the aorta: current status. Progr. Cardiovasc. Dis. *16*:87, 1973.

Index _____

Atrial septal defect (*Continued*)
single atrium in, 701
sinus venosus type, 403
therapy for, 417
Atrioventricular block. See *Heart block.*
Atrioventricular dissociation, 261
Atrioventricular junctional rhythm, 287
Atrioventricular node, physiological role of, 257
Atrioventricular valve incompetence, 553–578. See also *Mitral regurgitation.*
definition of, 553
Atrium, single, in trilocular heart, 702
Auscultation. See also *Heart sounds,* as well as specific sounds and murmurs.
special maneuvers in, 58
summary of, 56
Austin Flint murmur, 52
AV block. See *Heart block.*
AV node. See *Atrioventricular node.*

Bacterial endocarditis, 387–401. See also *Endocarditis, infective.*
Ballistocardiography, 119
Beriberi heart disease, 710
Biatrial abnormalities, in electrocardiogram, 85
Bing-Taussig syndrome, 693
Biventricular hypertrophy, electrocardiographic interpretation of, 89
Bleeding, excessive, after open heart surgery, 211
in cardiac catheterization, 136
Block. See specific term, as *Right bundle branch block.*
Blood pressure, control of, in ischemic heart disease, 607. See also *Hypertension.*
management of, 648
"Blue bloaters," 668
Bradyarrhythmias, diagnosis of, 270
Bradyarrhythmias, in conduction disturbances, management of, 307
Bradycardia, sinus, 273
Bypass, aortico-coronary, in ischemic heart disease, 608, 623

Calcification, aortic, 79
coronary, 78
myocardial, 79
pericardial, 79
radiographic interpretation of, 78
valvular, 78
Cardiac arrest, and syncope, 233
"Cardiac asthma," 20

Cardiac catheterization. See *Catheterization, cardiac.*
Cardiac contraction, mechanism of, 255
Cardiac cycle, phases of, 256
Cardiac disease, classification of, 315
nosology, etiology and special features of, 315–325
rarer forms of, 691–711
Cardiac emergencies, 244
Cardiac failure. See also *Left ventricular failure; Right ventricular failure.*
acute, as medical or surgical emergency, 244
congestive, 248
after open heart surgery, 211, 214
causes and mechanisms of, 217–230
causes of, 222, 226
chronic, 234
treatment of, 249
definition of, 217
development of, 218
evaluation of cardiac function in, 240
hemodynamics in, 238
history taking in, 231
in cor pulmonale, 669
in hypertensive disease, 661
in ischemic heart disease, 615
angiocardiography in, 618
cardiac catheterization in, 618
diagnosis of, 617
echocardiography in, 618
electrocardiographic features of, 617
radiographic features of, 617
surgical treatment for, 620
treatment for, 622
in myocardial infarction, 343
treatment of, 354
"intractable," management of, 252
left ventricular filling pressure and cardiac output in, 225
management of, 244–254
physical examination in, 232
physiological consequences of, 224, 226
recognition and evaluation of, 231–243
reversibility of, 228
significance of, 242
"Cardiac failure," vs. "heart failure," 217
Cardiac function, evaluation of, in cardiac failure, 240
Cardiac index, equation for, 126
Cardiac output, Fick formula for, 126
Cardiac reserve, 218
Cardiac rhythm, abnormal mechanisms of, 259
normal mechanisms of, 257
Cardiac size, 71
Cardiac tamponade, and pericarditis, 375–386
in catheterization, 135
Cardiac tumors, 703